Psychological Co-morbidities of Physical Illness

Sherry Pagoto
Editor

Psychological Co-morbidities of Physical Illness

A Behavioral Medicine Perspective

Springer

Editor
Sherry Pagoto
Department of Medicine
Division of Preventive and Behavioral Medicine
University of Massachusetts Medical School
Worcester, MA, USA
Sherry.pagoto@umassmed.edu

ISBN 978-1-4419-0030-2 e-ISBN 978-1-4419-0029-6
DOI 10.1007/978-1-4419-0029-6
Springer New York Dordrecht Heidelberg London

Library of Congress Control Number: 2011936222

Printed on acid-free paper

Springer is part of Springer Science+Business Media (www.springer.com)

Preface

Individuals with psychological disorders are disproportionately affected by chronic disease, which presents a significant health disparity that is underrecognized and underaddressed. Physical and psychological illnesses co-occur more often than not in clinical populations, and this co-occurrence is associated with greater impairment, lower adherence, poor treatment response, lower quality of life, increased healthcare costs, and higher mortality rates. This book is the first comprehensive resource regarding psychological co-morbidities of physical illness. It serves as both a handbook for clinicians who care for patients with co-morbidities as well as a call for research that increases our understanding of the connection between physical and psychological illness, with the ultimate goal of improving the health of people with psychological disorders.

A constellation of behavioral, pharmacological, and physiological factors play a role in the increased risk for disease among individuals with psychological disorders. Behavioral factors include higher rates of smoking, obesity, and unhealthy behaviors. Psychopharmacology has also been implicated given that many drugs promote weight gain and metabolic syndrome. Physiological processes of psychological distress, including hypothalamic-pituitary-adrenal axis dysfunction, inflammation, and autonomic dysfunction, can also manifest in the development of chronic disease. In addition to identifying the most prevalent psychological co-morbidities of physical illness, this book explores how behavioral, pharmacological, and physiological factors converge to put individuals with psychological disorders at greater risk for disease.

This book is firmly rooted in the philosophy of evidence-based practice and was designed to help narrow the existing research to practice gap. One of the most commonly cited reasons by clinicians for not using evidence-based treatments is that randomized clinical trials do not reflect their consumers who have multiple co-morbidities. Traditionally, randomized clinical trials, by having a disease-specific focus and excluding people with comorbid psychological disorders, have offered very few insights and discoveries regarding the treatment of co-morbidities or the underlying processes of comorbid physical and psychological illnesses. As a result, clinicians have very few resources that lend insight into the complex treatment decisions necessary for patients with co-morbidities. This book will assist both the clinician and the researcher by providing information regarding the prevalence of various psychological co-morbidities in populations with specific physical illnesses; physiological, pharmacological, and behavioral mechanisms of co-morbidities; and implications for assessment and treatment in these populations. Each chapter focuses on a physical illness and reviews research pertinent to the psychological co-morbidities associated with that illness concluding with clinical considerations specific to the comorbid population. Physical illnesses of focus include the largest contributors to mortality in our population, such as obesity, type 2 diabetes, tobacco dependence, cardiovascular disease, and cancer; as well as those that are associated with significant healthcare burden, including chronic pain, irritable bowel syndrome, HIV/AIDS, chronic obstructive pulmonary disease, multiple sclerosis, and dementia.

Although a significant body of research has specifically focused on psychological co-morbidities of physical illnesses, the research is distributed across disparate fields, including medicine, behavioral medicine, psychiatry, nursing, and mental health services. This book brings this research together, making it a valuable resource for professionals in each of these fields who may not otherwise be exposed to the vast array of findings, discoveries, and clinical information regarding psychological co-morbidities of physical illness.

This book also serves as a reference for clinicians, researchers, and trainees who work with comorbid populations in clinical, public health, and academic settings. The content is relevant to the work of psychologists, mental health providers, epidemiologists, social workers, nurses, nurse practitioners, primary care physicians, medical specialists, and other allied healthcare workers. Because patients with psychological and medical co-morbidities may be encountered in either mental health or medical settings, assessment and treatment issues are discussed from both perspectives. Psychological conditions can sometimes be overlooked in medical settings, just as physical illnesses can sometimes be overlooked in mental health settings. This book informs practitioners about common co-morbidities, the implications of the comorbidity, as well as how to assess and treat in that setting. Included are brief assessment tools, practical summaries of the treatment outcome literature, and discussion of challenging clinical issues. Finally, by bringing together the literature on psychological and physical co-morbidities, important unanswered clinical questions and avenues for future research are highlighted.

Worcester, MA, USA Sherry Pagoto

Contributors

Bradley M. Appelhans, PhD Departments of Preventive Medicine and Behavioral Sciences, Rush University Medical Center, Chicago, IL, USA

C. Andres Bedoya, PhD Massachusetts General Hospital/Harvard Medical School, Boston, MA, USA

Fenway Community Health, Boston, MA, USA

Carla Bejjani, MD Psychiatry and Behavioral Sciences, Baylor College of Medicine, Houston, TX, USA

Carol Curtin, MSW University of Massachusetts Medical School, Worcester, MA, USA

Kristine A. Donovan, PhD, MBA H. Lee Moffitt Cancer Center and Research Institute, Tampa, FL, USA

B. Van Dorsten, PhD Department of Physical Medicine and Rehabilitation, University of Colorado School of Medicine, Aurora, CO, USA

Sabrina A. Esbitt, BA Ferkauf Graduate School of Psychology, Yeshiva University, Bronx, NY, USA

Jeffrey S. Gonzalez, PhD Clinical Psychology Ph.D. Program with Health Emphasis, Ferkauf Graduate School of Psychology, Yeshiva University, Bronx, NY, USA

Diabetes Research Center, Albert Einstein College of Medicine, Bronx, NY, USA

Alexandra Hajduk, MPH University of Massachusetts Medical School, Worcester, MA, USA

Jared Israel, BA Massachusetts General Hospital/Harvard Medical School, Boston, MA, USA

Paul B. Jacobsen, PhD H. Lee Moffitt Cancer Center and Research Institute, Tampa, FL, USA

Chris W. Johnson, BA University of Massachusetts Medical School, Worcester, MA, USA

David Kalman, PhD University of Massachusetts Medical School, Worcester, MA, USA

Laurie Keefer, PhD Northwestern University, Feinberg School of Medicine, Division of Gastroenterology, Center for Psychosocial Research, Chicago, IL, USA

Jennifer L. Kiebles, PhD Northwestern University, Feinberg School of Medicine, Division of Gastroenterology, Center for Psychosocial Research, Chicago, IL, USA

Sun Kim, PhD, RN University of Massachusetts Medical School, Worcester, MA, USA

Monika Kolodziej, PhD University of Massachusetts Medical School, Worcester, MA, USA

Mark E. Kunik, MD, MPH VA HSR & D Houston Center of Excellence, Michael E. DeBakey Veterans Affairs Medical Center, Houston, TX, USA

Menninger Department of Psychiatry and Behavioral Sciences, Baylor College of Medicine, Houston, TX, USA

Veterans Affairs South Central Mental Illness Research, Education and Clinical Center, Houston, TX, USA

Elyse G. Kupperman, MA Ferkauf Graduate School of Psychology, Yeshiva University, Bronx, NY, USA

Susan McCrone, PhD, RN School of Nursing, West Virginia University, Morgantown, WV, USA

David C. Mohr, PhD Northwestern University, Feinberg School of Medicine, Department of Preventive Medicine, Chicago, IL, USA

Conall O'Cleirigh, PhD Massachusetts General Hospital/Harvard Medical School, Boston, MA, USA

Fenway Community Health, Boston, MA, USA

Patricia J. Osborne, MA Ferkauf Graduate School of Psychology, Yeshiva University, Bronx, NY, USA

Sherry Pagoto, PhD University of Massachusetts Medical School, Worcester, MA, USA

Division of Preventive and Behavioral Medicine, Department of Medicine, University of Massachusetts Medical School, Worcester, MA, USA

Christina Psaros, PhD Department of Psychiatry, Massachusetts General Hospital/Harvard Medical School, One Bowdoin Square, Boston, MA, USA

Heidi Putnam-Casdorph, PhD, RN West Virginia University, Morgantown, WV, USA

Steven A. Safren, PhD Massachusetts General Hospital/Harvard Medical School, Boston, MA, USA

Fenway Community Health, Boston, MA, USA

Havah E. Schneider, MA Ferkauf Graduate School of Psychology, Yeshiva University, Bronx, NY, USA

Kristin Schneider, PhD University of Massachusetts Medical School, Worcester, MA, USA

Tiffany H. Taft, PsyD Northwestern University, Feinberg School of Medicine, Division of Gastroenterology, Center for Psychosocial Research, Chicago, IL, USA

James N. Weisberg, PhD Department of Orthopedics, Emory University School of Medicine, Atlanta, GA, USA

Amanda L. Wheat, MS Department of Psychology, West Virginia University, Morgantown, WV, USA

Matthew C. Whited, PhD Department of Medicine, Division of Preventive and Behavioral Medicine, University of Massachusetts Medical School, Worcester, MA, USA

Douglas Ziedonis, MD, MPH Department of Psychiatry, University of Massachusetts Medical School, Worcester, MA, USA

Chapter 1
Psychological Co-morbidities of Obesity

Sherry Pagoto, Kristin Schneider, Bradley M. Appelhans, Carol Curtin, and Alexandra Hajduk

1.1 Introduction

The association between obesity and psychological disorders has gained attention as the prevalence of obesity has rapidly increased in recent decades. Prevalence of obesity in people with psychological disorders has grown as fast or faster than in the general population (Allison et al., 2009), which points to a growing health disparity in psychological-disordered populations. Not only are people with various psychological disorders disproportionately affected by obesity, but obesity appears to increase risk for various psychological disorders. The aim of this chapter is to provide a comprehensive overview of the associations between obesity and psychological disorders, potential mechanisms underlying these associations, and assessment and treatment of individuals with these co-morbidities, including clinical challenges. Gaps in the research literature will be identified and recommendations for future made.

1.2 Mood Disorders

Major depressive disorder, dysthymic disorder, and bipolar disorder are the primary mood disorders described in the DSM-IV-TR (American Psychiatric Association, 2000). This chapter will focus on major depressive disorder and bipolar disorder, because associations between these disorders and obesity have been documented in the literature.

S. Pagoto (✉)
University of Massachusetts Medical School, Worcester, MA, USA

Division of Preventive and Behavioral Medicine, Department of Medicine, University of Massachusetts Medical School, 55 Lake Avenue North S7-751, Worcester, MA 01655, USA
e-mail: sherry.pagoto@umassmed.edu

S. Pagoto (ed.), *Psychological Co-morbidities of Physical Illness: A Behavioral Medicine Perspective*, DOI 10.1007/978-1-4419-0029-6_1,

1.2.1 *Major Depressive Disorders*

1.2.1.1 Prevalence of Co-occurring Depression and Obesity

Major depressive disorder is characterized by periods of 2 weeks or more of depressed mood and/or anhedonia, in conjunction with other symptoms, including significant disturbance in appetite or sleep, psychomotor agitation or retardation, loss of energy, concentration problems, feelings of worthlessness or guilt, or suicidal ideation or intent (American Psychiatric Association, 2000). In the general US population, the prevalence of major depressive disorder is around 5–9% for women and 2–3% for men (American Psychiatric Association). An association between obesity and depression,[1] albeit modest at times, has been observed in both epidemiological and clinical studies. In a US nationally representative sample, a slightly but significantly higher percentage of obese adults (18.6%) met criteria for lifetime depression than nonobese adults (16.0%) (Simon et al., 2006). Another population-based study in the US reported that compared to normal-weight individuals, obese and morbidly obese individuals were 1.56 and 2.00 times, respectively, more likely to report depression in their lifetime and 1.52 and 1.91 times, respectively, more likely to endorse depression in the past year (Petry, Barry, Pietrzak, & Wagner, 2008).

Prevalence of depression seems to increase with increasing degrees of obesity. For example, in a US population-based sample, prevalence of lifetime depression in class I/II obesity (Body mass index (BMI) = 30–39.9) was 24.1% compared to 32.1% for class III obese (BMI ≥40) individuals. Differences were apparent for past year depression as well, with prevalence rates of 11.4% for class I/II obesity and 16.2% for class III obesity (Petry et al., 2008). Among weight loss treatment-seeking obese individuals, prevalence of depression is even higher, with 19–50% reporting a lifetime history of depression (Black, Goldstein, & Mason, 1992; Britz et al., 2000; Bulik, Sullivan, & Kendler, 2002). Although the relationship between depression and obesity has been found more often in women (Barry, Pietrzak, & Petry, 2008; Carpenter, Hasin, Allison, & Faith, 2000; Roberts, Deleger, Strawbridge, & Kaplan, 2003; Roberts, Kaplan, Shema, & Strawbridge, 2000) than men (Barry et al.), one study found that class III obesity was associated with depression in both sexes (Onyike et al., 2003). At higher levels of obesity, risk of depression appears to be comparable for men and women. Age might also be a factor in sex differences in the association between obesity and depression. In a prospective community-based cohort study of older adults aged 70–79, obesity and especially, abdominal obesity, predicted onset of significant depressive symptoms over 5 years in men but not women, controlling for SES (Vogelzangs et al., 2010).

Other studies found no significant association between obesity and depression. One longitudinal study examined the influence of obesity on depression incidence

[1] Major depressive disorder will be referred to as "depression" in this chapter, whereas "depressive symptoms" will be referred to where an actual diagnosis of major depressive disorder has not been formally made.

over 12 years using the Canadian National Population Health Survey and found no relationship between obesity and the development of depression in females, and that obesity actually protected against the development of depression in males (Gariepy, Wang, Lesage, & Schmitz, 2010). Although obesity did not significantly predict new cases of depression, the prevalence of depression at each time point was higher for obese individuals compared to nonobese individuals. Numerous physical and psychosocial factors were controlled for in this study, including sex, age, SES, marital status, physical activity, smoking status, perceived health status, social support, and childhood trauma; however, findings were the same in unadjusted models. Given the longitudinal nature of this study, results suggest that obesity is not a risk factor for depression. Another epidemiological study found that the association between obesity and depression in men or women was eliminated after controlling for stressful life events, medical conditions, and physical disability (Pickering, Grant, Chou, & Compton, 2007). Study results seem to vary depending on nature of sample and covariates included in the models.

Given the conflicting nature of the literature, two systematic reviews and one meta-analysis were performed to evaluate overall study findings on the association between obesity and depression (Atlantis & Baker, 2008; Blaine, 2008; Luppino et al., 2010). One systematic review of 4 prospective and 20 cross-sectional studies concluded that moderate support exists for an obesity-depression association (Atlantis & Baker, 2008). A systematic review and meta-analysis of longitudinal studies reported that obese individuals had a 55% increased risk of developing depression, and individuals with depression had a 58% increased risk of developing obesity (Luppino et al., 2010). Consistent results were reported in a second meta-analysis of longitudinal studies, such that risk for depression was significantly higher in obese compared to nonobese individuals (Blaine, 2008). Although there are some exceptions, evidence generally supports an association between depression and obesity.

1.2.1.2 Pathophysiology

Several mechanisms have been proposed to explain the relationship between obesity and depression, including hypothalamic-pituitary-adrenal (HPA) axis dysregulation, inflammation, antidepressant medication, and psychological factors.

Hypothalamic-Pituitary-Adrenal Axis Dysregulation

The HPA axis is a complex hormonal cascade that regulates the secretion of cortisol, a glucocorticoid hormone (Habib et al., 2000). Stress triggers neurons in the hypothalamus to secrete corticotrophin-releasing hormone (CRH) into the portal vasculature shared with the pituitary gland. CRH elicits secretion of adrenocorticotropic hormone (ACTH) from the anterior pituitary into the peripheral circulation, where it eventually stimulates the adrenal cortex to secrete cortisol. Circulating cortisol feeds back to the hypothalamus and pituitary to inhibit further HPA axis activation. Prolonged or frequent activation of the HPA axis due to chronic stress is believed to result in HPA axis dysregulation (Tsigos & Chrousos, 2002), which has been associated with both obesity and depression and thus, is a possible mechanism for the association. Numerous neural, hormonal, and immunological factors regulate the HPA axis and may play a role in the association between depression and obesity. This section will focus on the most well-studied components.

In addition to its role in regulating cortisol secretion, CRH helps to regulate a number of other behavioral, neuroendocrine, and autonomic responses during stress, including the suppression of appetite during the acute phase of stress (Dunn & Berridge, 1990; Mastorakos & Zapanti, 2004). Hypersecretion of CRH resulting from chronic stress may produce dysregulation of this component of the HPA axis. Individuals with depression demonstrate chronic hypersecretion of CRH (Tsigos & Chrousos, 2002) and increased CRH concentrations in cerebrospinal fluid (Raadsheer, Hoogendijk, Stam, Tilders, & Swaab, 1994). CRH hypersecretion is not only strongly associated with depression, but it also may influence obesity. One study reported that mice with CRH hypersecretion increased food intake, gained weight, and developed insulin resistance compared to those with normal CRH secretion (Coste, Murray, & Stenzel-Poore, 2001). The evidence on the role of CRH in depression has led to the development of CRH receptor antagonists for depression treatment, but clinical trials have not yet been conducted (Schule, Baghai, Eser, & Rupprecht, 2009). If CRH receptor antagonists demonstrate efficacy for depression, it would be worth exploring whether they can also decrease weight or adiposity.

As mentioned earlier, circulating cortisol feeds back to the hypothalamus and pituitary to suppress HPA axis activation (Bjorntorp, 2001). Impairment in this feedback mechanism, often referred to as glucocorticoid resistance, is associated with depression, perhaps playing a causal role (Anacker, Zunszain, Carvalho, & Pariante, 2011). Elevated circulating glucocorticoids (i.e., hypercortisolism) observed in depressed individuals can also contribute to the development of obesity (Tsigos & Chrousos, 2002). Hypercortisolism stimulates intake of carbohydrates and fat, and reduces energy expenditure (Kyrou, Chrousos, & Tsigos, 2006). Chronic hypercortisolism also promotes abdominal fat storage (Kyrou et al.; Weber-Hamann et al., 2002), which is highly correlated with obesity (Rosmond & Bjorntorp, 1998; Rosmond, Dallman, & Bjorntorp, 1998).

Hypercortisolism appears to contribute to overall obesity, not just abdominal fat storage, via leptin. Leptin affects the HPA axis by influencing cortisol production. Experimental studies with rats demonstrate that leptin sensitivity occurs following an adrenalectomy, and in this context, heightened administration of glucocorticoids leads to overeating and hence vulnerability to obesity (Bjorntorp, 2001). The higher leptin levels observed in obese individuals may result from desensitization to the effects of leptin (i.e., leptin resistance; Lu, 2007). This could increase risk for depression, as studies in rats suggest that leptin has antidepressant effects (c.f. Lu). More research is needed to confirm whether hypercortisolism can result in "leptin resistant" obesity, but leptin appears to be a potential mechanism linking depression and obesity.

Inflammatory Markers

Inflammatory markers are also associated with the HPA axis in that many stimulate its activation. Inflammatory markers such as tumor necrosis factor-α (TNF-α), interleukin-1β, interleukin-6 (IL-6), and C-reactive protein (CRP) have each been associated with obesity and depression (Rexrode, Pradhan, Manson, Buring, & Ridker, 2003). Obesity has been deemed a "low-grade inflammatory state," due in part to the high levels of inflammatory markers observed among the obese (c.f. Cancello & Clement, 2006). In turn, inflammation has been associated with depressive symptoms including anhedonia and increased sleep (Bower, Ganz, Aziz, & Fahey, 2002; Capuron, Ravaud, & Dantzer, 2000). A cross-sectional study of the relationship between depression, obesity, and inflammatory pathways found that increased inflammation resulting from obesity did not promote depression, but rather depression was associated with obesity, which promoted increased inflammation (Miller, Freedland, Carney, Stetler, & Banks, 2003). Longitudinal studies are needed to confirm the temporal relationship between depression, obesity, and inflammation.

Antidepressant Medication

Psychotropic medication has been implicated as a significant contributor to the obesity epidemic (McAllister et al., 2009) and likely plays a role in the association between depression and obesity. One population-based cross-sectional study of Norwegian adults found that use of selective serotonin reuptake inhibitors (SSRIs) was associated with total obesity and abdominal obesity (Raeder, Bjelland, Vollset, & Steen, 2006). Further analysis of the influence of specific SSRIs found that paroxetine was associated with total and abdominal obesity, but sertraline, fluoxetine, and fluvoxamine[2] were associated with abdominal but not total obesity. Citalopram was not associated with either total or abdominal obesity. A longitudinal study found an increased risk of obesity over 10 years among adults taking venlafaxine or an SSRI (Patten et al., 2009). Tricyclic antidepressants were not significantly associated with obesity risk in that study; however, two reviews have reported weight gain in individuals taking tricyclic antidepressants (Fava, 2000; Uher et al., 2011). Monoamine oxidase (MAO) inhibitors have also been associated with significant weight gain (Fava, 2000). That certain antidepressant medications are associated with weight gain could at least partially explain the association between obesity and depression.

Psychological Mechanisms

Several psychological factors characteristic of depression and/or obesity may explain their association. For example, weight stigmatization is a common experience among obese individuals (Puhl, Moss-Racusin, Schwartz, & Brownell, 2008). Weight stigma

[2] Given the low number of participants taking these medications, these three medications were categorized into one group.

can contribute to depression (Chen et al., 2007) and body dissatisfaction (Cargill, Clark, Pera, Niaura, & Abrams, 1999; Friedman, Reichmann, Costanzo, & Musante, 2002). Obesity is often perceived as unattractive and as a sign of poor self-control and/or laziness (Fabricatore & Wadden, 2004), and obese individuals commonly report experiencing stigma from loved ones, teachers, and healthcare professionals (Puhl & Brownell, 2006). Studies have found links between body dissatisfaction and depression in obese Caucasian males and females (Grilo & Masheb, 2005), obese adolescents (Goldfield et al., 2010), and Black and Hispanic women (Hrabosky & Grilo, 2007), suggesting that this association is true regardless of age, sex, and cultural background. Obesity stigma and negative body image are generally more predictive of depression in women than men (Puhl & Heuer, 2009), which may explain, in part, the weaker relationship observed between obesity and depression in men.

1.2.1.3 Clinical Care

Assessment

Given the high rate of depression among obese patients, assessing depression in obese patients in primary care, weight treatment settings, and in other medical settings would seem indicated and standard screening instruments should be used. Depression could have implications for further weight gain as well as ability to lose weight. In studies of weight loss program participants, depression has been associated with less weight loss (Pagoto et al., 2007) and higher risk for regain (Clark, Cargill, Medeiros, & Pera, 1996; Linde et al., 2004), although not all studies report an adverse effect of depression on weight loss outcomes. One trial reported no difference in weight loss in depressed and nondepressed weight loss program participants, but the fairly high drop-out rate (30% did not attend any weight loss groups) could have masked group differences (Ludman et al., 2009). Although depression is prevalent in bariatric surgery patients, depressive symptoms at baseline was not associated with 1-year weight loss outcomes following gastric bypass in one study (Ma et al., 2006), no association was found between a lifestime history of depressive disorders and 1-year weight loss outcomes following lap band surgery in another study (Semanscin-Doerr, Windover, Ashton, & Heinberg, 2010), and depression improved significantly following gastric bypass in a third study (Hayden, Dixon, Dixon, Shea, & O'Brien, 2011). The literature suggests that depression is not a predictor of outcome following weight loss surgery and should not therefore be considered a contraindication. Depression assessment appears to be critical prior to nonsurgical weight loss attempts given it has implications for outcome, but less so for surgical weight loss attempts.

Treatment

When depression is co-morbid with obesity, treatments that can impact both conditions are ideal and options include certain psychotherapies, antidepressant medications, and appetite-suppressing medications.

Psychotherapy

Several randomized controlled trials have tested the efficacy of psychotherapy on weight loss and depression in samples that were not selected for depression. In separate studies, both cognitive-behavioral therapy (CBT) and cognitive therapy (CT) were tested as adjuncts to dietary intervention and both studies found improved weight loss outcomes compared to diet-alone conditions (Rodriguez-Hernandez et al., 2009; Werrij et al., 2009). Although these studies found no overall differences in self-reported depression scores between conditions, one of the studies examined a subsample of participants with mild-to-severe depressive symptoms (Beck Depression Inventory scores ≥10) and found that the CBT condition was more successful at maintaining their weight loss relative to diet alone (Werrij et al.). Integrating components of cognitive and/or behavioral therapy into weight loss treatment has become commonplace and generally results in decreases in depressive symptoms within nondepressed samples (e.g., Andersen et al., 1999; Bacon et al., 2002; Carels, Darby, Cacciapaglia, & Douglass, 2004; Ello-Martin, Roe, Ledikwe, Beach, & Rolls, 2007; Malone, Alger-Mayer, & Anderson, 2005; Sbrocco, Nedegaard, Stone, & Lewis, 1999; Womble et al., 2004). In addition to being added as an adjunct to weight loss treatment, CBT has also been tested as the sole intervention for weight loss. One randomized controlled trial compared CBT to a modified version of CBT that focused on the psychological and physiological effects of obesity (Rapoport, Clark, & Wardle, 2000). Despite the fact that neither treatment included a traditional diet intervention, results demonstrated that both treatments produced modest weight loss, which was maintained at the 1-year follow-up (Rapoport et al.). CBT appears effective at reducing weight and depressive symptoms, but whether results generalize to samples who actually have a diagnosis of depression remains to be seen.

Major depressive disorder is often an exclusion criterion in weight loss trials, which limits our knowledge of weight loss outcomes in people who have depression. Two studies specifically recruited samples with depression to address this gap in the literature. One was a small nonrandomized study that examined whether behavioral activation treatment for depression combined with dietary counseling improved depression and facilitated weight loss in 14 obese women with depression (Pagoto, Bodenlos, et al., 2008). After 12 weeks of treatment, significant decreases in depression and weight were observed, with 72% of the sample in remission from depression by the end of treatment. Results suggest that targeting both depression and obesity in treatment may be helpful. Another study randomized 203 obese patients with depression to a behavioral weight loss intervention with or without CBT for depression (Linde et al., 2011). They found that the addition of CBT did not improve weight loss, but did result in slightly greater improvements in depressive symptoms, although both groups improved significantly. More research is clearly needed to determine the optimal behavioral approach to weight loss and depression when they co-occur, as well as whether it is necessary to treat depression to facilitate weight loss.

Antidepressant Medication

The effects of different antidepressants on body weight are variable. Generally, SSRIs are either weight neutral or cause weight gain (e.g., paroxetine). Early studies suggested that fluoxetine produced short-term weight loss, but effects were not sustained for 1 year or longer (Darga, Carroll-Michals, Botsford, & Lucas, 1991; Goldstein et al., 1994; Michelson et al., 1999). Buproprion, a noradrenaline and dopamine reuptake inhibitor, is an antidepressant that may facilitate weight loss. Two placebo-controlled randomized trials examined the efficacy of buproprion on depressive symptoms and weight loss (Croft et al., 2002; Jain et al., 2002). One trial recruited people with obesity and mild depressive symptoms and found that participants who received 26 weeks of bupropion plus a reduced calorie diet lost significantly more weight (4.4 kg) than participants who received placebo plus a reduced calorie diet (1.7 kg), although improvement in depressive symptoms did not differ between the conditions (Jain et al., 2002). The second trial examined the effect of sustained buproprion treatment in people with major depression and who had lost weight after an 8-week open-label phase of buproprion (Croft et al., 2002). Results showed that individuals taking buproprion were significantly more likely to maintain their weight loss during the subsequent 44 weeks of treatment than those taking the placebo (Croft et al., 2002). Buproprion has also been combined with naltrexone for weight loss given the effect of naltrexone on reducing food intake and tempering brain reward pathways. Results from placebo-controlled randomized trials demonstrated that the combination of buproprion and naltrexone resulted in significantly greater weight loss than placebo, buproprion alone, and naltrexone alone (Greenway et al., 2010; Greenway, Dunayevich, et al., 2009; Greenway, Whitehouse, et al., 2009; Wadden et al., 2011). None of these trials included or identified enough participants with depression to be able to evaluate the impact on depressive symptoms. Whether the combination of buproprion and naltrexone improves depression and facilitates weight loss among individuals with diagnosed depression should be examined.

Appetite Suppressants

Sibutramine, an appetite suppressant, and serotonin-norepinephrine-dopamine reuptake inhibitor gained significant interest as a promising obesity medication, particularly in people with depression (James et al., 2000; McNeely & Goa, 1998). Enthusiasm has since dissolved given studies showing sibutramine is not efficacious in the treatment of depression (Sharma & Henderson, 2008), can raise blood pressure in some people (McTigue et al., 2003), and increases risk for nonfatal myocardial infarction and nonfatal stroke per emerging data from the SCOUT trial (James et al., 2010). As a result of these findings, in 2010 the European Medicines Agency suspended its use as a weight loss agent in Europe (European Medicines Agency, 2010) and the US FDA followed shortly thereafter (U.S. Food and Drug Administration, 2010). Generally, the literature provides very little support for any medication that improves depressive symptoms and facilitates weight loss.

Issues in Treatment Decision Making

Because depression can lead to weight gain as well as interfere with weight loss attempts, treating depression using evidence-based approaches prior to an intensive behavioral weight loss program may be indicated (Fabricatore & Wadden, 2004). One clinical challenge is that some patients presenting for weight loss treatment may not be interested in depression treatment or may not want to wait until depressive symptoms remit before trying to lose weight. Some patients attribute their depression directly to their weight problems and believe that improvement in depression is contingent on a certain amount of weight loss. Such cognitions can be the source of significant resistance to depression treatments that do not directly address weight. For this reason, integrating weight loss strategies into depression treatment can be helpful. Cognitive strategies that challenge the belief that resolving depression is dependent on weight loss may be helpful, and behavioral strategies such as activity and mood monitoring can be used to increase the patient's awareness of activities that have a positive impact on their mood at their current weight. Exercise is another intervention that could impact both depression and weight. Several trials have now established the efficacy of exercise for treating depression (Blumenthal et al., 2007; Craft, Freund, Culpepper, & Perna, 2007; Dunn, Trivedi, Kampert, Clark, & Chambliss, 2005) and it has recently been recommended in National Institute of Health and Clinical Excellence guidelines as an evidence-based treatment for depression (National Institute of Health and Clinical Excellence, 2009). Exercise trials have not exclusively recruited obese samples or demonstrated a significant impact on weight loss; however, patients not interested in traditional depression treatments might consider an exercise intervention given the relevance to weight.

Clinicians treating obese patients with co-morbid depression should be aware of any psychotropic medications the patient may be taking, given that some have weight gain side effects. Patients on medications associated with weight gain should be encouraged to discuss the weight implications and alternatives with the prescribing provider. A concern regarding antidepressant medications in particular is that initial evidence suggests they are less effective in obese patients. An inpatient clinic-based study of 408 patients with depression reported that after 5 weeks of antidepressant treatment, 50% of lean individuals experienced a 50% reduction in depression rating scale symptoms, while only 17.4% of obese individuals experienced that same reduction (Kloiber et al., 2007). Whether obese individuals are slower to respond to antidepressant medication or whether they have less overall treatment response is unknown. Given the high rate of depression among obese patients, more controlled research is needed on the efficacy of antidepressant medications among obese individuals.

Considerations for Racial and Ethnic Minorities

Although racial and ethnic minorities have higher rates of obesity than Caucasians (Flegal, Carroll, Ogden, & Johnson, 2002; Hedley et al., 2004), obesity does not seem as strongly linked to depression. In a nationally representative sample of 9,125 participants from the National Co-morbidity Survey Replication, the prevalence of lifetime depression in obese vs. nonobese individuals was significantly greater among non-Hispanic Whites (24.4% vs. 18.9%), but not among African-American, Hispanic, and other racial and ethnic categories (Simon et al., 2006). However, the negative health consequences of co-occurring obesity and depression appear to be more detrimental for ethnic minorities than non-Hispanic Whites. One cross-sectional study examined the relationship between obesity, depression, race, and chronic disease risk in a sample of primary care patients and found that the influence of obesity and depression on diabetes and hypertension risk was greater for African-American patients, compared to non-Hispanic White participants (Stecker & Sparks, 2006). Obese African-Americans with depression were 12 times more likely to be diagnosed with hypertension and almost 15 times more likely to be diagnosed with diabetes, compared to lean non-Hispanic White participants without depression. Improving depression screening and treatment in racial and ethnic minorities with obesity may be important to curb the health disparities observed in obesity-related medical conditions.

1.2.2 Bipolar Disorder

Bipolar disorder is a mood disorder that is characterized by clinically distinct mood swings and accompanying shifts in activity levels. Patients with bipolar disorder typically experience bouts of depression and one or more episodes of mania or hypomania. Currently, bipolar disorder has two types: bipolar I disorder requires the occurrence of manic episodes that significantly interfere with functioning, often in addition to depressive episodes, while a diagnosis of bipolar II disorder requires the occurrence of major depressive episodes and at least one hypomanic episode (American Psychiatric Association, DSM-IV-TR, 2000). In the US, the prevalence of bipolar I disorder ranges from 0.4 to 1.6% and the prevalence of bipolar II disorder is 0.5% (American Psychiatric Association).

1.2.2.1 Prevalence of Co-occurring Bipolar Disorder and Obesity

Epidemiological studies suggest a link between obesity and bipolar disorder. A study of a nationally representative sample of adults found significantly higher lifetime prevalence of bipolar disorder in obese individuals (2.8%) compared to their lean counterparts (1.9%) (Simon et al., 2006). Studies using clinical samples with bipolar disorder report rates of obesity that range from 19 to 35% (Elmslie, Silverstone, Mann, Williams, & Romans, 2000; Fagiolini et al., 2002; Fagiolini, Kupfer, Houck, Novick, & Frank, 2003; McElroy et al., 2002). One study found that rates of obesity in individuals with bipolar disorder were higher (19 and 20%, in males and females respectively) than a reference group of age- and sex-matched controls (10 and 13%, in males and females, respectively; Elmslie et al., 2000). Other studies have shown elevated risk of obesity in females with bipolar disorder, but not males (Barry et al., 2008; Pickering et al., 2007). Taken together, the evidence favors an increased risk for obesity among adults with bipolar disorder.

1.2.2.2 Pathophysiology

Weight gain appears to occur at the onset of bipolar disorder, suggesting that factors related to the disorder or its treatment may be involved in the development of obesity (Shah, Shen, & El-Mallakh, 2006). Mechanisms explaining the association between bipolar disorder and obesity include psychopharmacology and HPA axis dysregulation, which will be discussed below. A third mechanism is lifestyle factors, including diet quality and physical activity levels, which may become disrupted by bipolar disorder. Lifestyle behaviors of individuals with severe mental illness (which includes bipolar disorder) are discussed at length in Sect. 1.5.2.2 of this chapter.

Psychopharmacology

One likely contributor to obesity among people with bipolar disorder is weight gain side effects from medications used to treat bipolar disorder. Weight gain, and often substantial weight gain, is a significant side effect of mood stabilizers, anticonvulsants, and antipsychotic medications, the three types of psychotropic medications used to treat bipolar disorder (Chen & Silverstone, 1990; McIntyre, 2002; Torrent et al., 2008). A complete discussion of weight gain side effects of antipsychotic medication can be found in Sect. 1.5.2.1 of this chapter. In terms of mood stabilizers and anticonvulsants, a review of the literature reported that lithium increased weight in 9.8–11.1% of participants across trials and valproate increased weight in 11.9–20.8% of participants across trials (Coryell, 2009). Another review reported that studies have shown lithium can cause 4.5–12 kg weight gain in the first year with leveling off thereafter (Torrent et al., 2008). Weight gain side effects of lithium have been attributed to slowed metabolism, increased appetite, fluid retention, and hypothyroidism, in some cases. The review also concluded that valproate, an anticonvulsant, has been associated with 3–10 kg weight gains over 1 year, but lamotrigine, another anticonvulsant, was not associated with significant weight gain in trials (Torrent et al.). The majority of medications used to treat bipolar disorder seem to have weight gain side effects, although not all patients are affected.

HPA Axis Dysregulation

Chronic stress and activation of the HPA axis have been observed during both manic and depressive episodes in individuals with bipolar disorder (Cassidy, Ritchie, & Carroll, 1998) and abnormalities in HPA axis functioning have been observed during active symptoms and remission (Watson, Gallagher, Ritchie, Ferrier, & Young, 2004). One study reported that individuals with bipolar disorder had higher cortisol levels compared to individuals with unipolar depression, regardless of whether symptoms were present or in remission (Rybakowski & Twardowska, 1999). Research into the impact of manic episodes on HPA axis functioning is sparse, but may have implications for the development of obesity.

1.2.2.3 Clinical Care

Assessment

If bipolar disorder is suspected in an obese patient presenting for weight management, referral to psychiatry for formal diagnostic assessment should follow. Because medication is typically necessary in the management of bipolar disorder, thorough assessment of medication status and adherence is necessary before proceeding to weight loss treatment. Untreated bipolar disorder could certainly have implications for success in behavioral weight management as well as for outcomes and postsurgical self-care in bariatric surgery patients. Little consensus exists on the psychological grounds on which to postpone or recommend against surgery, but bipolar disorder is one of the top reasons cited for recommending against surgery (Walfish, Vance, & Fabricatore, 2007), and initial evidence suggests that surgical weight loss outcomes may be worse in individuals with bipolar disorder (Semanscin-Doerr et al., 2010). However, worse weight loss outcome does not necessarily justify denial of surgery, as people with bipolar disorder might have even greater difficulty losing weight using nonsurgical means than people without mental illness. Key issues of surgical readiness are psychological stability. and ultimately, the ability to follow through with pre- and postsurgical care instructions, given that noncompliance can affect outcomes. Finally, suicidality should be evaluated in weight treatment-seeking patients with bipolar disorder, given that bipolar is associated with a suicide rate that is 20 times that of the general population (Simon, Hunkeler, Fireman, Lee, & Savarino, 2007).

Evidence-Based Treatment

Medication Augmentation and Switching

Weight gain is a common reason for medication discontinuation in bipolar disorder (Sachs & Rush, 2003). One approach to offsetting weight gain from mood stabilizing or antipsychotic medications is via supplemental medications that facilitate weight loss. One randomized controlled trial compared the effect of supplementing mood stabilizers or antipsychotics with either sibutramine or topiramate on weight (McElroy, Frye, et al., 2007). Participants were obese and met criteria for a bipolar disorder or schizoaffective disorder bipolar type and had experienced a recent weight gain attributed to their psychotropic medication. Results demonstrated that participants lost significant and comparable amounts of weight on sibutramine (4% of body weight) and topiramate (3% of body weight) over 24 weeks. However, the study had an 88% drop-out rate mostly due to worsened mood, side effects, and lack of weight loss, with no differences in drop-out between conditions.

Another approach to correcting medication-induced weight gain is medication switching, which involves switching from a medication with a high weight gain profile to one of a weight neutral or weight loss profile. Lamotrigine, an anticonvulsant medication with some initial efficacy data in the treatment of bipolar disorder but with a weight neutral profile, is one candidate for medication switching. Two double-blind placebo-controlled randomized trials comparing lamotrigine to lithium in participants with bipolar I disorder demonstrated that patients taking lamotrigine remained weight stable (Sachs et al., 2006) or lost weight (Bowden et al., 2006) after 1 year of treatment, while participants taking lithium gained weight. Symptom control was not reported in either trial, but unfortunately, the effectiveness of lamotrigine for acute mania is not well-supported. A thorough discussion of medication switching in the context of antipsychotic medication regimens can be found in Sect. 1.5.3.2, but generally, switches from olanzipine or risperidone to either ziprasione or aripiprazole have been found to reverse weight gains. Further research is needed to establish the optimal medication(s) for bipolar disorder in the context of obesity.

Research suggests that female sex, family history of obesity, and severe weight fluctuations during adulthood are risk factors for medication-induced weight gain in bipolar disorder and should be assessed during a medication consultation (Baptista, De Mendoza, Beaulieu, Bermudez, & Martinez, 2004; Fagiolini & Chengappa, 2007). In 2004, the American Diabetes Association, American Psychiatric Association, American Association of Clinical Endocrinologists, and the North American Association for the Study of Obesity made recommendations for the monitoring of patients taking antipsychotic medications (Bond, Kauer-Sant'Anna, Lam, & Yatham, 2010). These recommendations include taking a personal and family history of obesity and obesity-related medical conditions; regular monitoring of BMI, blood pressure, and metabolic indices; and lifestyle counseling for diet and physical activity. Providers should be aware that weight gain, particularly in weight-conscious patients, could lead to medication nonadherence and/or discontinuation, which has implications for management of bipolar disorder.

Behavioral Interventions

A full review of behavioral weight loss interventions in populations with severe mental illness can be found in Sect. 1.5.3.1. Generally, behavioral weight loss interventions have been shown to be efficacious in people with a range of severe mental illnesses including bipolar disorder (Poulin et al., 2007). Many of these studies included individuals with bipolar disorder, but none focused exclusively on this group. As such, the specific challenges to behavioral weight loss in individuals with bipolar disorder are not well-described.

In practice, few patients with bipolar disorder receive adequate weight counseling. A cohort chart review study of patients from a veterans' medical center who were diagnosed with bipolar disorder reported that 41% of patients received two diet and/or physical activity consultations (i.e., counseling contacts) and only 24% received more than two consultations (Goodrich, Lai, Lasky, Burghardt, & Kilbourne, 2010). When medications with weight gain side effects are prescribed, patients may benefit from concurrent enrollment in a weight gain prevention program to temper the effect of medication on weight. Intervention timing may play a key role in whether concurrent weight gain prevention treatment is effective. Stabilization of depressive and/or manic symptoms may be required prior to weight loss treatment to maximize outcomes.

1.2.3 Summary

Mood disorders in general appear to be linked to greater risk for obesity. Common physiological and psychological processes between mood disorders and obesity seem to account for the co-morbidity at least in part but psychotropic medications also appear to play a role. Mood disorders have negative implications for behavioral weight loss interventions, possibly due to the intensity and reliance on self-regulation. Surgical weight loss intervention outcomes are less impacted, however uncontrolled bipolar disorder could increase the risks of surgical interventions. More research is needed to understand how to prevent weight gain in these populations as well as more potent weight loss strategies, given the elevated rate of obesity.

1.3 Anxiety Disorders

Collectively, anxiety disorders are the most common psychological disorders with approximately 40 million American adults, or about 18.1% having an anxiety disorder in a given year (Kessler, Chiu, Demler, Merikangas, & Walters, 2005). Anxiety disorders encompass a range of diagnoses including generalized anxiety disorder (GAD), agoraphobia, panic disorder, specific phobia, social phobia, obsessive compulsive disorder (OCD), posttraumatic stress disorder (PTSD), acute stress disorder, anxiety due to a general medical condition, substance-induced anxiety disorder, and anxiety disorder not otherwise specified (American Psychiatric Association, 2000). Epidemiological studies have demonstrated an increased risk of obesity with GAD, panic disorder, specific phobia, social phobia, and PTSD (Petry et al., 2008; Scott et al., 2008; Simon et al., 2006). Although not an anxiety disorder in itself, a history of childhood sexual abuse, regardless of whether accompanied by PTSD, has also been shown to be associated with increased risk for obesity. The associations between anxiety disorders and obesity appear to be somewhat weaker than other psychological disorders reviewed in this chapter, and the literature is far less developed. This section will review the available literature on the prevalence of co-occurring anxiety disorders and obesity, the pathophysiology of the co-occurrence, assessment and treatment issues, and areas for future research.

1.3.1 Generalized Anxiety Disorder

The predominant features of GAD are excessive anxiety and worry, difficulty controlling worry, irritability, restlessness, disturbed sleep, muscle tension, and problems with concentration occurring for at least 6 months. Approximately 3% of the population in any given year will have GAD (Kessler et al., 2005) and the lifetime prevalence is 5% (American Psychiatric Association, 2000).

1.3.1.1 Prevalence of Co-morbid Anxiety Disorders and Obesity

Epidemiological research suggests an association between GAD and obesity. In a cross-sectional study using the National Epidemiologic Survey on Alcohol and Related Conditions (NESARC), being overweight, obese, or extremely obese was associated with significantly increased odds of having lifetime or past year GAD relative to normal-weight individuals (Petry et al., 2008). Lifetime prevalence of GAD was 3.85% among the overweight, 5.60% among the obese, and 8.26% among the extremely obese. Past year prevalence of GAD was 1.86% among the overweight, 2.77% among the obese, and 3.67% among the extremely obese. A prospective population-based study of 544 women observed that obesity was associated with a 6.27 increased risk of developing GAD over 30 years (Kasen, Cohen, Chen, & Must, 2008). However, findings from the National Co-morbidity Survey-Replication found higher prevalence of any lifetime anxiety disorder in obese adults, but not GAD specifically (Simon et al., 2006).

1.3.1.2 Pathophysiology and Treatment Implications

GAD might increase risk for obesity via physiological and/or behavioral mechanisms, but research is lacking in this area. Psychopharmacology for GAD may play a role in the connection to obesity because antidepressant medications are often used to treat GAD and some have weight gain side effects. A thorough discussion of antidepressants and weight gain can be found in section "Antidepressant Medication" of this chapter. Anxiolytics, also used in the treatment of GAD, generally do not cause weight gain. Potential implications of GAD on the treatment of obesity are unclear. No studies have examined whether people with GAD have worse weight loss outcomes in either surgical or behavioral weight loss interventions. However, high perceived stress has been associated with worse weight loss outcomes in behavioral weight loss interventions (Kim, Bursac, DiLillo, White, & West, 2009), and many individuals with GAD are likely to have elevated stress as a result of their anxiety symptoms. The role of chronic stress in the association between anxiety disorders and obesity requires further study.

1.3.2 Panic Disorder

Panic disorder is characterized by recurrent panic attacks that involve at least four physiological (e.g., sweating, heart palpitations) or psychological (e.g., fear of dying, derealization) symptoms and occur suddenly, often with no discernable precipitating factors (American Psychiatric Association, 2000). To meet criteria for panic disorder, the panic attacks must include 1 month of at least one of the following: (1) persistent fear of future attacks; (2) worry about consequences of attacks; or (3) altered behavior to cope with the fear of attacks. Panic disorder may or may not be accompanied by agoraphobia, which is excessive fear of not having access to help or being embarrassed in the event of a panic attack, which results in avoidance of situations like being out of the home alone, being around crowds, or traveling on buses or trains. Panic disorder affects approximately 2.7% of the population (American Psychiatric Association).

1.3.2.1 Prevalence of Co-morbid Panic Disorder and Obesity

Initial research provides evidence for an association between obesity and panic disorder. In a nationally representative sample, obese individuals (BMI 30–39.9) were between 1.4 and 1.8 times more likely than normal-weight individuals to have current or a lifetime history of panic disorder, and individuals with extreme obesity (BMI: ≥40) were between 1.7 and 2.6 times more likely to have current or a lifetime history of panic disorder (Petry et al., 2008). After controlling for psychotropic medication use, past year panic disorder was no longer associated with obesity and lifetime panic disorder was no longer associated with extreme obesity. A significant relationship was observed in another nationally representative sample, where the prevalence of lifetime panic disorder or agoraphobia was 7.1% among obese individuals and 5.6% among nonobese individuals; and the prevalence of past year panic disorder or agoraphobia was 4.6% among obese individuals and 3.1% among nonobese individuals; however, medication use was not controlled in that study (Simon et al., 2006). A third population-based study in Canadian adults found no relationship between lifetime or past year panic disorder and obesity, although the presence of panic attacks, both lifetime and past year, was significantly associated with an increased risk of obesity (Mather, Cox, Enns, & Sareen, 2009). Panic disorder appears to be associated with a slightly increased risk for obesity, although the role of medication as a mediator of this association should be investigated further.

1.3.2.2 Pathophysiology and Treatment

No studies have examined the mechanisms linking panic disorder and obesity. That some associations between panic disorder and obesity diminished when psychotropic medication use was accounted for implicates the role of psychotropic medication. The only study that controlled for medications did not provide data on the specific medications, so it is unclear which medications are implicated. Panic disorder is treated with either anxiolytics, which do not typically cause weight gain, or anti-depressant medications, some of which can cause weight gain. Simon et al. (2006) found that controlling for smoking status and co-morbid psychological disorders such as mood disorders and substance abuse did not affect the relationship between panic disorder and obesity, which would seem to rule out the possibility that the relationship is accounted for by these conditions. One possible area for exploration is the extent to which a sedentary lifestyle and exercise avoidance play a role in the development of obesity among individuals with panic disorder. Intense fear of physiological arousal is common in panic disorder which can result in avoidance of nonessential arousal via physical activities due to fear that it will trigger panic (Merom et al., 2008). Interestingly, exercise itself has been suggested as a treatment for panic disorder to help patients navigate this very challenge. Two randomized trials (Broocks et al., 1998; Merom et al., 2008) showed that exercise was effective at reducing symptoms in patients with panic disorder. Exercise interventions may be particularly indicated in obese individuals with panic disorder, given that it reduces panic and anxiety symptoms and is critical to weight loss maintenance (Jakicic, Marcus, Lang, & Janney, 2008). Identifying and overcoming anxiety- and panic-related challenges to exercise may be helpful to achieving and maintaining a healthy weight in obese patients with panic disorder.

1.3.3 Social Phobia

Social phobia refers to persistent and excessive anxiety specifically related to social situations such as public speaking or eating in front of people, such that the specific situations are avoided due to concern about embarrassment (American Psychiatric Association, 2000). Lifetime prevalence of social phobia ranges from 3 to 13% (American Psychiatric Association).

1.3.3.1 Prevalence of Co-morbid Social Phobia and Obesity

Several epidemiological studies have examined the association between social phobia and obesity with somewhat varied results. In a nationally representative sample of US adults, the prevalence of social phobia was higher among adults with obesity (lifetime: 5.86%; past year 3.39%) and morbid obesity (lifetime: 8.71%; past year 5.81%) compared to lean individuals (Petry et al., 2008). However, sex differences were reported in one nationally representative sample of Canadians, where social phobia was associated with a significantly greater risk of obesity (1.2 and 1.4 times greater lifetime and past year risk, respectively) in females only (Mather et al., 2009). Sex differences were also observed in a study that found that obese women, but not obese men, were at significantly greater risk for social phobia in the past year (1.8 times) and in their lifetime (1.7 times) (Barry et al., 2008).

Finally, two epidemiological studies of nationally representative samples did not find an association between social phobia and obesity in the lifetime or past year (Chou & Chi, 2005; Pickering et al., 2007). The evidence is modest for a heightened risk of social phobia in obesity, and possibly only true for women.

1.3.3.2 Pathophysiology and Treatment

Studies explaining the association between social phobia and obesity are lacking. In the context of obesity management, social phobia may become a challenge to developing healthy lifestyle habits. For example, patients with social phobia may have reluctance to join a gym, group-based weight loss programs (e.g., Weight Watchers), exercise classes, or any activities that involve group participation, given that anxiety may be generated by these activities. This may result in more sedentary lifestyles which could possibly lead to weight gain as well as increasing the difficulty of weight loss attempts. Further research on social phobia is also needed to determine the extent to which fear of eating in front of others, a characteristic of social phobia, may affect eating behavior. For example, patients with social phobia who conceal their eating may be prevented from eating in response to hunger to the extent that they must wait to eat until alone. One study demonstrated a significant association between social anxiety and eating pathology (Wonderlich-Tierney & Vander Wal, 2010). In the context of clinical weight management, the impact of social anxiety symptoms on eating behavior, physical activity, and adherence should be explored as part of the clinical assessment.

1.3.4 Specific Phobia

Specific phobia refers to excessive fear of a specific stimulus (e.g., heights, seeing blood, animals, or insects) that is recognized by the individual as irrational (American Psychiatric Association, 2000). Avoidance of the feared stimulus can be extensive and typically interferes with the individual's functioning. Lifetime prevalence of specific phobia is 12.5% (Kessler et al., 2005). Two studies using nationally representative samples support an association between specific phobia and obesity (Pickering et al., 2007) preported that specific phobia in the past year was significantly, but weakly, associated with obesity in men (1.2 times greater risk) and women (1.3 times greater risk) and Petry et al. (2008) observed that past year and lifetime-specific phobia were significantly associated with obesity and extreme obesity. Prevalence for past year and lifetime-specific phobia was, respectively, 6.48 and 8.57% in normal-weight individuals, 8.67 and 11.37% in obese individuals, and 11.96 and 15.15% in severely obese individuals (Petry et al.). Finally, in a study using the NESARC, obesity was associated with increased odds of specific phobia in both men and women, although overweight was associated with increased odds of specific phobia in women only (Barry et al., 2008). Very little research has examined the mechanisms by which specific phobia and obesity may be associated, and whether it is a direct relationship or if it is better accounted for by psychotropic medications, other psychiatric co-morbidities, or some other third factor.

1.3.5 Posttraumatic Stress Disorder

PTSD develops following a traumatic event and involves reexperiencing symptoms (e.g., flashbacks, recurrent dreams of event), avoidance behaviors (avoiding people, places or things that remind person of event), and hyperarousal (e.g., disturbed sleep, feeling on edge, and heightened startle response) (American Psychiatric Association, 1994). Traumatic events are those that may involve threat of death or a serious injury or threat to physical or psychological integrity of self or others and are associated with feelings of intense fear, helplessness, or horror. PTSD has a lifetime prevalence of 6.5% in the general U.S. population (Elhai, Grubaugh, Kashdan, & Frueh, 2008).

1.3.5.1 Prevalence of Co-morbid PTSD and Obesity

An association between PTSD and obesity has been observed in several studies. A population-based study in New Zealand showed that obesity is more strongly associated with PTSD than any of the mood and anxiety disorders (Scott et al., 2008). A longitudinal population-based study in Germany revealed that PTSD predicted obesity over 10 years in young adult females but not males (Perkonigg, Owashi, Stein, Kirschbaum, & Wittchen, 2009). In that study, only 4% of the sample was obese, and unlike other studies, neither mood nor other anxiety disorders were associated with obesity. In a population-based study of US adults, past year PTSD was associated with greater likelihood of obesity (OR = 1.51; 95% CI = 1.18, 1.95) and the association was similar among men and women (Pagoto, Lemon, et al., 2008). Finally, one study using a Veterans Administration patient database found that male veterans with PTSD had significantly higher rates of obesity compared to male veterans without PTSD (40% vs. 30%; Vieweg et al., 2007). These findings provide further support that the association between PTSD and obesity is evident in males. Of all the anxiety disorders, PTSD seems to have the strongest associations with obesity, although the reasons for the association remain unclear.

Childhood abuse is a common form of trauma among patients with PTSD. A history of childhood abuse, regardless of presence of PTSD, has been shown to be associated with obesity in adulthood. One large study of members of a health maintenance organization found that adults who reported having experienced childhood abuse (either verbal, physical, or sexual) were on average 0.6–4.0 kg heavier than adults who did not report such abuse and had a 6–39% increased risk for being obese (Williamson, Thompson, Anda, Dietz, & Felitti, 2002). In that study, PTSD and other psychological disorders were not assessed, so it is not known to what extent psychopathology stemming from abuse contributed to the association with higher weight. A subsequent study of 340 consecutive extremely obese bariatric surgery candidates found rates of childhood abuse that were 2–3 times higher than a normative sample, with 46% reporting emotional abuse, 32% reporting sexual abuse, and 29% reporting physical abuse (Grilo et al., 2005). Similar results were found in four other studies of bariatric surgery candidates that reported rates of childhood sexual abuse of 23% (Larsen & Geenen, 2005), 27% (Oppong, Nickels, & Sax, 2006), 27% (Clark et al., 2007), and over 30% (Wildes, Kalarchian, Marcus, Levine, & Courcoulas, 2008). In the latter study, childhood sexual abuse and other forms of childhood abuse and neglect were associated with increased rates of mood and anxiety disorders (Wildes et al.). Together, this literature suggests that histories of childhood sexual and other forms of abuse are fairly common in bariatric surgery candidates and may play a role in the development of extreme obesity in adulthood.

1.3.5.2 Pathophysiology of PTSD and Obesity

Neurobiological Mechanisms

PTSD may be associated with obesity via neurobiological processes. For example, PTSD is associated with alterations in the functioning of the HPA axis, a neurohormonal pathway that regulates the secretion of the appetite-suppressing hormone CRH and the glucocorticoid hormone cortisol (Mastorakos & Zapanti, 2004). Individuals with PTSD have lower circulating cortisol levels relative to healthy controls, though these findings are more robust in women and are also influenced by age, time since trauma, and other factors (de Kloet et al., 2006; Freidenberg et al., 2010; Meewisse, Reitsma, de Vries, Gersons, & Olff, 2007; Pervanidou & Chrousos, 2010). HPA axis functioning has also been linked to stress-related weight gain (Vicennati, Pasqui, Cavazza, Pagotto, & Pasquali, 2009) and stress-induced increases (Epel, Lapidus, McEwen, & Brownell, 2001; George, Khan, Briggs, & Abelson, 2010; Newman, O'Connor, & Conner, 2007) and decreases (Appelhans, Pagoto, Peters, & Spring, 2010; Mastorakos & Zapanti, 2004) in energy intake. The mechanisms of HPA axis involvement in both PTSD and obesity are still being elucidated.

It is worth considering the possibility that obesity might somehow confer increased risk for PTSD, or that both obesity and PTSD are caused by some third set of factors. For example, obesity and PTSD may both be influenced by genetic polymorphisms common to both conditions. Alternatively, both may be influenced by low socioeconomic status, which has been linked to greater risk for PTSD among those exposed to trauma (Brewin, Andrews, & Valentine, 2000) and higher adiposity (McLaren, 2007; Wang & Beydoun, 2007). To our knowledge, no studies have found that obesity is a prospective risk factor for exposure to severe trauma or the development of PTSD, though this possibility has yet to be ruled out.

Psychological Mechanisms

Several hypotheses have been put forth regarding the psychological mechanisms of the association between PTSD and obesity, although not all are well supported by data. The relationship between history of childhood sexual abuse and the development of obesity, especially extreme obesity, has also been discussed extensively. Depression, disordered eating, inhibitory control, and the extent to which obesity-promoting behaviors serve as avoidance behaviors (in the case of sexual abuse survivors) are factors discussed in the development of obesity among trauma survivors (Capuron et al., 2011; Gustafson & Sarwer, 2004).

Depression and Disordered Eating

Depression has been suggested as a plausible factor explaining the relationship between PTSD and obesity; however, very little research actually supports this contention. One study controlled for all mood disorders when examining the association between obesity and PTSD and found that this did not reduce the association (Scott et al., 2008). Similarly, another population-based study found that depression did not account for significant variance in the relationship between PTSD and obesity (Pagoto, Lemon, et al., 2008). These findings together would suggest that depression probably does not account for the association between PTSD and obesity.

Disordered eating could develop as an attempt to cope with trauma and possibly explain why PTSD is associated with increased risk for obesity. PTSD (Hudson, Hiripi, Pope, & Kessler, 2007), early life trauma (Allison, Grilo, Masheb, & Stunkard, 2007; Harrington, Crowther, Payne Henrickson, & Mickelson, 2006), and childhood sexual abuse (Gustafson & Sarwer, 2004) have all been associated with increased risk for binge-eating disorder (BED). However, BED does not appear to account for the relationship between PTSD and obesity, as evidenced by one cross-sectional population-based study which found that PTSD was related to increased odds of both BED and obesity, but BED did not attenuate the association between PTSD and obesity (Pagoto, Lemon, et al., 2008). Although causal links cannot be established in this cross-sectional study, these findings weaken the case for a prominent role of BED in explaining the association between PTSD and obesity. However, findings do not rule out the possibility that milder and more prevalent forms of eating pathology, including emotional eating and externally cued eating, could play a role in the development of obesity in trauma survivors with PTSD. Further research is certainly needed of the causal and temporal relationships between trauma, eating pathology, and obesity given their co-occurrence.

Inhibitory Control

PTSD has also been associated with weakened inhibitory control. Individuals with PTSD perform worse on behavioral tasks that measure the capacity to suppress inappropriate behavioral responses, a manifestation of inhibitory control largely mediated by the frontal cortex (Falconer et al., 2008; Lagarde, Doyon, & Brunet, 2010; Miller & Cohen, 2001; Simmonds, Pekar, & Mostofsky, 2008). Recent evidence suggests that the capacity for inhibitory control is critical to suppressing food intake in a modern environment characterized by frequent exposure to highly palatable food (Alonso-Alonso & Pascual-Leone, 2007; Appelhans, 2009; van den Bos & de Ridder, 2006). Supporting this notion are findings linking impulsivity and deficits in inhibitory control to obesity and poorer weight loss outcomes in behavioral treatment programs (Nederkoorn, Braet, Van Eijs, Tanghe, & Jansen, 2006; Nederkoorn, Jansen, Mulkens, & Jansen, 2007; Nederkoorn, Smulders, Havermans, Roefs, & Jansen, 2006; Pauli-Pott, Albayrak, Hebebrand, & Pott, 2010). Based on these findings, it is plausible that the neurobiological disruption of inhibitory control associated with PTSD may also confer vulnerability to overeating and obesity. Further research is certainly merited in this area.

Obesity-Promoting Behaviors as Anxiety Avoidance

Obesity has been purported to serve an adaptive avoidance function for some survivors of sexual abuse by preventing sexual attention and the anxiety generated by sexual feelings and experiences (Gustafson & Sarwer, 2004). In such individuals, activities that maintain obesity, including overeating and sedentary behavior, are proposed to function as avoidance behaviors that prevent the intense anxiety generated by sexual attention and intimacy. Individuals with histories of sexual abuse show reduced weight loss motivation, body dissatisfaction, and adherence to a weight loss attempt (Sarwer & Thompson, 2002). Further research on this topic is needed.

1.3.5.3 Clinical Considerations

A few studies have examined the impact of PTSD and/or childhood sexual abuse on outcomes of both behavioral and surgical interventions for obesity. Although high rates of PTSD and childhood sexual trauma are observed in bariatric patients, surgical outcomes do not appear to be affected. Veterans with PTSD stemming from service-related trauma lost comparable amounts of weight 1-year after bariatric surgery compared to those without PTSD (Ikossi, Maldonado, Hernandez-Boussard, & Eisenberg, 2010). Four studies reported that survivors of childhood sexual abuse did not demonstrate significantly worse bariatric surgery outcomes than patients without abuse histories for up to 1-year postsurgery (Buser, Dymek-Valentine, Hilburger, & Alverdy, 2004; Clark et al., 2007; Larsen & Geenen, 2005; Oppong et al., 2006), but one study did find that a history of sexual abuse correlated with less weight loss 1 year following bariatric surgery (Ray, Nickels, Sayeed, & Sax, 2003; Stefaniak, Babinska, Trus, & Vingerhoets, 2007) suggests that findings from studies using questionnaire measures of sexual abuse should be interpreted with caution because of the vast degree of underreporting of childhood sexual abuse via questionnaire measures. However, the only two studies (i.e., Buser et al., 2004; Clark et al., 2007) that used clinical interviews rather than questionnaires did not find differences in weight loss following surgery in people with a history of sexual abuse from those with no history. The majority of studies do not support a negative impact of sexual abuse history on surgical weight loss outcome. In one study of bariatric patients, the majority of patients (73%) with psychiatric hospitalizations following bariatric surgery had a history of childhood sexual abuse, which suggests that the identification and monitoring of these patients before and after bariatric surgery may be important even if weight loss outcomes are not affected (Clark et al.). Only one study examined whether behavioral weight loss outcomes might be affected by having a trauma history and results showed that weight loss at 6 months was significantly less among patients with a history of sexual abuse relative to patients without such a history (King, Clark, & Pera, 1996). More research is clearly needed to definitively determine whether history of childhood sexual abuse and PTSD in general is associated with obesity treatment failure.

1.3.6 Conclusion

Anxiety disorders seem to be associated with a modest increased risk for obesity; however, very little research has explored the reasons for the association. In a recent population-based cross-sectional study using the Canadian Community Health Survey, use of antidepressant and antipsychotic medications accounted for 32% of the association between anxiety disorders and obesity (Smits et al., 2010). Although antidepressants are often used to treat anxiety disorders, antipsychotic medications are not which suggests that findings could possibly reflect the presence of co-morbid psychiatric conditions. Another potential but unexplored mechanism is chronic stress, which may be elevated among individuals with anxiety disorders and may account for some of the relationship between anxiety disorders and obesity. The bulk of the literature has focused on the association between PTSD, childhood abuse, and obesity, and a variety of mechanisms have been proposed, but few tested. Some anxiety disorders may have significant implications for the management of obesity, especially to the extent that anxiety and stress affect appetite, eating behavior, and physical activity levels. More research is needed to establish whether anxiety disorders are associated with worse obesity treatment outcomes. PTSD does not appear to have an adverse effect on surgical weight loss outcomes, but may have implications for behavioral weight loss outcome; however, the latter has received very little research attention.

1.4 Eating Disorders

Eating disorders in the DSM-IV include anorexia nervosa, bulimia nervosa, and eating disorders not otherwise specified (American Psychiatric Association, 1994). Anorexia nervosa requires an underweight criterion and thus it cannot co-occur with obesity by definition. Bulimia nervosa does not appear to be significantly more prevalent among obese individuals than lean and overweight individuals (Bulik, Sullivan, & Kendler, 2000; Hudson et al., 2007; Wade, Bergin, Tiggemann, Bulik, & Fairburn, 2006) and, as such, will not be discussed in this chapter. In the DSM-IV, BED is a diagnostic criteria set requiring further study. Night eating syndrome (NES) is not addressed in the DSM-IV; however, provisional criteria have been developed elsewhere (Allison, Lundgren, O'Reardon, et al., 2010). BED (Allison et al., 2006; Grucza, Przybeck, & Cloninger, 2007; Hasler et al., 2004; Hudson et al., 2007) and NES (Adami, Campostano, Marinari, Ravera, & Scopinaro, 2002; Allison et al., 2006, 2007; Colles, Dixon, & O'Brien, 2007; Jarosz, Dobal, Wilson, & Schram, 2007) are highly co-morbid with obesity and will be the focus of this section.

1.4.1 Binge-Eating Disorder

The DSM-IV criteria for BED requires binge-eating episodes at least twice weekly for 6 months that last 2 h or less and involve the consumption of an amount of food that is much larger than what most people would consume in that period of time (American Psychiatric Association, 1994). The binge-eating episode must be characterized by a perceived lack of control and must also be associated with three or more of the following: rapid eating, eating until uncomfortably full, binge eating in the absence of hunger, eating alone, and feelings of disgust, guilt, or depressed mood following the episode. This pattern should be characterized by marked distress. The main distinguishing factor of BED from bulimia is the absence of compensatory strategies such as vomiting or laxative use. In the general population, rates of BED range between 1.0 and 3.5% (Hudson et al., 2007; Spitzer, Williams, Gibbon, & First, 1992; Spitzer et al., 1993).

1.4.1.1 Prevalence of Co-morbid BED and Obesity

BED and obesity are highly co-morbid in that the vast majority of people with BED are obese. In a community sample, about 70% of adults with BED were obese (Grucza et al., 2007). However, only a minority of obese people have BED. The prevalence of BED among overweight or obese adults ranges from 3 to 14.8% in population and community samples (Grucza et al.; Hudson et al., 2007). Much higher prevalence rates are generally observed in weight loss treatment-seeking samples, ranging from 4.2 to 33% (Allison et al., 2006; Pagoto et al., 2007; Ramacciotti et al., 2000). The only prospective study of the relationship between BED and weight status revealed that BED predicted greater odds of becoming overweight for males and females over 20 years, even after controlling for demographics and psychiatric co-morbidities (Hasler et al., 2004). Given the association between BED and obesity, some experts have questioned whether BED should even be considered a distinct disorder from obesity, but instead a subtype of obesity (Davis et al., 2008; Devlin, Goldfein, & Dobrow, 2003; Stunkard & Allison, 2003). However, a review of the validity and clinical utility of the BED diagnosis supports the distinction of BED as a separate disorder (Wonderlich, Gordon, Mitchell, Crosby, & Engel, 2009) and it has been recommended for inclusion in the DSM-V (American Psychiatric Association, 2010). BED is not only strongly associated with obesity, but also appears to be associated with elevated rates of obesity-related conditions such as the metabolic syndrome (Roehrig, Masheb, White, & Grilo, 2009) and type 2 diabetes (Hudson et al., 2010), making it an indicator of elevated health risk.

1.4.1.2 Pathophysiology of Co-morbid BED and Obesity

Research into the mechanisms underlying the co-morbidity of BED and obesity suggests bidirectional mechanisms. On the one hand, overconsumption during binge episodes can lead to weight gain. A prospective study of women with BED revealed an average weight gain of 4.2 kg over 5 years (Fairburn, Cooper, Doll, Norman, & O'Connor, 2000). Alternatively, obesity may precede BED (Davis et al., 2009). One study examining the onset of overweight and binge eating among overweight adults with BED revealed that 63% reported being overweight *before* they began binge eating, while only 15.8% reported that their binge eating predated overweight (Reas & Grilo, 2007).

Stress

Stress is a factor in the development of BED (Striegel-Moore et al., 2007) and obesity (Dallman, Pecoraro, & la Fleur, 2005; Vicennati et al., 2009), which suggests that it could be a common mechanism of the co-morbidity. Stress precipitates binge-eating episodes (Greeno & Wing, 1994; Torres & Nowson, 2007) and triggers the response of the HPA axis. The HPA axis is a complex hormonal cascade that regulates the secretion of the glucocorticoid hormone, cortisol (Habib et al., 2000). With the onset of stress, neurons in the hypothalamus secrete CRH into the portal vasculature shared with the pituitary gland. CRH elicits secretion of ACTH from the anterior pituitary into the peripheral circulation, where it eventually stimulates the adrenal cortex to secrete cortisol. Circulating cortisol feeds back to the hypothalamus and pituitary to inhibit further HPA axis activation. The response of the HPA axis to stress can stimulate the ingestion of high fat, high caloric foods (Epel et al., 2006; Gluck et al.; Oliver et al., 2000; Zellner et al., 2006) and consumption of these foods appears to temper the stress response by reducing CRH expression and ACTH release (Dallman, 2010; Foster et al., 2009; Pecoraro, Reyes, Gomez, Bhargava, & Dallman, 2004). Consuming high fat, high caloric foods may help to alleviate feelings of stress (Macht, 2008), and due to the involvement of glucocorticoids and CRH in memory and learning processes, could facilitate a learned association between eating and stress reduction (Dallman, 2010). Over time, regular use of food to alleviate stress is likely to result in weight gain. Women with BED demonstrate higher basal cortisol rates (Gluck, Geliebter, & Lorence, 2004; Pirke, Platte, Laessle, Seidl, & Fichter, 1992) and increased cortisol responses to stress (Gluck et al.), which could be indicative of chronic stress and HPA axis hyperactivity. If individuals with BED experience stress more consistently and consume high fat, high caloric foods in response to stress, they are at risk for obesity (Dallman et al., 2005; Vicennati et al., 2009), especially abdominal obesity (Dallman, Akana, Strack, Hanson, & Sebastian, 1995).

Neurobiological Mechanisms

Neurobiological mechanisms common to both obesity and eating disorders have been proposed in the literature recently. Berridge, Ho, Richard, & DiFeliceantonio, 2010 proposed that dysfunction in the reward pathways in the brain may explain the co-morbidity of obesity and BED. Neural activation of the mesolimbic dopamine system appears to drive "wanting" (motivation to consume food), while opioidergic processes in the nucleus accumbens and the ventral pallidum influence liking (the pleasure value of food) (Berridge et al.). One study provides preliminary evidence that the opioid system may be more influential in binge eating than obesity, as administration of naloxone, an opiate blocker, significantly reduced food consumption in individuals with BED compared to those without BED, but did not influence consumption by obese individuals, regardless of BED status (Drewnowski, Krahn, Demitrack, Nairn, & Gosnell, 1995). It is currently unclear whether dysfunction in these reward pathways increases the likelihood of subsequently developing BED and obesity, or if reward pathways become altered in response to repeated binge eating or excessive weight gain (Berridge et al.).

Psychological Factors

Psychological mechanisms put forth to explain the co-morbidity of BED and obesity include depression and a history of childhood abuse. Depression may partially explain the BED and obesity co-morbidity because depression is highly co-morbid with each. In one clinic-based study, 54% of weight treatment-seeking patients with BED also met criteria for depression (Pagoto, Lemon, et al., 2008). In that study, BED and depression were each associated with poorer weight loss outcomes following treatment, but having both disorders did not result in an additive increase in risk relative to either disorder alone. This suggests BED and depression may impede weight loss success to the same degree and possibly through common mechanisms.

A history of child abuse has also been shown to be a risk factor for BED (Fosse & Holen, 2006; Grilo, Masheb, & Wilson, 2001; Smolak & Murnen, 2002) and child abuse has also been associated with obesity (Johnson, Cohen, Kasen, & Brook, 2002; Rohde et al., 2008; Walker et al., 1999; Williamson et al., 2002). The mechanisms by which child abuse leads to BED or obesity have not been clearly established, but may involve an altered stress response as discussed above. Many of the mechanisms of co-morbid BED and obesity are likely interrelated, and the stress response appears to be one common denominator. For example, depression and child abuse are associated with each other (Dunkley, Masheb, & Grilo, 2010; Rohde et al., 2008) and increased cortisol secretion (Heim, Mletzko, Purselle, Musselman, & Nemeroff, 2008; Shea, Walsh, Macmillan, & Steiner, 2005). Additional research is needed to understand how these psychological mechanisms promote pathological eating and the extent to which they contribute to co-morbid BED and obesity.

1.4.1.3 Clinical Care

Assessment

Assessment of BED in obese patients who present weight loss and primary care settings may be important given that BED may have implications for weight loss success. Generally, evidence shows that binge eaters have more difficulty losing weight. A meta-analysis demonstrated a strong adverse effect of BED on weight loss outcomes (Blaine & Rodman, 2007). Participants with BED lost an average of 1.3 kg, whereas participants without BED lost 10.5 kg. Consistent with these results, a chart review study of patients in a hospital-based outpatient weight loss program found that only 16% of patients with BED met the 7% weight loss goal by the end of treatment compared to 38% of patients without BED (Pagoto et al., 2007). Binge eaters appear to lose less weight and have lower rates of clinically significant weight loss than their obese counterparts.

Assessment of BED can be challenging given that binging is a private behavior that is accompanied by shame. A clinical diagnosis can be made via the Structured Clinical Interview for DSM disorders (SCID) (Spitzer et al., 1992) or the Eating Disorder Examination (EDE) (Fairburn, Marcus, & Wilson, 1993), but clinical interviews are labor-intensive. It has been recommended that primary care providers routinely screen for binge eating and other eating disorders given that individuals with eating disorders are frequent consumers of healthcare services and that eating disorders are associated with substantial psychological and medical co-morbidities (Sim et al., 2010). Self-report questionnaires include the 32-item EDE-Questionnaire (EDE-Q) (Fairburn & Beglin, 1994) and the 27-item Questionnaire for Eating and Weight Patterns-Revised (QEWP-R) (Yanovski, Nelson, Dubbert, & Spitzer, 1993), both of which demonstrate adequate validity and reliability for the assessment of BED (Barnes, Masheb, White, & Grilo, 2011; Celio, Wilfley, Crow, Mitchell, & Walsh, 2004; de Zwaan et al., 1993; Elder et al., 2006; Goldfein, Devlin, & Kamenetz, 2005). A somewhat briefer instrument is the Binge Eating Scale (BES), a 16-item questionnaire that assesses the presence and severity of binge eating in obese people (Gormally, Black, Daston, & Rardin, 1982). The BES cannot be used to make a diagnosis of BED, but would certainly inform a clinician of whether further assessment and specialized treatment is necessary. Another challenge of assessment in BED is distinguishing between common overeating episodes (e.g., large holiday meal) and binge eating, which typically involve unusually large consumption and a significant degree of shame around the episode.

Current guidelines for bariatric surgery assessment recommend inclusion of BED measures (Blackburn et al., 2009). Although BED is not associated with a poorer weight loss outcome between 18 and 35 months after bariatric surgery, it is associated with higher frequency of binge-like episodes and vomiting after surgery, which can present significant health concerns (de Zwaan et al., 2010). Clinical guidelines do not identify BED as a contraindication for surgery, but instead a condition to be continuously monitored because remitted eating disorders can resurface following surgery in some patients (Blackburn et al., 2009).

Evidence-Based Treatment

Behavioral Treatments for BED and Obesity

The literature includes several treatment approaches to BED and obesity, including psychotherapy for BED, behavioral weight loss interventions, combination of psychotherapy and behavioral weight loss, and medication. The optimal approach to treatment should reduce both weight and binge eating.

A recent meta-analysis reported that the largest between group effects sizes for reduction in binge eating are for psychotherapy and self-help approaches (Vocks et al., 2010). The National Institute for Clinical Excellence (NICE) recommends CBT as a first-line treatment for adults with BED (National Institute for Clinical Excellence, 2004). Goals of CBT are to address the negative emotions that trigger binges, develop regular eating patterns, and identify the maladaptive cognitions that contribute to binge-eating episodes (Fairburn et al., 1993). In cases where CBT is ineffective, NICE guidelines recommend interpersonal psychotherapy (IPT) and dialectical behavior therapy (DBT) for BED (National Institute for Clinical Excellence, 2004). Theoretically, psychotherapy that effectively reduces binge eating would seem to promote weight loss to the extent that total calorie consumption is affected by eliminating binge episodes. However, CBT, IPT, or DBT for BED do not appear to facilitate significant weight loss (Brownley, Berkman, Sedway, Lohr, & Bulik, 2007; Hay, Bacaltchuk, Stefano, & Kashyap, 2009; Yager, 2008).

An alternative approach to reducing both binge eating and weight is via behavioral weight loss interventions, typically involving both dietary and physical activity counseling. One trial randomized obese binge eaters to CBT for BED or a behavioral weight loss program and found that CBT was more effective at reducing binge eating, but the behavioral weight loss program was more effective at reducing weight at 6 months (Munsch et al., 2007). Group differences vanished by 1 year. Another trial randomized obese binge eaters to self-help versions of CBT and behavioral weight loss and found that the CBT condition was superior to behavioral weight loss on binge eating, but the conditions did not differ on weight loss outcomes (Grilo & Masheb, 2005). Weight loss may not have been significant because self-help versions of behavioral weight loss programs have not typically been as effective as self-guided interventions. These studies would suggest that behavioral weight loss interventions alone do not appear to be very effective for reducing binge eating in obese binge eaters, although they may help to facilitate some weight loss.

Another treatment approach involves combining CBT and behavioral weight loss, given that each appears to be effective in reducing its corresponding target. In a meta-analysis of BED trials, combination treatments had the highest within group (but not between group) effect sizes on a broad range of outcomes including weight and binge eating (Vocks et al., 2010). Randomized trials of combination treatments either compare them to conditions involving CBT alone or behavioral weight loss treatment alone. In terms of the former, three randomized trials found that the combination resulted in greater weight loss and reductions in binge-eating episodes than CBT alone (Fossati et al., 2004; Painot, Jotterand, Kammer, Fossati, & Golay, 2001). In terms of the latter, two trials found that while the combination improved binge-eating outcomes, it did not outperform a behavioral weight loss condition on weight loss outcomes (de Zwaan, Mitchell, & Crosby, 2005; Devlin et al., 2005; McElroy, Frye, et al., 2007; McElroy, Hudson, et al., 2007). The combination of CBT and behavioral weight loss treatment deserves further study. Future studies might explore whether a simultaneous or sequential treatment approach is optimal for both binge eating and weight loss outcomes (Devlin, 2001).

Pharmacotherapy

Several medication classes have been examined as a potential treatment for BED, and two meta-analyses provide support for medium effect sizes on binge-eating outcomes (Reas & Grilo, 2008; Vocks et al., 2010). One of these meta-analyses found that psychotherapy for BED combined with topiramate (e.g., Claudino et al., 2007) or orlistat (e.g., Golay et al., 2005) resulted in greater weight loss outcomes than psychotherapy plus placebo, but no significant effect for fluoxetine (Reas & Grilo, 2008). Zonisamide has recently been tested as an adjunct to CBT for BED as well. A randomized controlled trial that randomized participants to 6 months of CBT or CBT plus zonisamide reported that the combination resulted in greater weight loss and decreased binge eating at 1 year (Ricca, Castellini, Lo Sauro, Rotella, & Faravelli, 2009). A serious consideration though is that 50% of participants randomized to the CBT plus zonisamide condition failed to complete the study (20% dropped due to medication side effects). In general, combining topiramate, orlistat, or zonisamide with evidence-based psychotherapy for BED may offer benefits on weight loss and binge eating beyond that observed with psychotherapy alone, although the benefits may be limited to patients who can tolerate the medications. Also, high placebo response rates have been observed in medication studies as noted in a recent meta-analysis, which may raise questions about the specificity of effects of medication (Vocks et al., 2010). Further study is clearly needed.

Issues in Treatment Decision Making

Predictors of Treatment Response

Binge eating severity (Agras et al., 1995; Agras, Telch, Arnow, Eldredge, & Marnell, 1997; Loeb, Wilson, Gilbert, & Labouvie, 2000; Peterson et al., 2000) and psychiatric co-morbidities (Masheb & Grilo, 2008; Wilfley et al., 2000) are strong predictors of attrition and poor weight treatment outcome. Studies have not yet addressed whether improving upon factors that predict poor treatment outcome actually improves outcomes. For example, treating co-morbid depression and/or anxiety disorders prior to treatment might increase efficacy.

One positive predictor of treatment outcome appears to be early response to treatment (Grilo, White, Masheb, Rothschild, & Burke-Martindale, 2006). In a randomized trial of 16 weeks of four different treatments (i.e., fluoxetine, placebo, CBT plus fluoxetine, and CBT plus placebo), participants who decreased binge-eating episodes by 65% or more in the first 4 weeks of treatment (early treatment responders) were more likely to achieve remission than late treatment responders, regardless of treatment condition. Moreover, early responders in the CBT condition lost more weight by the end of treatment. Although the study did not identify characteristics of early treatment responders, results suggest that early treatment response could be a cue to clinicians to determine whether treatment should be augmented.

Ethnic and Racial Issues

The presentation of BED may differ across ethnic groups. A study comparing African-American and Caucasian women with BED reported that African-American women endorsed significantly more binge episodes and less weight concern, eating concern, shape concern, and dietary restraint (Pike, Dohm, Striegel-Moore, Wilfley, & Fairburn, 2001). These differences in clinical presentation could have treatment implications, although this has not yet been explored. Further investigation of the manifestation of BED in ethnic and racial groups could enhance treatment in populations who typically receive less treatment for eating pathology than Caucasians (Marques et al., 2011).

1.4.2 Night Eating Syndrome

1.4.2.1 Prevalence

An international consortium of NES researchers was convened to establish a consensus for NES diagnostic criteria (Allison, Lundgren, Moore, et al., 2010; Allison, Lundgren, O'Reardon, et al., 2010). Core criteria include consumption of at least 25% of daily energy intake in the evening (i.e., prior to sleep) and at least two episodes of nocturnal eating (i.e., waking up during the night and eating) per week for at least 3 months, as well as awareness of the evening and nocturnal eating episodes. Criteria for NES also include at least three of the following: (1) lack of desire to eat in the morning or skipping breakfast 4 or more times/week; (2) strong urge to eat after dinner and before sleep onset and/or during the night; (3) insomnia during four or more nights per week; (4) belief that eating assists with initiating or returning to sleep; or (5) frequent depressed mood or worsened mood in the evening (Allison, Lundgren, Moore, et al.; Allison, Lundgren, O'Reardon, et al.). NES is distinct from sleep-related eating disorders, which involve involuntary nocturnal eating (similar to sleep walking), because NES requires awareness of nocturnal eating episodes (Allison, Lundgren, Moore, et al.; Allison, Lundgren, O'Reardon, et al.). Although features of NES may overlap with BED, the amount of food consumed during night eating episodes does not need to be considered abnormally large as the average consumption during evening or nocturnal eating episodes of individuals with NES is approximately 350 kcal (Birketvedt et al., 1999).

NES was first identified in obese individuals (Stunkard, Grace, & Wolff, 1955), but it is unclear whether the prevalence increases with increasing BMI. Two population-based studies reported that the prevalence of NES ranged from 1.5 to 35.8% depending on the criteria used, but neither found an association of NES with BMI (Rand, Macgregor, & Stunkard, 1997; Striegel-Moore, Franko, Thompson, Affenito, & Kraemer, 2006). On the other hand, a Swedish population-based study of NES that used a broader classification of NES then what has since been defined by Allison and colleagues (Allison, Lundgren, Moore, et al., 2010; Allison, Lundgren, O'Reardon, et al., 2010) reported that prevalence was 2 times as great in obese than nonobese individuals (Tholin et al., 2009). Research on weight loss treatment-seeking overweight and obese individuals reported that the prevalence of NES ranged from 3.8 to 64.0%, with only 4 out of 12 studies reporting NES prevalence below 10% (Adami et al., 2002; Allison et al., 2006, 2007; Aronoff et al., 2001; Ceru-Bjork et al., 2001; Colles et al., 2007; Gluck et al., 2001; Jarosz et al., 2007; Napolitano et al., 2001; Stunkard, 1959; Stunkard et al., 1955, 1996). The variability in prevalence rates is likely due to varying criteria, measures, and samples (de Zwaan, Burgard, Schenck, & Mitchell, 2003; Striegel-Moore et al., 2006). Further research is needed to create reliable and valid assessment instruments so that more accurate prevalence estimates can be made

1.4.2.2 Pathophysiology

That NES contributes to the development of obesity is supported by one prospective study showing that individuals with NES gained significantly more weight (Mean = 6.2 kg) over an average of 3.4 years compared to individuals without NES (Mean = 1.7 kg) (Gluck, Venti, Salbe, & Krakoff, 2008). More research is needed to determine whether NES precedes obesity or whether obesity precedes NES (Howell,

Schenck, & Crow, 2009). Candidate mechanisms linking obesity and NES include circadian system disruption and HPA axis dysregulation.

Circadian Rhythm Disruption

Disruption in circadian rhythm is one of the most compelling mechanisms linking NES and obesity. Circadian rhythms involve the external and internal synchronization of behavioral and physiological processes. External synchronization involves the influence of environmental factors, such as exposure to sunlight, while internal synchronization involves the influence of internal processes, such as body temperature regulation or metabolism (Laposkya, Bassb, Kohsakac, & Turek, 2008). Individuals with NES display sleeping patterns that are desynchronized with their eating patterns. Two studies demonstrated that although NES was not associated with alterations in sleep onset and offset, it was associated with delayed food consumption (O'Reardon, Ringel, et al., 2004; Rogers et al., 2006). Individuals with NES also wake more frequently during the night (Birketvedt et al., 1999) and sleep fewer hours (O'Reardon, Ringel, et al., 2004; Rogers et al., 2006) compared to individuals without NES. This pattern of abnormal sleep timing, delayed food consumption, and interrupted sleep is indicative of a circadian disruption, which has also been shown to negatively impact metabolism (Laposkya et al., 2008) and has been implicated in the development of obesity (Garaulet, Ordovás, & Madrid, 2010). Metabolism is affected such that circadian disruption decreases leptin levels and increases ghrelin levels, resulting in increased food intake, weight gain and, potentially over time, obesity (Garaulet et al.). One study examined hormone profiles of NES patients and found elevated ghrelin levels compared to matched controls, but no significant differences in leptin (Allison et al., 2005). Other evidence suggests that obesity can cause circadian disruption, thereby contributing to the development of NES. For example, animal studies with genetically and high fat diet-induced obese mice showed that obesity altered the expression of genes involved in circadian rhythms (Ando et al., 2005; Kaneko et al., 2009). More research is needed to elucidate the exact nature of the circadian disruption that is associated with obesity and NES.

Hypothalamic Pituitary Adrenal Axis

HPA axis functioning is also impacted by circadian disruption. Two HPA axis hormones, cortisol and ACTH, rise sharply in the morning and decline during the day (Stone et al., 2001; Van Cauter & Refetoff, 1985). For individuals with NES, decreased sleep could stimulate the HPA axis not unlike what is observed during a stress response (Balbo, Leproult, & Van Cauter, 2010). Chronic stimulation of the HPA axis can manifest in higher basal cortisol, which has been observed in NES (Birketvedt et al., 1999; Gluck et al., 2004), although not universally (Allison et al., 2005). If NES is associated with HPA axis hyperactivity, the resulting increased cortisol secretion could stimulate food intake and lead to obesity.

1.4.2.3 Clinical Care

Assessment

Few valid and reliable assessment instruments for NES exist given that consensus on NES criteria has only recently been reached. The 14-item Night Eating Questionnaire (Allison et al., 2008) is recommended for use as a screening tool given that acceptable reliability and validity has been established (Allison et al.). Development of a quick and valid screening instrument could be helpful in settings where screening time is limited; however, NES can be superficially assessed by inquiring about evening hyperphagia, nocturnal consumption, and insomnia as these are core symptoms of NES and are likely indicative of the syndrome (Sim et al., 2010).

Evidence-Based Treatment

Treatment research for NES, particularly when it is co-morbid with obesity, is in its infancy. Pharmacotherapy includes SSRIs and behavioral approaches include weight loss treatment and CBT.

Pharmacotherapy

SSRIs have been shown to improve NES symptoms and stimulate weight loss. Three trials demonstrated that the SSRI sertraline decreased nocturnal awakenings and night eating (O'Reardon et al., 2006; O'Reardon, Stunkard, et al., 2004; Stunkard et al., 2006). The first was a 12-week open-label nonblind trial in which 17 patients with NES were treated with NES (O'Reardon, Stunkard, et al., 2004). Results showed significant improvements in awakenings, ingestion, and total intake and 5 of 17 subjects were remitted. In a second trial, participants with NES were encouraged to seek sertraline from their primary care physician via web-, mail-, and phone-based intervention contacts. Of the 50 that participated, data on 41 completers who initiated sertraline under their physicians revealed significant improvements in awakenings, ingestion, and total intake of a similar magnitude as reported in the previous trial (Stunkard et al., 2006). The third study randomized 34 overweight and obese participants with NES to sertraline or placebo and found that sertraline participants had greater improvements in NES symptoms and lost significantly more weight after 8 weeks (Mean = −2.9 kg) compared to placebo participants (Mean = −0.30 kg) (O'Reardon et al., 2006). Initial findings are encouraging, but larger randomized trials with longer follow-up periods would more strongly support the effectiveness of sertraline and other SSRIs for NES and obesity.

Behavioral Approaches

Weight loss treatment has shown some efficacy in treating NES while simultaneously facilitating weight loss. A 21-day inpatient weight loss program that included a low-calorie diet, exercise, and psychoeducational groups followed by outpatient follow-up found that only 22.8% met criteria for NES at 6 months and average weight loss was 2.7 kg (Dalle Grave, Calugi, Ruocco, & Marchesini, 2011). Whether outpatient weight loss programs would also be efficacious has not yet been tested.

CBT may also hold promise for the treatment of NES by addressing the eating, sleep disturbance, and mood symptoms characteristic of NES. One single-group study of people with NES tested the effect of ten sessions of CBT for NES, which targeted NES symptoms and provided weight loss skills. Results revealed decreases in nocturnal food consumption, NES symptoms, awakenings, total calories, weight and depression symptoms (Allison, Lundgren, Moore, et al., 2010; Allison, Lundgren, O'Reardon, et al., 2010). Randomized trials are needed to demonstrate efficacy of CBT for NES compared to usual care or active treatment conditions.

Issues in Treatment Decision Making

A key issue in NES is whether it interferes with weight loss treatment success. Research is limited on this question and preliminary evidence is mixed. One study of outpatient weight loss patients reported that patients with NES lost 40% less weight than patients without NES after 1 month of treatment (Gluck et al., 2001). However, a 4-week weight loss treatment study reported that neither a clinician diagnosis of NES, nor scores on the NEQ were associated with weight loss at the end of treatment (Vander Wal, Waller, Klurfeld, McBurney, & Dhurandhar, 2005). Similarly, a study of inpatient weight loss treatment found no differences in weight loss after a 21-day inpatient program and at the 6-month follow-up between individuals with NES and matched controls (Dalle Grave et al., 2011). A review of bariatric surgery outcomes also reported mixed evidence with some studies reporting no differences in weight loss between individuals with and without NES and some reporting less weight loss among individuals with NES (Colles & Dixon, 2006). Further research is needed, but from a clinical standpoint, weight loss and night eating should be closely monitored in individuals with NES who are participating in a weight loss program.

Other clinical issues include psychiatric co-morbidities, which appear to be prevalent among individuals with NES and may have treatment implications. Binge-eating disorder, depression, anxiety disorders, and possibly substance abuse are common co-morbidities (Vinai et al., 2008). Trauma histories also appear to be more common among patients with NES. One cross-sectional study reported that a history of childhood emotional abuse and physical neglect were significantly greater in individuals with NES compared to a noneating disordered control group of overweight and obese individuals (Allison et al., 2007). Traumatic experiences could trigger physiological changes that increase risk of NES and obesity. For example, children with a history of abuse sometimes report frequent night awakenings and greater nocturnal activity than nonabused control children and children diagnosed with depression (Glod, Teicher, Hartman, & Harakal, 1997). To the extent that disrupted sleep is a risk factor for nocturnal consumption and obesity, childhood trauma could be a predisposing factor to NES and obesity.

1.4.2.4 Conclusion

BED and NES are the eating disorders of most concern among individuals with obesity. The majority of people with BED are obese (Grucza et al., 2007), and NES is associated with obesity, but diagnostic criteria for the latter have only recently been defined, making prevalence rates difficult to interpret. BED is a significant clinical concern for obese patients (and possibly NES as well) because such patients have higher rates of obesity-related diseases (Hudson et al., 2010). The treatment outcome literature for BED is more developed than it is for NES with the most promising therapeutic options including the combination of CBT and weight loss treatment and the combination of antidepressant medication and psychotherapy. Psychotherapy treatments which are effective at reducing binge eating do not result in weight loss without adjunctive weight loss treatment. Research is needed to determine whether psychotherapies halt continued weight gain or if eating pathology continues in a form that affects energy balance, but does not meet the threshold for binge eating. Intervention research for NES is much needed and similar therapeutic approaches to BED (e.g., CBT) may be effective, although dysregulated sleep habits should be directly addressed in treatment. Given the impact on health risk and ability to lose weight, eating disorders in the context of obesity should be a treatment priority.

1.5 Psychotic Disorders

1.5.1 Prevalence of Psychotic Disorders and Co-morbid Obesity

The psychotic disorders (e.g., schizophrenia, schizoaffective disorder, and psychotic depression) are generally characterized by a constellation of symptoms including hallucinations, delusions, disordered thinking, social withdrawal, and cognitive deficits. Patients experience great difficulty with social, occupational, and independent functioning and typically require pharmacologic intervention to address disabling symptoms.

The prevalence of schizophrenia in the United States is approximately 1.1% and affects males and females evenly. Individuals with schizophrenia are disproportionately affected by obesity, a co-morbidity that has increased over the past two decades with the widespread use of second-generation antipsychotic (SGAs) medications, which can cause weight gain. The National Health Interview Survey reported higher mean BMI among women with and without schizophrenia (27.4 vs. 24.5), but no differences between men with and without schizophrenia (26.1 vs. 25.6) (Allison et al., 1999). However, sex differences were not found in a nationally representative sample of Finnish adults over 30 years old, where people with schizophrenia were over 2 times more likely to have obesity and abdominal obesity than people without schizophrenia (mean BMIs = 28.9 vs. 26.8) after controlling for sex, education, medication, diet, and smoking (Saarni et al., 2009). The role of SGAs was suggested by findings from a nationally representative sample of French adults, where obesity rates were elevated in patients with schizophrenia who were taking SGAs relative to the general population, but were not elevated in those who were not taking SGAs (Limosin, Gasquet, Leguay, Azorin, & Rouillon, 2008). In a sample of adult Medicaid recipients, sex differences were only apparent among SGA users (Daumit et al., 2003). The prevalence of obesity was elevated in both men and women with severe mental illness (including schizophrenia, bipolar disorder, depression, and substance disorder) compared to a NHANES-III comparison group adjusted for age, sex, race, and tobacco use. Obesity prevalence in women with and without severe mental illness was 60% vs. 28.5%, and in men, 29% vs. 17.7%, respectively. The association between SGA use and obesity was observed in men only, such that men taking SGAs were 4 times more likely to be obese than nonusers.

Participants in the Clinical Antipsychotic Trials of Intervention Effectiveness (CATIE), the largest national trial of antipsychotic medication effectiveness in people with schizophrenia ($N = 1,460$), had a mean BMI of 29.9 at baseline, with females (Mean = 32.8, SD = 7.8) higher than males (Mean = 28.8, SD = 6.4; McEvoy et al., 2005). Abdominal obesity in this sample was also elevated in both females and males, with 74% of females and 37% of males having waist circumference in the criterion range for metabolic syndrome, both of which were significantly greater than NHANES III subjects. Obesity appears to be a significant clinical issue among people with psychotic disorders, especially those taking certain antipsychotic medications.

1.5.2 Pathophysiology

As noted, the high rate of obesity among persons with psychotic disorders has been attributed to SGAs, also known as atypical antipsychotic medications, many of which have weight gain side effects. Studies have also shown that lifestyle factors such as poor dietary habits and low rates of physical activity have contributed to the development of obesity in this population.

1.5.2.1 Second-Generation Antipsychotic Medication

The role of pharmacological treatments for psychotic disorders in the development of obesity is quite significant. Studies of preschizophrenic and first-episode cohorts have revealed that patients with schizophrenia have lower BMIs than average at the onset of their illness and subsequent treatment, but BMI increases following onset which strongly suggests a role of medication in the development of obesity (Verma, Subramaniam, Liew, & Poon, 2009). Weight gain from SGAs can range from 0.5 to 5.0 kg in the first 10 weeks of treatment (Allison & Casey, 2001), with continued but slower gains for months and sometimes 1–2 years until plateau occurs (Rummel-Kluge et al., 2010). A recent head-to-head meta-analysis revealed that olanzipine and clozipine have the highest weight gain profiles, followed by risperidone, sertindole, and quetipine which have moderate weight gain profiles, followed by aripiprazole and amisulpride which have neutral to low weight gain profiles, and finally ziprasidone with a neutral weight gain profile (Rummel-Kluge et al., 2010).

The exact pathway by which SGAs cause weight gain is not known, but multiple factors are implicated given that SGAs have effects on both the endocrine system and neurotransmitters that affect appetite and weight regulation (Baptista, Reyes, & Hernandez, 1999). Some individuals may be more prone to SGA-associated weight gain than others, per studies revealing concordance in SGA-induced weight gain among twins, high heritability of weight gain, and certain polymorphisms in the leptin protein and serotonin- and cannibus-receptor genes associated with SGA-induced weight gain (Gregoor et al., 2009; Tiwari et al., 2010). Further research is needed to understand the mechanisms of weight gain in SGAs given that such information could guide the development of newer medications that do not cause weight gain and other metabolic problems.

Obesity and other metabolic side effects resulting from SGAs can have serious consequences to mortality in people with psychotic disorders. One study estimated and then compared the mortality consequences of clozapine on suicide prevention and weight gain (Fontaine et al., 2001). Results showed that clozapine prevents 492 suicides/100,000 patients over 10 years, but at the same time, medication-induced weight gain of 22 lb results in 416 deaths/100,000 over 10 years among those with BMI >27. According to these estimates, the mortality benefit is nearly canceled out by the mortality cost. Mortality stemming from obesity is likely related to the development of obesity-related diseases including type 2 diabetes and cardiovascular disease (CVD). The reader is referred to Chaps. 2 and 3 of this book on type 2 diabetes and CVD for a complete discussion of these disorders in the context of schizophrenia.

1.5.2.2 Lifestyle Factors

Although very few studies have evaluated the lifestyle habits, i.e., dietary intake and physical activity, of people with schizophrenia, available data suggest that they have poorer lifestyle habits than the general population, which may put them at higher risk for obesity (Amani, 2007). Poor lifestyle habits are seen in both institutionalized (Faulkner, Gorczynski, & Cohn, 2009) and community-living patients (Strassnig, Brar, & Ganguli, 2003). Institutional settings have been characterized as "obesogenic" such that they often contain soda-filled vending machines, limit access to water (often to prevent water intoxication), limit access to stairs, have buffet-style meals, have high availability of high-fat and high-sugar foods and low availability of fresh produce and lean meats, are located in low-income neighborhoods that have limited access to healthier food choices, and have staff that are reluctant to restrict food choices so as not to infringe upon patient autonomy (Faulkner et al., 2009).

Poor lifestyle habits are also evident in community-dwelling adults with schizophrenia. Using 24-h dietary recall data, two studies compared diets of community-dwelling adults with schizophrenia to matched controls using the NHANES database and reported that adults with schizophrenia consume significantly greater total fat and calories (Strassnig et al., 2003; Strassnig, Singh Brar, & Ganguli, 2005). Another study comparing general practice patients with and without severe mental illness found that patients with severe mental illness were less physically active and consumed less fiber and more saturated fat in their diets (Osborn, Nazareth, & King, 2007). The limitation of these studies is that the validity of dietary and physical activity recall is not well-established in individuals with severe mental illness, who may have more substantial challenges accurately recalling relative to the general population due to possible cognitive limitations. Regardless, the diets and physical activity patterns of people with schizophrenia appear to increase their risk for obesity.

1.5.3 Treatment

Four approaches to weight loss for people with schizophrenia have been discussed in the literature. First, lifestyle interventions that include nutrition, physical activity, and behavioral modification for weight loss are recommended as a first-line treatment for obesity. The second, medication switching, involves switching the patient from an SGA with a high weight gain profile to one with a low weight gain profile. Third, pharmacological approaches which entail adding medications known to reduce weight to the SGA regimen have been tested in the literature, albeit with limited success. Finally, bariatric surgery is not well studied in patients with schizophrenia and there is debate about whether or not schizophrenia is a contraindication for bariatric surgery.

1.5.3.1 Lifestyle Interventions

Lifestyle intervention is one of the eight psychosocial treatment recommendations put forth by the Schizophrenia Patient Outcomes Research Team in 2009 (Dixon et al., 2010). Two systematic reviews of randomized trials of lifestyle interventions concluded that they were effective in preventing and reducing antipsychotic medication-induced weight gain in adults with schizophrenia (Alvarez-Jimenez, Hetrick, Gonzalez-Blanch, Gleeson, & McGorry, 2008; Gabriele, Dubbert, & Reeves, 2009). Alvarez-Jimenez et al. (2008) reviewed ten studies focused on either weight gain prevention at the initiation of an SGA regimen or weight loss following SGA-induced weight gain. Interventions involving cognitive-behavior therapy for weight loss or lifestyle interventions (nutrition with and without physical activity) were equally effective. Interventions lasted between 8 weeks and 6 months. Individually delivered interventions had somewhat better outcomes than group-delivered interventions. The weighted mean difference across all ten studies was −2.56 kg weight loss, which the authors equated to a 2.5–4% difference from baseline weight. Two caveats pertaining to the studies included in this systematic review are the short duration of follow-up (2–3 months) and the infrequent use of intention to treat analyses. Gabriele et al. (2009) reviewed 16 studies focused specifically on atypical antipsychotic-induced weight gain, 6 non-RCTs and 10 RCTs. Conclusions were consistent with the previous review such that lifestyle interventions are effective in both preventing and treating atypical antipsychotic weight gain. However, they reported that 4 studies showed no differences in weight loss between intervention and control conditions, but these studies had smaller sample sizes and shorter duration than the 12 studies that reported significant effects.

Three studies have been conducted since these reviews and evaluated the outcomes of lifestyle intervention programs conducted within actual clinical settings, thus no randomization or control groups were employed. Weight losses were generally consistent in these samples (range of mean losses from 2.1 to 2.7 kg over 12–48 weeks), although completion rates were somewhat lower than those in the randomized trials (ranging from unreported to 77%) (Chen, Chen, & Huang, 2009; Lee, Choi, & Kwon, 2008; Lindenmayer et al., 2009). One program tested the Solutions for Wellness program, a 36-week manualized lifestyle intervention developed by Eli Lilly, in 275 inpatients in Connecticut (Lindenmayer et al.). The program resulted in mean weight losses of 2.2 kg over 36 weeks among the 72% of enrollees who completed follow-up assessments. Significant reductions were also observed in triglycerides, glucose, and rates of metabolic syndrome. The Solutions for Wellness manual is publicly available at http://www.treatmentteam.com. The two other programs were conducted in public clinical programs in Korea (Lee et al., 2008) and Taiwan (Chen et al., 2009). The Korean program was a 12-week group-based lifestyle intervention for outpatients with schizophrenia or schizoaffective disorder across 33 clinical centers in South Korea (Lee et al., 2008). Outcomes were available for the 232 patients who completed 8 or more sessions and mean weight loss was 2.64 kg. The total number of enrollees was not reported. The Taiwanese study evaluated 33 outpatients with schizophrenia or schizoaffective disorder following a 10-week group-based weight control program and found weight losses of 2.1 and 2.7 kg at 10- and 48-weeks, respectively, among the 77% who complied with the program (Chen et al., 2009). Declines in triglycerides, psychotic symptoms, depression, and anxiety, as well as improvements in quality of life were also observed.

The magnitude of weight loss via lifestyle interventions in the schizophrenia population is somewhat less than what is observed in nonmentally ill populations where 3–5 kg mean weight losses over 1 year are typical (McTigue et al., 2003). However, the impact of SGAs on weight losses should be taken into account. Weight loss of even modest proportions might indicate that the intervention is arresting SGA-induced weight gain, an important and clinically relevant outcome.

Clinical Challenges

A number of clinical challenges may be encountered when assisting patients with schizophrenia in weight control. First, dietary reporting may be less accurate in this population, which can make dietary assessment and intervention more difficult. In one study, women with schizophrenia were more likely to underreport dietary consumption via 24-h recalls than nonpsychiatric controls (77% vs. 50%) (Khazaal, Rothen, Moriniere Trombert, Fresard, & Zullino, 2007). Very little is known about the dietary intake of people with schizophrenia and valid and reliable measures in this population are lacking. Another treatment challenge is that people with schizophrenia and obesity have elevated rates of binge eating. In one study, 35% of a sample of outpatients with schizophrenia and obesity met criteria for BED compared to 10% of obese nonpsychiatric controls (Khazaal, Fresard, Borgeat, & Zullino, 2006). Further, 60% reported binge-eating symptomatology vs. 30% in obese nonpsychiatric controls. Binge eating can be a significant barrier to weight loss and should be assessed at the outset of treatment so that it can be targeted directly (see Sect. 1.4). Another challenge is that patients with schizophrenia may have cognitive deficits that increase the challenge of tasks like dietary self-monitoring, calorie counting, portion sizing, and label reading. In these cases, setting more concrete goals may be helpful, such as daily servings of foods that are high-calorie (e.g., 1 can of soda/day) and low-calorie (e.g., 3 fruits/day). The use of meal replacements can also simplify portion control and self-monitoring. Finally, weight loss may be fairly slow given that the patient's efforts are competing with medication side effects. This can result in frustration and demoralization, which can impact adherence. For this reason, focusing patients on goals other than weight can be helpful. For example, the patient might set goals for pedometer steps, minutes of exercise, calories, and/or servings of certain foods.

1.5.3.2 Medication Switching

To the extent that weight gain can be directly tied to the onset of a medication regimen, switching to a medication with a lower probability of weight gain can be an effective strategy to halt or reverse medication-induced weight gain (McElroy, 2009). If weight gain began before the onset of medication, lifestyle is a likely factor which may reduce the efficacy of a medication switch. Weiden, Simpson, Potkin, and O'Sullivan (2003) and Weiden (2007) recommend a "watchful waiting" period to determine the course of weight change after beginning a new antipsychotic medication regimen. In the event of a relatively small weight gain or eventual weight gain reversal, the disadvantages of medication switching may outweigh the benefits. An important indicator for the need to switch is the magnitude of weight gain, the degree of patient distress over weight gain, and/or the development of eating pathology, which could impact medication adherence and ultimately lead to relapse (Weiden).

A primary concern regarding medication switching is the risk that symptom control may be compromised. An alternative to switching might seem to be to simply reduce the dosage of the current medication, but this is likely to be ineffective because weight gain variability within the range of optimal dosing is negligible (Weiden, 2007). Data from the CATIE study revealed that patients randomized to a medication switch did not exhibit differences in psychotic symptom severity, quality of life, depression, neurocognition, or neurological side effects compared to those randomized to a continued regimen condition (Rosenheck et al., 2009). In fact, the only difference observed between groups was in weight, with weight gain observed in those switching to olanzipine and weight loss observed in those switching to ziprasidone, perphenazine, or quetiapine. These findings suggest that the benefits of medication switching could significantly outweigh the risks.

Medication switching is a fairly common practice with about 25–50% of patients being prescribed medication changes within 1 year of treatment (Weiden et al., 2003). About 30% of these changes are attributed to side effects. Olanzipine and clozipine, the SGAs with the greatest weight gain profiles, are the most often switched medications. Randomized trials and observational studies evaluating the impact of medication switching on weight and other metabolic side effects show support for weight loss following certain medication switches. An early short-term study reported weight changes of −1.3 to −1.8 kg over the course of 6 weeks following a switch from either olanzipine and risperidone to ziprasidone, with accompanying improvements in positive and negative symptoms (Weiden et al.). Participants were then followed in a 52-week extension study to observe the longer term impact on weight and psychiatric symptoms. Participants who were switched from olanzipine to ziprasidone lost 10.3% of body weight (mean weight loss of 9.8 kg) over the year, those switched from risperidone to ziprasidone lost 7.8% of body weight (mean weight loss of 6.9 kg), but those switched from conventional antipsychotic medications to ziprasidone did not show significant weight changes over the year. Switching to ziprasidone had neutral or beneficial effects on positive and negative symptoms. Discontinuation rates were not different across groups but were significant, ranging from 58 to 64%. Finally, an observational study of patients with schizophrenia who were switched from either olanzipine or risperidone to ziprasidone revealed a weight loss of 5.1 kg over 6 months with significant improvements in psychotic symptom indices (Montes et al., 2007). Overall, results of randomized trials and observational studies consistently reveal significant weight loss following switches from olanzipine or risperidone to ziprasidone, with no evidence for worsening of symptoms or functioning.

Evidence from two randomized trials supports efficacy for weight loss from switches to aripiprazole, one of the newer SGAs. A short-term trial randomized 311 male patients with schizophrenia to three different switching approaches to aripiprazole (i.e., complete switch, switch with tapering, titrated switch with tapering) and observed −1.3 to −1.7 kg weight loss over 8 weeks (Casey et al., 2003). The other somewhat longer study randomized 173 olanzipine-treated patients with schizophrenia to either continuation of olanzipine or switch to aripiprazole for 16 weeks and found significant group differences in weight change with a gain of 1.4 kg in the continuation group and loss of 1.8 kg in the aripiprazole group (Newcomer et al., 2008). The aripiprazole group had higher discontinuation rates than the olanzipine group (36% vs. 26%) and slightly lower symptom improvement scores. The remaining studies are observational and involve small samples, but findings are consistent. An uncontrolled cohort study reported weight losses of −3 to −4.4 kg, respectively, over 1 year in 53 overweight patients with schizophrenia when aripiprozale was used in addition to or instead of clozapine or olanzipine (Schorr et al., 2008). The discontinuation rate in that cohort was 45%. In a retrospective chart review, 24 outpatients with schizophrenia were switched to aripiprazole and exhibited decreases in weight of 5.3 kg over 6 months (Spurling, Lamberti, Olsen, Tu, & Tang, 2007). Finally, a 1-year open-label study of 32 inpatients and outpatients with schizophrenia who were switched to aripiprazole from their previous regimens (primarily olanzipine and risperidone) reported 4 kg weight loss with only 25% of participants experiencing a two point or more increase in severity on the Clinical Global Impression severity scale (Takeuchi, Uchida, Suzuki, Watanabe, & Kashima, 2010). A small open-label study revealed that switching from aripiprozale to ziprasidone in insufficient responders produced both weight loss and symptom improvement over 12 weeks (Kim et al., 2010), which suggests that ziprasidone can be helpful even when aripiprozale is not. The literature thus far provides strong support for medication switches from clozapine, olanzipine, and risperidone to either ziprasione or aripiprazole.

1.5.3.3 Adjunctive Pharmacological Intervention

Although medication switching can be effective at reversing medication-induced weight gain, discontinuation rates following a switch have been reported to range from 26 up to 64%. Also, some patients might prefer not to change their medication, thus alternative approaches to weight gain prevention and reversal are needed. Medications that have weight loss effects can be added to the current regimen to prevent or reverse SGA-associated weight gain. Adjunctive weight loss medications that have been tested in populations with psychotic disorders include orlistat, H2 receptor agonists (i.e., nizatidine, ranitidine and famotidine), topirimate, betahistine, fluoxetine, fluvoxetine, reboxetine, sibutramine, phenopropanolamine, amantidine, and antidiabetic agents (i.e., metformin and rosiglitazone; Baptista et al., 2008). Three reviews have been published in recent years that summarize this literature. In 2007, Faulkner, Cohn, and Remington (2007) published a systematic review of adjunctive pharmacological treatments for antipsychotic medication-induced weight gain and reported that trials for amantidine, famotidine, fluoxetine, fluvoxetine, metformin, topiramate, reboxetine, sibutramine, phenopropanolamine, and nizatidine revealed weight changes from −1.17 to −3.85 kg. Given the modest amount of weight reduction from these medications combined with associated side effects, the review concluded that the evidence is insufficient to support the use of pharmacological adjuncts for weight management in schizophrenia. In 2008, Baptista et al. (2008) found evidence for weight gain prevention for topiramate, reboxetine, and fluvoxetine, as well as evidence for weight gain reversal for metformin, amantidine, and topiramate. Mixed results were found for sibutramine and nizatidine. In 2010, Ellinger, Ipema, and Stachnik (2010) published a review of the evidence for metformin and topiramate. Weight loss observed in trials for metformin and topiramate ranged from −2 to 3 kg and −4 to 5 kg, respectively, over 10–12 weeks. They reported that while data are limited, both metformin and topiramate may be effective in the treatment and prevention of SGA-induced weight gain; however, a larger evidence base (8 trials vs. 3 trials), a better safety profile, and less interference of symptom control were observed for metformin compared to topiramate. The authors caution that the recent FDA warning regarding increased suicidal behavior resulting from topiramate is a significant clinical consideration in the decision to use topiramate as a weight loss adjunctive medication for people with schizophrenia. The review concluded that the evidence for pharmacological treatments for weight management remains modest; however, adjunctive medications may be a consideration in cases where lifestyle interventions (nutrition and/or physical activity) have not been effective.

1.5.3.4 Bariatric Surgery

At this time, no randomized trials have tested the efficacy and safety of bariatric surgery in patients with schizophrenia. In one study, 86% of bariatric program staff surveyed cited uncontrolled schizophrenia as a definite contraindication to bariatric surgery (Bauchowitz et al., 2005). Although uncontrolled schizophrenia could clearly present concerns about safety and surgical outcomes, patients with well-controlled schizophrenia may benefit from bariatric surgery with no more than usual risk (Hamoui, Kingsbury, Anthone, & Crookes, 2004). Medical records were reviewed in five patients with schizophrenia who underwent bariatric surgery and outcomes were compared to nonpsychotic patients. Comparable weight losses at 6 months were reported, length of hospitalization was not different between the groups, and no serious complications were reported. Patients in that study were stabilized on SGAs, did not have active psychotic symptoms at the presurgery evaluation, and were living at home and independently performing activities of daily living. Patients were removed from antipsychotic medication 1 day prior to surgery to a few days following surgery with one patient reporting psychotic symptoms during that time. Results may not generalize to lower functioning people with schizophrenia, but do support the need for further research on surgical weight loss in well controlled, high-functioning patients with schizophrenia. Further research may also be needed to determine what degree of symptom control is necessary for a patient with schizophrenia to have a successful surgical outcome.

1.5.4 Summary

High rates of obesity are observed in adults with schizophrenia. Some SGAs cause significant weight gain and have contributed to obesity rates in this population. Clozipine, risperidone, and olanzipine have the most significant weight gain profiles. Patients with SGA-associated weight gain appear to benefit from switching to weight neutral SGAs, with the strongest data existing for ziprasidone and aripiprozale. Lifestyle factors including poor diet and sedentary lifestyle also contribute to unhealthy weight in patients with schizophrenia, and intensive lifestyle interventions appear to have efficacy in reducing weight and preventing weight gain. More research is needed on efficacy of bariatric surgery in patients with psychotic disorders as the only existing study found that high-functioning patients with schizophrenia achieve weight losses comparable to patients without severe mental illness following bariatric surgery. Integrating healthy weight programs into mental health care may have the most potential for impact on people with schizophrenia given that mental health is the most common healthcare point of contact for this population.

1.6 Attention Deficit Hyperactivity Disorder

The DSM-IV defines Attention Deficit Hyperactivity Disorder (ADHD) as a disorder characterized by a persistent pattern of inattention and/or hyperactivity-impulsivity that is more frequent and severe than is typically observed in individuals at a comparable level of development (American Psychiatric Association, 1994). Symptoms must have persisted for at least 6 months and have been present before the age of 7 years. The DSM-IV describes three subtypes of ADHD. The Inattentive Type is characterized by failure to pay attention to details, frequent careless mistakes in school, work, or other activities, difficulty sustaining attention, difficulty listening, failure to follow through on instructions, difficulty organizing tasks, avoidance and/or dislike of tasks that require sustained mental effort, losing things, distractibility, and forgetfulness in daily activities. The Hyperactive-Impulsive Type is characterized by fidgetiness, restlessness, difficulty engaging in activities quietly, acts as if "driven by a motor," excessive talking, interrupting, and difficulty awaiting turn. Those with the Combined Type of ADHD satisfy criteria for both subtypes. ADHD has been shown to persist into adulthood in 50% of cases (Lara et al., 2009) and affects about 4.4% of US adults (Kessler et al., 2006).

1.6.1 Prevalence

Four population-based studies examined the association between ADHD and risk for obesity, three of which were conducted in children and/or adolescents. Studies of children report mixed findings with one showing an association between ADHD and obesity (Lam & Yang, 2007), one showing no association (Bandini, Curtin, Hamad, Tybor, & Must, 2005), and a third showing that the association is moderated by medication status, such that unmedicated children with ADHD were more likely to be obese than children without ADHD and medicated children with ADHD were more likely to be underweight (Waring & Lapane, 2008). The only population study of adults examining the association between ADHD and risk for obesity used the Collaborative Psychiatric Epidemiology Surveys (Pagoto et al., 2009), a nationally representative, population-based study of US households ($N=6,735$).

Adult ADHD diagnoses were made via structured clinical interviews, including verification of childhood symptoms via retrospective assessment of the Diagnostic Interview Schedule for DSM-IV and current symptomatology. Adult ADHD was associated with greater likelihood of overweight (odds ratio (OR) = 1.58; 95% confidence interval (CI) = 1.05, 2.38) and obesity (OR = 1.81; 95% CI = 1.14, 2.64). Among adults with ADHD, the prevalence of overweight and obesity was 33.9 and 29.4%, respectively, compared to 28.8 and 21.6% among persons with no history of ADHD. Results were similar when adjusting for demographics, psychotropic medication, and depression.

Other studies have examined the prevalence of ADHD in obese samples and found unusually high rates of ADHD (Cortese et al., 2008). Three studies were in adults and one in adolescents, and all were retrospective studies in clinical weight loss treatment settings. Findings suggested a higher than expected prevalence of ADHD in obese patients, ranging from 13.3 to 57.7%; this is in stark contrast to the prevalence of ADHD in the general population, estimated to be 3–5% (Kessler et al., 2006). Similar findings were reported in a more recent retrospective chart review study of ADHD in weight loss clinic patients (Pagoto et al., 2010). Of 63 weight loss program enrollees, 30% endorsed symptoms consistent with ADHD. These data suggest that ADHD appears to affect a significant portion of treatment-seeking obese patients.

1.6.2 Pathophysiology of ADHD and Obesity

Very little research has explored the pathophysiology of the association between ADHD and obesity, although shared pathways have been alluded to in several papers (Bazar, Yun, Lee, Daniel, & Doux, 2006; Cortese et al., 2008; Davis et al., 2008). Hypotheses put forth suggest that overconsumption of food may contribute to ADHD (Bazar et al., 2006), cognitive hyperstimulation may lead to obesity (Bazar et al.), sleep problems associated with ADHD may contribute to the development of obesity (Cortese et al., 2008), and that ADHD and obesity have certain shared genetic pathways (Agranat-Meged et al., 2008; Davis et al., 2009). Although data exist to support possible shared genetic pathways between ADHD and obesity, these hypotheses have not yet been empirically substantiated but merit further exploration. One consistent finding in the literature is of elevated rates of eating pathology, including BED, among people with ADHD (Cortese, Bernardina, & Mouren, 2007; Davis et al., 2008; Mikami, Hinshaw, Patterson, & Lee, 2008; Nazar et al., 2008; Pagoto et al., 2007). In fact, the population-based study that established an increased risk of obesity among adults with ADHD reported that BED fully accounted for the relationship between ADHD and obesity (Pagoto et al.). Through mechanisms that have yet to be elucidated, ADHD appears to involve appetitive dysregulation which may have implications for the development of obesity. Recent research has alluded to neurobiological mechanisms in ADHD that may contribute to energy imbalance and obesity. Specifically, inattention, reward sensitivity, and impulsivity seem to be related to problems regulating food intake among persons with ADHD. These are discussed as distinct psychobiological traits below, although they are related and often co-occur in individuals with ADHD.

1.6.2.1 Inattention and Weight Regulation

Inattention, a hallmark of ADHD, refers to distractibility, reduced ability to sustain attention, and susceptibility to interference, and it can impact myriad areas of life (Arnsten, 2006). The prefrontal cortex (PFC) is implicated in attentional deficits in ADHD, as evidenced by studies indicating lower PFC volume, particularly on the right side of the brain (Casey et al., 1997; Castellanos et al., 1996). Interestingly, lower right PFC volume has been implicated in obesity as well (Alonso-Alonso & Pascual-Leone, 2007). Inattention might influence the ability to regulate weight by causing irregular eating habits and reducing dietary adherence. Inattention might also affect awareness of internal hunger and satiety cues, especially when the individual is engaged in other activities (Fleming & Levy, 2002; Schweickert, Strober, & Moskowitz, 1997). Inattention may interfere with behaviors critical to successful weight loss, such as meal planning, implementation of specific behavioral skills (e.g., use of shopping lists), and follow-through with planned exercise. In some studies, the inattentive type of ADHD has been found to be more prevalent than the hyperactive/impulsive type in obese samples (Agranat-Meged et al., 2005; Altfas, 2002; Fleming, Levy, & Levitan, 2005).

1.6.2.2 Reward Sensitivity and Weight Regulation

Reward sensitivity is a biologically based personality trait originally described by Gray (1987) in the context of the Behavioral Inhibition System/Behavioral Activation System (BIS/BAS) psychobiological model of personality. BAS refers to the reward system and BIS to the punishment system. Highly sensitive BAS or "reward sensitivity" describes individuals who are especially sensitive to rewards in their environment. Diminished reward sensitivity describes individuals who are especially insensitive to rewards in their environment and is sometimes likened to anhedonia, or the inability to experience pleasure. BAS is primarily responsible for *appetitive motivation*, such that reward sensitivity is said to mediate responses to appetitive stimuli, including drugs, food, and sex (Gray & McNaughton, 2000). Dopaminergic (DA) processes are central to reward sensitivity (Derryberry & Tucker, 1991; Reuter, Schmitz, Corr, & Hennig, 2006) with greater sensitivity to reward at the behavioral level being associated with either a hyper- or hypo-responsive DA system (Cohen, Young, Baek, Kessler, & Ranganath, 2005; Depue & Collins, 1999; Evans et al., 2006). Recent evidence has emerged of diminished reward sensitivity in ADHD (particularly those with Inattentive Type) (Volkow et al., 2009). Because palatable foods enhance dopamine activation, eating might serve a "self-medicating" function for some individuals with ADHD (Bowirrat & Oscar-Berman, 2005). However, while some studies suggest that obesity is associated with diminished reward sensitivity (Blum et al., 1996; Comings & Blum, 2000; Davis, Strachan, & Berkson, 2004; Pagoto, Spring, Cook, McChargue, & Schneider, 2006), one study supports a curvilinear relationship where lean individuals have moderate reward sensitivity, overweight and slightly obese individuals have high reward sensitivity, and morbid-to-severe obese individuals have very low reward sensitivity (Davis & Fox, 2008). Given that ADHD is generally characterized by diminished reward sensitivity, obese adults with ADHD may have lower reward sensitivity relative to their obese counterparts without ADHD. Further research is certainly needed to elucidate the role of reward sensitivity, ADHD, and obesity.

1.6.2.3 Impulsivity

Impulsivity, although a multifaceted construct, can be characterized as action without foresight (Winstanley, Eagle, & Robbins, 2006). Although obese individuals are not more impulsive than others in general, impulsivity can affect eating behavior (Applehans, 2009) and people high in impulsivity may be prone to overeating, weight gain (Guerrieri, Nederkoorn, & Jansen, 2007; Nederkoorn, Guerrieri, Roefs, & Jansen, 2008), and obesity (Nederkoorn, Braet, et al., 2006; Nederkoorn, Smulders, et al., 2006). Among 228 adolescent girls with ADHD, impulsivity was a much stronger predictor of eating pathology than inattention, although both inattentive and impulsive ADHD subtypes were equally likely to be obese (Mikami et al., 2008). This suggests that impulsivity might play a role in the observed association between ADHD and BED (Biederman et al., 2006; Ivan, Azarbad, Corsica, & Hood, 2009; Pagoto et al., 2009). Greater impulsivity may be associated with greater difficulty inhibiting the consumption of high-energy dense palatable foods, especially in response to stress and other cues, as described by Lowe in a recent review (Lowe, van Steenburgh, Ochner, & Coletta, 2009). The increasingly obesogenic environment may be particularly challenging for people high in impulsivity, given the omnipresence of food cues. Supporting this contention is a study that showed that impulsivity was associated with greater food consumption in an environment characterized by high food variety, but not in an environment characterized by monotonous foods (Guerrieri, Nederkoorn, & Jansen, 2008). This impulsivity by environment interaction suggests that persons with ADHD might be disproportionately vulnerable to developing obesity in an obesogenic environment. Impulsive individuals also appear to be more vulnerable to internal cues, as evidenced in a study that found that impulsive individuals consumed more food than their less impulsive counterparts under conditions of hunger, but not under conditions of satiety (Nederkoorn, Guerrieri, Havermans, Roefs, & Jansen, 2009). These findings suggest that restrictive diets might be especially challenging for people with ADHD and high impulsivity, and at least one study has reported an association between impulsivity and weight loss treatment failure (Nederkoorn et al., 2007). Further research is needed to understand how impulsivity affects weight regulation among individuals with ADHD and obesity.

1.6.2.4 Depression

Depression is highly co-morbid with both obesity (Simon et al., 2006) and ADHD (Kessler et al., 2006) which might suggest a mediating role for depression in the association between ADHD and obesity. The literature so far has not supported a mediating role of depression. Two epidemiological studies of ADHD and obesity found that controlling for depression did not attenuate the relationship (Pagoto et al., 2009; Waring & Lapane, 2008). Similarly, in a clinic study comparing adults with and without ADHD who participated in a weight loss program, both groups had similar rates of depression, and although ADHD was associated with worse weight loss outcomes, depression did not attenuate the weight loss difference between groups (Pagoto et al., 2010). These data suggest that ADHD has a unique impact on weight that is not accounted for by depression.

1.6.3 Clinical Care

1.6.3.1 Assessment

Because ADHD is fairly prevalent in weight treatment settings and appears to have implications for weight treatment success, screening for ADHD in weight treatment settings may be necessary. One retrospective chart review study of 215 clinical weight loss program patients found that 27% of patients met criteria for ADHD and 42% of those with BMI above 40 (Altfas, 2002). Patients with ADHD lost half the weight of their counterparts without ADHD, in spite of attending more clinic visits. Likewise, a second retrospective chart review study of clinical weight loss program patients found that 30% scored positive on an ADHD screener and these patients lost 40% less weight during a 4-month treatment program than individuals who scored negative on the screener. These two studies suggest that people with ADHD should be identified in weight loss settings because of the possible need for extra assistance during a weight loss attempt. A brief screener that is likely the most feasible measure in clinical settings is the Adult ADHD Symptom Rating Scale (ASRS), a 6-item scale that has been shown to be a reliable and valid scale for identifying adult ADHD and shows a high internal consistency and high concurrent validity with the rater-administered ADHD rating scale (Adler et al., 2006). Patients who screen positive for ADHD or in whom ADHD is suspected should be referred for a diagnostic evaluation by a qualified diagnostician who has expertise in ADHD assessment. The diagnosis is typically made using an extensive clinical interview, including review of current symptoms and the presence of symptoms in childhood by the age of 7. Adults must meet the DSM-IV symptom criteria of ADHD, and functional impairment as a result of these symptoms must be present in two or more settings (e.g., work, home, socially), both historically and currently.

1.6.3.2 Treatment

To date, randomized trials for the treatment of obesity in people with ADHD have not been conducted; however, medication trials for the treatment of ADHD have reported weight loss effects. To the extent that medications for ADHD cause weight loss make them a promising treatment option for individuals with ADHD and obesity.

ADHD Medication

Psychotropic medications used for the treatment of ADHD include psychostimulants, selective norepinephrine-reuptake inhibitors (SNRIs), and selective serotonin reuptake inhibitors (SSRIs). Psychostimulants and SNRIs can have weight- and appetite-suppressing side effects which may be helpful for obese patients with ADHD. Although no study has tested ADHD medications specifically for the indication of weight loss in samples with ADHD, a clinical observational study found that severely obese patients with ADHD who received stimulants for their ADHD lost 12% of their weight over 466 days relative to a 2% weight gain in ADHD controls who refused or discontinued medication (Levy, Fleming, & Klar, 2009). No formal weight loss program was provided to patients in this study which suggest that treating ADHD may be a first step toward weight loss among individuals with ADHD and obesity. What remains unclear is if the weight loss effect of stimulants is related to ADHD symptom control or a direct effect of the medication or some combination. Two studies have shown that the stimulant, methylphenidate, reduces energy intake acutely (Goldfield, Lorello, & Doucet, 2007; Leddy et al., 2004), but whether this results in weight change has never been tested. A review of pharmacological treatments for ADHD suggests that the effect of stimulants on weight is small and short-lived (Biederman & Spencer, 2008), which raises doubt about the ability of stimulants to have a prolonged effect on weight in the absence of additional weight loss treatment. Stimulants have also been associated with significant adverse events, including increased blood pressure and heart rate (Hammerness et al., 2009) as well as sudden death in a small number of patients (Conway, Wong, O'Connell, & Warren, 2008). As such, stimulants may be contraindicated in patients with symptomatic CVD or known structural cardiac abnormalities. This raises concerns about broad use in obese patients, many of whom have significant cardiovascular risk factors.

Atomoxetine is an SNRI with empirical support for the treatment of ADHD (Faraone & Glatt, 2010) and some patients experience a weight loss side effect. Two studies have tested atomoxetine for the indication of weight loss in obese adults who did not have ADHD. A randomized placebo- controlled trial of atomoxetine in 30 obese women revealed a 3.6 kg weight loss over 12 weeks compared to 0.1 kg weight gain in the placebo group (Gadde, Yonish, Wagner, Foust, & Allison, 2006). Withdrawal rates in the atomoxetine condition were twice that of placebo (40% vs. 20%), but only one atomoxetine withdrawal was attributed to side effects. The second trial randomized 40 people with BED to 10 weeks of atomoxetine or placebo and found significant reductions in both binge eating and weight (McElroy, Hudson, et al., 2007). The atomoxetine condition lost 2.7 kg on average compared to no weight change in the placebo condition. These studies support a short-term weight loss effect of atomoxetine in obese adults. Obese adults with ADHD who are unmedicated might benefit from atomoxetine via reductions in ADHD symptoms and weight. Longer term weight loss studies of samples of obese adults with ADHD are needed.

Psychological Interventions

Although medication is the first-line treatment for ADHD, it may not be preferred by some patients and may be contraindicated for people with certain health conditions. Furthermore, 20–50% of adults with ADHD are nonresponders to pharmacotherapy (Wender, 1998; Wilens, Spencer, & Biederman, 2002). A psychological intervention that could have applicability for ADHD in the context of obesity is CBT for ADHD which provides patients with strategies and coping skills to manage or overcome functional impairments (Hesslinger et al., 2002; Rostain & Ramsay, 2006; Safren, 2006; Stevenson, Whitmont, Bornholt, Livesey, & Stevenson, 2002). This approach may be especially indicated in the context of weight loss treatment, given the focus on building self-management skills and the importance of self-management to weight control. Two studies support the efficacy of CBT for ADHD on ADHD symptoms (Safren et al., 2005, 2010). Weight management skills could be incorporated into CBT to help patients with ADHD who have difficulties with their weight, although this approach has not yet been tested empirically.

1.6.4 Issues in Treatment Decision Making

In weight loss and/or nutrition clinical settings, the clinician should note that people with ADHD may experience greater than average difficulty with organization, self-monitoring, planning, follow-through on goals, and consistency. One study of clinical weight loss patients reported that patients who screened positive for ADHD rated weight loss strategies, such as dietary self-monitoring, as much more difficult than their counterparts who screened negative (Pagoto et al., 2010). Extra support and guidance may be needed to ensure follow-through and consistency. The same study found that obese patients screening positive for ADHD made on average ten short-lived (less than 3 days long) weight loss attempts per year and five weight loss attempts that lasted greater than 3 days/year, while obese patients screening negative only reported about two short-lived attempts and just over two longer attempts each year (Pagoto et al., 2010). Deficits in working memory and persistence in ADHD can manifest in poor follow-through with intentions, plans, and goals (Barkley, 1997). This, combined with a greater tendency toward impulsivity and difficulty sustaining effort, might result in poor adherence and greater susceptibility to the lure of gimmick diets that promise fast weight loss.

Clinicians in other settings (e.g., primary care, mental health) where adults with ADHD are encountered should be aware that obesity management may require more intensive support and guidance for these patients with ADHD. When ADHD is suspected, referral for assessment and treatment will be helpful even when obesity is the presenting concern.

1.6.5 Summary

ADHD appears to be associated with a greater risk for obesity, but the reasons for this association have not been well studied. People with ADHD have higher rates of eating pathology including BED which likely contributes to the increased risk for obesity. Features of ADHD such as inattention and impulsivity might also have implications for poor eating habits and lower diet quality. Further research is needed to understand whether people with ADHD are also at higher risk for obesity-related diseases such as type 2 diabetes and CVD. Adults with ADHD who are obese have greater difficulty losing weight than those who do not have ADHD. Very little research has addressed weight management in the context of ADHD, although it appears that pharmacological treatments for ADHD may facilitate weight loss. Clinicians encountering adults with ADHD and obesity who are seeking treatment for their obesity should keep in mind the impact of ADHD symptoms on eating behavior, appetite, physical activity, and the ability to follow through on a structured weight loss plan. Controlling ADHD symptoms may be a necessary first step in such patients given the potential for symptoms to impede a weight loss attempt, as is the case with many psychiatric co-morbidities of obesity.

References

Adami, G. F., Campostano, A., Marinari, G. M., Ravera, G., & Scopinaro, N. (2002). Night eating in obesity: A descriptive study. *Nutrition, 18*(7–8), 587–589.

Adler, L. A., Spencer, T., Faraone, S., Kessler, R. C., Howes, M. J., Biederman, J., et al. (2006). Validity of pilot Adult ADHD Self-Report Scale (ASRS) to rate adult ADHD symptoms. *Annals of Clinical Psychiatry, 18*(3), 145–148.

Agranat-Meged, A., Deitcher, C., Goldzweig, G., Leibenson, L., Stein, M., & Galili-Weisstub, E. (2005). Childhood obesity and attention deficit/hyperactivity disorder: A newly described co-morbidity in obese hospitalized children. *The International Journal of Eating Disorders, 37*(4), 357–359.

Agranat-Meged, A., Ghanadri, Y., Eisenberg, I., Ben Neriah, Z., Kieselstein-Gross, E., & Mitrani-Rosenbaum, S. (2008). Attention deficit hyperactivity disorder in obese melanocortin-4-receptor (MC4R) deficient subjects: A newly described expression of MC4R deficiency. *American Journal of Medical Genetics. Part B, Neuropsychiatric Genetics, 147B*(8), 1547–1553.

Agras, W. S., Telch, C. F., Arnow, B., Eldredge, K., Detzer, M. J., Henderson, J., et al. (1995). Does interpersonal therapy help patients with binge eating disorder who fail to respond to cognitive-behavioral therapy? *Journal of Consulting and Clinical Psychology, 63*(3), 356–360.
Agras, W. S., Telch, C. F., Arnow, B., Eldredge, K., & Marnell, M. (1997). One-year follow-up of cognitive-behavioral therapy for obese individuals with binge eating disorder. *Journal of Consulting and Clinical Psychology, 65*(2), 343–347.
Allison, K. C., Ahima, R. S., O'Reardon, J. P., Dinges, D. F., Sharma, V., Cummings, D. E., et al. (2005). Neuroendocrine profiles associated with energy intake, sleep, and stress in the night eating syndrome. *The Journal of Clinical Endocrinology and Metabolism, 90*(11), 6214–6217.
Allison, D. B., & Casey, D. E. (2001). Antipsychotic-induced weight gain: A review of the literature. *The Journal of Clinical Psychiatry, 62*(Suppl 7), 22–31.
Allison, D. B., Fontaine, K. R., Heo, M., Mentore, J. L., Cappelleri, J. C., Chandler, L. P., et al. (1999). The distribution of body mass index among individuals with and without schizophrenia. *The Journal of Clinical Psychiatry, 60*(4), 215–220.
Allison, K., Grilo, C. M., Masheb, R., & Stunkard, A. J. (2007). High self-reported rates of neglect and emotional abuse by persons with binge eating disorder and night eating syndrome. *Behaviour Research and Therapy, 45*(12), 2874–2883.
Allison, K. C., Lundgren, J. D., Moore, R. H., O'Reardon, J. P., & Stunkard, A. J. (2010). Cognitive behavior therapy for night eating syndrome: A pilot study. *American Journal of Psychotherapy, 64*(1), 91–106.
Allison, K. C., Lundgren, J. D., O'Reardon, J. P., Geliebter, A., Gluck, M. E., Vinai, P., et al. (2010). Proposed diagnostic criteria for night eating syndrome. *The International Journal of Eating Disorders, 43*(3), 241–247.
Allison, K. C., Lundgren, J. D., O'Reardon, J. P., Martino, N. S., Sarwer, D. B., Wadden, T. A., et al. (2008). The Night Eating Questionnaire (NEQ): Psychometric properties of a measure of severity of the night eating syndrome. *Eating Behaviors, 9*(1), 62–72.
Allison, D. B., Newcomer, J. W., Dunn, A. L., Blumenthal, J. A., Fabricatore, A. N., Daumit, G. L., et al. (2009). Obesity among those with mental disorders: A National Institute of Mental Health meeting report. *American Journal of Preventive Medicine, 36*(4), 341–350.
Allison, K. C., Wadden, T. A., Sarwer, D. B., Fabricatore, A. N., Crerand, C. E., Gibbons, L. M., et al. (2006). Night eating syndrome and binge eating disorder among persons seeking bariatric surgery: Prevalence and related features. *Obesity (Silver Spring), 14*(Suppl 2), 77S–82S.
Alonso-Alonso, M., & Pascual-Leone, A. (2007). The right brain hypothesis for obesity. *Journal of the American Medical Association, 297*(16), 1819–1822.
Altfas, J. R. (2002). Prevalence of attention deficit/hyperactivity disorder among adults in obesity treatment. *BMC Psychiatry, 2*, 9.
Alvarez-Jimenez, M., Hetrick, S. E., Gonzalez-Blanch, C., Gleeson, J. F., & McGorry, P. D. (2008). Non-pharmacological management of antipsychotic-induced weight gain: Systematic review and meta-analysis of randomised controlled trials. *The British Journal of Psychiatry, 193*(2), 101–107.
Amani, R. (2007). Is dietary pattern of schizophrenia patients different from healthy subjects? *BMC Psychiatry, 7*, 15.
American Psychiatric Association. (1994). *Diagnostic and statistical manual of mental disorders*. Washington, DC: American Psychiatric Association.
American Psychiatric Association. (2000). *Diagnostic and statistical manual of mental disorders*. Washington, DC: American Psychiatric Association.
American Psychiatric Association. (2010). *DSM-5 proposed diagnostic criteria for binge eating disorder*. Retrieved August, 2010 from http://www.dsm5.org/ProposedRevisions/Pages/proposedrevision.aspx?rid=372#.
Anacker, C., Zunszain, P. A., Carvalho, L. A., & Pariante, C. M. (2011). The glucocorticoid receptor: Pivot of depression and of antidepressant treatment? *Psychoneuroendocrinology, 36*(3), 415–425.

Andersen, R. E., Wadden, T. A., Bartlett, S. J., Zemel, B., Verde, T. J., & Franckowiak, S. C. (1999). Effects of lifestyle activity vs structured aerobic exercise in obese women: A randomized trial. *Journal of the American Medical Association, 281*(4), 335–340.

Ando, H., Yanagihara, H., Hayashi, Y., Obi, Y., Tsuruoka, S., Takamura, T., et al. (2005). Rhythmic messenger ribonucleic acid expression of clock genes and adipocytokines in mouse visceral adipose tissue. *Endocrinology, 146*(12), 5631–5636.

Appelhans, B. M. (2009). Neurobehavioral inhibition of reward-driven feeding: Implications for dieting and obesity. *Obesity (Silver Spring), 17*(4), 640–647.

Appelhans, B. M., Pagoto, S. L., Peters, E. N., & Spring, B. J. (2010). HPA axis response to stress predicts short-term snack intake in obese women. *Appetite, 54*(1), 217–220.

Applehans, B. (2009). Neurobehavioral Inhibition of reward-driven feeding: Implications for dieting and obesity. *Obesity, 17*, 640–647.

Arnsten, A. F. (2006). Fundamentals of attention-deficit/hyperactivity disorder: Circuits and pathways. *The Journal of Clinical Psychiatry, 67*(Suppl 8), 7–12.

Atlantis, E., & Baker, M. (2008). Obesity effects on depression: Systematic review of epidemiological studies. *International Journal of Obesity (London), 32*(6), 881–891.

Bacon, L., Keim, N. L., Van Loan, M. D., Derricote, M., Gale, B., Kazaks, A., et al. (2002). Evaluating a 'non-diet' wellness intervention for improvement of metabolic fitness, psychological well-being and eating and activity behaviors. *International Journal of Obesity and Related Metabolic Disorders, 26*(6), 854–865.

Balbo, M., Leproult, R., & Van Cauter, E. (2010). Impact of sleep and its disturbances on hypothalamo-pituitary-adrenal axis activity. *International Journal of Endocrinology, 2010*, 759234.

Bandini, L. G., Curtin, C., Hamad, C., Tybor, D. J., & Must, A. (2005). Prevalence of overweight in children with developmental disorders in the continuous national health and nutrition examination survey (NHANES) 1999-2002. *The Journal of Pediatrics, 146*(6), 738–743.

Baptista, T., De Mendoza, S., Beaulieu, S., Bermudez, A., & Martinez, M. (2004). The metabolic syndrome during atypical antipsychotic drug treatment: Mechanisms and management. *Metabolic Syndrome and Related Disorders, 2*(4), 290–307.

Baptista, T., ElFakih, Y., Uzcategui, E., Sandia, I., Talamo, E., Araujo de Baptista, E., et al. (2008). Pharmacological management of atypical antipsychotic-induced weight gain. *CNS Drugs, 22*(6), 477–495.

Baptista, T., Reyes, D., & Hernandez, L. (1999). Antipsychotic drugs and reproductive hormones: Relationship to body weight regulation. *Pharmacology, Biochemistry, and Behavior, 62*(3), 409–417.

Barkley, R. A. (1997). Behavioral inhibition, sustained attention, and executive functions: Constructing a unifying theory of ADHD. *Psychological Bulletin, 121*(1), 65–94.

Barnes, R. D., Masheb, R. M., White, M. A., & Grilo, C. M. (2011). Comparison of methods for identifying and assessing obese patients with binge eating disorder in primary care settings. *The International Journal of Eating Disorders, 44*(2), 157–163.

Barry, D., Pietrzak, R. H., & Petry, N. M. (2008). Gender differences in associations between body mass index and DSM-IV mood and anxiety disorders: Results from the National Epidemiologic Survey on alcohol and related conditions. *Annals of Epidemiology, 18*(6), 458–466.

Bauchowitz, A. U., Gonder-Frederick, L. A., Olbrisch, M. E., Azarbad, L., Ryee, M. Y., Woodson, M., et al. (2005). Psychosocial evaluation of bariatric surgery candidates: A survey of present practices. *Psychosomatic Medicine, 67*(5), 825–832.

Bazar, K. A., Yun, A. J., Lee, P. Y., Daniel, S. M., & Doux, J. D. (2006). Obesity and ADHD may represent different manifestations of a common environmental oversampling syndrome: A model for revealing mechanistic overlap among cognitive, metabolic, and inflammatory disorders. *Medical Hypotheses, 66*(2), 263–269.

Berridge, K. C., Ho, C. Y., Richard, J. M., & DiFeliceantonio, A. G. (2010). The tempted brain eats: Pleasure and desire circuits in obesity and eating disorders. *Brain Research, 1350*, 43–64.

Biederman, J., Monuteaux, M. C., Mick, E., Spencer, T., Wilens, T. E., Klein, K. L., et al. (2006). Psychopathology in females with attention-deficit/hyperactivity disorder: A controlled, five-year prospective study. *Biological Psychiatry, 60*(10), 1098–1105.

Biederman, J., & Spencer, T. J. (2008). Psychopharmacological interventions. *Child and Adolescent Psychiatric Clinics of North America, 17*(2), 439–458, xi.

Birketvedt, G. S., Florholmen, J., Sundsfjord, J., Osterud, B., Dinges, D., Bilker, W., et al. (1999). Behavioral and neuroendocrine characteristics of the night-eating syndrome. *Journal of the American Medical Association, 282*, 657–663.

Bjorntorp, P. (2001). Do stress reactions cause abdominal obesity and comorbidities? *Obesity Reviews, 2*(2), 73–86.

Black, D. W., Goldstein, R. B., & Mason, E. E. (1992). Prevalence of mental disorder in 88 morbidly obese bariatric clinic patients. *The American Journal of Psychiatry, 149*(2), 227–234.

Blackburn, G. L., Hutter, M. M., Harvey, A. M., Apovian, C. M., Boulton, H. R., Cummings, S., et al. (2009). Expert panel on weight loss surgery: executive report update. *Obesity, 17*(5), 842–862.

Blaine, B. (2008). Does depression cause obesity?: A meta-analysis of longitudinal studies of depression and weight control. *Journal of Health Psychology, 13*(8), 1190–1197.

Blaine, B., & Rodman, J. (2007). Responses to weight loss treatment among obese individuals with and without BED: A matched-study meta-analysis. *Eating and Weight Disorders, 12*(2), 54–60.

Blum, K., Braverman, E. R., Wood, R. C., Gill, J., Li, C., Chen, T. J., et al. (1996). Increased prevalence of the Taq I A1 allele of the dopamine receptor gene (DRD2) in obesity with co-morbid substance use disorder: A preliminary report. *Pharmacogenetics, 6*(4), 297–305.

Blumenthal, J. A., Babyak, M. A., Doraiswamy, P. M., Watkins, L., Hoffman, B. M., Barbour, K. A., et al. (2007). Exercise and pharmacotherapy in the treatment of major depressive disorder. *Psychosomatic Medicine, 69*(7), 587–596.

Bond, D. J., Kauer-Sant'Anna, M., Lam, R. W., & Yatham, L. N. (2010). Weight gain, obesity, and metabolic indices following a first manic episode: Prospective 12-month data from the Systematic Treatment Optimization Program for Early Mania (STOP-EM). *Journal of Affective Disorders, 124*(1–2), 108–117.

Bowden, C. L., Calabrese, J. R., Ketter, T. A., Sachs, G. S., White, R. L., & Thompson, T. R. (2006). Impact of lamotrigine and lithium on weight in obese and nonobese patients with bipolar I disorder. *The American Journal of Psychiatry, 163*(7), 1199–1201.

Bower, J. E., Ganz, P. A., Aziz, N., & Fahey, J. L. (2002). Fatigue and proinflammatory cytokine activity in breast cancer survivors. *Psychosomatic Medicine, 64*(4), 604–611.

Bowirrat, A., & Oscar-Berman, M. (2005). Relationship between dopaminergic neurotransmission, alcoholism, and reward deficiency. *American Journal of Medical Genetics, 132*, 29–37.

Brewin, C. R., Andrews, B., & Valentine, J. D. (2000). Meta-analysis of risk factors for posttraumatic stress disorder in trauma-exposed adults. *Journal of Consulting and Clinical Psychology, 68*(5), 748–766.

Britz, B., Siegfried, W., Ziegler, A., Lamertz, C., Herpertz-Dahlmann, B. M., Remschmidt, H., et al. (2000). Rates of psychiatric disorders in a clinical study group of adolescents with extreme obesity and in obese adolescents ascertained via a population based study. *International Journal of Obesity and Related Metabolic Disorders, 24*(12), 1707–1714.

Broocks, A., Bandelow, B., Pekrun, G., George, A., Meyer, T., Bartmann, U., et al. (1998). Comparison of aerobic exercise, clomipramine, and placebo in the treatment of panic disorder. *The American Journal of Psychiatry, 155*(5), 603–609.

Brownley, K. A., Berkman, N. D., Sedway, J. A., Lohr, K. N., & Bulik, C. M. (2007). Binge eating disorder treatment: A systematic review of randomized controlled trials. *The International Journal of Eating Disorders, 40*(4), 337–348.

Bulik, C. M., Sullivan, P. F., & Kendler, K. S. (2000). An empirical study of the classification of eating disorders. *The American Journal of Psychiatry, 157*(6), 886–895.

Bulik, C. M., Sullivan, P. F., & Kendler, K. S. (2002). Medical and psychiatric morbidity in obese women with and without binge eating. *The International Journal of Eating Disorders, 32*(1), 72–78.
Buser, A., Dymek-Valentine, M., Hilburger, J., & Alverdy, J. (2004). Outcome following gastric bypass surgery: Impact of past sexual abuse. *Obesity Surgery, 14*(2), 170–174.
Cancello, R., & Clement, K. (2006). Is obesity an inflammatory illness? Role of low-grade inflammation and macrophage infiltration in human white adipose tissue. *British Journal of Obstetrics and Gynaecology, 113*(10), 1141–1147.
Capuron, L., Poitou, C., Machaux-Tholliez, D., Frochot, V., Bouillot, J. L., Basdevant, A., et al. (2011). Relationship between adiposity, emotional status and eating behaviour in obese women: Role of inflammation. *Psychological Medicine, 41*(7), 1517–1528.
Capuron, L., Ravaud, A., & Dantzer, R. (2000). Early depressive symptoms in cancer patients receiving interleukin 2 and/or interferon alfa-2b therapy. *Journal of Clinical Oncology, 18*(10), 2143–2151.
Carels, R. A., Darby, L. A., Cacciapaglia, H. M., & Douglass, O. M. (2004). Reducing cardiovascular risk factors in postmenopausal women through a lifestyle change intervention. *Journal of Women's Health (Larchmt), 13*(4), 412–426.
Cargill, B. R., Clark, M. M., Pera, V., Niaura, R. S., & Abrams, D. B. (1999). Binge eating, body image, depression, and self-efficacy in an obese clinical population. *Obesity Research, 7*(4), 379–386.
Carpenter, K., Hasin, D., Allison, D., & Faith, M. (2000). Relationships between obesity and DSM-IV major depressive disorder, suicide ideation, and suicide attempts: Results from a general population study. *American Journal of Public Health, 90*(2), 251–257.
Casey, D. E., Carson, W. H., Saha, A. R., Liebeskind, A., Ali, M. W., Jody, D., et al. (2003). Switching patients to aripiprazole from other antipsychotic agents: A multicenter randomized study. *Psychopharmacology (Berlin), 166*(4), 391–399.
Casey, B. J., Castellanos, F. X., Giedd, J. N., Marsh, W. L., Hamburger, S. D., Schubert, A. B., et al. (1997). Implication of right frontostriatal circuitry in response inhibition and attention-deficit/hyperactivity disorder. *Journal of the American Academy of Child and Adolescent Psychiatry, 36*(3), 374–383.
Cassidy, F., Ritchie, J. C., & Carroll, B. J. (1998). Plasma dexamethasone concentration and cortisol response during manic episodes. *Biological Psychiatry, 43*(10), 747–754.
Castellanos, F. X., Giedd, J. N., Marsh, W. L., Hamburger, S. D., Vaituzis, A. C., Dickstein, D. P., et al. (1996). Quantitative brain magnetic resonance imaging in attention-deficit hyperactivity disorder. *Archives of General Psychiatry, 53*(7), 607–616.
Celio, A. A., Wilfley, D. E., Crow, S. J., Mitchell, J., & Walsh, B. T. (2004). A comparison of the binge eating scale, questionnaire for eating and weight patterns-revised, and eating disorder examination questionnaire with instructions with the eating disorder examination in the assessment of binge eating disorder and its symptoms. *The International Journal of Eating Disorders, 36*(4), 434–444.
Chen, E. Y., Bocchieri-Ricciardi, L. E., Munoz, D., Fischer, S., Katterman, S., Roehrig, M., et al. (2007). Depressed mood in class III obesity predicted by weight-related stigma. *Obesity Surgery, 17*(5), 669–671.
Chen, C. K., Chen, Y. C., & Huang, Y. S. (2009). Effects of a 10-week weight control program on obese patients with schizophrenia or schizoaffective disorder: A 12-month follow up. *Psychiatry and Clinical Neurosciences, 63*(1), 17–22.
Chen, Y., & Silverstone, T. (1990). Lithium and weight gain. *International Clinical Psychopharmacology, 5*(3), 217–225.
Chou, K. L., & Chi, I. (2005). Prevalence of depression among elderly Chinese with diabetes. *International Journal of Geriatric Psychiatry, 20*(6), 570–575.
Clark, M. M., Cargill, B. R., Medeiros, M. L., & Pera, V. (1996). Changes in self-efficacy following obesity treatment. *Obesity Research, 4*(2), 179–181.
Clark, M. M., Hanna, B. K., Mai, J. L., Graszer, K. M., Krochta, J. G., McAlpine, D. E., et al. (2007). Sexual abuse survivors and psychiatric hospitalization after bariatric surgery. *Obesity Surgery, 17*(4), 465–469.

Claudino, A. M., de Oliveira, I. R., Appolinario, J. C., Cordas, T. A., Duchesne, M., Sichieri, R., et al. (2007). Double-blind, randomized, placebo-controlled trial of topiramate plus cognitive-behavior therapy in binge-eating disorder. *The Journal of Clinical Psychiatry, 68*(9), 1324–1332.

Cohen, M. X., Young, J., Baek, J. M., Kessler, C., & Ranganath, C. (2005). Individual differences in extraversion and dopamine genetics predict neural reward responses. *Brain Research. Cognitive Brain Research, 25*(3), 851–861.

Colles, S. L., & Dixon, J. B. (2006). Night eating syndrome: Impact on bariatric surgery. *Obesity Surgery, 16*(7), 811–820.

Colles, S. L., Dixon, J. B., & O'Brien, P. E. (2007). Night eating syndrome and nocturnal snacking: Association with obesity, binge eating and psychological distress. *International Journal of Obesity (London), 31*(11), 1722–1730.

Comings, D. E., & Blum, K. (2000). Reward deficiency syndrome: Genetic aspects of behavioral disorders. *Progress in Brain Research, 126*, 325–341.

Conway, J., Wong, K. K., O'Connell, C., & Warren, A. E. (2008). Cardiovascular risk screening before starting stimulant medications and prescribing practices of Canadian physicians: Impact of the Health Canada advisory. *Pediatrics, 122*(4), e828–e834.

Cortese, S., Angriman, M., Maffeis, C., Isnard, P., Konofal, E., Lecendreux, M., et al. (2008). Attention-deficit/hyperactivity disorder (ADHD) and obesity: A systematic review of the literature. *Critical Reviews in Food Science and Nutrition, 48*(6), 524–537.

Cortese, S., Bernardina, B. D., & Mouren, M. C. (2007). Attention deficit/hyperactivity disorder (ADHD) and binge eating. *Nutrition Reviews, 65*(9), 404–411.

Cortese, S., Isnard, P., Frelut, M. L., Michel, G., Quantin, L., Guedeney, A., et al. (2007). Association between symptoms of attention-deficit/hyperactivity disorder and bulimic behaviors in a clinical sample of severely obese adolescents. *International Journal of Obesity (London), 31*(2), 340–346.

Coryell, W. (2009). Maintenance treatment in bipolar disorder: A reassessment of lithium as the first choice. *Bipolar Disorders, 11*(Suppl 2), 77–83.

Coste, S. C., Murray, S. E., & Stenzel-Poore, M. P. (2001). Animal models of CRH excess and CRH receptor deficiency display altered adaptations to stress. *Peptides, 22*(5), 733–741.

Craft, L. L., Freund, K. M., Culpepper, L., & Perna, F. M. (2007). Intervention study of exercise for depressive symptoms in women. *Journal of Women's Health (Larchmt), 16*(10), 1499–1509.

Croft, H., Houser, T. L., Jamerson, B. D., Leadbetter, R. A., Bolden-Watson, C., Donahue, R., et al. (2002). Effect on body weight of bupropion sustained-release in patients with major depression treated for 52 weeks. *Clinical Therapeutics, 24*(4), 662–672.

Dalle Grave, R., Calugi, S., Ruocco, A., & Marchesini, G. (2011). NES and weight loss outcome in obese patients. *International Journal of Eating Disorders, 44*(2), 150–156.

Dallman, M. F. (2010). Stress-induced obesity and the emotional nervous system. *Trends in Endocrinology and Metabolism, 21*(3), 159–165.

Dallman, M. F., Akana, S. F., Strack, A. M., Hanson, E. S., & Sebastian, R. J. (1995). The neural network that regulates energy balance is responsive to glucocorticoids and insulin and also regulates HPA axis responsivity at a site proximal to CRF neurons. *Annals of the New York Academy of Sciences, 771*, 730–742.

Dallman, M. F., Pecoraro, N. C., & la Fleur, S. E. (2005). Chronic stress and comfort foods: Self-medication and abdominal obesity. *Brain, Behavior, and Immunity, 19*, 275–280.

Darga, L. L., Carroll-Michals, L., Botsford, S. J., & Lucas, C. P. (1991). Fluoxetine's effect on weight loss in obese subjects. *The American Journal of Clinical Nutrition, 54*(2), 321–325.

Daumit, G. L., Clark, J. M., Steinwachs, D. M., Graham, C. M., Lehman, A., & Ford, D. E. (2003). Prevalence and correlates of obesity in a community sample of individuals with severe and persistent mental illness. *The Journal of Nervous and Mental Disease, 191*(12), 799–805.

Davis, C., & Fox, J. (2008). Sensitivity to reward and body mass index (BMI): Evidence for a non-linear relationship. *Appetite, 50*(1), 43–49.

Davis, C., Levitan, R. D., Kaplan, A. S., Carter, J., Reid, C., Curtis, C., et al. (2008). Reward sensitivity and the D2 dopamine receptor gene: A case-control study of binge eating disorder. *Progress in Neuro-Psychopharmacology & Biological Psychiatry, 32*(3), 620–628.

Davis, C., Patte, K., Levitan, R. D., Carter, J., Kaplan, A. S., Zai, C., et al. (2009). A psychogenetic study of associations between the symptoms of binge eating disorder and those of attention deficit (hyperactivity) disorder. *Journal of Psychiatric Research, 43*(7), 687–696.

Davis, C., Strachan, S., & Berkson, M. (2004). Sensitivity to reward: Implications for overeating and overweight. *Appetite, 42*(2), 131–138.

de Kloet, C. S., Vermetten, E., Geuze, E., Kavelaars, A., Heijnen, C. J., & Westenberg, H. G. (2006). Assessment of HPA-axis function in posttraumatic stress disorder: Pharmacological and non-pharmacological challenge tests, a review. *Journal of Psychiatric Research, 40*(6), 550–567.

de Zwaan, M., Burgard, M. A., Schenck, C. H., & Mitchell, J. E. (2003). Night time eating: A review of the literature. *European Eating Disorders Review, 11*, 7–24.

de Zwaan, M., Hilbert, A., Swan-Kremeier, L., Simonich, H., Lancaster, K., Howell, L. M., et al. (2010). Comprehensive interview assessment of eating behavior 18-35 months after gastric bypass surgery for morbid obesity. *Surgery for Obesity and Related Diseases, 6*(1), 79–85.

de Zwaan, M., Mitchell, J. E., & Crosby, R. D. (2005). Short-term cognitive behavioral treatment does not improve outcome of a comprehensive very-low-calorie diet program in obese women with binge eating disorder. *Behavior Therapy, 36*, 89–99.

de Zwaan, M., Mitchell, J. E., Specker, S. M., Pyle, R. L., Mussell, M. P., & Seim, H. C. (1993). Diagnosing binge eating disorder: Level of agreement between self-report and expert-rating. *The International Journal of Eating Disorders, 14*(3), 289–295.

Depue, R. A., & Collins, P. F. (1999). Neurobiology of the structure of personality: Dopamine, facilitation of incentive motivation, and extraversion. *The Behavioral and Brain Sciences, 22*(3), 491–517; discussion 518–569.

Derryberry, D., & Tucker, D. M. (1991). The adaptive base of the neural hierachy: Elementary motivational controls on network function. In R. Dienstbier (Ed.), *Neraska symposim on motivation: Vol 38 Perspectives on motivation* (pp. 289–342). Lincoln, NE: University of Nebraska Press.

Devlin, M. J. (2001). Binge-eating disorder and obesity. A combined treatment approach. *The Psychiatric Clinics of North America, 24*(2), 325–335.

Devlin, M. J., Goldfein, J. A., & Dobrow, I. (2003). What is this thing called BED? Current status of binge eating disorder nosology. *The International Journal of Eating Disorders, 34*(Suppl), S2–S18.

Devlin, M. J., Goldfein, J. A., Petkova, E., Jiang, H., Raizman, P. S., Wolk, S., et al. (2005). Cognitive behavioral therapy and fluoxetine as adjuncts to group behavioral therapy for binge eating disorder. *Obesity Research, 13*(6), 1077–1088.

Dixon, L. B., Dickerson, F., Bellack, A. S., Bennett, M., Dickinson, D., Goldberg, R. W., et al. (2010). The 2009 schizophrenia PORT psychosocial treatment recommendations and summary statements. *Schizophrenia Bulletin, 36*(1), 48–70.

Drewnowski, A., Krahn, D. D., Demitrack, M. A., Nairn, K., & Gosnell, B. A. (1995). Naloxone, an opiate blocker, reduces the consumption of sweet high-fat foods in obese and lean female binge eaters. *The American Journal of Clinical Nutrition, 61*(6), 1206–1212.

Dunkley, D. M., Masheb, R. M., & Grilo, C. M. (2010). Childhood maltreatment, depressive symptoms, and body dissatisfaction in patients with binge eating disorder: The mediating role of self-criticism. *The International Journal of Eating Disorders, 43*(3), 274–281.

Dunn, A. J., & Berridge, C. W. (1990). Physiological and behavioral responses to corticotropin-releasing factor administration: Is CRF a mediator of anxiety or stress responses? *Brain Research. Brain Research Reviews, 15*(2), 71–100.

Dunn, A. L., Trivedi, M. H., Kampert, J. B., Clark, C. G., & Chambliss, H. O. (2005). Exercise treatment for depression: Efficacy and dose response. *American Journal of Preventive Medicine, 28*(1), 1–8.

Elder, K. A., Grilo, C. M., Masheb, R. M., Rothschild, B. S., Burke-Martindale, C. H., & Brody, M. L. (2006). Comparison of two self-report instruments for assessing binge eating in bariatric surgery candidates. *Behaviour Research and Therapy, 44*(4), 545–560.

Elhai, J. D., Grubaugh, A. L., Kashdan, T. B., & Frueh, B. C. (2008). Empirical examination of a proposed refinement to DSM-IV posttraumatic stress disorder symptom criteria using the National Co-morbidity Survey Replication data. *The Journal of Clinical Psychiatry, 69*(4), 597–602.

Ellinger, L. K., Ipema, H. J., & Stachnik, J. M. (2010). Efficacy of metformin and topiramate in prevention and treatment of second-generation antipsychotic-induced weight gain. *The Annals of Pharmacotherapy, 44*(4), 668–679.

Ello-Martin, J. A., Roe, L. S., Ledikwe, J. H., Beach, A. M., & Rolls, B. J. (2007). Dietary energy density in the treatment of obesity: A year-long trial comparing 2 weight-loss diets. *The American Journal of Clinical Nutrition, 85*(6), 1465–1477.

Elmslie, J. L., Silverstone, J. T., Mann, J. I., Williams, S. M., & Romans, S. E. (2000). Prevalence of overweight and obesity in bipolar patients. *The Journal of Clinical Psychiatry, 61*(3), 179–184.

Epel, E., Lapidus, R., McEwen, B., & Brownell, K. (2001). Stress may add bite to appetite in women: A laboratory study of stress-induced cortisol and eating behavior. *Psychoneuroendocrinology, 26*(1), 37–49.

Epel, E. S., Lin, J., Wilhelm, F. H., Wolkowitz, O. M., Cawthon, R., Adler, N. E., et al. (2006). Cell aging in relation to stress arousal and cardiovascular disease risk factors. *Psychoneuroendocrinology, 31*(3), 277–287.

European Medicines Agency. (2010). *Weight-loss medicine associated with increased risk of cardiovascular events to be removed from all markets in the European Union*. Retrieved November 12, 2010 from http://www.ema.europa.eu/docs/en_GB/document_library/Press_release/2010/01/WC500069995.pdf.

Evans, A. H., Lawrence, A. D., Potts, J., MacGregor, L., Katzenschlager, R., Shaw, K., et al. (2006). Relationship between impulsive sensation seeking traits, smoking, alcohol and caffeine intake, and Parkinson's disease. *Journal of Neurology, Neurosurgery, and Psychiatry, 77*(3), 317–321.

Fabricatore, A. N., & Wadden, T. A. (2004). Psychological aspects of obesity. *Clinics in Dermatology, 22*(4), 332–337.

Fagiolini, A., & Chengappa, K. N. (2007). Weight gain and metabolic issues of medicines used for bipolar disorder. *Current Psychiatry Reports, 9*(6), 521–528.

Fagiolini, A., Frank, E., Cherry, C. R., Houck, P. R., Novick, D. M., Buysse, D. J., et al. (2002). Clinical indicators for the use of antidepressants in the treatment of bipolar I depression. *Bipolar Disorders, 4*(5), 277–282.

Fagiolini, A., Kupfer, D. J., Houck, P. R., Novick, D. M., & Frank, E. (2003). Obesity as a correlate of outcome in patients with bipolar I disorder. *The American Journal of Psychiatry, 160*(1), 112–117.

Fairburn, C., & Beglin, S. J. (1994). Assessment of eating disorders: Interview or self-report questionnaire? *The International Journal of Eating Disorders, 16*, 363–370.

Fairburn, C. G., Cooper, Z., Doll, H. A., Norman, P., & O'Connor, M. (2000). The natural course of bulimia nervosa and binge eating disorder in young women. *Archives of General Psychiatry, 57*(7), 659–665.

Fairburn, C. G., Marcus, M. D., & Wilson, G. T. (1993). Cognitive-behavioral therapy for binge eating and bulimia nervosa: A comprehensive treatment manual. In C. G. Fairburn, M. D. Marcus, & G. T. Wilson (Eds.), *Binge eating: Nature, assessment, and treatment*. New York, NY: Guilford.

Falconer, E., Bryant, R., Felmingham, K. L., Kemp, A. H., Gordon, E., Peduto, A., et al. (2008). The neural networks of inhibitory control in posttraumatic stress disorder. *Journal of Psychiatry & Neuroscience, 33*(5), 413–422.

Faraone, S. V., & Glatt, S. J. (2010). A comparison of the efficacy of medications for adult attention-deficit/hyperactivity disorder using meta-analysis of effect sizes. *The Journal of Clinical Psychiatry, 71*(6), 754–763.

Faulkner, G., Cohn, T., & Remington, G. (2007). Interventions to reduce weight gain in schizophrenia. *Cochrane Database of Systematic Reviews* (1), CD005148.

Faulkner, G. E., Gorczynski, P. F., & Cohn, T. A. (2009). Psychiatric illness and obesity: Recognizing the "obesogenic" nature of an inpatient psychiatric setting. *Psychiatric Services, 60*(4), 538–541.

Fava, M. (2000). Weight gain and antidepressants. *The Journal of Clinical Psychiatry, 61*(Suppl 11), 37–41.

Flegal, K. M., Carroll, M. D., Ogden, C. L., & Johnson, C. L. (2002). Prevalence and trends in obesity among US Adults, 1999-2000. *Journal of the American Medical Association, 288*(14), 1723–1727.

Fleming, J., & Levy, L. D. (2002). Eating disorders in women with ADHD. In P. O. Quinn & K. G. Nadeua (Eds.), *Gender issues and ADHD: Research, diagnosis and treatment.* Silver Spring, MD: Advantage Books.

Fleming, J. P., Levy, L. D., & Levitan, R. D. (2005). Symptoms of attention deficit hyperactivity disorder in severely obese women. *Eating and Weight Disorders, 10*(1), e10–e13.

Fontaine, K. R., Heo, M., Harrigan, E. P., Shear, C. L., Lakshminarayanan, M., Casey, D. E., et al. (2001). Estimating the consequences of anti-psychotic induced weight gain on health and mortality rate. *Psychiatry Research, 101*(3), 277–288.

Fossati, M., Amati, F., Painot, D., Reiner, M., Haenni, C., & Golay, A. (2004). Cognitive-behavioral therapy with simultaneous nutritional and physical activity education in obese patients with binge eating disorder. *Eating and Weight Disorders, 9*(2), 134–138.

Fosse, G. K., & Holen, A. (2006). Childhood maltreatment in adult female psychiatric outpatients with eating disorders. *Eating Behaviors, 7*(4), 404–409.

Foster, M. T., Warne, J. P., Ginsberg, A. B., Horneman, H. F., Pecoraro, N. C., Akana, S. F., et al. (2009). Palatable foods, stress, and energy stores sculpt corticotropin-releasing factor, adrenocorticotropin, and corticosterone concentrations after restraint. *Endocrinology, 150*(5), 2325–2333.

Freidenberg, B. M., Gusmano, R., Hickling, E. J., Blanchard, E. B., Bremner, J. D., & Frye, C. (2010). Women with PTSD have lower basal salivary cortisol levels later in the day than do men with PTSD: A preliminary study. *Physiology and Behavior, 99*(2), 234–236.

Friedman, K. E., Reichmann, S. K., Costanzo, P. R., & Musante, G. J. (2002). Body image partially mediates the relationship between obesity and psychological distress. *Obesity Research, 10*(1), 33–41.

Gabriele, J. M., Dubbert, P. M., & Reeves, R. R. (2009). Efficacy of behavioural interventions in managing atypical antipsychotic weight gain. *Obesity Reviews, 10*(4), 442–455.

Gadde, K. M., Yonish, G. M., Wagner, H. R., II, Foust, M. S., & Allison, D. B. (2006). Atomoxetine for weight reduction in obese women. A preliminary randomised controlled trial. *International Journal of Obesity, 30*(7), 1138–1142.

Garaulet, M., Ordovás, J. M., & Madrid, J. A. (2010). The chronobiology, etiology and pathophysiology of obesity. *International Journal of Obesity, 34*(12), 1667–1683.

Gariepy, G., Wang, J., Lesage, A. D., & Schmitz, N. (2010). The longitudinal association from obesity to depression: Results from the 12-year National Population Health Survey. *Obesity, 18*(5), 1033–1038.

George, S. A., Khan, S., Briggs, H., & Abelson, J. L. (2010). CRH-stimulated cortisol release and food intake in healthy, non-obese adults. *Psychoneuroendocrinology, 35*(4), 607–612.

Glod, C. A., Teicher, M. H., Hartman, C. R., & Harakal, T. (1997). Increased nocturnal activity and impaired sleep maintenance in abused children. *Journal of the American Academy of Child and Adolescent Psychiatry, 36*(9), 1236–1243.

Gluck, M. E., Geliebter, A., & Lorence, M. (2004). Cortisol stress response is positively correlated with central obesity in obese women with binge eating disorder (BED) before and after cognitive-behavioral treatment. *Annals of the New York Academy of Sciences, 1032*, 202–207.

Gluck, M. E., Geliebter, A., & Satov, T. (2001). Night eating syndrome is associated with depression, low self-esteem, reduced daytime hunger, and less weight loss in obese outpatients. *Obesity Research, 9*(4), 264–267.

Gluck, M. E., Venti, C. A., Salbe, A. D., & Krakoff, J. (2008). Nighttime eating: Commonly observed and related to weight gain in an inpatient food intake study. *The American Journal of Clinical Nutrition, 88*(4), 900–905.

Golay, A., Laurent-Jaccard, A., Habicht, F., Gachoud, J. P., Chabloz, M., Kammer, A., et al. (2005). Effect of orlistat in obese patients with binge eating disorder. *Obesity Research, 13*, 1701–1708.

Goldfein, J. A., Devlin, M. J., & Kamenetz, C. (2005). Eating Disorder Examination-Questionnaire with and without instruction to assess binge eating in patients with binge eating disorder. *The International Journal of Eating Disorders, 37*(2), 107–111.

Goldfield, G. S., Lorello, C., & Doucet, E. (2007). Methylphenidate reduces energy intake and dietary fat intake in adults: A mechanism of reduced reinforcing value of food? *The American Journal of Clinical Nutrition, 86*(2), 308–315.

Goldfield, G. S., Moore, C., Henderson, K., Buchholz, A., Obeid, N., & Flament, M. F. (2010). Body dissatisfaction, dietary restraint, depression, and weight status in adolescents. *The Journal of School Health, 80*(4), 186–192.

Goldstein, D. J., Rampey, A. H., Jr., Enas, G. G., Potvin, J. H., Fludzinski, L. A., & Levine, L. R. (1994). Fluoxetine: A randomized clinical trial in the treatment of obesity. *International Journal of Obesity and Related Metabolic Disorders, 18*(3), 129–135.

Goodrich, D. E., Lai, Z., Lasky, E., Burghardt, A. R., & Kilbourne, A. M. (2010). Access to weight loss counseling services among patients with bipolar disorder. *Journal of Affective Disorders, 126*(1–2), 75–79.

Gormally, J., Black, S., Daston, S., & Rardin, D. (1982). The assessment of binge eating severity among obese persons. *Addictive Behaviors, 7*, 47–55.

Gray, J. A. (1987). The neuropsychology of emotion and personality. In S. M. Stahl, S. D. Iverson, & E. C. Goodman (Eds.), *Cognitive neurochemistry* (pp. 171–190). Oxford, UK: Oxford University Press.

Gray, J. A., & McNaughton, N. (2000). *The neuropsychology of anxiety*. Oxford, England: Oxford University Press.

Greeno, C. G., & Wing, R. R. (1994). Stress-induced eating. *Psychological Bulletin, 115*(3), 444–464.

Greenway, F. L., Dunayevich, E., Tollefson, G., Erickson, J., Guttadauria, M., Fujioka, K., et al. (2009). Comparison of combined bupropion and naltrexone therapy for obesity with monotherapy and placebo. *The Journal of Clinical Endocrinology and Metabolism, 94*(12), 4898–4906.

Greenway, F. L., Fujioka, K., Plodkowski, R. A., Mudaliar, S., Guttadauria, M., Erickson, J., et al. (2010). Effect of naltrexone plus bupropion on weight loss in overweight and obese adults (COR-I): A multicentre, randomised, double-blind, placebo-controlled, phase 3 trial. *The Lancet, 376*(9741), 595–605.

Greenway, F. L., Whitehouse, M. J., Guttadauria, M., Anderson, J. W., Atkinson, R. L., Fujioka, K., et al. (2009). Rational design of a combination medication for the treatment of obesity. *Obesity (Silver Spring), 17*(1), 30–39.

Gregoor, J. G., van der Weide, J., Mulder, H., Cohen, D., van Megen, H. J., Egberts, A. C., et al. (2009). Polymorphisms of the LEP- and LEPR gene and obesity in patients using antipsychotic medication. *Journal of Clinical Psychopharmacology, 29*(1), 21–25.

Grilo, C. M., & Masheb, R. M. (2005). A randomized controlled comparison of guided self-help cognitive behavioral therapy and behavioral weight loss for binge eating disorder. *Behaviour Research and Therapy, 43*(11), 1509–1525.

Grilo, C. M., Masheb, R. M., Brody, M., Toth, C., Burke-Martindale, C. H., & Rothschild, B. S. (2005). Childhood maltreatment in extremely obese male and female bariatric surgery candidates. *Obesity Research, 13*(1), 123–130.

Grilo, C. M., Masheb, R. M., & Wilson, G. T. (2001). Different methods for assessing the features of eating disorders in patients with binge eating disorder: A replication. *Obesity Research, 9*(7), 418–422.

Grilo, C. M., White, M. A., Masheb, R. M., Rothschild, B. S., & Burke-Martindale, C. H. (2006). Relation of childhood sexual abuse and other forms of maltreatment to 12-month postoperative outcomes in extremely obese gastric bypass patients. *Obesity Surgery, 16*(4), 454–460.

Grucza, R. A., Przybeck, T. R., & Cloninger, C. R. (2007). Prevalence and correlates of binge eating disorder in a community sample. *Comprehensive Psychiatry, 48*(2), 124–131.

Guerrieri, R., Nederkoorn, C., & Jansen, A. (2007). How impulsiveness and variety influence food intake in a sample of healthy women. *Appetite, 48*(1), 119–122.

Guerrieri, R., Nederkoorn, C., & Jansen, A. (2008). The interaction between impulsivity and a varied food environment: Its influence on food intake and overweight. *International Journal of Obesity (London), 32*(4), 708–714.

Gustafson, T. B., & Sarwer, D. B. (2004). Childhood sexual abuse and obesity. *Obesity Reviews, 5*(3), 129–135.

Habib, K. E., Weld, K. P., Rice, K. C., Pushkas, J., Champoux, M., Listwak, S., et al. (2000). Oral administration of a corticotropin-releasing hormone receptor antagonist significantly attenuates behavioral, neuroendocrine, and autonomic responses to stress in primates. *Proceedings of the National Academy of Sciences of the United States of America, 97*(11), 6079–6084.

Hammerness, P., Wilens, T., Mick, E., Spencer, T., Doyle, R., McCreary, M., et al. (2009). Cardiovascular effects of longer-term, high-dose OROS methylphenidate in adolescents with attention deficit hyperactivity disorder. *Journal of Pediatrics, 155*(1), 84–89, 89 e1.

Hamoui, N., Kingsbury, S., Anthone, G. J., & Crookes, P. F. (2004). Surgical treatment of morbid obesity in schizophrenic patients. *Obesity Surgery, 14*(3), 349–352.

Harrington, E., Crowther, J., Payne Henrickson, H., & Mickelson, K. (2006). The relationships among trauma, stress, ethnicity, and binge eating. *Cultural Diversity and Ethnic Minority Psychology, 12*(2), 212–229.

Hasler, G., Pine, D. S., Gamma, A., Milos, G., Ajdacic, V., Eich, D., et al. (2004). The associations between psychopathology and being overweight: A 20-year prospective study. *Psychological Medicine, 34*(6), 1047–1057.

Hay, P. P., Bacaltchuk, J., Stefano, S., & Kashyap, P. (2009). Psychological treatments for bulimia nervosa and binging. *Cochrane Database of Systematic Reviews* (4), CD000562.

Hayden, M. J., Dixon, J. B., Dixon, M. E., Shea, T. L., & O'Brien, P. E. (2011). Characterization of the improvement in depressive symptoms following bariatric surgery. *Obesity Surgery, 21*(3), 328–335.

Hedley, A. A., Ogden, C. L., Johnson, C. L., Carroll, M. D., Curtin, L. R., & Flegal, K. M. (2004). Prevalence of overweight and obesity among US children, adolescents, and adults, 1999-2002. *Journal of the American Medical Association, 291*(23), 2847–2850.

Heim, C., Mletzko, T., Purselle, D., Musselman, D. L., & Nemeroff, C. B. (2008). The dexamethasone/corticotropin-releasing factor test in men with major depression: Role of childhood trauma. *Biological Psychiatry, 63*(4), 398–405.

Hesslinger, B., Tebartz van Elst, L., Nyberg, E., Dykierek, P., Richter, H., Berner, M., et al. (2002). Psychotherapy of attention deficit hyperactivity disorder in adults – a pilot study using a structured skills training program. *European Archives of Psychiatry and Clinical Neuroscience, 252*(4), 177–184.

Howell, M. J., Schenck, C. H., & Crow, S. J. (2009). A review of nighttime eating disorders. *Sleep Medicine Reviews, 13*(1), 23–34.

Hrabosky, J. I., & Grilo, C. M. (2007). Body image and eating disordered behavior in a community sample of Black and Hispanic women. *Eating Behaviors, 8*(1), 106–114.

Hudson, J. I., Hiripi, E., Pope, H. G., Jr., & Kessler, R. C. (2007). The prevalence and correlates of eating disorders in the National Co-morbidity Survey Replication. *Biological Psychiatry, 61*(3), 348–358.

Hudson, J. I., Lalonde, J. K., Coit, C. E., Tsuang, M. T., McElroy, S. L., Crow, S. J., et al. (2010). Longitudinal study of the diagnosis of components of the metabolic syndrome in individuals with binge-eating disorder. *The American Journal of Clinical Nutrition, 91*(6), 1568–1573.

Ikossi, D. G., Maldonado, J. R., Hernandez-Boussard, T., & Eisenberg, D. (2010). Post-traumatic stress disorder (PTSD) is not a contraindication to gastric bypass in veterans with morbid obesity. *Surgical Endoscopy, 24*(8), 1892–1897.

Ivan, I., Azarbad, L., Corsica, J., & Hood, M. (2009). Does binge eating mediate the relationship between ADHD characteristics and obesity severity? *Obesity, 17*(Suppl 2), S286.

Jain, A. K., Kaplan, R. A., Gadde, K. M., Wadden, T. A., Allison, D. B., Brewer, E. R., et al. (2002). Bupropion SR vs. placebo for weight loss in obese patients with depressive symptoms. *Obesity Research, 10*(10), 1049–1056.

Jakicic, J. M., Marcus, B. H., Lang, W., & Janney, C. (2008). Effect of exercise on 24-month weight loss maintenance in overweight women. *Archives of Internal Medicine, 168*(14), 1550–1559; discussion 1559–1560.

James, W. P., Astrup, A., Finer, N., Hilsted, J., Kopelman, P., Rossner, S., et al. (2000). Effect of sibutramine on weight maintenance after weight loss: A randomised trial. STORM Study Group. Sibutramine Trial of Obesity Reduction and Maintenance. *The Lancet, 356*(9248), 2119–2125.

James, W. P., Caterson, I. D., Coutinho, W., Finer, N., Van Gaal, L. F., Maggioni, A. P., et al. (2010). Effect of sibutramine on cardiovascular outcomes in overweight and obese subjects. *The New England Journal of Medicine, 363*(10), 905–917.

Jarosz, P. A., Dobal, M. T., Wilson, F. L., & Schram, C. A. (2007). Disordered eating and food cravings among urban obese African American women. *Eating Behaviors, 8*(3), 374–381.

Johnson, J. G., Cohen, P., Kasen, S., & Brook, J. S. (2002). Childhood adversities associated with risk for eating disorders or weight problems during adolescence or early adulthood. *The American Journal of Psychiatry, 159*(3), 394–400.

Kaneko, K., Yamada, T., Tsukita, S., Takahashi, K., Ishigaki, Y., Oka, Y., et al. (2009). Obesity alters circadian expressions of molecular clock genes in the brainstem. *Brain Research, 1263*, 58–68.

Kasen, S., Cohen, P., Chen, H., & Must, A. (2008). Obesity and psychopathology in women: A three decade prospective study. *International Journal of Obesity (London), 32*(3), 558–566.

Kessler, R. C., Adler, L., Barkley, R., Biederman, J., Conners, C. K., Demler, O., et al. (2006). The prevalence and correlates of adult ADHD in the United States: Results from the National Co-morbidity Survey Replication. *The American Journal of Psychiatry, 163*(4), 716–723.

Kessler, R. C., Chiu, W. T., Demler, O., Merikangas, K. R., & Walters, E. E. (2005). Prevalence, severity, and co-morbidity of 12-month DSM-IV disorders in the National Co-morbidity Survey Replication. *Archives of General Psychiatry, 62*(6), 617–627.

Khazaal, Y., Fresard, E., Borgeat, F., & Zullino, D. (2006). Binge eating symptomatology in overweight and obese patients with schizophrenia: A case control study. *Annals of General Psychiatry, 5*, 15.

Khazaal, Y., Rothen, S., Moriniere Trombert, N., Fresard, E., & Zullino, D. F. (2007). Dietary underreporting in women with schizophrenia requiring dietary intervention: A case control study. *Eating and Weight Disorders, 12*(4), e83–e85.

Kim, K. H., Bursac, Z., DiLillo, V., White, D. B., & West, D. S. (2009). Stress, race, and body weight. *Health Psychology, 28*(1), 131–135.

Kim, S. W., Shin, I. S., Kim, J. M., Bae, K. Y., Yang, S. J., & Yoon, J. S. (2010). Effectiveness of switching from aripiprazole to ziprasidone in patients with schizophrenia. *Clinical Neuropharmacology, 33*(3), 121–125.

King, T. K., Clark, M. M., & Pera, V. (1996). History of sexual abuse and obesity treatment outcome. *Addictive Behaviors, 21*(3), 283–290.

Kloiber, S., Ising, M., Reppermund, S., Horstmann, S., Dose, T., Majer, M., et al. (2007). Overweight and obesity affect treatment response in major depression. *Biological Psychiatry, 62*(4), 321–326.

Kyrou, I., Chrousos, G. P., & Tsigos, C. (2006). Stress, visceral obesity, and metabolic complications. *Annals of the New York Academy of Sciences, 1083*, 77–110.

Lagarde, G., Doyon, J., & Brunet, A. (2010). Memory and executive dysfunctions associated with acute posttraumatic stress disorder. *Psychiatry Research, 177*(1–2), 144–149.

Lam, L. T., & Yang, L. (2007). Overweight/obesity and attention deficit and hyperactivity disorder tendency among adolescents in China. *Internation Journal of Obesity (London), 31*(4), 584–590.

Laposkya, A. D., Bassb, J., Kohsakac, A., & Turek, F. W. (2008). Sleep and circadian rhythms: Key components in the regulation of energy metabolism. *FEBS Letters, 582*, 142–151.

Lara, C., Fayyad, J., de Graaf, R., Kessler, R. C., Aguilar-Gaxiola, S., Angermeyer, M., et al. (2009). Childhood predictors of adult attention-deficit/hyperactivity disorder: Results from the World Health Organization World Mental Health Survey Initiative. *Biological Psychology, 65*(1), 46–54.

Larsen, J. K., & Geenen, R. (2005). Childhood sexual abuse is not associated with a poor outcome after gastric banding for severe obesity. *Obesity Surgery, 15*(4), 534–537.

Leddy, J. J., Epstein, L. H., Jaroni, J. L., Roemmich, J. N., Paluch, R. A., Goldfield, G. S., et al. (2004). Influence of methylphenidate on eating in obese men. *Obesity Research, 12*(2), 224–232.

Lee, S. J., Choi, E. J., & Kwon, J. S. (2008). A naturalistic multicenter trial of a 12-week weight management program for overweight and obese patients with schizophrenia or schizoaffective disorder. *The Journal of Clinical Psychiatry, 69*(4), 555–562.

Levy, L. D., Fleming, J. P., & Klar, D. (2009). Treatment of refractory obesity in severely obese adults following management of newly diagnosed attention deficit hyperactivity disorder. *International Journal of Obesity, 33*, 326–334.

Limosin, F., Gasquet, I., Leguay, D., Azorin, J. M., & Rouillon, F. (2008). Body mass index and prevalence of obesity in a French cohort of patients with schizophrenia. *Acta Psychiatrica Scandinavica, 118*(1), 19–25.

Linde, J. A., Jeffery, R. W., Levy, R. L., Sherwood, N. E., Utter, J., Pronk, N. P., et al. (2004). Binge eating disorder, weight control self-efficacy, and depression in overweight men and women. *International Journal of Obesity and Related Metabolic Disorders, 28*(3), 418–425.

Linde, J. A., Simon, G. E., Ludman, E. J., Ichikawa, L. E., Operskalski, B. H., Arterburn, D., et al. (2011). A randomized controlled trial of behavioral weight loss treatment versus combined weight loss/depression treatment among women with co-morbid obesity and depression. *Annals of Behavioral Medicine, 41*(1), 119–130.

Lindenmayer, J. P., Khan, A., Wance, D., Maccabee, N., Kaushik, S., & Kaushik, S. (2009). Outcome evaluation of a structured educational wellness program in patients with severe mental illness. *The Journal of Clinical Psychiatry, 70*(10), 1385–1396.

Loeb, K. L., Wilson, G. T., Gilbert, J. S., & Labouvie, E. (2000). Guided and unguided self-help for binge eating. *Behaviour Research and Therapy, 38*(3), 259–272.

Lowe, M. R., van Steenburgh, J., Ochner, C., & Coletta, M. (2009). Neural correlates of individual differences related to appetite. *Physiology and Behavior, 97*(5), 561–571.

Lu, X. Y. (2007). The leptin hypothesis of depression: A potential link between mood disorders and obesity? *Current Opinion in Pharmacology, 7*(6), 648–652.

Ludman, E., Simon, G. E., Ichikawa, L. E., Operskalski, B. H., Arterburn, D., Linde, J. A., et al. (2009). Does depression reduce the effectiveness of behavioral weight loss treatment? *Behavioral Medicine, 35*(4), 126–134.

Luppino, F. S., de Wit, L. M., Bouvy, P. F., Stijnen, T., Cuijpers, P., Penninx, B. W., et al. (2010). Overweight, obesity, and depression. A systematic review and meta-analysis of longitudinal studies. *Archives of General Psychiatry, 67*(3), 220–229.

Ma, Y., Pagoto, S. L., Olendzki, B. C., Hafner, A. R., Perugini, R. A., Mason, R., et al. (2006). Predictors of weight status following laparoscopic roux-en-y gastric bypass. *Obesity Surgery, 16*(9), 1227–1231.

Macht, M. (2008). How emotions affect eating: A five-way model. *Appetite, 50*, 1–11.

Malone, M., Alger-Mayer, S. A., & Anderson, D. A. (2005). Medication associated with weight gain may influence outcome in a weight management program. *The Annals of Pharmacotherapy, 39*(7–8), 1204–1208.

Marques, L., Alegria, M., Becker, A. E., Chen, C. N., Fang, A., Chosak, A., et al. (2011). Comparative prevalence, correlates of impairment, and service utilization for eating disorders across US ethnic groups: Implications for reducing ethnic disparities in health care access for eating disorders. *International Journal of Eating Disorders, 44*(5), 412–420.

Masheb, R. M., & Grilo, C. M. (2008). Examination of predictors and moderators for self-help treatments of binge-eating disorder. *Journal of Consulting and Clinical Psychology, 76*(5), 900–904.

Mastorakos, G., & Zapanti, E. (2004). The hypothalamic-pituitary-adrenal axis in the neuroendocrine regulation of food intake and obesity: The role of corticotropin releasing hormone. *Nutritional Neuroscience, 7*(5–6), 271–280.

Mather, A. A., Cox, B. J., Enns, M. W., & Sareen, J. (2009). Associations of obesity with psychiatric disorders and suicidal behaviors in a nationally representative sample. *Journal of Psychosomatic Research, 66*(4), 277–285.
McAllister, E. J., Dhurandhar, N. V., Keith, S. W., Aronne, L. J., Barger, J., Baskin, M., et al. (2009). Ten putative contributors to the obesity epidemic. *Critical Reviews in Food Science and Nutrition, 49*(10), 868–913.
McElroy, S. L. (2009). Obesity in patients with severe mental illness: Overview and management. *The Journal of Clinical Psychiatry, 70*(Suppl 3), 12–21.
McElroy, S. L., Frye, M. A., Altshuler, L. L., Suppes, T., Hellemann, G., Black, D., et al. (2007). A 24-week, randomized, controlled trial of adjunctive sibutramine versus topiramate in the treatment of weight gain in overweight or obese patients with bipolar disorders. *Bipolar Disorders, 9*(4), 426–434.
McElroy, S. L., Frye, M. A., Suppes, T., Dhavale, D., Keck, P. E., Jr., Leverich, G. S., et al. (2002). Correlates of overweight and obesity in 644 patients with bipolar disorder. *The Journal of Clinical Psychiatry, 63*(3), 207–213.
McElroy, S. L., Hudson, J. I., Capece, J. A., Beyers, K., Fisher, A. C., & Rosenthal, N. R. (2007). Topiramate for the treatment of binge eating disorder associated with obesity: A placebo-controlled study. *Biological Psychiatry, 61*(9), 1039–1048.
McEvoy, J. P., Meyer, J. M., Goff, D. C., Nasrallah, H. A., Davis, S. M., Sullivan, L., et al. (2005). Prevalence of the metabolic syndrome in patients with schizophrenia: Baseline results from the Clinical Antipsychotic Trials of Intervention Effectiveness (CATIE) schizophrenia trial and comparison with national estimates from NHANES III. *Schizophrenia Research, 80*(1), 19–32.
McIntyre, R. S. (2002). Psychotropic drugs and adverse events in the treatment of bipolar disorders revisited. *The Journal of Clinical Psychiatry, 63*(Suppl 3), 15–20.
McLaren, L. (2007). Socioeconomic status and obesity. *Epidemiologic Reviews, 29*, 29–48.
McNeely, W., & Goa, K. L. (1998). Sibutramine. A review of its contribution to the management of obesity. *Drugs, 56*(6), 1093–1124.
McTigue, K., Harris, R., Hemphill, M. B., Bunton, A. J., Lux, L. J., Sutton, S., et al. (2003). *Systematic evidence review. Screening and interventions for overweight and obesity in adults.* Research Triangle Park, NC: Agency for Healthcare Research and Quality, U.S. Department of Health and Human Services.
Meewisse, M. L., Reitsma, J. B., de Vries, G. J., Gersons, B. P., & Olff, M. (2007). Cortisol and post-traumatic stress disorder in adults: Systematic review and meta-analysis. *The British Journal of Psychiatry, 191*, 387–392.
Merom, D., Phongsavan, P., Wagner, R., Chey, T., Marnane, C., Steel, Z., et al. (2008). Promoting walking as an adjunct intervention to group cognitive behavioral therapy for anxiety disorders – a pilot group randomized trial. *Journal of Anxiety Disorders, 22*(6), 959–968.
Michelson, D., Amsterdam, J. D., Quitkin, F. M., Reimherr, F. W., Rosenbaum, J. F., Zajecka, J., et al. (1999). Changes in weight during a 1-year trial of fluoxetine. *The American Journal of Psychiatry, 156*(8), 1170–1176.
Mikami, A. Y., Hinshaw, S. P., Patterson, K. A., & Lee, J. C. (2008). Eating pathology among adolescent girls with attention-deficit/hyperactivity disorder. *Journal of Abnormal Psychology, 117*(1), 225–235.
Miller, E. K., & Cohen, J. D. (2001). An integrative theory of prefrontal cortex function. *Annual Review of Neuroscience, 24*, 167–202.
Miller, G. E., Freedland, K. E., Carney, R. M., Stetler, C. A., & Banks, W. A. (2003). Pathways linking depression, adiposity, and inflammatory markers in healthy young adults. *Brain, Behavior, and Immunity, 17*(4), 276–285.
Montes, J. M., Rodriguez, J. L., Balbo, E., Sopelana, P., Martin, E., Soto, J. A., et al. (2007). Improvement in antipsychotic-related metabolic disturbances in patients with schizophrenia switched to ziprasidone. *Progress in Neuro-Psychopharmacology & Biological Psychiatry, 31*(2), 383–388.
Munsch, S., Biedert, E., Meyer, A., Michael, T., Schlup, B., Tuch, A., et al. (2007). A randomized comparison of cognitive behavioral therapy and behavioral weight loss treatment for overweight individuals with binge eating disorder. *The International Journal of Eating Disorders, 40*(2), 102–113.

Napolitano, M. A., Head, S., Babyak, M. A., & Blumenthal, J. A. (2001). Binge eating disorder and night eating syndrome: Psychological and behavioral characteristics. *The International Journal of Eating Disorders, 30*(2), 193–203.

National Institute for Clinical Excellence. (2004). *NICE guidelines for eating disorders*. Retrieved August, 2010 from http://www.nice.org.uk/nicemedia/live/10932/29220/29220.pdf.

National Institute of Health and Clinical Excellence. (2009). *NICE guidelines for depression care*. Retrieved March 21, 2010 from http://www.nice.org.uk/nicemedia/pdf/Depression_Update_FULL_GUIDELINE.pdf.

Nazar, B. P., Pinna, C. M., Coutinho, G., Segenreich, D., Duchesne, M., Appolinario, J. C., et al. (2008). Review of literature of attention-deficit/hyperactivity disorder with co-morbid eating disorders. *Revista Brasileira de Psiquiatria, 30*(4), 384–389.

Nederkoorn, C., Braet, C., Van Eijs, Y., Tanghe, A., & Jansen, A. (2006). Why obese children cannot resist food: The role of impulsivity. *Eating Behaviors, 7*(4), 315–322.

Nederkoorn, C., Guerrieri, R., Havermans, R. C., Roefs, A., & Jansen, A. (2009). The interactive effect of hunger and impulsivity on food intake and purchase in a virtual supermarket. *International Journal of Obesity (London), 33*(8), 905–912.

Nederkoorn, C., Guerrieri, R., Roefs, A., & Jansen, A. (2008). Effects of impulsivity on food purchase and weight gain over time. *Appetite, 51*, 752.

Nederkoorn, C., Jansen, E., Mulkens, S., & Jansen, A. (2007). Impulsivity predicts treatment outcome in obese children. *Behaviour Research and Therapy, 45*(5), 1071–1075.

Nederkoorn, C., Smulders, F. T., Havermans, R. C., Roefs, A., & Jansen, A. (2006). Impulsivity in obese women. *Appetite, 47*(2), 253–256.

Newcomer, J. W., Campos, J. A., Marcus, R. N., Breder, C., Berman, R. M., Kerselaers, W., et al. (2008). A multicenter, randomized, double-blind study of the effects of aripiprazole in overweight subjects with schizophrenia or schizoaffective disorder switched from olanzapine. *The Journal of Clinical Psychiatry, 69*(7), 1046–1056.

Newman, E., O'Connor, D. B., & Conner, M. (2007). Daily hassles and eating behaviour: The role of cortisol reactivity status. *Psychoneuroendocrinology, 32*(2), 125–132.

O'Reardon, J. P., Allison, K. C., Martino, N. S., Lundgren, J. D., Heo, M., & Stunkard, A. J. (2006). A randomized, placebo-controlled trial of sertraline in the treatment of night eating syndrome. *The American Journal of Psychiatry, 163*(5), 893–898.

O'Reardon, J. P., Ringel, B. L., Dinges, D. F., Allison, K. C., Rogers, N. L., Martino, N. S., et al. (2004). Circadian eating and sleeping patterns in the night eating syndrome. *Obesity Research, 12*(11), 1789–1796.

O'Reardon, J. P., Stunkard, A. J., & Allison, K. C. (2004). Clinical trial of sertraline in the treatment of night eating syndrome. *Eating Disorders, 35*(1), 16–26.

Oliver, G., Wardle, J., & Gibson, E. L. (2000). Stress and food choice: A laboratory study. *Psychosomatic Medicine, 62*(6), 853–865.

Onyike, C. U., Crum, R. M., Lee, H. B., Lyketsos, C. G., & Eaton, W. W. (2003). Is obesity associated with major depression? Results from the Third National Health and Nutrition Examination Survey. *American Journal of Epidemiology, 158*(12), 1139–1147.

Oppong, B. A., Nickels, M. W., & Sax, H. C. (2006). The impact of a history of sexual abuse on weight loss in gastric bypass patients. *Psychosomatics, 47*(2), 108–111.

Osborn, D. P., Nazareth, I., & King, M. B. (2007). Physical activity, dietary habits and coronary heart disease risk factor knowledge amongst people with severe mental illness: A cross sectional comparative study in primary care. *Social Psychiatry and Psychiatric Epidemiology, 42*(10), 787–793.

Pagoto, S. L., Bodenlos, J. S., Kantor, L., Gitkind, M., Curtin, C., & Ma, Y. (2007). Association of major depression and binge eating disorder with weight loss in a clinical setting. *Obesity, 15*(11), 2557–2559.

Pagoto, S. L., Curtin, C., Bandini, L. G., Anderson, S. E., Schneider, K., Bodenlos, J. S., et al. (2010). Weight loss following a clinic-based weight loss program among adults with attention deficit/hyperactivity disorder symptoms. *Eating and Weight Disorders, 15*, e166–e172.

Pagoto, S. L., Bodenlos, J. S., Schneider, K. L., Olendzki, B. C., Spates, C. R., & Ma, Y. (2008). Initial investigation of behavioral activation therapy for co-morbid major depressive disorder and obesity. Psychotherapy: Theory, Research, Practice, *Training, 45*(3), 410–415.

Pagoto, S. L., Curtin, C., Lemon, L., Bandini, L. G., Schneider, K., Bodenlos, J. S., et al. (2009). Association between adult attention deficit/hyperactivity disorder and obesity in the US population. *Obesity, 17*(3), 539–544.

Pagoto, S. L., Lemon, S. C., Schneider, K., Bodenlos, J. S., & Ma, Y. (2008). Association of post-traumatic stress disorder and obesity in a nationally representative sample. *Obesity, 16*(Suppl 1), S94.

Pagoto, S. L., Schneider, K. L., Oleski, J. L., Luciani, J. M., Bodenlos, J. S., & Whited, M. C., (2011). Male inclusion in randomized controlled trials of lifestyle weight loss interventions. *Obesity (Silver Spring)*, [Epub ahead of print].

Pagoto, S. L., Spring, B., Cook, J. W., McChargue, D., & Schneider, K. (2006). High BMI and reduced frequency and enjoyment of pleasant events. *Personality and Individual Differences, 40*(7), 1421–1431.

Painot, D., Jotterand, S., Kammer, A., Fossati, M., & Golay, A. (2001). Simultaneous nutritional cognitive–behavioural therapy in obese patients. *Patient Education and Counseling, 42*(1), 47–52.

Patten, S. B., Williams, J. V., Lavorato, D. H., Brown, L., McLaren, L., & Eliasziw, M. (2009). Major depression, antidepressant medication and the risk of obesity. *Psychotherapy and Psychosomatics, 78*(3), 182–186.

Pauli-Pott, U., Albayrak, O., Hebebrand, J., & Pott, W. (2010). Does inhibitory control capacity in overweight and obese children and adolescents predict success in a weight-reduction program? *European Child & Adolescent Psychiatry, 19*(2), 135–141.

Pecoraro, N. C., Reyes, F., Gomez, F., Bhargava, A., & Dallman, M. F. (2004). Chronic stress promotes palatable feeding, which reduces signs of stress: Feedforward and feedback effects of chronic stress. *Endocrinology, 145*(8), 3754–3762.

Perkonigg, A., Owashi, T., Stein, M. B., Kirschbaum, C., & Wittchen, H. U. (2009). Posttraumatic stress disorder and obesity: Evidence for a risk association. *American Journal of Preventive Medicine, 36*(1), 1–8.

Pervanidou, P., & Chrousos, G. P. (2010). Neuroendocrinology of post-traumatic stress disorder. *Progress in Brain Research, 182*, 149–160.

Peterson, C. B., Crow, S. J., Nugent, S., Mitchell, J. E., Engbloom, S., & Mussell, M. P. (2000). Predictors of treatment outcome for binge eating disorder. *The International Journal of Eating Disorders, 28*(2), 131–138.

Petry, N. M., Barry, D., Pietrzak, R. H., & Wagner, J. A. (2008). Overweight and obesity are associated with psychiatric disorders: Results from the National Epidemiologic Survey on alcohol and related conditions. *Psychosomatic Medicine, 70*(3), 288–297.

Pickering, R. P., Grant, B. F., Chou, S. P., & Compton, W. M. (2007). Are overweight, obesity, and extreme obesity associated with psychopathology? Results from the national epidemiologic survey on alcohol and related conditions. *The Journal of Clinical Psychiatry, 68*(7), 998–1009.

Pike, K. M., Dohm, F. A., Striegel-Moore, R. H., Wilfley, D. E., & Fairburn, C. G. (2001). A comparison of black and white women with binge eating disorder. *The American Journal of Psychiatry, 158*(9), 1455–1460.

Pirke, K. M., Platte, P., Laessle, R., Seidl, M., & Fichter, M. M. (1992). The effect of a mental challenge test of plasma norepinephrine and cortisol in bulimia nervosa and in controls. *Biological Psychiatry, 32*(2), 202–206.

Poulin, M. J., Chaput, J. P., Simard, V., Vincent, P., Bernier, J., Gauthier, Y., et al. (2007). Management of antipsychotic-induced weight gain: Prospective naturalistic study of the effectiveness of a supervised exercise programme. *The Australian and New Zealand Journal of Psychiatry, 41*(12), 980–989.

Puhl, R. M., & Brownell, K. D. (2006). Confronting and coping with weight stigma: An investigation of overweight and obese adults. *Obesity (Silver Spring), 14*(10), 1802–1815.

Puhl, R. M., & Heuer, C. A. (2009). The stigma of obesity: A review and update. *Obesity (Silver Spring), 17*(5), 941–964.

Puhl, R. M., Moss-Racusin, C. A., Schwartz, M. B., & Brownell, K. D. (2008). Weight stigmatization and bias reduction: Perspectives of overweight and obese adults. *Health Education Research, 23*(2), 347–358.

Raadsheer, F. C., Hoogendijk, W. J., Stam, F. C., Tilders, F. J., & Swaab, D. F. (1994). Increased numbers of corticotropin-releasing hormone expressing neurons in the hypothalamic paraventricular nucleus of depressed patients. *Neuroendocrinology, 60*(4), 436–444.

Raeder, M. B., Bjelland, I., Vollset, S. E., & Steen, V. M. (2006). Obesity, dyslipidemia, and diabetes with selective serotonin reuptake inhibitors: The Hordaland Health Study. *The Journal of Clinical Psychiatry, 67*, 1974–1982.

Ramacciotti, C. E., Coli, E., Passaglia, C., Lacorte, M., Pea, E., & Dell'Osso, L. (2000). Binge eating disorder: Prevalence and psychopathological features in a clinical sample of obese people in Italy. *Psychiatry Research, 94*(2), 131–138.

Rand, C. S., Macgregor, A. M., & Stunkard, A. J. (1997). The night eating syndrome in the general population and among postoperative obesity surgery patients. *The International Journal of Eating Disorders, 22*(1), 65–69.

Rapoport, L., Clark, M., & Wardle, J. (2000). Evaluation of a modified cognitive-behavioural programme for weight management. *International Journal of Obesity and Related Metabolic Disorders, 24*(12), 1726–1737.

Ray, E. C., Nickels, M. W., Sayeed, S., & Sax, H. C. (2003). Predicting success after gastric bypass: The role of psychosocial and behavioral factors. *Surgery, 134*(4), 555–563; discussion 563–564.

Reas, D. L., & Grilo, C. M. (2007). Timing and sequence of the onset of overweight, dieting, and binge eating in overweight patients with binge eating disorder. *The International Journal of Eating Disorders, 40*(2), 165–170.

Reas, D. L., & Grilo, C. M. (2008). Review and meta-analysis of pharmacotherapy for binge-eating disorder. *Obesity (Silver Spring), 16*(9), 2024–2038.

Reuter, M., Schmitz, A., Corr, P., & Hennig, J. (2006). Molecular genetics support Gray's personality theory: The interaction of COMT and DRD2 polymorphisms predicts the behavioural approach system. *The International Journal of Neuropsychopharmacology, 9*(2), 155–166.

Rexrode, K. M., Pradhan, A., Manson, J. E., Buring, J. E., & Ridker, P. M. (2003). Relationship of total and abdominal adiposity with CRP and IL-6 in women. *Annals of Epidemiology, 13*(10), 674–682.

Ricca, V., Castellini, G., Lo Sauro, C., Rotella, C. M., & Faravelli, C. (2009). Zonisamide combined with cognitive behavioral therapy in binge eating disorder: A one-year follow-up study. *Psychiatry (Edgmont), 6*(11), 23–28.

Roberts, R. E., Deleger, S., Strawbridge, W. J., & Kaplan, G. A. (2003). Prospective association between obesity and depression: Evidence from the Alameda County Study. *International Journal of Obesity and Related Metabolic Disorders, 27*(4), 514–521.

Roberts, R. E., Kaplan, G. A., Shema, S. J., & Strawbridge, W. J. (2000). Are the obese at greater risk for depression? *American Journal of Epidemiology, 152*(2), 163–170.

Rodriguez-Hernandez, H., Morales-Amaya, U. A., Rosales-Valdez, R., Rivera-Hinojosa, F., Rodriguez-Moran, M., & Guerrero-Romero, F. (2009). Adding cognitive behavioural treatment to either low-carbohydrate or low-fat diets: Differential short-term effects. *The British Journal of Nutrition, 102*(12), 1847–1853.

Roehrig, M., Masheb, R. M., White, M. A., & Grilo, C. M. (2009). The metabolic syndrome and behavioral correlates in obese patients with binge eating disorder. *Obesity (Silver Spring), 17*(3), 481–486.

Rogers, N. L., Dinges, D. F., Allison, K. C., Maislin, G., Martino, N., O'Reardon, J. P., et al. (2006). Assessment of sleep in women with night eating syndrome. *Sleep, 29*(6), 814–819.

Rohde, P., Ichikawa, L., Simon, G. E., Ludman, E. J., Linde, J. A., Jeffery, R. W., et al. (2008). Associations of child sexual and physical abuse with obesity and depression in middle-aged women. *Child Abuse & Neglect, 32*(9), 878–887.

Rosenheck, R. A., Davis, S., Covell, N., Essock, S., Swartz, M., Stroup, S., et al. (2009). Does switching to a new antipsychotic improve outcomes? Data from the CATIE trial. *Schizophrenia Research, 107*(1), 22–29.

Rosmond, R., & Bjorntorp, P. (1998). Endocrine and metabolic aberrations in men with abdominal obesity in relation to anxio-depressive infirmity. *Metabolism, 47*(10), 1187–1193.
Rosmond, R., Dallman, M. F., & Bjorntorp, P. (1998). Stress-related cortisol secretion in men: Relationships with abdominal obesity and endocrine, metabolic and hemodynamic abnormalities. *The Journal of Clinical Endocrinology and Metabolism, 83*(6), 1853–1859.
Rostain, A. L., & Ramsay, J. R. (2006). A combined treatment approach for adults with ADHD – results of an open study of 43 patients. *Journal of Attention Disorders, 10*(2), 150–159.
Rummel-Kluge, C., Komossa, K., Schwarz, S., Hunger, H., Schmid, F., Lobos, C. A., et al. (2010). Head-to-head comparisons of metabolic side effects of second generation antipsychotics in the treatment of schizophrenia: A systematic review and meta-analysis. *Schizophrenia Research, 123*(2–3), 225–233.
Rybakowski, J. K., & Twardowska, K. (1999). The dexamethasone/corticotropin-releasing hormone test in depression in bipolar and unipolar affective illness. *Journal of Psychiatric Research, 33*(5), 363–370.
Saarni, S. E., Saarni, S. I., Fogelholm, M., Heliovaara, M., Perala, J., Suvisaari, J., et al. (2009). Body composition in psychotic disorders: A general population survey. *Psychological Medicine, 39*(5), 801–810.
Sachs, G., Bowden, C., Calabrese, J. R., Ketter, T., Thompson, T., White, R., et al. (2006). Effects of lamotrigine and lithium on body weight during maintenance treatment of bipolar I disorder. *Bipolar Disorders, 8*(2), 175–181.
Sachs, G. S., & Rush, A. J. (2003). Response, remission, and recovery in bipolar disorders: What are the realistic treatment goals? *The Journal of Clinical Psychiatry, 64*(Suppl 6), 18–22; discussion 28.
Safren, S. A. (2006). Cognitive-behavioral approaches to ADHD treatment in adulthood. *The Journal of Clinical Psychiatry, 67*(Suppl 8), 46–50.
Safren, S. A., Otto, M. W., Sprich, S., Winett, C. L., Wilens, T. E., & Biederman, J. (2005). Cognitive-behavioral therapy for ADHD in medication-treated adults with continued symptoms. *Behaviour Research and Therapy, 43*(7), 831–842.
Safren, S. A., Sprich, S., Mimiaga, M. J., Surman, C., Knouse, L., Groves, M., et al. (2010). Cognitive behavioral therapy vs relaxation with educational support for medication-treated adults with ADHD and persistent symptoms: A randomized controlled trial. *Journal of the American Medical Association, 304*(8), 875–880.
Sarwer, D. B., & Thompson, J. K. (2002). Obesity and body image disturbance. In T. Wadden & A. J. Stunkard (Eds.), *Handbook of obesity treatment* (pp. 447–464). New York, NY: Guilford.
Sbrocco, T., Nedegaard, R. C., Stone, J. M., & Lewis, E. L. (1999). Behavioral choice treatment promotes continuing weight loss: Preliminary results of a cognitive-behavioral decision-based treatment for obesity. *Journal of Consulting and Clinical Psychology, 67*(2), 260–266.
Schorr, S. G., Slooff, C. J., Postema, R., Van Oven, W., Schilthuis, M., Bruggeman, R., et al. (2008). A 12-month follow-up study of treating overweight schizophrenic patients with aripiprazole. *Acta Psychiatrica Scandinavica, 118*(3), 246–250.
Schule, C., Baghai, T. C., Eser, D., & Rupprecht, R. (2009). Hypothalamic-pituitary-adrenocortical system dysregulation and new treatment strategies in depression. *Expert Review of Neurotherapeutics, 9*(7), 1005–1019.
Schweickert, L. A., Strober, M., & Moskowitz, A. (1997). Efficacy of methylphenidate in bulimia nervosa co-morbid with attention-deficit hyperactivity disorder: A case report. *The International Journal of Eating Disorders, 21*(3), 299–301.
Scott, K. M., Bruffaerts, R., Simon, G. E., Alonso, J., Angermeyer, M., de Girolamo, G., et al. (2008). Obesity and mental disorders in the general population: Results from the world mental health surveys. *International Journal of Obesity (London), 32*(1), 192–200.
Semanscin-Doerr, D. A., Windover, A., Ashton, K., & Heinberg, L. J. (2010). Mood disorders in laparoscopic sleeve gastrectomy patients: Does it affect early weight loss? *Surgery for Obesity and Related Diseases, 6*(2), 191–196.

Shah, A., Shen, N., & El-Mallakh, R. S. (2006). Weight gain occurs after onset of bipolar illness in overweight bipolar patients. *Annals of Clinical Psychiatry, 18*(4), 239–241.

Sharma, B., & Henderson, D. C. (2008). Sibutramine: Current status as an anti-obesity drug and its future perspectives. *Expert Opinion on Pharmacotherapy, 9*(12), 2161–2173.

Shea, A., Walsh, C., Macmillan, H., & Steiner, M. (2005). Child maltreatment and HPA axis dysregulation: Relationship to major depressive disorder and post traumatic stress disorder in females. *Psychoneuroendocrinology, 30*(2), 162–178.

Sim, L. A., McAlpine, D. E., Grothe, K. B., Himes, S. M., Cockerill, R. G., & Clark, M. M. (2010). Identification and treatment of eating disorders in the primary care setting. *Mayo Clinic Proceedings, 85*(8), 746–751.

Simmonds, D. J., Pekar, J. J., & Mostofsky, S. H. (2008). Meta-analysis of Go/No-go tasks demonstrating that fMRI activation associated with response inhibition is task-dependent. *Neuropsychologia, 46*(1), 224–232.

Simon, G. E., Hunkeler, E., Fireman, B., Lee, J. Y., & Savarino, J. (2007). Risk of suicide attempt and suicide death in patients treated for bipolar disorder. *Bipolar Disorders, 9*(5), 526–530.

Simon, G. E., Von Korff, M., Saunders, K., Miglioretti, D. L., Crane, P. K., van Belle, G., et al. (2006). Association between obesity and psychiatric disorders in the US adult population. *Archives of General Psychiatry, 63*(7), 824–830.

Smits, J. A., Rosenfield, D., Mather, A. A., Tart, C. D., Henriksen, C., & Sareen, J. (2010). Psychotropic medication use mediates the relationship between mood and anxiety disorders and obesity: Findings from a nationally representative sample. *Journal of Psychiatric Research, 44*(15), 1010–1016.

Smolak, L., & Murnen, S. K. (2002). A meta-analytic examination of the relationship between child sexual abuse and eating disorders. *The International Journal of Eating Disorders, 31*(2), 136–150.

Spitzer, R. L., Williams, J. B., Gibbon, M., & First, M. B. (1992). The Structured Clinical Interview for DSM-III-R (SCID). I: History, rationale, and description. *Archives of General Psychiatry, 49*(8), 624–629.

Spitzer, R. L., Yanovski, S., Wadden, T., Wing, R., Marcus, M. D., Stunkard, A., et al. (1993). Binge eating disorder: Its further validation in a multisite study. *The International Journal of Eating Disorders, 13*(2), 137–153.

Spurling, R. D., Lamberti, J. S., Olsen, D., Tu, X., & Tang, W. (2007). Changes in metabolic parameters with switching to aripiprazole from another second-generation antipsychotic: A retrospective chart review. *The Journal of Clinical Psychiatry, 68*(3), 406–409.

Stecker, T., & Sparks, S. (2006). Prevalence of obese patients in a primary care setting. *Obesity, 14*, 373–376.

Stefaniak, T., Babinska, D., Trus, M., & Vingerhoets, A. (2007). The impact of history of sexual abuse on weight loss in gastric bypass patients. *Psychosomatics, 48*(3), 270–271.

Stevenson, C. S., Whitmont, S., Bornholt, L., Livesey, D., & Stevenson, R. J. (2002). A cognitive remediation programme for adults with attention deficit hyperactivity disorder. *The Australian and New Zealand Journal of Psychiatry, 36*(5), 610–616.

Stone, A. A., Schwartz, J. E., Smyth, J., Kirschbaum, C., Cohen, S., Hellhammer, D., et al. (2001). Individual differences in the diurnal cycle of salivary free cortisol: A replication of flattened cycles for some individuals. *Psychoneuroendocrinology, 26*(3), 295–306.

Strassnig, M., Brar, J. S., & Ganguli, R. (2003). Nutritional assessment of patients with schizophrenia: A preliminary study. *Schizophrenia Bulletin, 29*(2), 393–397.

Strassnig, M., Singh Brar, J., & Ganguli, R. (2005). Dietary fatty acid and antioxidant intake in community-dwelling patients suffering from schizophrenia. *Schizophrenia Research, 76*(2–3), 343–351.

Striegel-Moore, R. H., Dohm, F. A., Kraemer, H. C., Schreiber, G. B., Taylor, C. B., & Daniels, S. R. (2007). Risk factors for binge-eating disorders: An exploratory study. *The International Journal of Eating Disorders, 40*(6), 481–487.

Striegel-Moore, R. H., Franko, D. L., Thompson, D., Affenito, S., & Kraemer, H. (2006). Night eating: Prevalence and demographic correlates. *Obesity, 14*, 139–147.

Stunkard, A. J. (1959). Eating patterns and obesity. *The Psychiatric Quarterly, 33*, 284–295.
Stunkard, A. J., & Allison, K. C. (2003). Two forms of disordered eating in obesity: Binge eating and night eating. *International Journal of Obesity and Related Metabolic Disorders, 27*(1), 1–12.
Stunkard, A. J., Allison, K. C., Lundgren, J. D., Martino, N. S., Heo, M., Etemad, B., et al. (2006). A paradigm for facilitating pharmacotherapy at a distance: Sertraline treatment of the night eating syndrome. *The Journal of Clinical Psychiatry, 67*(10), 1568–1572.
Stunkard, A., Berkowitz, R., Wadden, T., Tanrikut, C., Reiss, E., & Young, L. (1996). Binge eating disorder and the night-eating syndrome. *International Journal of Obesity and Related Metabolic Disorders, 20*(1), 1–6.
Stunkard, A. J., Grace, W. J., & Wolff, H. G. (1955). The night-eating syndrome; a pattern of food intake among certain obese patients. *The American Journal of Medicine, 19*(1), 78–86.
Takeuchi, H., Uchida, H., Suzuki, T., Watanabe, K., & Kashima, H. (2010). Changes in metabolic parameters following a switch to aripiprazole in Japanese patients with schizophrenia: One-year follow-up study. *Psychiatry and Clinical Neurosciences, 64*(1), 104–106.
Tholin, S., Lindroos, A., Tynelius, P., Akerstedt, T., Stunkard, A. J., Bulik, C. M., et al. (2009). Prevalence of night eating in obese and nonobese twins. *Obesity (Silver Spring), 17*(5), 1050–1055.
Tiwari, A. K., Zai, C. C., Likhodi, O., Lisker, A., Singh, D., Souza, R. P., et al. (2010). A common polymorphism in the cannabinoid receptor 1 (CNR1) gene is associated with antipsychotic-induced weight gain in Schizophrenia. *Neuropsychopharmacology, 35*(6), 1315–1324.
Torrent, C., Amann, B., Sanchez-Moreno, J., Colom, F., Reinares, M., Comes, M., et al. (2008). Weight gain in bipolar disorder: Pharmacological treatment as a contributing factor. *Acta Psychiatrica Scandinavica, 118*(1), 4–18.
Torres, S. J., & Nowson, C. A. (2007). Relationship between stress, eating behavior, and obesity. *Nutrition, 23*(11–12), 887–894.
Tsigos, C., & Chrousos, G. P. (2002). Hypothalamic-pituitary-adrenal axis, neuroendocrine factors and stress. *Journal of Psychosomatic Research, 53*(4), 865–871.
U.S. Food and Drug Administration. (2010). *Meridia (sibutramine): Market withdrawal due to risk of serious cardiovascular events*. Retrieved January 3, 2011 from http://www.fda.gov/Safety/MedWatch/SafetyInformation/SafetyAlertsforHumanMedicalProducts/ucm228830.htm.
Uher, R., Mors, O., Hauser, J., Rietschel, M., Maier, W., Kozel, D., et al. (2011). Changes in body weight during pharmacological treatment of depression. *International Journal of Neuropsychopharmacology, 14*(3), 367–375.
Van Cauter, E., & Refetoff, S. (1985). Evidence for two subtypes of Cushing's disease based on the analysis of episodic cortisol secretion. *The New England Journal of Medicine, 312*(21), 1343–1349.
van den Bos, R., & de Ridder, D. (2006). Evolved to satisfy our immediate needs: Self-control and the rewarding properties of food. *Appetite, 47*(1), 24–29.
Vander Wal, J. S., Waller, S. M., Klurfeld, D. M., McBurney, M. I., & Dhurandhar, N. V. (2005). Night eating syndrome: Evaluation of two screening instruments. *Eating Behaviors, 6*(1), 63–73.
Verma, S. K., Subramaniam, M., Liew, A., & Poon, L. Y. (2009). Metabolic risk factors in drug-naive patients with first-episode psychosis. *The Journal of Clinical Psychiatry, 70*(7), 997–1000.
Vicennati, V., Pasqui, F., Cavazza, C., Pagotto, U., & Pasquali, R. (2009). Stress-related development of obesity and cortisol in women. *Obesity (Silver Spring), 17*(9), 1678–1683.
Vieweg, W. V., Julius, D. A., Bates, J., Quinn, J. F., III, Fernandez, A., Hasnain, M., et al. (2007). Posttraumatic stress disorder as a risk factor for obesity among male military veterans. *Acta Psychiatrica Scandinavica, 116*(6), 483–487.
Vinai, P., Allison, K. C., Cardetti, S., Carpegna, G., Ferrato, N., Masante, D., et al. (2008). Psychopathology and treatment of night eating syndrome: A review. *Eating and Weight Disorders, 13*(2), 54–63.
Vocks, S., Tuschen-Caffier, B., Pietrowsky, R., Rustenbach, S. J., Kersting, A., & Herpertz, S. (2010). Meta-analysis of the effectiveness of psychological and pharmacological treatments for binge eating disorder. *The International Journal of Eating Disorders, 43*(3), 205–217.

Vogelzangs, N., Kritchevsky, S. B., Beekman, A. T., Brenes, G. A., Newman, A. B., Satterfield, S., et al. (2010). Obesity and onset of significant depressive symptoms: Results from a prospective community-based cohort study of older men and women. *The Journal of Clinical Psychiatry, 71*(4), 391–399.

Volkow, N. D., Wang, G. J., Kollins, S. H., Wigal, T. L., Newcorn, J. H., Telang, F., et al. (2009). Evaluating dopamine reward pathway in ADHD: Clinical implications. *Journal of American Medical Association, 302*(10), 1084–1091.

Wadden, T. A., Foreyt, J. P., Foster, G. D., Hill, J. O., Klein, S., O'Neil, P. M., et al. (2011). Weight loss with naltrexone SR/bupropion SR combination therapy as an adjunct to behavior modification: The COR-BMOD trial. *Obesity, 19*(1), 110–120.

Wade, T. D., Bergin, J. L., Tiggemann, M., Bulik, C. M., & Fairburn, C. G. (2006). Prevalence and long-term course of lifetime eating disorders in an adult Australian twin cohort. *The Australian and New Zealand Journal of Psychiatry, 40*(2), 121–128.

Walfish, S., Vance, D., & Fabricatore, A. N. (2007). Psychological evaluation of bariatric surgery applicants: Procedures and reasons for delay or denial of surgery. *Obesity Surgery, 17*(12), 1578–1583.

Walker, E. A., Gelfand, A., Katon, W. J., Koss, M. P., Von Korff, M., Bernstein, D., et al. (1999). Adult health status of women with histories of childhood abuse and neglect. *The American Journal of Medicine, 107*(4), 332–339.

Wang, Y., & Beydoun, M. A. (2007). The obesity epidemic in the United States – gender, age, socioeconomic, racial/ethnic, and geographic characteristics: A systematic review and meta-regression analysis. *Epidemiologic Reviews, 29*, 6–28.

Waring, M. E., & Lapane, K. L. (2008). Overweight in children and adolescents in relation to attention-deficit/hyperactivity disorder: Results from a national sample. *Pediatrics, 122*(1), e1–e6.

Watson, S., Gallagher, P., Ritchie, J. C., Ferrier, I. N., & Young, A. H. (2004). Hypothalamic-pituitary-adrenal axis function in patients with bipolar disorder. *The British Journal of Psychiatry, 184*, 496–502.

Weber-Hamann, B., Hentschel, F., Kniest, A., Deuschle, M., Colla, M., Lederbogen, F., et al. (2002). Hypercortisolemic depression is associated with increased intra-abdominal fat. *Psychosomatic Medicine, 64*(2), 274–277.

Weiden, P. J. (2007). Switching antipsychotics as a treatment strategy for antipsychotic-induced weight gain and dyslipidemia. *The Journal of Clinical Psychiatry, 68*(Suppl 4), 34–39.

Weiden, P. J., Simpson, G. M., Potkin, S. G., & O'Sullivan, R. L. (2003). Effectiveness of switching to ziprasidone for stable but symptomatic outpatients with schizophrenia. *The Journal of Clinical Psychiatry, 64*(5), 580–588.

Wender, P. H. (1998). Pharmacotherapy of attention-deficit/hyperactivity disorder in adults. *The Journal of Clinical Psychiatry, 59*(Suppl 7), 76–79.

Werrij, M. Q., Jansen, A., Mulkens, S., Elgersma, H. J., Ament, A. J., & Hospers, H. J. (2009). Adding cognitive therapy to dietetic treatment is associated with less relapse in obesity. *Journal of Psychosomatic Research, 67*(4), 315–324.

Wildes, J. E., Kalarchian, M. A., Marcus, M. D., Levine, M. D., & Courcoulas, A. P. (2008). Childhood maltreatment and psychiatric morbidity in bariatric surgery candidates. *Obesity Surgery, 18*(3), 306–313.

Wilens, T. E., Spencer, T. J., & Biederman, J. (2002). A review of the pharmacotherapy of adults with attention-deficit/hyperactivity disorder. *Journal of Attention Disorders, 5*(4), 189–202.

Wilfley, D. E., Friedman, M. A., Dounchis, J. Z., Stein, R. I., Welch, R. R., & Ball, S. A. (2000). Co-morbid psychopathology in binge eating disorder: Relation to eating disorder severity at baseline and following treatment. *Journal of Consulting and Clinical Psychology, 68*(4), 641–649.

Williamson, D. F., Thompson, T. J., Anda, R. F., Dietz, W. H., & Felitti, V. (2002). Body weight and obesity in adults and self-reported abuse in childhood. *International Journal of Obesity and Related Metabolic Disorders, 26*(8), 1075–1082.

Winstanley, C. A., Eagle, D. M., & Robbins, T. W. (2006). Behavioral models of impulsivity in relation to ADHD: Translation between clinical and preclinical studies. *Clinical Psychology Review, 26*(4), 379–395.

Womble, L. G., Wadden, T. A., McGuckin, B. G., Sargent, S. L., Rothman, R. A., & Krauthamer-Ewing, E. S. (2004). A randomized controlled trial of a commercial internet weight loss program. *Obesity Research, 12*(6), 1011–1018.

Wonderlich, S. A., Gordon, K. H., Mitchell, J. E., Crosby, R. D., & Engel, S. G. (2009). The validity and clinical utility of binge eating disorder. *The International Journal of Eating Disorders, 42*(8), 687–705.

Wonderlich-Tierney, A. L., & Vander Wal, J. S. (2010). The effects of social support and coping on the relationship between social anxiety and eating disorders. *Eating Behaviors, 11*(2), 85–91.

Yager, J. (2008). Binge eating disorder: The search for better treatments. *The American Journal of Psychiatry, 165*(1), 4–6.

Yanovski, S. Z., Nelson, J. E., Dubbert, B. K., & Spitzer, R. L. (1993). Association of binge eating disorder and psychiatric co-morbidity in obese subjects. *The American Journal of Psychiatry, 150*(10), 1472–1479.

Zellner, D. A., Loaiza, S., Gonzalez, Z., Pita, J., Morales, J., Pecora, D., et al. (2006). Food selection changes under stress. *Physiology and Behavior, 87*(4), 789–793.

Chapter 2
Psychological Issues in Adults with Type 2 Diabetes

Jeffrey S. Gonzalez, Sabrina A. Esbitt, Havah E. Schneider, Patricia J. Osborne, and Elyse G. Kupperman

2.1 Introduction

The global epidemic of type 2 diabetes is a major public health problem, with the world prevalence among adults estimated to be 6.4% for 2010. By 2030, it is expected that the burden of diabetes will affect more than 439 million adults worldwide or 7.7% of the global population. Over the next 20 years, the developed world will see an increase of 20% in the number of adults living with diabetes and developing countries will see an increase of 69% (Shaw, Sicree, & Zimmet, 2010). As the prevalence of diabetes rises, so too does the importance of improving the treatment outcomes and the prevention of complications among those affected.

In this chapter, we focus on type 2 diabetes mellitus (T2DM) in adult populations, although we occasionally draw on data from the literature on type 1 diabetes mellitus (T1DM) where literature is lacking for patients with T2DM. T2DM is the most common type of diabetes, accounting for approximately 90% of diabetes cases in the United States and is usually diagnosed in adulthood, although child and adolescent cases are becoming more common. While T1DM involves an absolute insulin deficiency caused by an autoimmune response that destroys pancreatic beta cells, resulting in a total insulin deficiency, T2DM involves a combination of insulin resistance and relative insulin deficiency (Fowler, 2007) and may not require treatment

J.S. Gonzalez (✉)
Clinical Psychology Ph.D. Program with Health Emphasis,
Ferkauf Graduate School of Psychology, 1300 Morris Park Avenue, Bronx, NY 10461, USA

Diabetes Research Center, Albert Einstein College of Medicine, Bronx, NY, USA
e-mail: jeffrey.gonzalez@einstein.yu.edu

S. Pagoto (ed.), *Psychological Co-morbidities of Physical Illness: A Behavioral Medicine Perspective*, DOI 10.1007/978-1-4419-0029-6_2,

with external insulin, especially at early stages. In either case, the goal of treatment of diabetes is to achieve strict control of blood sugar (glucose) levels. Obesity is associated with insulin resistance and this may be the reason that obesity is more common among patients with T2DM and is associated with worse diabetes control and treatment outcomes. As such, lifestyle factors related to diet and exercise are important in the management of glucose levels in T2DM in addition to treatment adherence to prescribed medications that act to lower blood sugar levels. The ability to successfully manage T2DM is largely dependent upon patient adherence to an intensive set of self-care behaviors (Anderson, 1995) involving adherence to prescribed medications, monitoring of blood glucose, adherence to dietary and physical activity recommendations, preventive foot care, attendance at medical appointments, and regular screening for complications. Self-care in diabetes is extremely important in the prevention of poor health outcomes. Adherence to treatment guidelines helps achieve good diabetes control, reduces cardiovascular risk, and decreases risk of complications and mortality (American Diabetes Association [ADA], 2009; Hartz et al., 2006; Ho et al., 2006). Self-care activities, such as increasing physical activity and maintaining healthy nutrition, can slow disease progression (Glasgow, Boles, McKay, Feil, & Barrera, 2003; Newman, Steed, & Mulligan, 2004; Norris, Engelgau, & Venkat Narayan, 2001). However, diabetes self-care places a significant burden of time and effort on patients; it has been estimated that approximately 2 h/day are required to meet the ADA-recommended guidelines for self-care for patients taking oral medications for diabetes (Russell, Suh, & Safford, 2005). A meta-analysis by DiMatteo, Lepper, and Croghan (2000) demonstrated that patients with diabetes, like patients with other chronic illnesses, exhibit suboptimal adherence to medical recommendations (Ingersoll & Cohen, 2008). Deficiencies in self-care often result from patients' inability to appreciate the long-term benefits of adherence, such as a reduction in the risk of diabetes-related complications and a tendency to focus on the short-term disadvantages of self-care activities, such as medication side effects and lifestyle disruption (Rubin, 2005). Nationally representative data show that less than half of patients with diabetes are able to meet goals for glycemic control, and when control of blood pressure and cholesterol is also taken into account, fewer than 10% of patients are achieving recommended levels of glycemic control and optimal control over cardiovascular disease risk factors as recommended by the ADA (Saydah, Fradkin, & Cowie, 2004).

We emphasize the importance of treatment adherence in determining the health outcomes of patients with T2DM and highlight the difficulties that many patients have in achieving diabetes treatment goals as a context in which to consider the role of psychopathology in patients with T2DM. Below we review: (1) the evidence for higher prevalence of various psychological problems in patients with diabetes as compared to the general population, (2) the association between various psychological problems and diabetes treatment outcomes, including an examination of potential mechanisms, and (3) assessment and treatment issues related to addressing these psychological problems and the impact they may have on diabetes outcomes. At the outset of this review, we would like to urge clinicians to bear in mind that the treatment of diabetes requires changes in health behavior and intensive self-management of treatment. These are difficult tasks for most patients with T2DM, and those who are suffering from psychological problems are likely to have even greater difficulty. Therefore, clinicians have an important opportunity to address health behavior and treatment adherence in their approaches to psychopathology in patients with diabetes. Such an approach may improve not only the psychological outcomes of treatment, but may also have a beneficial impact on health outcomes.

2.2 Depression

2.2.1 Epidemiology

Major depressive disorder (MDD) is a highly prevalent and serious illness, with lifetime prevalence of 17% and a point prevalence of 7% in the general US population (Kessler, Berglund, et al., 2005; Kessler, Chiu, Demler, & Walters, 2005). It is among the most serious health problems in the country, associated with substantial suffering, lost productivity, and loss of life (Klerman & Weissman, 1989, 1992; Stewart, Ricci, Chee, Hahn, & Morganstein, 2003). Individuals with MDD experience reduced functioning and decreased quality of life, as well as higher health care utilization and costs, and disability (Bijl & Ravelli, 2000; Eren, Erdi, & Mehmet, 2008; Katon et al., 2003; Katz, 1996; Pennix et al., 1998; Pennix, Leveille, Ferrucci, van Eijk, & Guralnik, 1999; Spitzer et al., 1995). Furthermore, depression is more prevalent in patients with chronic illness in general and diabetes in particular; meta-analyses of the available literature suggest that the point prevalence of depression in diabetes patients is nearly twice as high as the prevalence found in nondiabetic adults (Ali, Stone, Peters, Davies, & Khunti, 2006; Anderson, Freedland, & Clouse, 2001). Most of the studies included in these meta-analyses did not focus on the assessment of MDD, but rather on elevated symptoms of depression. Those studies that used structured diagnostic interviews tended to find somewhat lower prevalence rates (Ali et al.; Anderson et al.). A large scale, international, population-based survey of diabetes patients in 17 countries used a structured diagnostic interview to assess the presence of various mental disorders and found the overall odds of MDD to be 40% greater in participants with diabetes compared to those without diabetes. The overall odds of dysthymia were approximately 30% greater, but this difference did not reach statistical significance (Lin et al., 2008). Fisher et al. (2008) evaluated over 500 T2DM patients with a structured clinical interview and found prevalence rates of MDD and dysthymia to be 60% and 7% higher, respectively, relative to community adults assessed with the same diagnostic interview. The results reported by Fisher et al. also show that the prevalence of elevated depressive affect and distress was much higher than the prevalence of any mood disorder and these subclinical conditions tended to be more persistent over time.

Although aggregate studies tend to find that the point prevalence of clinically significant depression is twice as high in diabetes patients as in patients without diabetes, studies using the strongest methods of assessment suggest that the prevalence of MDD is more likely to be on the order of 40–60% more prevalent. Differences in prevalence rates for dysthymia, though less often evaluated, appear to be less significant. Meta-analyses of the literature have shown that depression is consistently associated with hyperglycemia (Lustman, Anderson, et al., 2000), risk of diabetes complications (de Groot, Anderson, Freedland, Clouse, & Lustman, 2001), and diabetes treatment nonadherence (Gonzalez, Peyrot, et al., 2008). Several studies have also linked depression to increased risk for mortality (Black, Markides, & Ray, 2003; Katon et al., 2005, 2008; Zhang et al., 2005). Importantly, subclinical symptoms of depression and distress tend to be very common in patients with diabetes, are persistent over time, and are more closely related to diabetes control than mood disorders per se (Fisher et al., 2008). Subclinical symptoms of depression are also associated with treatment nonadherence (Gonzalez et al., 2007) and risk of complications and mortality (Black et al., 2003) in patients with T2DM.

2.2.2 *Pathophysiology*

Diabetes and depression appear to have a consistent bidirectional relationship, with depression often preceding the development of T2DM in adults (Mezuk, Eaton, Albrecht, & Golden, 2008). If these relationships are causal, it is possible that depression and diabetes may be related through either biological or behavioral pathways. Biological pathways through which depression may impact diabetes and its complications include hormonal abnormalities, alterations in glucose transport function, and increased immuno-inflammatory activation (Golden, 2007; Musselman, Betan, Larsen, & Phillips, 2003). The available literature does not yet provide definitive answers about whether biological processes associated with depression may mediate the relationship between depression and diabetes outcomes or whether negative health behaviors associated with depression such as inactivity, poor diet, smoking, and nonadherence to treatment recommendations and self-care may be important explanatory factors. These same biobehavioral factors may be involved in explaining the risk of developing T2DM in depressed individuals. An additional important health behavior that may be implicated in the relationship between depression and diabetes is cigarette smoking; individuals with depression and other mood disorders smoke at higher rates than the general population (McClave et al., 2009; Mueser & McGurk, 2004; Spangler, Summerson, Bell, & Konen, 2001; Ziedonis, Williams, Smelson, 2003) and smoking is associated with insulin resistance, reduced insulin secretion responses, increased central adiposity, and the development of T2DM (ADA, 2004; Willi, Bodenmann, Ghali, Faris, & Cornuz, 2007). At this point, it is not clear whether the relationship between diabetes and depression is causal or whether the association may be explained by shared environmental and genetic factors, confounding between depression and severity of diabetes or other co-morbid illnesses, etc. Nevertheless, the consistency of the relationship between depression and worse diabetes treatment outcomes has led to an increased focus on improving the recognition and treatment of depression in patients with diabetes in the hopes that such treatment may also improve health outcomes of patients with T2DM.

2.2.3 *Clinical Care*

2.2.3.1 Assessment and Diagnostic Issues

Assessment of depression in diabetes patients can be challenging both to mental health professionals and medical staff. Confounding between physical symptoms known to be associated with diabetes and those that are part of the diagnostic criteria for MDD (e.g., concentration difficulties, appetite disturbance and weight changes, sleep disturbance, fatigue) complicates the diagnosis of MDD in patients with diabetes and may lead to mistakenly identifying diabetes-related symptoms as symptoms of depression. Various self-report measures have been used to assess depression in patients with diabetes including the Beck Depression Inventory (Beck, Steer, & Brown, 1996), the Centers for Epidemiologic Studies Depression Scale (CESD; Radloff, 1977), and the PHQ-9 (Kroenke, Spitzer, & Williams, 2001). While the potential for confounding between diabetes-related symptoms and scores on these scales has not often been examined, an early study did suggest that the BDI could effectively discriminate between diabetes patients with and without MDD, regardless of whether the total score, the somatic items, or the cognitive items were used (Lustman, Clouse, Griffith, & Carney, 1997). It is recommended that a careful assessment of depression in diabetes should include the use of a structured clinical interview as data have shown that approximately 70% of T2DM patients who score above the cutoff for clinically significant depression on the CESD do not meet criteria for MDD or dysthymia based on a structured clinical interview. Furthermore, 34% of those who met criteria based on a structured clinical interview did not reach the CESD cutoff (Fisher et al., 2007). It is important to note that even those patients who fall short of meeting criteria for a formal diagnosis of a mood disorder, but who nevertheless report significant symptoms of depression may be at elevated risk for worse diabetes outcomes (Black et al., 2003; Fisher et al., 2007; Gonzalez et al., 2007). Therefore, recognizing and providing treatment for subclinical presentations of depression is recommended.

An additionally important assessment issue is differentiating symptoms of depression that are directly associated with living with the burden of diabetes from those that may be more independent of diabetes. Fisher and colleagues have published several studies suggesting that diabetes-specific distress may be more closely related to problems with diabetes treatment adherence and worse diabetes control than distress assessed by generic depression instruments, such as the CESD (Fisher et al., 2007, 2008, 2010). Thus, measuring symptoms of distress that are specific reactions to living with diabetes may have clinical importance. Even general symptoms of depression are closely tied to aspects of living with diabetes. For example, patients on insulin therapy consistently report higher levels of depression than those who are not taking insulin (e.g., Gonzalez et al., 2007; Katon, Von Korff, et al., 2004). Two studies of patients with diabetic peripheral neuropathy have compellingly demonstrated how aspects of the illness itself, including objective indicators of neuropathy severity, symptoms such as unsteadiness and pain, limitations in activities of daily living, and changes in role functioning, are linked to generic symptoms of depression, both cross-sectionally and longitudinally (Vileikyte et al., 2005, 2009). These findings underscore the importance of a comprehensive assessment of depressive symptoms that carefully evaluates the relationship between these symptoms and important aspects of living with diabetes. The patient's perspective on these relationships may have implications for the selection of treatments that address the burden of diabetes vs. those that treat depression with less focus on the context of diabetes.

2.2.3.2 Evidence-Based Treatment

Various randomized trials of treatments for depression have been conducted in patients with diabetes (for a review see Markowitz, Gonzalez, Wilkinson, & Safren, 2011). These interventions have included cognitive-behavioral therapy (CBT) and a variety of other approaches and, while overall these interventions have shown promise in successfully reducing the severity of depression, results on glycemic control and treatment adherence have been much less promising. However, there is good reason to suspect that treating depression may be necessary, but not sufficient in order to improve diabetes outcomes for depressed diabetes patients. Meta-analyses of depression's relationship to hyperglycemia (Lustman, Anderson, et al., 2000), diabetes complications (de Groot et al., 2001), and diabetes treatment nonadherence (Gonzalez, Peyrot, et al., 2008) suggest that while the relationships between depression and these important diabetes outcomes are robust, they are also in the small to medium range. Thus, even if the relationships between depression and these outcomes are causal, amelioration of depression may result in only modest improvements in these diabetes-related outcomes. It is clear that treatment adherence and lifestyle modifications are perhaps the strongest determinants of diabetes treatment outcomes and interventions aimed at improving self-management of diabetes patients have consistent effects on glycemic control (Norris et al., 2004). Patients with diabetes and depression may need comprehensive treatment that targets adherence to this demanding regimen in addition to treatment for their depression. Intervention approaches that integrate adherence training and support for changing health behaviors with strategies aimed at treating depression may capitalize on the consistent relationship between depression and nonadherence and may result in greater improvements in diabetes control than interventions that focus on depression alone.

Safren and colleagues have developed a psychological treatment model for the integration of CBT with adherence counseling for patients with chronic illness, CBT for adherence and depression (CBT-AD; Safren, Gonzalez, & Soroudi, 2008a, 2008b; Soroudi et al., 2008). The integration of adherence training with cognitive-behavioral techniques in CBT-AD is based on the belief that the strategies employed in CBT for depression (e.g., activity scheduling and mood monitoring, cognitive restructuring) have important applications in facilitating successful treatment adherence in patients with chronic illness (e.g., increasing physical activity, monitoring behavior change, correcting maladaptive beliefs about the illness, and treatment). It is also based on the belief that there is often a bidirectional relationship between depression and the management of medical illness and interventions that improve patients' ability to successfully manage their illness that will result in an improved sense of self-efficacy and mastery, which will in turn improve patients' cognitions and underlying negative mood states. Each session of the treatment focuses on the difficulties that the patient is having with disease management, the symptoms of depression that the patient is experiencing, and how these two problems influence each other. The strategies employed are presented to the patient as equally applicable to the difficulties of illness management as to the symptoms of depression.

CBT-AD is an individually delivered program consisting of six modules addressing motivational enhancement and orientation to the program, adherence counseling, behavioral activation, cognitive restructuring, problem solving, and relaxation training. The sequencing of modules and the number of sessions spent on each module is flexible, though it is intended to take approximately 10–12 sessions in total. This approach has been shown to be successful in a recent two-arm randomized crossover trial comparing CBT-AD to enhanced usual care in 45 depressed individuals with HIV/AIDS. Results showed that those who received CBT-AD achieved significantly greater improvements in medication adherence and depression relative to the control group, with control participants who crossed-over to CBT-AD after the acute outcome assessment achieving similar improvements in both depression and adherence outcomes. Treatment gains for those in the intervention group were generally maintained at 6- and 12-month follow-up assessments (Safren et al., 2009).

CBT-AD is currently being evaluated in an ongoing randomized controlled trial in depressed patients with T2DM (NIH 1R01 MH078571). While outcome data are not yet available, data from an open phase pilot of five depressed T2DM patients have been completed (Gonzalez et al., 2010). This study provides preliminary evidence for a successful adaptation of CBT-AD, originally developed for patients with HIV, for patients with T2DM. CBT-AD appears to have been acceptable to all patients and successful in improving diabetes self-care and depression. All participants experienced an improvement in depressive symptoms and four of five patients demonstrated improvements in both depression and glycemic control. All participants reported improvement in self-reported glucose testing and all participants reported either a maintenance or improvement in self-reported medication adherence. These results are promising in suggesting that interventions that target both adherence and depression may maximize treatment benefits for diabetes patients.

Pharmacological interventions for depression have been recommended for patients with diabetes, both to reduce depression and improve glycemic control. Selective serotonin reuptake inhibitors (SSRIs) are the most commonly prescribed antidepressants because of their safety profile and their efficacy (MacGillivray et al., 2003; Sclar, Robinson, Skaer, & Galin, 1998). They have been recommended in depressed patients with diabetes, because they may lower glucose levels and result in weight loss in addition to their antidepressant properties (Goodnick, Henry, & Buki, 1995). Fluoxetine, for example, can improve glycemic control (Goodnick, 2001), but not all studies are supportive of this (Lustman, Freedland, et al., 2000). Bupropion, a norepinephrine/dopamine reuptake inhibitor, is as effective for in the treatment of depression as the SSRIs (Thase et al., 2005) and has shown favorable effects on weight in patients with obesity and depressive symptoms (Jain et al., 2002) and may improve glycemic control in patients with diabetes (Lustman, Williams, Sayuk, Nix, & Clouse, 2007). Other effective antidepressant medications, however, have been linked to side effects that are particularly undesirable in patients with diabetes. For example, monoamine oxidase inhibitors (MAOIs) can cause weight gain and tricyclic antidepressants (TCAs) can cause hyperglycemia, both of which can be problematic in individuals without diabetes but are especially counterproductive and even dangerous in patients with diabetes (Goodnick et al., 1995). Atypical antipsychotics, some of which are now approved for and have been shown to be effective in the treatment of depression (Philip, Carpenter, Tyrka, & Price, 2008), cannot only cause weight gain (Allison et al., 1999), but can worsen glycemic control in patients with diabetes and cause glycemic abnormalities (including the development of diabetes) in patients without a preexisting diagnosis (Haddad & Sharma, 2007).

2.2.3.3 Issues in Treatment Decision-Making

The current literature supports the utility for both psychosocial and pharmacological interventions for depression in patients with diabetes. Clinical intervention with depressed diabetes patients may be strengthened by an integrative approach that simultaneously treats depression and diabetes treatment nonadherence from a behavioral perspective. Accumulating evidence suggests that even subclinical presentations of depression and distress can be associated with worse treatment outcomes; therefore, approaches that target symptoms of depression that fall short of a formal diagnosis appear warranted. In these cases, it may be especially helpful to evaluate whether a conceptualization that considers these symptoms secondary to the burden of diabetes (e.g., diabetes distress) is clinically useful.

2.3 Anxiety Disorders

2.3.1 Epidemiology

Nationally representative surveys suggest that the prevalence of anxiety disorders may be as high as 18.1%, affecting approximately 40 million US adults (Kessler, Berglund, et al., 2005; Kessler, Chiu, et al., 2005). While there appears to be a higher prevalence of anxiety disorders in patients with diabetes than the general population, prevalence estimates are not well established and anxiety has received much less research attention than depression in diabetes patients. The available literature gives varying estimates, most probably due to differences in measurement methods and sampling. One large-scale study including more than 200,000 participants from the United States Behavioral Risk Factor Surveillance System assessed for lifetime prevalence of anxiety diagnosis by asking patients whether a healthcare provider had ever diagnosed them with an anxiety disorder. Results showed that the age-adjusted prevalence of lifetime diagnosis of anxiety was 19.5% in people with either type 1 or 2 diabetes and 10.9% in those without diabetes respectively. After adjustment for educational level, marital status, employment status, current smoking, leisure-time physical activity, and body mass index, people with diabetes still had a 20% higher prevalence of lifetime diagnosis of anxiety than those without (Li et al., 2008). While the measurement methods used to assess lifetime prevalence of anxiety disorders in this study were rather limited, similar estimates finding increased 12-month prevalence relative to those without diabetes were found using a structured clinical interview in a large community sample from 17 countries: patients with diabetes were 20% more likely to have an anxiety disorder in the last 12 months than those without diabetes (Lin et al., 2008).

Generalized Anxiety Disorder (GAD) appears to be the most common anxiety disorder in patients with diabetes with reviews suggesting point-prevalence rates between 13 and 14% (Grigsby, Anderson, Freedland, Clouse, & Lustman, 2002; Mitsonis, Dimopoulous, & Psarra, 2009). This is markedly higher than the 3% rate found in community studies (e.g., Kessler, Chiu, et al., 2005). Grigsby et al. (2002) also found that the prevalence of specific phobia was substantially higher than the rates found in community samples – 21.6% vs. 8.7%, but this estimate was based on only two studies. Reviews suggest that the rates of other anxiety disorders in patients with diabetes are comparable to those found in the general population, though few studies are available (Grigsby et al., 2002; Mitsonis et al., 2009). However, some recent studies report significantly elevated rates of other anxiety disorders. For example, Lin et al. (2008), using a structured clinical interview in a large sample, showed that patients with diabetes are 50% more likely to have Panic Disorder and 30% more likely to have Post-Traumatic Stress Disorder (PTSD) or Social Phobia than those without the disease. Fisher et al. (2008) found 85% higher rates of Panic Disorder and 123% higher rates of GAD relative to national estimates, using structured clinical interviews (Fisher et al.).

Research also suggests elevated prevalence of symptoms of anxiety. For example, Friedman, Vila, Timsit, Boitard, and Mouren-Simeoni (1998) reported that 48.6% of its sample of 69 outpatients had anxiety symptoms, and that two thirds had at least one episode of anxiety (Friedman et al.). Another study of 1,458 attendees of a diabetes education program determined that 49% of its sample reported anxiety symptoms (Peyrot & Rubin, 1997). Finally, two recent reviews, which included studies that used mixed type 1 and 2 diabetes samples, found elevated rates of anxiety symptoms in 40–42% of patients (Grigsby et al., 2002; Mitsonis et al., 2009). This increased prevalence may be related to fears of self-injecting or self-testing. One study found that approximately 9% of insulin-treated diabetes patients reported self-injecting-related anxiety symptoms (Mollema, Snoek, Heine, & van der Ploeg, 2001). Another study of 115 type 1 and 2 patients found that 28% of its sample reported elevated injection anxiety scores on a self-report questionnaire. In addition, 14% avoided injections because of anxiety (Zambanini, Newson, Maisey, & Feher, 1999). Thus, specific features of diabetes treatment and self-management may be associated with increased symptoms of anxiety.

While exact prevalence is unknown, fear of hypoglycemia, or low blood sugars, is another common fear in patients taking insulin (Polonsky, Davis, Jacobson, & Anderson, 1992; Pramming, Thorsteinsson, Bendtson, & Binder, 1991; Weinger & Lee, 2006). Hypoglycemia is often associated with unpleasant symptoms, such as tremors, profuse sweating, cognitive dysfunction, and irritability. If blood glucose drops to dangerously low levels, loss of consciousness, seizures, and death can occur. Patients sometimes try to avoid hypoglycemia at all costs and may prefer to keep blood glucose at high levels to avoid the risk of low blood sugars (Weinger & Lee). Fear of hypoglycemia is especially prevalent in patients with past hypoglycemic experiences (Green, Feher, & Catalan, 2000; Polonsky, 2002; Weinger & Lee, 2006) and can reach levels of intensity that have led some investigators to draw parallels to PTSD. For example, one study found that 25% of its sample of T1DM patients met criteria for PTSD related to hypoglycemia because of avoidance and intrusive thoughts related to hypoglycemia (Myers, Boyer, Herbert, Barakat, & Scheiner, 2007). Patients may also present with subclinical symptoms of anxiety related to hypoglycemia that may not represent disorder, but may still negatively impact diabetes self-management (Myers et al.; Wild et al., 2007).

There is also evidence to suggest that anxiety is associated with problems with disease management, worse clinical outcomes, and decreased functioning and quality of life, even at subclinical levels. For example, a meta-analysis of 11 studies showed a nonsignificant trend for an overall relationship between anxiety and hyperglycemia. When the analysis was limited to studies that used diagnostic interviews for anxiety, the effect size between anxiety and hyperglycemia was in the medium range and significant (Anderson et al., 2002). Panic episodes have been associated with worse diabetes control, increased diabetic complications and symptoms, greater disability, and lower self-rated health and functioning in a sample of over 4,000 patients with diabetes, even after controlling for the effects of co-morbid depression (Ludman et al., 2006). Diabetes-specific manifestations of anxiety may also be associated with worse outcomes. For example, insulin-treated adult diabetes patients with severe fear of self-injecting or self-testing had higher levels of diabetes-related distress, poorer general well-being, and poorer treatment adherence than those who did not have such fears (Mollema, Snoek, Ader, Heine, & van der Ploeg, 2001).

2.3.2 *Pathophysiology*

The development of anxiety symptoms in patients with diabetes may arise from a number of underlying causes. While research on the biobehavioral mechanisms between anxiety and diabetes is generally lacking, plausible mechanisms linking anxiety and diabetes include reactions to the stress associated with the self-management of diabetes and underlying biological changes that may be associated with both anxiety and glycemic control.

Diabetes-related stress, including feeling overwhelmed by diabetes and its care, feeling discouraged with the treatment plan, and feeling fearful of the future, may contribute to symptoms of anxiety (Weinger & Lee, 2006). The stress of dealing with diabetes may impact patients' psychosocial functioning and quality of life, which may also increase the risk for developing anxiety symptoms (Weinger & Jacobson, 2001). Certain aspects of the diabetes self-care regimen, such as frequent self-testing of blood glucose and insulin injections, may also lead to the development or exacerbation of anxiety symptoms, such as phobias, intrusive worry, and avoidance (Green et al., 2000; Mollema, Snoek, Ader, et al., 2001; Mollema, Snoek, Heine, & van der Ploeg, 2001; Polonsky et al., 1992; Pramming et al., 1991; Zambanini et al., 1999). For example, the anticipation before or avoidance of activities such as self-testing may contribute to problematic anxiety, panic disorder, or GAD. Diabetes patients may experience short-term, episodic stress related to self-care activities, or more long-term, chronic stress related to living with a chronic illness, which may eventually develop into anxiety symptoms or a chronic anxiety disorder (Petrak et al., 2005).

Further, patients may develop anxiety symptoms due to fears of hypoglycemia, complications, or mortality. Some patients may be able to better manage diabetes-related stress or general life stress than others, based on their coping skills: use of maladaptive coping could increase the risk for anxiety in patients with diabetes (Sultan, Epel, Sachon, Vaillant, & Hartemann-Heurtier, 2008; Tuncay, Musabak, Gok, & Kutlu, 2008; Weinger & Lee, 2006). Studies suggest that patients who use a variety of coping mechanisms, including both task-based coping and emotion-based coping, have better emotion regulation and diabetes control (Sultan et al., 2008). Conversely, emotion-based coping, such as anxious and angry styles, is associated with poor glycemic control (Peyrot, McMurry, & Kruger, 1999; Yi, Yi, Vitaliano, & Weinger, 2008). Patients who experience diabetes-related stress may become entrenched in a vicious cycle – anxiety and avoidance related to their self-care may cause them to be less adherent to their treatment regimen, which may in turn affect their blood glucose control or cause complications – thus leading to even greater levels of anxiety. Finally, psychiatric illness such as anxiety disorders often co-occurs with tobacco and other substance use, highlighting a potential pathway between anxiety and worse diabetes outcomes (Spangler et al., 2001).

Physiological mechanisms are also plausible in explaining the link between diabetes and anxiety and the principal candidate is overactivation of the hypothalamic-pituitary-adrenal (HPA) axis and sympathetic nervous system. Models that have been proposed to account for neuroendocrine pathways between depression and diabetes also have relevance for anxiety (Golden, 2007). Studies have suggested that co-morbid anxiety may play an important role in the HPA-axis dysregulation seen in patients with depression (Young, Abelson, & Cameron, 2004). Elevated cortisol has been shown to inhibit insulin function (Ehlert, Gaab, & Heinrichs, 2001) and cortisol levels appear to be dysregulated in patients with anxiety disorders (e.g., Chaudieu et al., 2008).

As with depression, there is little understanding of these mechanisms and questions remain as to the directionality and causal nature of the relationships between anxiety and diabetes. However, as anxiety seems to be a risk factor for potential problems with diabetes management and worse treatment outcomes, clinical intervention has the potential to result in mental and physical health benefits for patients.

2.3.3 Clinical Care

2.3.3.1 Assessment and Diagnostic Issues

Proper identification and diagnosis of anxiety is necessary so that appropriate treatments may be implemented, but the task of accurate assessment of problems with anxiety is complicated by the context of diabetes. Problems with anxiety may be undertreated or misdiagnosed because they may resemble physiologic changes associated with hypoglycemic episodes, for example (Boyle, Allan, & Millar, 2004; Jacobson, 1996; Polonsky et al., 1992). Both patients and clinicians may have difficulty distinguishing between hypoglycemia and anxiety symptoms such as dizziness, shakiness, lack of coordination, and heart palpitations. Other physiological explanations for anxiety, such as a thyroid disorder, should be ruled out and consultation with the patient's healthcare provider(s) should be sought (Aina & Susman, 2006). If physical symptoms are present, providers should be sure to ask about behavioral and emotional issues, as these should distinguish diabetes-related physical symptoms from an anxiety disorder (Jacobson, 1996). In addition, anxiety disorders often co-occur with other psychiatric disorders – the co-morbidity between anxiety and depression, for example, appears to be higher in people with diabetes than in the general population (Fisher et al., 2008).

Given the potential difficulty in assessing anxiety in patients with diabetes, several assessment tools should be used, including structured clinical interviews, diabetes-specific anxiety measures, as well as the patient's self-report, to make an accurate diagnosis. It is important to note that anxiety poses a significant risk for suicide and co-morbid anxiety and depression is associated with an even greater risk (Keller & Hanks, 1995; Kessler, Borges, & Walters, 1999). For example, panic disorder is associated with a 7% risk of suicide in the general population, but if co-morbid depression exists, this risk increases to 23.6%. Likewise, MDD without anxiety was associated with a 7.9% risk of suicide, but when co-morbid anxiety was present, this risk increased to 19.8% (Keller & Hanks, 1995).

A number of formal screening tools may have utility in working with diabetes patients. These include the Hospital Anxiety and Depression Scale (HADS; Zigmond & Snaith, 1983) and Generalized Anxiety Disorder (GAD-7) Scale (Spitzer, Kroenke, Williams, & Lowe, 2006). Given the relatively high rates of anxiety disorders in patients with diabetes, formal evaluation using structured clinical interviews may be warranted for those patients who report symptoms of anxiety. The focus on psychopathology should be supplemented with an assessment of diabetes-specific distress and screening for fears related to hypoglycemia, self-monitoring of blood glucose, and self-injection with insulin. Standardized scales may facilitate this diabetes-focused assessment, including the Diabetes Distress Scale (Polonsky et al., 2005), the Diabetes Quality of Life questionnaire (Burroughs, Desikan, Waterman, Gilin, & McGill, 2004), the Hypoglycemia Fear Survey (Cox, Irvine, Gonder-Frederick, Nowacek, & Butterfield, 1987), and the Diabetes Fear of Injection and Self-Testing Questionnaire (Snoek, Mollema, Heine, Bouter, & van der Ploeg, 1997). It is also recommended to assess the frequency of patients' self-monitoring blood glucose levels and adherence to insulin regimens, if prescribed, as well as any barriers to adherence. Consultation with diabetes care providers is important in order to identify problems with treatment adherence.

2.3.3.2 Evidence-Based Treatment

A meta-analysis of the literature on psychological interventions in patients with T2DM suggests that a variety of psychological interventions have been utilized, and overall, these interventions have been effective in reducing symptoms of psychological distress and in improving glycemic control (Ismail, Winkley, & Rabe-Hesketh, 2004). While this overall evaluation is promising, important questions as to which approaches are likely to be most effective remain unanswered. We review a variety of approaches below, but note that the empirical literature provides little guidance at this time as to which approaches are likely to be most effective with which patient presentations.

Education programs such as those focused on self-care or living with a diabetes diagnosis may reduce the risk for anxiety symptoms or help to alleviate existing symptoms. Group education programs including a coping skills component have been shown to be useful in reducing stress and improving both coping skills and diabetes control (Grey, Boland, Davidson, Li, & Tamborlane, 2000; Karlsen, Idsoe, Dirdal, Hanestad, & Bru, 2004; Rubin, Peyrot, & Saudek, 1993).

A recent review of ten studies evaluating the efficacy of stress management interventions in adults with diabetes suggests that, overall, these approaches may not only be helpful in reducing stress, anxiety, and related negative emotions, but may also be effective in improving glycemic control (Soo & Lam, 2009). While results across studies were variable, several studies showed promise in improving diabetes control. For example, T2DM patients who completed a program consisting of five group-based sessions involving training in progressive muscle relaxation, guided imagery, and instruction in behavioral and cognitive skills to recognize and reduce stress showed improvement in glycemic control over 12 months, relative to control patients. Surprisingly, no differences in stress or anxiety were observed (Surwit et al., 2002). Individually delivered, biofeedback-assisted relaxation training was found to reduce symptoms of anxiety and depression, muscle tension, and improve diabetes control in a small trial of 30 patients with diabetes with T2DM (McGinnis, McGrady, Cox, & Grower-Dowling, 2005). Henry, Wilson, Bruce, Chisholm, and Rawling (1997) tested a group-based 6-session program including relaxation training, cognitive restructuring, and training in problem-solving skills and found improvements in anxiety symptoms, stress, and some evidence of a small effect on diabetic control in a small sample of 19 adults with T2DM (Henry et al.). There is also early evidence that mindfulness-based stress management may be successfully applied in patients with T2DM (Whitebird, Kreitzer, & O'Connor, 2009). The one trial of mindfulness-based stress management conducted to date involved an uncontrolled pilot study of 14 patients with T2DM and found improvements in diabetes control, decreased symptoms of depression, anxiety, and general psychological distress after completion of a mindfulness program (Rosenzweig, Reibel, Greeson, Jasser, & McMearty, 2007).

Given the association between hypoglycemia, self-injecting, and anxiety symptoms, providers may need to focus on self-monitoring and self-injecting routines with patients on insulin. Cognitive distortions regarding self-monitoring of blood glucose or injections, avoidance of these behaviors, and associated feelings of worry and fear may be effectively addressed using a cognitive-behavioral approach. This could involve challenging maladaptive and inaccurate beliefs through the provision of education and cognitive restructuring and addressing behavioral avoidance through exposure, self-monitoring, and other in-session and at home "behavioral experiments" to improve patient adherence to the self-care regimen while at the same time reducing avoidance and anxiety. Clinicians should collaboratively review blood glucose records with patients at each clinic visit, in order to determine patterns of how eating and physical activity are related to blood glucose levels. They may also wish to discuss physical symptoms and glycemic control in order to help the patient better recognize how physical symptoms are related to high or low blood glucose levels. Clinicians should also be prepared to evaluate whether patients are becoming maladaptively focused or obsessive about glucose monitoring as too great of an emphasis on blood glucose monitoring has actually been linked with increased anxiety (O'Kane, Bunting, Copeland, & Coates, 2008). In this work, it is crucial to consult with the patient's diabetes care provider(s) to become thoroughly familiar with the patient's individual self-management plan and the rationale for the frequency of monitoring of blood glucose.

The relationship between patients and their social support system (including their healthcare team) may also play a role in the prevention or amelioration of anxiety symptoms (Harris & Lustman, 1998; Jacobson, 1996; Weinger, 2007; Weinger & Lee, 2006). Patient satisfaction with the support obtained from family members, and the patients' relationships with their treatment providers, should be evaluated and strategies for strengthening these relationships should be applied. These may include role-plays to assist the patient in rehearsing questions for their care providers, assertiveness training, and psychoeducation about effective communication. Group-based patient groups may be available to the patient at local diabetes treatment centers and the clinician should explore these options for augmenting treatment.

Regarding specific psychotherapy approaches to anxiety disorders in the context of diabetes, very little is known. Case reports have suggested possible efficacy of cognitive-behavioral interventions for anxiety disorders such as specific phobias relating to hypoglycemia and panic disorders in patients with diabetes (Boyle et al., 2004; Green et al., 2000), but randomized clinical trials are lacking. Boyle et al. (2004), found that an intervention consisting of behavioral experiments, reduction of safety behaviors, and reframing of maladaptive/irrational thoughts and beliefs led to reductions in both a fear of hypoglycemia and panic attacks in a 37-year-old woman with a diabetes-related anxiety disorder. Green et al. (2000) described the treatment of an adult male with T1DM who had poor diabetes control due to an excessive fear of hypoglycemia and who was diagnosed with agoraphobia and panic disorder. He also developed increasing fears of diabetes complications and death as his diabetes control deteriorated and these fears often led to anxious rumination at night and difficulty sleeping. Treatment consisted of graded exposure exercises, self-monitoring of episodes of hypoglycemia and panic, instruction in the use of relaxation techniques, and cognitive restructuring. The authors do not report the length of treatment, but did report that the patient became able to cope with feared situations, became less fearful of hypoglycemia and was better able to differentiate these episodes from panic attacks, became less anxious, and achieved improved glycemic control. After treatment, he no longer exhibited avoidance behaviors related to fear of hypoglycemia (Green et al.).

As with psychotherapy interventions, we are unaware of any randomized trial testing the efficacy of pharmacological agents in treating anxiety disorders in patients with diabetes. However, fludiazepam was shown to be successful in reducing anxiety symptoms and improving lipid profiles in 20 patients with T2DM (Okada et al., 1994). One randomized trial reported an evaluation of alprazolam and found a benefit in glycemic control in poorly controlled patients with diabetes, but relatively few participants had an anxiety disorder and no treatment effects were found on symptoms of anxiety (Lustman et al. 1995). It should be noted that patients with diabetes should be closely monitored on psychotropic medications that may cause weight gain as this may complicate their diabetes control and increase their risks for complications. Also, beta-blockers are useful to reduce some symptoms of anxiety, but should be used with great caution in patients on insulin because they block the adrenergic symptoms of hypoglycemia (Jacobson, 1996).

2.3.3.3 Issues in Treatment Decision-Making

Patients with T2DM may present with a variety of problems related to anxiety and each presentation may require a distinct treatment approach. Subclinical symptoms may need to be treated differently than formal disorders, co-morbid anxiety and depression may need to be treated differently than anxiety alone, and patients for whom problems with anxiety are secondary to problems with diabetes may need interventions that focus on diabetes self-management with an interdisciplinary approach, including collaboration with diabetes educators, dietitians, and physicians providing diabetes care. A careful comprehensive assessment and case conceptualization that addresses the interplay between anxiety, diabetes, and other psychological or physical co-morbidities is an essential first part of treatment. Based on this initial conceptualization, clinicians can choose a tailored set of treatment elements from a variety of interventions that may be effective, including educational, behavioral, supportive, psychotherapeutic, and psychopharmacological approaches. Although there is little information available regarding treatment sequencing and appropriate blending of therapeutic approaches, we emphasize that treatments that target problems with anxiety and problems with diabetes self-management are likely to have a greater impact than those that target these problems in isolation.

2.4 Eating Disorders

2.4.1 Epidemiology

Disordered patterns of eating appear to be more prevalent in individuals with diabetes than nondiabetic individuals but it should be noted that few investigations have been conducted and most have been based on either small or nonrepresentative samples, or both. Therefore, statements about prevalence must be made with caution. Most of the literature has focused on the co-morbidity in adolescent female populations with T1DM (Papelbaum et al., 2005); we extrapolate from this literature when appropriate.

Data from the National Co-morbidity Survey Replication (NCS-R) suggest the prevalence of binge-eating disorder (BED) is 2.0% in the national population (Hudson, Hiripi, Pope, & Kessler, 2007). One study of 3,000 primary care patients from family practice and internal medicine clinics found that individuals with diabetes were 2.4 times more likely to have either bulimia nervosa or BED than those without diabetes. Post-hoc analyses revealed that diabetes was associated with significantly increased odds of BED, but the relationship to bulimia nervosa was not significant. No other medical illness was associated with increased risk of these eating disorders, but the overall prevalence of these disorders was high (7%) in this primary care sample (Goodwin, Hoven, & Spitzer, 2003). Other estimates on the prevalence of BED in patients with T2DM vary considerably. In a small convenience sample ($n=43$) of adult T2DM patients, the prevalence of BED was 25.6% based on the Structured Clinical Interview for the DSM-IV (Crow, Kendall, Praus, & Thuras, 2001). A Brazilian study examining prevalence of eating disorders using structured clinical interviews in a sample ($n=70$) of adult T2DM patients found that 10% had BED (Papelbaum et al., 2005). Other studies found low rates of prevalence. One study of overweight patients with T2DM found that the prevalence of BED in females ($n=80$) was 2.5%, and that no men ($n=76$) met criteria for BED. This study also compared the prevalence of BED in the diabetes sample to that of a sample of patients without diabetes. The prevalence of BED was also no different between the two samples (Mannucci et al., 2002). A study of 215 women found no difference in bingeing between T2DM patients and controls. However, a nonsignificant trend towards more bingeing in the diabetes group was found (Carroll, Tiggemann, & Wade, 1999). Similarly, in a study of 845 older adult T2DM patients, the prevalence of BED was only 1.4% (Allison et al., 2007). Although another study found that BED was the most diagnosed eating disorder in overweight and obese sample of people with diabetes, the prevalence rates were still relatively low. The lifetime prevalence of BED in the female sample ($n=168$) was 7.1% and 4.5% in the male sample ($n=154$; Herpertz, Albus, et al., 1998). In a study of more than 5,000 overweight and obese T2DM middle-aged and older patients, 11.7% reported at least one bingeing episode, as assessed by self-report questionnaire. These patients were younger and more likely to be female, white, and college-educated than their nonbinge-eating counterparts. However, only 123 (2.6%) met diagnostic criteria for BED (Gorin et al., 2008). One study of female T2DM patients found that 21% reported engaging in binge eating at least weekly, but did not assess BED, per se (Kenardy, Mensch, Bowen, Green, & Walton, 2002). In contrast, another study of 125 women with T2DM found that bingeing was endorsed by 9.4% of patients (Carroll et al., 1999). Finally, a French study of adult T2DM patients ($n=51$) found that 27% of men and 11% of women exhibited binge eating or overeating (Ryan, Gallanagh, Livingstone, Gaillard, & Ritz, 2008). Due to the small sample sizes of most studies and the variability of methods used to assess binge eating, questions remain about the heterogeneity and generalizability of these estimates.

Data from the NCS-R suggest the prevalence of anorexia to be 0.6% in the US population (Hudson et al., 2007) and the presence of anorexia nervosa in adults with T2DM appears to be minimal (Herpertz, Albus, et al., 1998). Prevalence estimates for bulimia in type 2 patients also appear to be similar to those in the national population. In the NCS-R sample, lifetime bulimia prevalence is 1.1% (Hudson et al., 2007), and reports have found similar prevalence estimates in people with T2DM (Herpertz, Albus, et al., 1998). However, the prevalence of these disorders is especially understudied.

Insulin omission is designated as "misuse of medications for weight loss" in the DSM-IV and, depending on the severity, may qualify as eating disorder-NOS (American Psychiatric Association [APA], 2000). Omitting or reducing insulin to induce glycosuria, where glucose is excreted through the urine causing weight loss, is a form of calorie purging and has significant health consequences for diabetes patients. A study of 8,484 adult T2DM patients on insulin found that nearly 25% of patients exhibited insulin nonadherence based on outpatient pharmacy refill data (Cramer & Pugh, 2005). While relatively little attention has been paid to reasons for intentional insulin nonadherence, concerns about weight gain represent one possible factor associated with nonadherence. For example, in a sample of 100 adults with T2DM, 22% reported that they feared that taking insulin would cause weight gain and would therefore be unwilling to take insulin (Larkin et al., 2008). Insulin omission also appears to be more common among patients with eating disorders than those without, based on research in T1DM adolescent females (Nielsen, Emborg, & Molbak, 2002; Takii et al, 2008).

Another eating disorder prevalent among people with diabetes is Night-Eating Syndrome, which is characterized by greater than 25% of caloric intake occurring after the evening meal, and/or waking up at least 3 times/week to eat at night (Schenck, 2006). In a study of 714 type 1 and type 2 patients, Morse, Ciechanowski, Katon, and Hirsch (2006) found that 9.7% reported night-eating behaviors and these patients were more likely to be less adherent with diet, exercise, and glucose monitoring. They were also more likely to be obese, to have worse diabetes control, and to have more diabetes complications than patients without night-eating behaviors (Morse et al.).

Negative health outcomes also appear to be associated with other types of eating disorders and related problems in patients with diabetes. For example, studies show that patients who restrict their insulin have poorer metabolic control (Battaglia, Alemzadeh, Katte, Hall, & Perlmuter, 2006; Daneman et al., 2002) and higher rates of nephropathy (Crow, Keel, & Kendall, 1998; Kelly, Howe, Hendler, & Lipman, 2005; Takii et al., 2008). Furthermore, retinopathy (Crow et al., 1998; Daneman et al., 2002; Kelly et al., 2005; Takii et al., 2008), diabetic ketoacidosis (DKA) (Kelly et al., 2005) and other microvascular complications (Kelly et al.; Peveler et al., 2005; Takii et al., 2008) are more prevalent and more severe in people who deliberately restrict their insulin intake. Moreover, insulin omission was shown to increase the relative risk of mortality by 3.2-times in a study of 234 adult women with T1DM. Women who restricted their insulin use were also more likely to die younger than women who did not and were more likely to experience nephropathy and foot problems over the follow-up (Goebel-Fabbri et al., 2008). The relationship between BED and worse diabetes outcomes is less clear. Crow et al. (2001) found that BED was not related to poor diabetes outcome, but Carroll et al. (1999) found BED to be a significant predictor of poor glucose control. Further research may be needed given the few studies examining the effects of BED in diabetes.

Subthreshold variants of eating disorders, such as occasional binge-eating episodes, engaging in extreme dietary restraint or excessive exercise, and when self-evaluation is greatly influenced by shape and weight, appear to be more common in people with diabetes than people without (Colton, Olmsted, Daneman, Rydall, & Rodin, 2004). They are also associated with poorer glycemic control (Mannucci et al., 2002; Peveler et al., 2005) and higher rates of retinopathy and nephropathy (Cantwell & Steel, 1996; Rydall, Rodin, Olmsted, & Devenyi, 1997) as compared to individuals with diabetes who exhibit normal eating behavior. In addition, maladaptive eating attitudes, such as excessive concern with eating, weight, and body shape, have also been shown to significantly correlate with poorer glycemic control (Mannucci et al., 2002). These studies suggest that diabetes control can be affected by poor body image issues and eating behaviors, even in patients without a diagnosable eating disorder.

2.4.2 Pathophysiology

There are various possible explanations for the relationship between eating disorders and diabetes. Several studies have shown that family dysfunction predicts the development of maladaptive eating behaviors in females with and without T1DM (Neumark-Sztainer et al., 2002; Rodin et al., 2002). One study of adolescent females with T1DM studied the relationship between family dysfunction and maladaptive eating behaviors in diabetes. Family dysfunction, as defined by negative familial communication regarding weight and shape, was related to maladaptive eating attitudes and behaviors. Notably, this relationship was moderated by body image dissatisfaction (Kichler, Foster, & Opipari Arrigan, 2008). Moreover, in a review of the relevant literature, Daneman et al. (2002) found that eating disturbances were associated with self-reported family functioning, and more severe eating problems were linked to greater levels of family dysfunction in girls with T1DM. Those with eating disturbances reported significantly poorer relationships and that their parents were not responsive to their needs, leading to greater feelings of anger and hopelessness toward their parents. Additionally, they found that family environment and maternal weight and shape concerns were interrelated with eating disturbances in young women with T1DM. Daneman et al. postulate that individual, family, and societal factors interact with diabetes-specific vulnerabilities and lead to core features of eating disorders, such as body dissatisfaction, drive for thinness, and dietary restraint. These features then lead to disordered eating behaviors, resulting in diabetes-specific outcomes (such as hyperglycemia and complications). The extent to which these etiological factors may be relevant for adults with T2DM is not clear, but Ismail (2008) suggests a theoretical model of potential pathways between disordered eating behaviors and T2DM. She postulates that cultural factors (such as beliefs about diabetes, insulin, and body image) and vulnerability factors (such as social adversity) may lead to overeating and obesity, which is a risk factor for developing diabetes. Overweight people with diabetes often suffer from depression, which is associated with poor diabetes self-care, further increasing the risk of sub-optimal diabetes control.

Furthermore, various aspects of diabetes and its treatment may increase the risk of eating disorders, such as dietary restraint and a focus on portion control, calorie monitoring, and carbohydrate counting (Papelbaum et al., 2005; Rodin & Daneman, 1992). Chronic dieting, rigid restraint of eating, and perceptions of "forbidden foods" may also contribute to the development of eating disorders (Polivy & Herman, 1985). Other maladaptive behaviors, such as vomiting, using laxatives, or omitting insulin, also have important clinical implications (Rodin, Craven,

Littlefield, & Murray, 1991; Rydall et al., 1997; Steel, Young, Lloyd, & Clarke, 1987) and may compromise adherence to treatment, self-management, and result in worse treatment outcomes.

2.4.3 *Clinical Care*

2.4.3.1 Assessment

Diabetes management often includes careful focus on the quality and quantity of food eaten. This may complicate the evaluation of abnormal behaviors and concerns used to diagnose eating disorders (Rubin & Peyrot, 2001). Possible diabetes-related clues to underlying eating disorder include unexplained episodes of DKA (when there is no glucose for the body to use as energy so it begins to break down fat and muscle, changing the body's chemical balance, which has potentially life-threatening consequences), frequent episodes of hypoglycemia, or easy control in inpatient settings of blood glucose levels that were previously difficult to manage in outpatient settings (Tierney, Deaton, & Whitehead, 2009). Additionally, clinicians should note when patients frequently request changing meal plans to accommodate low-fat, low-carbohydrate, or other diets, refuse to be weighed at clinic visits, exhibit anxiety upon being weighed, or frequently complain about their body weight or shape. These behaviors may have important implications in the context of diabetes management.

There are a variety of tools to assess for eating disorders in the general population. Several generic tools for the assessment of eating disorders have been modified for specific use in people with diabetes (Neumark-Sztainer et al., 2002). The Eating Disorder Examination (EDE) is a standardized interview, designed to measure the current level of eating disorder psychopathology (Cooper & Fairburn, 1987). It is commonly used to assess eating disorders in populations with diabetes (Allison et al., 2007; Gorin et al., 2008; Kenardy et al., 2002; Mannucci et al., 2002) and is the gold standard for assessing binge eating (Fairburn & Beglin, 1994; Grilo, Masheb, & Wilson, 2001). Another screening tool commonly used in populations with diabetes is the Eating Attitudes Test (EAT). The EAT is a 40-question measure of eating attitudes and is predictive of disordered eating behaviors (Garner & Garfinkel, 1979). A shortened form of the EAT-40, the EAT-26, is often used because it minimizes responder burden and is still has high validity and reliability (Berland, Thompson, & Linton, 1986). The Eating Disorder Inventory (Garner, Olmsted, & Polivy, 1983) is a 64-item self-report questionnaire that assesses psychological and behavioral traits common in anorexia and bulimia and has been used in patients with diabetes (Herpertz, Wagener, et al., 1998; Kenardy et al., 2002).

Assessment of insulin misuse and nonadherence is also important for T2DM patients treated with insulin. Some indicators of insulin misuse may include poor metabolic control in spite of adequate diet and insulin regimen or episodes of DKA. Clinically, it would be important to assess patient concerns about insulin and the associated risk of weight gain, especially in cases where the patient reports less than optimal adherence to the insulin regimen. Such an assessment should include evaluation of frequency of missed or skipped doses, modifying doses to take fewer units than recommended by the patient's physician, and patient reported reasons for omission or nonadherence. Specific probing for concerns about weight gain may be clinically useful, especially in the context of already reported concern about body weight or shape or other maladaptive attitudes toward eating. Patients who are not taking insulin and have resisted the prescription of insulin by a provider should also be interviewed about their perceptions regarding the negative consequences of insulin, as fears of weight gain have been shown to be a possible reason for resistance to insulin therapy (Larkin et al., 2008). In each of these cases, consultation with the patient's diabetes care provider(s) would be important.

2.4.3.2 Evidence-Based Treatment

It has been suggested that eating disorders in women with diabetes may be more difficult to treat than in those without diabetes but this view is speculative and based on select cases reported in the literature (Daneman et al., 2002). Although many studies have investigated the efficacy of weight-loss programs in people with T2DM, few interventions for treating eating disorders in people with diabetes have been investigated (Snoek & Skinner, 2002). Additionally, of the limited published psychotherapy intervention studies addressing disordered eating in patients with diabetes, most lack methodological rigor (Rubin & Peyrot, 2001).

One study investigated the efficacy of CBT and nonprescriptive therapy (NPT), a treatment designed to have no theoretical or empirical support in eating disorders, as interventions for binge eating in patients with diabetes. The study was a 10-week randomized control trial of 24 women with T2DM and BED. Assessments were done at posttreatment and at 6-month follow-up. CBT and NPT both appeared to effective treatments, though CBT appeared to provide more sustained change, as there were significantly fewer relapses in CBT condition. Across treatments, decreases in bingeing were associated with improved diabetes control (Kenardy et al., 2002). While this investigation shows promise for the successful treatment of BED in patients with diabetes, no other studies were found investigating other possible treatments for people with T2DM and other eating disorders. Until more research is conducted in this area, it is appropriate to apply the current literature on treating eating disorders in the general population to that of the diabetic population.

Various treatments for anorexia nervosa, including psychotherapeutic and pharmacological interventions, are available and have empirical support for their efficacy. While a review of these treatments is beyond the scope of the present chapter, recent reviews are available (Bulik, Berkman, Brownley, Sedway, & Lohr, 2007) and suggest that cognitive-behavioral, interpersonal, and pharmacological approaches can be helpful. In the context of T2DM, it is important to modify the application of these interventions to take into consideration the importance of weight loss to improve treatment outcomes. Thus, weight loss should be incorporated as a goal of treatment in work with patients with BED, for example. The importance of treatment adherence and careful attention to the possible relationship between insulin restriction or omission and disordered eating should also be given important consideration. Consultation with the diabetes treatment provider(s) should be sought and collaboration with a dietitian with expertise in the management of diabetes may be beneficial.

2.4.3.3 Issues in Treatment Decision-Making

The current literature gives little guidance for the selection of the most appropriate treatments for eating disorders in the context of T2DM. Interventions that have been empirically supported in nondiabetes populations appear applicable, but there may be a further need to consider even subclinical presentations of maladaptive eating behaviors and attitudes as necessitating treatment given their association with worse treatment outcomes in the context of T2DM. As in the treatment of other psychological problems in patients with T2DM, consideration of the associations between maladaptive patterns of eating behaviors and attitudes about weight and body image on the one hand and insulin omission and other aspects of diabetes treatment adherence on the other may result in more accurate case conceptualizations and more effective treatments.

2.5 Psychotic Disorders and Bipolar Disorders

2.5.1 Epidemiology

T2DM is more prevalent among individuals with serious and persistent mental illnesses such as bipolar disorder and schizophrenia than in the general population (Citrome et al., 2005; Parks, Svendsen, Singer, Foti, & Mauer, 2006). Estimates from a range of national and international epidemiological studies have shown the prevalence of diabetes in patients with schizophrenia to be 1.5–2.5 times greater than that found in the general population, with the difference being particularly striking among younger patients (Parks et al.; Rouillon & Sorbara, 2005). The point prevalence of schizophrenia itself is estimated at 0.5%, lifetime prevalence at around 1%, and annual incidence around 0.2% (APA, 2000; Eaton et al., 2008; Mueser & McGurk, 2004). Due to the comparative rarity of the diagnoses, individuals with schizoaffective, schizophreniform, and other psychotic illnesses are often included as part of a larger sample of individuals with psychotic disorders. The true prevalence of diabetes among individuals with psychotic disorders may be grossly underestimated due to the silent nature of diabetes and the myriad of other, more immediately pressing medical, economic, and social problems people with psychotic disorders face (Bushe & Holt, 2004; Mueser & Gingerich, 2006; Mueser & McGurk, 2004; Parks et al., 2006).

A number of studies have shown that the prevalence of T2DM is also increased among patients with bipolar disorders. For example, a retrospective chart review study of patients between the ages of 50 and 74 found T2DM in 26% of patients with bipolar I (Regenold, Thapar, Marano, Gavirneni, & Kondapavuluru, 2002). An examination of a sample of more than 4,000 VA patients with bipolar disorder found the prevalence of diabetes to be over 17% (Kilbourne et al, 2004). According to the NCS-R, the 12-month prevalence of bipolar I and II disorders is 2.6% (Kessler, Chiu, et al., 2005). Bipolar patients with diabetes have been found to be older, more chronically ill, present with rapid cycling, and have an overall lower level of global functioning than patient with bipolar disorder but without diabetes; they were also found to have higher rates of long-term disability and were also more likely to have higher BMIs (Ruzickova, Slaney, Garnham, & Alda, 2003). Individuals with serious and persistent mental illnesses die on average 25 years younger than the general population due to illnesses such as diabetes and cardiovascular disease (American Diabetes Association, American Psychiatry Association, & American Association of Clinical Endocrinologists, 2006; Parks et al., 2006; Pratt, Dey, & Cohen, 2007).

2.5.2 *Pathophysiology*

There are many possible reasons for the co-morbidity of serious and persistent mental illness and T2DM, reasons that are likely interactive and interconnected (Rouillon & Sorbara, 2005). Antipsychotic medication, particularly newer atypical antipsychotics, have been associated with metabolic disturbance and higher rates of diabetes (Bushe & Holt, 2004; Mueser & McGurk, 2004). This is particularly important given the dramatic increase in the prescription of atypical antipsychotics over the last decade (Domino & Swartz, 2008). Some atypical antipsychotics as well as conventional antipsychotics have been associated with higher rates of diabetes and metabolic dysregulation both independently and through certain medication side effects, such as weight gain, insulin resistance, decreased physical activity, and metabolic syndrome (Barnett et al., 2007; Basu & Meltzer, 2006; Bushe & Holt, 2004; Folnegovic-Smalc, Jukic, Kozumplik, Mimica, & Uzun, 2004; Kohen, 2004; Mueser & McGurk, 2004; Parks et al., 2006; Sernyak, Leslie, Alarcon, Losonczy, & Rosenheck, 2002, but see Holt & Peveler, 2006; Koro et al., 2002; Smith et al., 2008). However, the association between schizophrenia, diabetes, and diabetic risk appears to be independent of medication regimen, which could be explained by physiological abnormalities co-occurring with the disease, socioeconomic and other environmental correlates of schizophrenia, or a combination of these factors (Bushe & Holt, 2004; Holt, Peveler, & Byrne, 2004).

Individuals receiving medication for the treatment of bipolar disorder also frequently experience weight gain (Elmslie, Silverstone, Mann, Williams, & Romans, 2000). Mood stabilizers such as lithium and anticonvulsants are often the first line of pharmacological treatment for bipolar disorder. Numerous studies have found associations between lithium treatment and weight gain, but how lithium precipitates weight gain is unclear (Kupka et al., 2002). Lithium may stimulate the hypothalamus and thus appetite, which can increase caloric consumption, and may may increase thirst, which can increase fluid retention. Lithium has also been associated with reduced thyroid functioning, which can effect glucose regulation (Kupka et al., 2002). Among individuals taking lithium, thyroid dysfunction has been found to be as high as 47%, with females 5 times more likely to develop this side effect than males (Kupka et al.; Livingstone & Rampes, 2006). Hypothyroidism may also be related to increased likelihood of rapid mood cycling between manic and depressive episodes and severity of depression among patients with bipolar disorder (APA, 2002; Livingstone & Rampes, 2006). Valproic acid can increase levels of testosterone in women and increase the likelihood of developing polycystic ovary syndrome, which can result in obesity as well as endocrine disruption (Joffe et al., 2006).

Poor diet, physical inactivity, smoking, and poor treatment adherence – independent risk factors for T2DM and its complications – are also more common among individuals with schizophrenia (Barnett et al., 2007; Dinan, 2004; El-Mallakh, 2006, 2007; Holt et al., 2004; Kohen, 2004; Kreyenbuhl et al., 2008; McIntyre et al., 2005; Peet, 2004; Piette, Heisler, Ganoczy, McCarthy, & Valenstein, 2007; Rouillon & Sorbara, 2005; Weiss et al., 2006). Risk factors for T2DM and schizophrenia may overlap, including obesity, sedentary lifestyle, lower socioeconomic status, a family history of diabetes, race/ethnicity, poverty, and excess stress (Black, 2002; Centers for Disease Control [CDC], 2005; Kreyenbuhl et al., 2008; Mueser & McGurk, 2004). Individuals with schizophrenia may have impaired glucose metabolism even before they develop schizophrenia, and historical surveys of the co-morbidity literature show an association between schizophrenia and diabetes before the use of neuroleptics and antipsychotics became common among treatments for schizophrenia (Bushe & Holt, 2004; Citrome et al., 2005; Dixon et al., 2000; Kohen, 2004). Individuals with schizophrenia have been found to have more than 3 times the intra-abdominal fat as matched healthy controls and are also at higher risk for developing features of metabolic syndrome – both risk factors for insulin resistance and diabetes (ADA, 2004; Thakore, 2005). Citrome et al. (2005) note that patients with schizophrenia often have increased visceral fat even in the absence of antipsychotic treatment, and visceral and intra-abdominal fat is associated with insulin resistance and metabolic syndrome, both significant risk factors for T2DM. In addition, researchers involved in the National Institute of Mental Health Clinical Antipsychotic Trials of Intervention Effectiveness (CATIE) study, which recruited 1,460 participants from over 57 catchment areas, found that metabolic syndrome was present in over 40% of the sample. Men and women from the CATIE sample were 138 and 251% more likely to develop metabolic syndrome than a matched sample, respectively (McEvoy et al., 2005). The frequency of metabolic syndrome among people with schizophrenia could be related to blood glucose increases, central abdominal obesity, and disordered lipid metabolism (increasing cortisol production), and any or all of these could be influenced by medication effects, physiological traits concurrent with schizophrenia, or health behaviors such as sedentary lifestyle, food choice, and smoking (Holt et al., 2004; McEvoy et al., 2005). Seventy- to ninety-percent of patients with schizophrenia smoke, compared to less than 30%

of the overall population, and smoking has been implicated in insulin dysregulation (Diwan et al. 1998; Mueser & McGurk, 2004).

People with bipolar disorder are also more likely to be overweight or obese than the general population and are 2–3 times more likely to experience the metabolic syndrome (Elmslie, Silverstone, Mann, Williams, & Romans, 2000; Livingstone & Rampes, 2006; Pendlebury & Holt, 2008). Wang et al. (2006) examined overweight and obesity in 377 participants enrolled in the Systematic Treatment Enhancement Program for Bipolar Disorder study and the majority (55%) of participants were overweight or obese. Eating disorders such as BED are also more prevalent among individuals with bipolar disorder than the overall population and may also increase risk for the development of metabolic disturbances and diabetes (McIntyre et al., 2005). Socioeconomic factors that may increase the risk of diabetes and worse diabetes outcomes among individuals with bipolar disorder include poverty, limited access to health care, and higher rates of unemployment (McIntyre et al.).

Chronic and severe physical and psychological stress resulting from the hardships of serious mental illness may contribute to insulin resistance (Musselman et al., 2003). Stress results in the release of hormones such as glucocorticoids, growth hormone, catecholamines, and glucagon, which raise levels of blood glucose through a variety of metabolic pathways. The impact of stress and hormones, as well as increased immune system activation on glucose metabolism, has been more extensively studied in major depression than in bipolar or psychotic disorders, but as major depressive episodes are a central feature of bipolar and highly co-morbid with schizophrenia, similar risks may be present.

Both schizophrenia and T2DM have been found to have familial inheritance traits, and researchers who study individuals with T2DM and schizophrenia have found multiple links between the two conditions (Bellivier, 2005; Fernandez-Egea, Bernardo, et al., 2008; Fernandez-Egea, Miller, Bernardo, Donner, & Kirkpatrick, 2008; Rouillon & Sorbara, 2005). Research has also found that specific genetic loci and alleles may increase risk of developing bipolar disorder or schizophrenia, indicating that the polygenetic bases of schizophrenia are substantially shared with bipolar disorder, which is itself highly hereditable (Carroll & Owen, 2009; McGuffin et al., 2003; Purcell et al., 2009). This shared genetic risk for both bipolar disorder and schizophrenia is intriguing, as schizophrenia has been found to present an independent risk factor for the development of diabetes, controlling for multiple physiologic and behavioral risk factors, implicating a shared genetic risk for both illnesses (Bellivier, 2005; Fernandez-Egea, Miller, et al., 2008; Rouillon & Sorbara, 2005). Indeed, some researchers have found defects on genes that influence both neurochemicals implicated in schizophrenia as well as metabolic control (Bellivier, 2005).

Individuals with serious mental illnesses such as bipolar disorder or psychotic disorders also have higher rates of tobacco usage than the general population (Diaz et al., 2009; Diwan, Castine, Pomerleau, Meador-Woodruff, & Dalack, 1998). Additionally, the rate of substance and alcohol use among individuals with schizophrenia or bipolar disorder is higher than the general population; individuals with schizophrenia have been found to be more than 7.5 times more likely to report current or past substance abuse (Phillips & Johnson, 2001). These behaviors can compromise diabetes control and increase the risk for cardiovascular complications of diabetes (Haire-Joshu, Glasgow, & Tibbs, 2004; Himelhoch et al., 2009; McCreadie, 2003; Mueser & McGurk, 2004). Diseases of the pancreas and liver from alcohol abuse can also contribute to the risk of developing diabetes as well as the development of diabetic complications (McIntyre et al., 2005).

2.5.3 *Clinical Care*

2.5.3.1 Assessment

Up to 60–70% of cases of T2DM in individuals with serious and persistent mental illness may go undiagnosed (Pendlebury & Holt, 2008). Thus, screening for diabetes and diabetes risk factors is important in these patients, even when diabetes is not identified as part of the medical history. Mental health providers should be aware of the risk for T2DM in the patients they treat and whether T2DM is part of the patient's medical history. In the treatment of patients with co-morbid psychotic or bipolar disorders and T2DM, health behaviors should be carefully assessed, including lifestyle factors such as activity level, diet, smoking, drug and alcohol use, eating disorders, and treatment adherence. Adherence to dietary and exercise recommendations should be carefully assessed with the context of the client's resources and limitations in mind; many clients may not have adequate resources and assessing vulnerabilities and matching patients with the appropriate supportive services may be beneficial (El-Mallakh, 2006, 2007).

Although it seems reasonable to expect that patients with severe mental illness may have more problems with diabetes treatment adherence, few studies have examined this relationship and the existing literature suggests that this may not be the case. For example, adherence to medications for T2DM was better among diabetic individuals with schizophrenia as compared to those without schizophrenia in a study of diabetes patients in ongoing care in a VA health system. However, overall adherence was quite low in this sample (Kreyenbuhl et al., 2008). Piette et al. (2007) assessed treatment adherence in individuals with co-morbid schizophrenia, diabetes, and hypertension and found that adherence was better for oral medications for diabetes and hypertension than for antipsychotic medications. While little is known about the role of depressed mood in explaining the relationship between severe mental illness and worse diabetes outcomes, research documenting that depression symptoms are consistently associated with diabetes treatment nonadherence (Gonzalez, Peyrot, McCarl, et al., 2008) suggests that depressed mood should be carefully assessed in patients with psychotic or bipolar disorders. Supporting this, Kreyenbuhl et al. (2008) found that although schizophrenia was associated with better diabetes medication adherence, depression was associated with worse adherence. Individuals with schizophrenia have been found to have difficulties with treatment adherence for schizophrenia (Mueser & Gingerich, 2006; Parks, Svendsen, Singer,

Foti, & Mauer, 2006; Piette et al., 2007); thus, treatment adherence to psychotropic medications should also be carefully assessed, as control of the psychotic disorder will likely be a necessary condition for addressing diabetes risk. Knowledge about diabetes and its management should also be carefully assessed as patients may have not received adequate education about diabetes because of other treatment priorities or may have been less able to process information because of cognitive deficits.

Careful attention to diabetes risk factors is particularly important in patients treated with atypical antipsychotic medications. These patients should be referred for evaluation of blood glucose levels 4 months after starting an antipsychotic medication, then yearly if no problems are found (ADA, 2004; Gough and Peveler, 2004; Marder et al., 2002; McEvoy et al., 2005). As lithium treatment poses risk for reduction in thyroid function and weight gain, these patients should also be referred for evaluation of T2DM risk. After baseline assessment, thyroid function should be monitored after 3 months of lithium treatment and every 6–12 months after (Goldberg, 2008).

2.5.3.2 Evidence-Based Treatment

Preventing weight gain and reducing weight in those who are already overweight are two important priorities in the management of diabetes in patients suffering from psychotic or bipolar disorders. Education should be provided regarding nutrition and exercise and appropriate patients should be referred to programs to facilitate healthy lifestyle change, particularly if they are starting on atypical antipsychotics or lithium. Clients may be encouraged to chart and monitor their own weight over time. Family members or other caregivers should be made aware of the additional risks the patient faces for metabolic and cardiovascular illness (ADA, 2004; Marder et al., 2002; McEvoy et al., 2005). Lifestyle therapies tailored to individuals with schizophrenia addressing such issues as exercise, portion control, nutritional interventions, and other nonpharmacological interventions have been shown to be effective in controlled clinical trials of individuals with schizophrenia (Citrome & Vreeland, 2008).

Thomas, Raymondet, Charbonnel, and Vaiva (2005) offered a series of recommendations developed by psychiatrists and endocrinologists, encouraging collaboration between endocrinologists and mental health providers in the treatment of their patients. Diabetes information should be tailored to the family and the patient, with a focus on capitalizing on family support for lifestyle changes and treatment adherence. Concrete steps, such as articulating weight loss goals and developing specific behavioral modification strategies, should be outlined for patients and their families. Even modest improvements in nutrition can be beneficial for the metabolic health outcomes of individuals with schizophrenia (Thomas et al.).

Treatment for individuals with bipolar disorder is not significantly different than that for those with psychotic disorders – increased monitoring of risk factors and emphasis on prevention and lifestyle interventions are recommended (McIntyre et al., 2005). Primary goals for treatment of individuals with bipolar disorder are to reduce psychiatric symptoms, improve functioning, and reduce overall risk of mortality. Much of the weight gained by individuals with bipolar disorder during treatment may be gained during depressive stages, which may indicate that stabilizing mood symptoms is a first priority in controlling risk factors for diabetes and diabetic complications (Fagiolini et al., 2002). Again, we note that symptoms of depression have been associated with worse treatment adherence in diabetes and, thus, difficulty with treatment adherence should be carefully monitored in these patients, especially during depressive episodes. Pretreatment diet and exercise counseling are preferred for preventing treatment-related weight gain (Livingstone & Rampes, 2006).

While there are few well-controlled studies on weight management for individuals with schizophrenia which would allow for concrete guidelines for behavioral treatment of diabetes and modifiable diabetes risk factors, a variety of behavioral and supportive interventions including nutritional education, weight-loss counseling, group support and activities, and psychoeducation regarding challenges to dietary adherence have repeatedly been found to either result in weight loss or reduce or prevent weight gain compared to individuals not receiving similar interventions (Bushe, Haddad, Peveler, & Pendlebury, 2005; Loh, Meyer, & Leckband, 2008).

McKibbin et al. (2006) conducted a randomized controlled trial to examine the feasibility and efficacy of their Diabetes Awareness and Rehabilitation Training (DART) group lifestyle intervention for adults over 40 years of age with co-morbid schizophrenia and diabetes. The DART intervention is a 24-week manualized intervention based on social learning theory that addresses comprehensive diabetes self-care (nutrition, exercise, monitoring blood sugar, physician communication, foot care) and utilized behavioral techniques to assess and reinforce achievable lifestyle goals. Measures of diabetes knowledge as well as physiological assessments were taken at baseline and at 6 months. Comparing outcomes to a usual care plus information control group, they found that intervention was both feasible (90% adherence rate) and resulted in positive health outcomes. Patients in the DART group lost an average of 5 lb, while those in the control group gained a mean of 6 lb; significant interactions were also found for reductions in triglycerides, improvements in diabetes knowledge, diabetes self-efficacy, and self-reported physical activity but not for fasting plasma glucose or HbA1c.

In their review of behaviorally based interventions for weight management among individual with schizophrenia, Loh et al. (2008) found that the average length of treatment for studies that resulted in either significant weight loss or significant between-group differences was 6 months. Successful interventions consisted of behavioral modification, caloric restriction, and/or psychoeducation. Interventions with external incentives such as token systems were the most intensive in terms of utilization of resources and also most effective (Loh et al.).

The 2009 Schizophrenia Patient Outcomes Research Team (PORT) recommendations for weight loss interventions for individuals with schizophrenia recommend that comprehensive weight loss efforts should persist for at least 3 months to result in weight loss, which is likely to be small in size (Kreyenbuhl, Buchanan, Dickerson, & Dixon, 2010). Research including individuals with bipolar disorder has found similar results, namely that attendance at programs that involve social support, regular weigh-ins, as well as educational components can lead to weight loss and the prevention of weight gain (Pendlebury & Holt, 2008). Metformin, an oral medication used in the treatment of T2DM, has also been used to facilitate weight loss among individuals on antipsychotic treatment and improve weight loss outcomes on its own as well as for individuals engaged in healthy lifestyle interventions. Focusing on treatment adherence to metformin in these patients could result in multiple health benefits (Carrizo et al., 2009; Wu et al., 2008).

Regarding smoking cessation, the most recent PORT guidelines recommend bupropion therapy for 10–12 weeks (Kreyenbuhl et al., 2010) as a first-line treatment. As bupropion may also result in weight loss, decrease depression, and improve glucose control in T2DM, multiple benefits may be derived from this treatment for patients (Lustman et al., 2007). Smoking cessation programs that offer psychosocial support and nicotine replacement therapy should also be considered, although high attrition rates from many studies reflect the challenge of smoking cessation in general and especially among individuals with a co-morbid psychiatric illness (Kreyenbuhl et al., 2010; Lucksted, McGuire, Postrado, Kreyenbuhl, & Dixon, 2004; McEvoy & Allen, 2003; Weinberger & George, 2009; Ziedonis & George, 1997). Motivation has been found to be a key barrier to smoking cessation and psychoeducation regarding the risks of smoking is important to enhance motivation for quitting.

2.5.3.3 Issues in Treatment Decision-Making

Careful attention to the potential risks and benefits related to diabetes risk for medication regimens, monitoring of metabolic symptoms, integrative and comprehensive patient care, improving treatment adherence, and therapeutic lifestyle change are all key components of care for individuals with psychotic and bipolar disorders who are either at high risk for diabetes or who are already diagnosed with T2DM. Improved efficacy of and adherence to psychotropic medication may be essential for the ability to sustain lifestyle changes necessary to impact metabolic risks for these patients. These medications often prevent a lifetime of severe disability and their benefits may outweigh even serious metabolic risks (Llorente & Uruita, 2006). Thus, treatment adherence to psychotropic medications and to treatment for T2DM should be included as targets of behavioral interventions.

2.6 Substance Use Disorders

2.6.1 Epidemiology

While it does not appear that substance abuse or alcohol abuse rates are higher in T2DM patients than in the general population, it is important to briefly mention these disorders for at least three reasons. First, substance and/or alcohol use disorders complicate diabetes care, increase the risk of complications, and increase health care costs (Banerjea et al., 2008). Second, substance use disorders are commonly co-morbid with other psychological problems and may be prevalent in diabetes patients seeking psychological care. Third, these disorders are quite prevalent in the US population – more than 22 million people (8.9% of the population) aged 12 or older met DSM-IV criteria for substance dependence or abuse in 2008 (Substance Abuse and Mental Health Services Administration [SAMHSA], 2009). Of them, 3.1 million had alcohol and drug abuse disorders, 3.9 million had a substance use disorder but not an alcohol use disorder, and 15.2 million had alcohol use disorders but not substance use disorders. Furthermore, cigarette smoking is the leading cause of preventable death in the United States, and in 2008, 20.6% of adults were current smokers (CDC, 2008).

2.6.2 Pathophysiology

Substance use can impact diabetes self-care, interfering with treatment adherence and blood glucose monitoring (especially dangerous for those with insulin-dependent diabetes), and also by masking the symptoms of poor diabetes control and compilations such as severe hyperglycemia (Lee, Greenfield, & Campbell, 2009). Specific substances may have metabolic impacts. For example, ecstasy can precipitate ketoacidosis in users through its antidiuretic effects; heroin can result in alterations in glucose metabolism and hyperinsulinaemia; cocaine can result in elevated levels of cortisol and corticotropin (Lee et al., 2009; Seymour, Gilman, & Quin, 1996; Sheldon & Quin, 2005). Marijuana's effects on increased appetite may also indirectly influence glycemic control (Lee et al., 2009). Cigarette smoking increases the likelihood of developing diabetic risk factors, T2DM, and poorer diabetes treatment outcomes (ADA, 2004; CDC, 2008; Haire-Joshu et al., 2004; Willi et al., 2007). Cigarette smoking has also been associated with increased morbidity among diabetes due to cardiovascular disease and macrovascular complications, as well as increased likelihood of diabetic complications such as peripheral neuropathy (Haire-Joshu et al., 2004).

The impact of alcohol consumption on diabetes is complex, both metabolically and behaviorally. Moderate alcohol use has been associated with decreased risk of T2DM, but heavy alcohol use has been associated with increased risks (Banerjea et al., 2008; Ravert, 2009). When blood sugar levels are low, alcohol can induce hypoglycemia; as alcohol can impair judgment and reduce an individual's awareness of low blood sugar, heavier drinking can greatly increase the risk of negative diabetic consequences and complications (Ravert). Heavy alcohol use has been associated with higher rates of T2DM among lean men and with increased prevalence of diabetes overall, and also been linked to higher levels of abdominal obesity, controlling for BMI (Johnson, Bazargan, & Cherpitel, 2001; Risérus & Ingelsson, 2007). The association between alcohol intake and abdominal obesity specifically, as opposed to overall obesity, reflects the particular risk central adiposity poses for the development of diabetes in heavy alcohol drinkers. Long-term alcohol abuse can also result in pancreatitis, a disease of the pancreas and which can present as acute or chronic progressive disease in which the pancreas is irreversibly damaged, resulting in impaired endocrine and exocrine function as well as disabling pain

(Nair, Lawler, & Miller, 2007). In adults, alcoholism is the cause of 70% of all cases of chronic pancreatitis and more than 40% of individuals with chronic pancreatitis will develop T2DM. Most adults who develop chronic pancreatitis will develop diabetes within 5 years of onset (Nair et al.). In addition, some treatments for chronic pancreatitis, such as surgical removal of portions or the entire pancreas, may lead to the development of diabetes.

2.6.3 Clinical Care

2.6.3.1 Assessment

Among individuals with alcohol and/or substance disorders, less than 10% received the treatment they required for their disorder in a given year (SAMHSA, 2009). Indeed, among a population drawn for the Veterans Health Administration, disparities in diabetes care were found to be more pronounced when patients had a substance use disorder, increasing in a dose response effect with the addition of additional co-morbid mental health diagnoses (Clark, Weir, Ouellette, Zhang, & Baxter, 2009). Patients with T2DM that use alcohol and/or drugs have been found to receive lower quality of care, above and beyond patient underutilization of preventative and primary care resources of increased ER visits (Frayne et al., 2005). Clinicians should thoroughly assess for current and past substance and alcohol use as part of standard diabetes care, especially in those who are in poor control or have other co-morbid mental health illnesses (ADA, 2004). Recognition of the potential unhealthy effects on glycemic control associated with even moderate use is important in assessing treatment adherence and health behaviors that may impact diabetes treatment. Adolescents and young adults may be at greater risk for engaging in substance use, as are individuals with a former history of drug, alcohol, or tobacco use/misuse, and clinicians are advised to remain aware of the possibility of relapse and provide support and resources if relapse or initiation of use occurs (ADA).

2.6.3.2 Evidence-Based Treatment

Psychoeducation regarding the impact of tobacco, substance, and alcohol use on physical health may motivate patients to address their substance use issues and significant positive health benefits for both metabolic and psychiatric well-being can occur when patients are successful in reducing or discontinuing use (de Leon, Susce, Diaz, Rendon, & Velásquez, 2005). Among clients struggling with alcohol or substance misuse, treatment, especially insulin regimens, should be tailored to fit client's actual lifestyle to the extent feasible so as to maximize the likelihood of treatment adherence and reduce the risk of life-threatening complications (Lee et al., 2009).

As per the ADA's review of smoking and diabetes (2004), a number of specific recommendations can be made. Intensive smoking cessation interventions, such as attendance of cessation group or counseling, have been found to be most effective, but patients are less likely to engage in these treatments, due to factors such as time, cost, resources, and motivation (ADA, 2004; Haire-Joshu et al., 2004). All interventions regarding smoking cessation and diabetes should highlight the impact of cigarette smoking on diabetes management and quit aids, such as appropriate prescriptions for pharmacologic interventions and supportive community resources should be available to assist interested patients in cutting down or quitting. The patient's cessation attempts should be monitored and follow-up care, particularly within the first 2 weeks of the quit date, has also been found to improve cessation outcomes among individuals with diabetes (Haire-Joshu et al.). Finally, while fear of gaining weight may present an unfortunate deterrent to quitting smoking, actual weight gain following smoking cessation can pose at least an increased short-term risk of developing diabetes. Weight gain often occurs during and after a smoking cessation attempt, and smokers, especially heavier smokers, tend to have greater central adiposity than nonsmokers (Healton, Vallone, McCausland, Xiao, & Green, 2006; Willi et al., 2007).

2.6.3.3 Issues in Treatment Decision-Making

A large body of research has explored best practices for treating substance or alcohol use disorders and co-morbid illness in psychiatric illness, the details of which are beyond the scope of this chapter (Riggs, Levin, Green, & Vocci, 2008). As other psychiatric disorders are frequently co-morbid with substance use and have been found to co-occur at higher rates among diabetics than the general population, healthcare practitioners faced with these multiple co-morbidities should consider the implications for psychiatric treatment on diabetes outcomes when planning treatment, as serious mental health issues may often need to be addressed first or in tandem with substance or alcohol use cessation. In a National Epidemiologic Survey on Alcohol and Related Conditions, during the same 12-month period almost 20% of participants with any substance use disorder had at least one mood disorder and almost 18% had at least one anxiety disorder, with rates higher for dependence than abuse (Grant et al., 2003). Even more prevalent were co-morbid alcohol use and psychiatric illness; 40.7% of those with an alcohol use disorder had at least one current mood disorder during the same 12-month time period, and more than 33% had at least one anxiety disorder. Treatment of psychological issues may be essential to both successful substance or alcohol misuse treatment and improvement and stabilization of co-morbid diabetes.

As stated previously, smoking and psychiatric illness often co-occur; individuals with mental illness are approximately twice as likely to smoke as those without mental illness (Lasser et al., 2000). As psychiatric illness may have particular implications for individuals with diabetes and its care, including presenting an increased risk factor for the development of diabetes, metabolic disturbance, and complications from diabetes, it is of vital importance that healthcare professionals attend to co-morbid psychological issues that may underlie an individual's tobacco use when addressing smoking cessation and diabetes self-care (Kreyenbuhl et al., 2010; Lucksted et al., 2004; McEvoy & Allen, 2003; Ziedonis et al., 2003). As psychological issues often fuel substance use disorders and compromise both substance cessation and diabetes self-care and predict increased risk of relapse after quitting, it is vital to address mental health as a part of drug, alcohol, or smoking cessation as well as diabetes care (Haire-Joshu et al., 2004; Spangler et al., 2001).

2.7 Cultural Considerations: Diabetes, Race, and Ethnicity

2.7.1 Epidemiology

The problem of racial disparities in the US healthcare system is well documented. Approximately 14% of Hispanics and 12% of African Americans are affected by diabetes compared with 7% of non-Hispanic Whites (Bonds et al., 2003; Harris et al., 1998). Ethnic and racial disparities are also seen in rates of diabetes complications – African Americans and Hispanics have more diabetes-associated nephropathy, retinopathy, and diabetes-related amputations than non-Hispanic Whites (Bonds et al., 2003). Bonds et al. utilized data from the Insulin Resistance Atherosclerosis Study and compared process and outcome measures of diabetes care among African Americans, Hispanics, and non-Hispanic Whites; although the rates of treatment for diabetes and its associated co-morbidities were found to be similar across all three ethnic groups, African Americans and Hispanics had significantly worse control of hypertension and African Americans had worse control of diabetes than non-Hispanic Whites.

The literature is sparse regarding diabetes and mental illness in ethnic and racial minority populations. Studies have shown that greater than 25% of ethnic or racial minority individuals with diabetes reach criteria for MDD, and far more display high levels of depressive symptoms at rates above those found in non-Hispanic Whites (Fisher, Chesla, Mullan, Skaff, & Kanter, 2001; Lustman, Anderson, et al., 2000). Risk factors for increased incidence of depression often overlap with those for developing T2DM. These factors may be more common among individuals more likely to experience disparities in heathcare access and quality, including ethnic/racial minority status, lower SES, unemployment, multiple medical co-morbidities, complications from diabetes, female gender, lower quality of life, and the experience of negative life events or chronic stress (Fisher et al., 2001).

A recent epidemiologic study by Li et al. (2009) utilized a general measure of nonspecific psychological distress to estimate the prevalence of serious psychological distress (SPD) among US adults and found the prevalence of SPD highest among Hispanics (11.8%) and Native Americans (14.7%), individuals with low levels of income (17.3%) and education (15.6%), as well as individuals with T1DM (11.1%) or T2DM (11.5%) who are currently using insulin (Li et al.). Hispanics are also more likely to report higher levels of anxiety compared with Whites and higher levels of diabetes-related distress when compared with African Americans (Li et al.,

2008; Kahn et al., 2008; Spencer et al., 2006). The diabetes distress-anxiety association among Hispanics may be especially concerning for both mental and physical health outcomes, as the incidence of type 2 diabetes is projected to increase in the coming years among this rapidly growing segment of the US population (Li et al., 2008).

As discussed previously, risk factors for the development of T2DM and schizophrenia may overlap, including obesity, sedentary lifestyle, lower socioeconomic status, a family history of diabetes, race/ethnicity, poverty, and stress (Black, 2002; CDC, 2005; Mueser & McGurk, 2004). For example, African Americans are more likely to fall into lower economic brackets and rates of both diabetes and schizophrenia diagnoses are found to be higher among African Americans compared to Whites (Black, 2002; CDC, 2005; El-Mallakh, 2006; Mueser & McGurk, 2004). The overrepresentation of socioeconomic burdens among ethnic minority populations may also play a role in the expression of other types of disorders and distress in minority patients with diabetes.

The literature regarding the prevalence of eating disorders and T2DM in minority populations, to our knowledge, is nonexistent. In the general population, cultural beliefs and attitudes have been identified as significant contributing factors in the development of eating disorders (Ismail, 2008). Rates of these disorders appear to vary among different racial/ethnic and national groups, change across time as cultures evolve, and some, such as BED, may be more prevent among individuals who experience social adversity and depression (Ismail; Miller & Pumariega, 2001). As poor diet is a key component in overweight and obesity and increased dietary vigilance is an essential component of self-care for diabetes, research into the ways race, ethnicity, and culture interact with diabetes to impact eating attitudes and disordered eating would help to bridge this knowledge gap.

2.7.2 Clinical Care

Racial, ethnic, and socioeconomic disparities in treatment access, utilization, and quality exist in both mental health and diabetes care. In their examination of data from the Behavioral Risk Factor Surveillance System, Li et al. (2010) found that people with diabetes were less likely to be treated for mental health issues than those without. Among adults with diabetes and mental health problems, individuals who were of a non-White race/ethnicity, 65 years of age or older, lacked health insurance, had less than a high school education, or were unemployed were also less likely to receive treatment for mental health needs (Li et al.). The high prevalence of undertreatment may be due to the lack of recognition of mental health problems among these populations and disparities in availability of care or quality of care. The National Co-morbidity Study found that lack of perceived need, situational barriers, financial barriers, perceived lack of effectiveness, thinking the problem would get better by itself, and wanting to solve the problem on one's own are the major reasons for failing to seek treatment for serious mental illness (Kessler et al., 2001). In a prospective epidemiological cohort study of 69,068 patients regarding the use of antidepressants, African Americans with diabetes were much less likely to report taking antidepressant medication than Whites (Osborn et al., 2010). The high prevalence of undertreatment among African Americans and Hispanics with diabetes may suggest racial/ethnic disparities in access to medical care or quality of care.

Reducing medical and mental health treatment disparities is a goal of many state and national public health initiatives, as well as Healthy People 2020 (U.S. Department of Health and Human Services, 2010). As in all facets of diabetes care, screening and treatment of diabetes patients with mental illnesses should be culturally sensitive. Including evaluative components in diabetes and mental health interventions targeted to assess the effectiveness of these programs for diverse patient populations may help improve overall quality of care for patients experiencing mental and physical health disparities. Ultimately, there is no one "cookie cutter" approach to diabetes care or mental health treatment – mental health intervention programs should take into account patients' cultural backgrounds, access to health care, social and economic resources, native languages, as well as health and illness beliefs. There remains a paucity of evidence-based information regarding the treatment of mental health problems in ethnic/racial minority patients in general (Schraufnagel, Wagner, Miranda, & Roy-Byrne, 2006) and even less of this work has been done in patients with diabetes in particular. However, the few studies that have been conducted suggest that empirically supported approaches can be successfully adapted for minority groups. For example, one notable, well-controlled, randomized trial of 267 low-income, English- and Spanish-speaking, White and minority women (Blacks and Latinas) with current major depression demonstrated compared three conditions of treatment: antidepressant medication, manual-guided CBT, or referral to community mental health services (Miranda et al., 2003). Both the medication intervention and the CBT intervention reduced depressive symptoms significantly more than the community referral. Each intervention also had impacts on role functioning, and English- and Spanish-speaking patients responded equally well to each of the treatments. Results of this trial showed that augmentation of treatment with case management resulted in improved retention across all ethnic groups. Interestingly, augmenting the CBT intervention with supplemental case management was shown to improve response for Spanish-speaking depressed patients, but not for English-speaking patients. A recent preliminary report also suggests that a case-management approach to diabetes and depression can be effective in improving depression, self-management, and glycemic outcomes in elderly African Americans with depression and type 2 diabetes (Bogner & de Vries, 2010). This approach included an individualized program to improve adherence to oral hypoglycemic agents and antidepressants and employed a care-manager to facilitate communication between patients and physicians and to address depression and problems with diabetes self-management with sensitivity to cultural issues. Patients randomized to this intervention demonstrated improvements in depression symptom severity, adherence to oral hypoglycemics, adherence to antidepressants, and HbA1c post-intervention as compared to those receiving usual care.

2.8 General Conclusion

The literature reviewed in this chapter highlights the potential for worse treatment outcomes in T2DM patients with co-morbid psychological problems. We have emphasized the importance of careful assessment of psychological disorders in patients with attention to the context of the goals and challenges of living with T2DM. Interventions for psychological problems, even those that may not meet diagnostic thresholds, have the potential to not only improve the mental health and quality of life of patients with T2DM, but may also have important impacts on diabetes treatment outcomes, health, and longevity. For these interventions to be maximally effective, we believe a comprehensive approach that integrates the treatment of psychological problems with interventions aimed at improving health behaviors and diabetes treatment adherence is necessary. Thus far, remarkably few examples of these types of interventions are available in the literature. We sincerely hope that this chapter will encourage clinicians to think carefully about their ability to address the tremendous behavioral challenges facing individuals with co-morbid T2DM and psychopathology and look forward to future research on such integrative interventions that can more thoroughly evaluate the empirical support for our recommendations.

References

Aina, Y., & Susman, J. L. (2006). Understanding comorbidity with depression and anxiety disorders. *The Journal of the American Osteopathic Association, 5*(2), 9–14.

Ali, S., Stone, M., Peters, J., Davies, M., & Khunti, K. (2006). The prevalence of comorbid depression in adults with type 2 diabetes: A systematic review and meta-analysis. *Diabetic Medicine, 23*, 1165–1173.

Allison, K. C., Crow, S. J., Reeves, R. R., West, D. S., Foreyt, J. P., DiLillo, V. G., et al. (2007). Binge eating disorder and night eating syndrome in adults with type 2 diabetes. *Obesity (Silver Spring), 15*(5), 1287–1293.

Allison, D., Mentore, J., Heo, M., Chandler, L., Cappelleri, J., Infante, M., et al. (1999). Antipsychotic-induced weight gain: A comprehensive research synthesis. *The American Journal of Psychiatry, 156*(11), 1686–1696.

American Diabetes Association. (2004). Smoking and diabetes. *Diabetes, 27*(Suppl 1), 74–75.

American Diabetes Association. (2009). Standards of medical care in diabetes – 2009. *Diabetes Care, 32*(Suppl 1), 13–61.

American Psychiatric Association. (2000). *Diagnostic and statistical manual of mental disorders (Revised 4th ed.)*. Washington, DC: Author.

American Psychiatric Association. (2002). *Practice guideline for the treatment of patients with bipolar disorder (revised)*. Washington, DC: Author.

Americans Diabetes Association, American Psychiatry Association, & American Association of Clinical Endocrinologists. (2006). Consensus development conference on antipsychotic drugs and obesity and diabetes. *The Journal of Clinical Psychiatry, 65*, 267–272.

Anderson, R. M. (1995). Patient empowerment and the traditional medical model. A case of irreconcilable differences? *Diabetes Care, 18*, 412–415.

Anderson, R. J., Freedland, K. E., & Clouse, R. E. (2001). The prevalence of comorbid depression in adults with diabetes: A meta-analysis. *Diabetes Care, 24*, 1069–1078.

Anderson, R. J., Grigsby, A. B., Freedland, K. E., de Groot, M., McGill, J. B., Clouse, R. E., et al. (2002). Anxiety and poor glycemic control: A meta-analytic review of the literature. *International Journal of Psychiatry in Medicine, 32*(3), 235–247.

Banerjea, R., Sambamoorthi, U., Smelson, D., & Pogach, L. (2008). Expenditures in mental illness and substance use disorders among veteran clinic users with diabetes. *The Journal of Behavioral Health Services & Research, 35*(3), 290–303.

Barnett, A. H., Mackin, P., Chaudhry, I., Farooqi, A., Gadsby, R., Heald, A., et al. (2007). Minimising metabolic and cardiovascular risk in schizophrenia: Diabetes, obesity and dyslipidaemia. *Journal of Psychopharmacology, 21*(4), 357–373.

Basu, A., & Meltzer, H. Y. (2006). Differential trends in prevalence of diabetes and unrelated general medical illness for schizophrenia patients before and after the atypical antipsychotic era. *Schizophrenia Research, 86*(1–3), 99–109.

Battaglia, M. R., Alemzadeh, R., Katte, H., Hall, P. L., & Perlmuter, L. C. (2006). Brief report: Disordered eating and psychosocial factors in adolescent females with type 1 diabetes mellitus. *Journal of Pediatric Psychology, 31*(6), 552–556.

Beck, A. T., Steer, R. A., & Brown, G. K. (1996). *Beck Depression Inventory (BDI)-II manual*. San Antonio, TX: The Psychological Corporation.

Bellivier, F. (2005). Schizophrenia, antipsychotics and diabetes: Genetic aspects. *European Psychiatry, 4*, 335–339.

Berland, N. W., Thompson, J. K., & Linton, P. H. (1986). Correlation between the EAT-26 and the EAT-40, the eating disorders inventory, and the restrained eating inventory. *The International Journal of Eating Disorders, 5*(3), 569–574.

Bijl, R. V., & Ravelli, A. (2000). Current and residual functional disability associated with psychopathology: Findings from the Netherlands Mental Health Survey and Incidence Study (NEMESIS). *Psychological Medicine, 30*, 657–668.

Black, S. A. (2002). Diabetes, diversity, and disparity: What do we do with the evidence? *American Journal of Public Health, 92*(4), 543–548.

Black, S. A., Markides, K. S., & Ray, L. A. (2003). Depression predicts increased incidence of adverse health outcomes in older Mexican Americans with type 2 diabetes. *Diabetes Care, 26*, 2822–2828.

Bogner, H., & de Vries, H. (2010). Integrating type 2 diabetes mellitus and depression treatment among African Americans: A randomized controlled pilot trial. *The Diabetes Educator, 36*, 284–292.

Bonds, D. E., Zaccaro, D. J., Karter, A. J., Selby, J. V., Saad, M., & Goff, D. C. (2003). Ethnic and racial differences in diabetes care. *Diabetes Care, 26*, 1040–1046.

Boyle, S., Allan, C., & Millar, K. (2004). Cognitive-behavioural interventions in a patient with an anxiety disorder related to diabetes. *Behaviour Research and Therapy, 42*(3), 357–366.

Bulik, C. M., Berkman, N. D., Brownley, K. A., Sedway, J. A., & Lohr, K. N. (2007). Anorexia nervosa treatment: A systematic review of randomized controlled trials. *The International Journal of Eating Disorders, 40*(4), 310–320.

Burroughs, T. E., Desikan, R., Waterman, B. M., Gilin, D., & McGill, J. (2004). Development and validation of the Diabetes Quality of Life Brief Clinical Inventory. *Diabetes Spectrum, 17*, 41–49.

Bushe, C., Haddad, P., Peveler, R., & Pendlebury, J. (2005). The role of lifestyle interventions and weight management in schizophrenia. *Journal of Psychopharmacology, 19*(Suppl 6), 28–35.

Bushe, C., & Holt, R. (2004). Prevalence of diabetes and impaired glucose tolerance in patients with schizophrenia. *The British Journal of Psychiatry, 184*(Suppl 47), 67–71.

Cantwell, R., & Steel, J. M. (1996). Screening for eating disorders in diabetes mellitus. *Journal of Psychosomatic Research, 40*(1), 15–20.

Carrizo, E., Fernandez, V., Connell, L., Sandia, I., Prieto, D., Mogollon, J., et al. (2009). Extended release metformin for metabolic control assistance during prolonged clozapine administration:

A 14-week, double-blind, parallel group, placebo-controlled study. *Schizophrenia Research, 113*, 19–26.
Carroll, L., & Owen, M. (2009). Genetic overlap between autism, schizophrenia and bipolar disorder. *Genome Medicine, 1*(10), 102.
Carroll, P., Tiggemann, M., & Wade, T. (1999). The role of body dissatisfaction and bingeing in the self-esteem of women with type II diabetes. *Journal of Behavioral Medicine, 22*(1), 59–74.
Centers for Disease Control and Prevention. (2005). *National diabetes fact sheet: General information and national estimates on diabetes in the United States, 2005*. Retrieved October 10th, 2009 from http://www.cdc.gov/Diabetes/pubs/pdf/ndfs_2005.pdf.
Centers for Disease Control and Prevention. (2008). Smoking-attributable mortality, years of potential life lost, and productivity losses – United States, 2000–2004. *Morbidity and Mortality Weekly Report, 57*(45), 1227–1232. Retrieved February 21st, 2009 from http://www.cdc.gov/mmwr/preview/mmwrhtml/mm5745a3.htm.
Chaudieu, I., Beluche, I., Norton, J., Boulenger, J. P., Ritchie, K., & Ancelin, M. L. (2008). Abnormal reactions to environmental stress in elderly persons with anxiety disorders: Evidence from a population study of diurnal cortisol changes. *Journal of Affective Disorders, 106*(3), 307–313.
Citrome, L., Blonde, L., & Damatarca, C. (2005). Metabolic issues in patients with severe mental illness. *Southern Medical Journal, 98*(7), 714–720.
Citrome, L., & Vreeland, B. (2008). Schizophrenia, obesity, and antipsychotic medications: What can we do? *Postgraduate Medicine, 120*(2), 18–33.
Clark, R., Weir, S., Ouellette, R., Zhang, J., & Baxter, J. (2009). Beyond health plans: Behavioral health disorders and quality of diabetes and asthma care for Medicaid beneficiaries. *Medical Care, 47*(5), 545–552.
Colton, P., Olmsted, M., Daneman, D., Rydall, A., & Rodin, G. (2004). Disturbed eating behavior and eating disorders in preteen and early teenage girls with type 1 diabetes: A case controlled study. *Diabetes Care, 27*(7), 1654–1659.
Cooper, Z., & Fairburn, C. G. (1987). Eating disorder examination (EDE): A semi-structured interview for the assessment of the specific psychopathology of eating disorders. *The International Journal of Eating Disorders, 6*(6), 1–8.
Cox, D. J., Irvine, A., Gonder-Frederick, L., Nowacek, G., & Butterfield, J. (1987). Fear of hypoglycemia: Quantification, validation, and utilization. *Diabetes Care, 10*(5), 617–621.
Cramer, J. A., & Pugh, M. J. (2005). The influence of insulin use on glycemic control: How well do adults follow prescriptions for insulin? *Diabetes Care, 28*(1), 78–83.
Crow, S. J., Keel, P. K., & Kendall, D. (1998). Eating disorders and insulin-dependent diabetes mellitus. *Psychosomatics, 39*(3), 233–243.
Crow, S. J., Kendall, D., Praus, B., & Thuras, P. (2001). Binge eating and other psychopathology in patients with type II diabetes mellitus. *The International Journal of Eating Disorders, 30*(2), 222–226.
Daneman, D., Rodin, G., Jones, J. M., Colton, P., Rydall, A., Maharaj, S. I., et al. (2002). Eating disorders in adolescent girls and young adult women with type 1 diabetes. *Diabetes Spectrum, 15*, 83–105.
de Groot, M., Anderson, R., Freedland, K. E., Clouse, R. E., & Lustman, P. J. (2001). Association of depression and diabetes complications: A meta-analysis. *Psychosomatic Medicine, 63*, 619–630.
de Leon, J., Susce, M., Diaz, F., Rendon, D., & Velásquez, D. (2005). Variables associated with alcohol, drug, and daily smoking cessation in patients with severe mental illnesses. *The Journal of Clinical Psychiatry, 66*(11), 1447–1455.
Diaz, F., James, D., Botts, S., Maw, L., Susce, M., & de Leon, J. (2009). Tobacco smoking behaviors in bipolar disorder: A comparison of the general population, schizophrenia, and major depression. *Bipolar Disorders, 11*(2), 154–165.
DiMatteo, M. R., Lepper, H. S., & Croghan, T. W. (2000). Depression is a risk factor for noncompliance with medical treatment: Meta-analysis of the effects of anxiety and depression on patient adherence. *Archives of Internal Medicine, 160*, 2101–2107.

Dinan, T. G. (2004). Stress and the genesis of diabetes mellitus in schizophrenia. *The British Journal of Psychiatry, 184*(Suppl 47), 72–75.

Diwan, A., Castine, M., Pomerleau, C., Meador-Woodruff, J., & Dalack, G. (1998). Differential prevalence of cigarette smoking in patients with schizophrenic vs mood disorders. *Schizophrenia Research, 33*(1–2), 113–118.

Dixon, L., Weiden, P., Delahanty, J., Goldberg, R., Postrado, L., Luckstead, A., et al. (2000). Prevalence and correlates of diabetes in national schizophrenia samples. *Schizophrenia Bulletin, 26*, 903–912.

Domino, M., & Swartz, M. (2008). Who are the new users of antipsychotic medications? *Psychiatric Services, 59*(5), 507–514.

Eaton, W., Martins, S., Nestadt, G., Bienvenu, O., Clarke, D., & Alexandre, P. (2008). The burden of mental disorders. *Epidemiologic Reviews, 30*, 1–14.

Ehlert, U., Gaab, J., & Heinrichs, M. (2001). Psychoneuroendocrinological contributions to the etiology of depression, posttraumatic stress disorder, and stress-related bodily disorders: The role of the hypothalamus–pituitary–adrenal axis. *Biological Psychology, 57*, 141–152.

El-Mallakh, P. (2006). Evolving self-care in individuals with schizophrenia and diabetes mellitus. *Archives of Psychiatric Nursing, 20*(2), 55–64.

El-Mallakh, P. (2007). Doing my best: Poverty and self-care among individuals with schizophrenia and diabetes mellitus. *Archives of Psychiatric Nursing, 21*(1), 49–60.

Elmslie, J. L., Silverstone, J. T., Mann, J. I., Williams, S. M., & Romans, S. E. (2000). Prevalence of overweight and obesity in bipolar patients. *The Journal of Clinical Psychiatry, 61*(3), 179–184.

Eren, I., Erdi, O., & Mehmet, S. (2008). The effect of depression on quality of life of patients with type II diabetes mellitus. *Depression and Anxiety, 25*, 98–106.

Fagiolini, A., Frank, E., Houck, P. R., Mallinger, A. G., Swartz, H. A., Buysse, D. J., et al. (2002). Prevalence of obesity and weight change during treatment in patients with bipolar disorder. *The Journal of Clinical Psychiatry, 63*, 528–533.

Fairburn, C. G., & Beglin, S. J. (1994). Assessment of eating disorders: Interview or self-report questionnaire? *The International Journal of Eating Disorders, 16*(4), 363–370.

Fernandez-Egea, E., Bernardo, M., Parellada, E., Justicia, A., Garcia-Rizo, C., Esmatjes, E., et al. (2008). Glucose abnormalities in the siblings of people with schizophrenia. *Schizophrenia Research, 103*(1–3), 110–113.

Fernandez-Egea, E., Miller, B., Bernardo, M., Donner, T., & Kirkpatrick, B. (2008). Parental history of type 2 diabetes in patients with nonaffective psychosis. *Schizophrenia Research, 98*(1–3), 302–306.

Fisher, L., Chesla, C. A., Mullan, J. T., Skaff, M. M., & Kanter, R. A. (2001). Contributions to depression in Latino and European-American patients with type 2 diabetes. *Diabetes Care, 24*, 1751–1757.

Fisher, L., Mullan, J., Arean, P., Glasgow, R., Hessler, D., & Masharani, U. (2010). Diabetes distress but not clinical depression or depressive symptoms is associated with glycemic control in both cross sectional and longitudinal analyses. *Diabetes Care, 33*, 23–28.

Fisher, L., Skaff, M. M., Mullan, J. T., Arean, P., Glasgow, R., & Masharani, U. (2008). A longitudinal study of affective and anxiety disorders, depressive affect and diabetes distress in adults with type 2 diabetes. *Diabetic Medicine, 25*(9), 1096–1101.

Fisher, L., Skaff, M. M., Mullan, J. T., Arean, P., Mohr, D., Masharani, U., et al. (2007). Clinical depression versus distress among patients with type 2 diabetes: Not just a question of semantics. *Diabetes Care, 30*(3), 542–548.

Folnegovic-Smalc, V., Jukic, V., Kozumplik, O., Mimica, N., & Uzun, S. (2004). Olanzapine use in a patient with schizophrenia and the risk of diabetes. *European Psychiatry, 19*(1), 62–64.

Fowler, M. J. (2007). Diabetes: Magnitude and mechanisms. *Clinical Diabetes, 25*(1), 25–28.

Frayne, S., Halanych, J., Miller, D., Wang, F., Lin, H., Pogach, L., et al. (2005). Disparities in diabetes care: Impact of mental illness. *Archives of Internal Medicine, 165*(22), 2631–2638.

Friedman, S., Vila, G., Timsit, J., Boitard, C., & Mouren-Simeoni, M. C. (1998). Anxiety and depressive disorders in an adult insulin-dependent diabetic mellitus (IDDM) population:

Relationships with glycaemic control and somatic complications. *European Psychiatry, 13*(6), 295–302.
Garner, D. M., & Garfinkel, P. E. (1979). Eating attitudes test. *Psychological Medicine, 9*(2), 273–279.
Garner, D. M., Olmsted, M. P., & Polivy, J. (1983). Eating disorder inventory. Development and validation of a multidimensional eating disorder inventory for anorexia nervosa and bulimia. *The International Journal of Eating Disorders, 2*(2), 15–34.
Glasgow, R. E., Boles, S. M., McKay, G., Feil, E. G., & Barrera, M., Jr. (2003). The D-Net diabetes self-management program: Long-term implementation, outcomes, and generalization results. *Preventive Medicine, 36*, 410–419.
Goebel-Fabbri, A., Firkan, J., Franko, D., Pearson, K., Anderson, B., & Weinger, K. (2008). Insulin restriction and associated morbidity and mortality in women with type 1 diabetes. *Diabetes Care, 31*, 415–419.
Goldberg, J. F. (2008, October 31). *Management of hypothyroidism in patients on lithium prophylaxis for bipolar disorder*. Retrieved January 28, 2010 from http://www.medscape.com/viewarticle/581200.
Golden, S. H. (2007). A review of the evidence for a neuroendocrine link between stress, depression and diabetes mellitus. *Current Diabetes Reviews, 3*(4), 252–259.
Gonzalez, J. S., McCarl, L., Wexler, D., Cagliero, E., Delahanty, L., Soper, T., et al. (2010). Cognitive behavioral therapy for adherence and depression (CBT-AD) in type 2 diabetes. *Journal of Cognitive Psychotherapy, 24*(4), 329–343.
Gonzalez, J. S., Peyrot, M., McCarl, L., Collins, E., Serpa, L., Mimiaga, M., et al. (2008). Depression and diabetes treatment nonadherence: A meta-analysis. *Diabetes Care, 31*, 2398–2403.
Gonzalez, J. S., Safren, S. A., Cagliero, E., Wexler, D. J., Delahanty, L., Wittenberg, E., et al. (2007). Depression, self-care, and medication adherence in type 2 diabetes: Relationships across the full range of symptom severity. *Diabetes Care, 30*, 2222–2227.
Gonzalez, J. S., Safren, S. A., Cagliero, E., Wexler, D. J., Meigs, J. B., & Grant, R. W. (2008). Symptoms of depression prospectively predict poorer self-care and medication adherence in patients with type 2 diabetes. *Diabetic Medicine, 25*, 1102–1107.
Goodnick, P. J. (2001). Use of antidepressants in treatment of comorbid diabetes mellitus and depression as well as in diabetic neuropathy. *Annals of Clinical Psychiatry, 13*, 31–41.
Goodnick, P. J., Henry, J. H., & Buki, V. M. (1995). Treatment of depression in patients with diabetes mellitus. *The Journal of Clinical Psychiatry, 56*, 128–136.
Goodwin, R. D., Hoven, C. W., & Spitzer, R. L. (2003). Diabetes and eating disorders in primary care. *The International Journal of Eating Disorders, 33*(1), 85–91.
Gorin, A. A., Niemeier, H. M., Hogan, P., Coday, M., Davis, C., DiLillo, V. G., et al. (2008). Binge eating and weight loss outcomes in overweight and obese individuals with type 2 diabetes: Results from the look AHEAD trial. *Archives of General Psychiatry, 65*(12), 1447–1455.
Gough, S., & Peveler, R. (2004). Diabetes and its prevention: Pragmatic solutions for people with schizophrenia. *The British Journal of Psychiatry, 184*, 106–111.
Grant, R., Hamrick, H., Sullivan, C., Dubey, A., Chueh, H., Cagliero, E., et al. (2003). Impact of population management with direct physician feedback on care of patients with type 2 diabetes. *Diabetes Care, 26*(8), 2275–2280.
Green, L., Feher, M., & Catalan, J. (2000). Fears and phobias in people with diabetes. *Diabetes/Metabolism Research and Reviews, 16*(4), 287–293.
Grey, M., Boland, E. A., Davidson, M., Li, J., & Tamborlane, W. V. (2000). Coping skills training for youth with diabetes mellitus has long-lasting effects on metabolic control and quality of life. *The Journal of Pediatrics, 137*(1), 107–113.
Grigsby, A. B., Anderson, R. J., Freedland, K. E., Clouse, R. E., & Lustman, P. J. (2002). Prevalence of anxiety in adults with diabetes: A systematic review. *Journal of Psychosomatic Research, 53*(6), 1053–1060.
Grilo, C. M., Masheb, R. M., & Wilson, G. T. (2001). Different methods for assessing the features of eating disorders in patients with binge eating disorder: A replication. *Obesity Research, 9*(7), 418–422.

Haddad, P., & Sharma, S. (2007). Adverse effects of atypical antipsychotics: Differential risk and clinical implications. *CNS Drugs, 21*(11), 911–936.

Haire-Joshu, D., Glasgow, R., & Tibbs, T. (2004). Smoking and diabetes. *Diabetes Care, 27*(Suppl 1), 74–75.

Harris, M. I., Flegal, K. M., Cowie, C. C., Eberhardt, M. S., Goldstein, D. E., Little, R. R., et al. (1998). Prevalence of diabetes, impaired fasting glucose, and impaired glucose tolerance in U.S. adults: The Third National Health and Nutrition Examination Survey, 1988-1994. *Diabetes Care, 21*, 518–524.

Harris, M. A., & Lustman, P. J. (1998). The psychologist in diabetes care. *Clinical Diabetes, 16*, 91–93.

Hartz, A., Kent, S., James, P., Xu, Y., Kelly, M., & Daly, J. (2006). Factors that influence improvement for patients with poorly controlled type 2 diabetes. *Diabetes Research and Clinical Practice, 74*, 227–232.

Healton, C. G., Vallone, D., McCausland, K. L., Xiao, H., & Green, M. P. (2006). Smoking, obesity, and their co-occurrence in the United States: Cross sectional analysis. *British Medical Journal, 333*(7557), 25–26.

Henry, J. L., Wilson, P. H., Bruce, D. G., Chisholm, D. J., & Rawling, P. J. (1997). Cognitive-behavioural stress management for patients with non-insulin dependent diabetes mellitus. *Psychology, Health & Medicine, 2*(2), 109–118.

Herpertz, S., Albus, C., Wagener, R., Kocnar, M., Wagner, R., Henning, A., et al. (1998). Comorbidity of diabetes and eating disorders. Does diabetes control reflect disturbed eating behavior? *Diabetes Care, 21*(7), 1110–1116.

Herpertz, S., Wagener, R., Albus, C., Kocnar, M., Wagner, R., Best, F., et al. (1998). Diabetes mellitus and eating disorders: A multicenter study on the comorbidity of the two diseases. *Journal of Psychosomatic Research, 44*(3–4), 503–515.

Himelhoch, S., Leith, J., Goldberg, R., Kreyenbuhl, J., Medoff, D., & Dixon, L. (2009). Care and management of cardiovascular risk factors among individuals with schizophrenia and type 2 diabetes who smoke. *General Hospital Psychiatry, 31*(1), 30–32.

Ho, P., Rumsfeld, J., Masoudi, F., McClure, D., Plomondon, M., Steiner, J., et al. (2006). Effect of medication nonadherence on hospitalization and mortality among patients with diabetes mellitus. *Archives of Internal Medicine, 166*(17), 1836–1841.

Holt, R., & Peveler, R. (2006). Association between antipsychotic drugs and diabetes. *Diabetes, Obesity & Metabolism, 8*(2), 125–135.

Holt, R., Peveler, R., & Byrne, C. (2004). Schizophrenia, the metabolic syndrome and diabetes. *Diabetic Medicine, 21*(6), 515–523.

Hudson, J. I., Hiripi, E., Pope, H. G., Jr., & Kessler, R. C. (2007). The prevalence and correlates of eating disorders in the national comorbidity survey replication. *Biological Psychiatry, 61*(3), 348–358.

Ingersoll, K. S., & Cohen, J. (2008). The impact of medication regimen factors on adherence to chronic treatment: A review of literature. *Journal of Behavioral Medicine, 31*(3), 213–224.

Ismail, K. (2008). Eating disorders and diabetes. *Psychiatry, 7*(4), 179–182.

Ismail, K., Winkley, K., & Rabe-Hesketh, S. (2004). Systematic review and meta-analysis of randomised controlled trials of psychological interventions to improve glycaemic control in patients with type 2 diabetes. *The Lancet, 363*, 1589–1597.

Jacobson, A. M. (1996). The psychological care of patients with insulin dependent diabetes mellitus. *The New England Journal of Medicine, 334*(19), 1249–1253.

Jain, A. K., Kaplan, R. A., Gadde, K. M., Wadden, T. A., Allison, D. B., Brewer, E. R., et al. (2002). Bupropion SR vs. placebo for weight loss in obese patients with depressive symptoms. *Obesity Research, 10*(10), 1049–1056.

Joffe, H., Cohen, L., Suppes, T., Hwang, C., Molay, F., Adams, J., et al. (2006). Longitudinal follow-up of reproductive and metabolic features of valproate-associated polycystic ovarian syndrome features: A preliminary report. *Biological Psychiatry, 60*(12), 1378–1381.

Johnson, K., Bazargan, M., & Cherpitel, C. (2001). Alcohol, tobacco, and drug use and the onset of type 2 diabetes among inner-city minority patients. *The Journal of the American Board of Family Practice, 14*(6), 430–436.

Kahn, L. S., Fox, C. H., McIntyre, R. S., Tumiel-Berhalter, L., Berdine, D. E., & Lyle, H. (2008). Assessing the prevalence of depression among individuals with diabetes in Medicaid managed-care program. *International Journal of Psychiatry in Medicine, 38*, 13–29.
Karlsen, B., Idsoe, T., Dirdal, I., Hanestad, B. R., & Bru, E. (2004). Effects of a group-based counseling programme on diabetes-related stress, coping, psychological well-being and metabolic control in adults with type 1 or type 2 diabetes. *Patient Education and Counseling, 53*(3), 299–308.
Katon, W., Fan, M., Unützer, J., Taylor, J., Pincus, H., & Schoenbaum, M. (2008). Depression and diabetes: A potentially lethal combination. *Journal of General Internal Medicine, 23*, 1571–1575.
Katon, W. J., Lin, E. H., Russo, J., Von Korff, M., Ciechanowski, P., Simon, G., et al. (2004). Cardiac risk factors in patients with diabetes mellitus and major depression. *Journal of General Internal Medicine, 19*, 1192–1199.
Katon, W. J., Rutter, C., Simon, G., Lin, E. H., Ludman, E., Ciechanowski, P., et al. (2005). The association of comorbid depression with mortality in patients with type 2 diabetes. *Diabetes Care, 28*, 2668–2672.
Katon, W., Von Korff, M., Ciechanowski, P., Russo, J., Lin, E., Simon, G., et al. (2004). Behavioral and clinical factors associated with depression among individuals with diabetes. *Diabetes Care, 27*(4), 914–920.
Katon, W., Von Korff, M., Lin, E., Simon, G., Ludman, E., Bush, T., et al. (2003). Improving primary care treatment of depression among patients with diabetes mellitus: The design of the Pathways Study. *General Hospital Psychiatry, 25*, 158–168.
Katz, I. R. (1996). On the inseparability of mental and physical health in aged persons: Lessons from depression and medical comorbidity. *The American Journal of Geriatric Psychiatry, 4*, 1–16.
Keller, M. B., & Hanks, D. L. (1995). Anxiety symptom relief in depression treatment outcomes. *The Journal of Clinical Psychiatry, 56*(Suppl 6), 22–29.
Kelly, S., Howe, C., Hendler, J., & Lipman, T. (2005). Disordered eating behaviors in youth with type 1 diabetes. *The Diabetes Educator, 31*, 572–583.
Kenardy, J., Mensch, M., Bowen, K., Green, B., & Walton, J. (2002). Group therapy for binge eating in type 2 diabetes: A randomized trial. *Diabetic Medicine, 19*(3), 234–239.
Kessler, R. C., Berglund, P. A., Bruce, M. L., Koch, J. R., Lask, E. M., Leaf, P. J., et al. (2001). The prevalence and correlates of untreated serious mental illness. *Health Services Research, 36*, 987–1007.
Kessler, R. C., Berglund, P., Demler, O., Jin, R., Merikangas, K. R., & Walters, E. E. (2005). Lifetime prevalence and age-of-onset distributions of DSM-IV disorders in the National Comorbidity Survey Replication. *Archives of General Psychiatry, 62*(6), 593–602.
Kessler, R. C., Borges, G., & Walters, E. E. (1999). Prevalence of and risk factors for lifetime suicide attempts in the National Comorbidity Survey. *Archives of General Psychiatry, 56*, 617–626.
Kessler, R. C., Chiu, W. T., Demler, O., & Walters, E. E. (2005). Prevalence, severity, and comorbidity of 12-month DSM-IV disorders in the National Comorbidity Survey Replication. *Archives of General Psychiatry, 62*(6), 617–627.
Kichler, J. C., Foster, C., & Opipari Arrigan, L. (2008). The relationship between negative communication and body image dissatisfaction in adolescent females with type 1 diabetes mellitus. *Journal of Health Psychology, 13*(3), 336–347.
Kilbourne, A. M., Cornelius, J. R., Han, X., Pincus, H. A., Shad, M., Salloum, I., et al. (2004). Burden of general medical conditions among individuals with bipolar disorder. *Bipolar Disorders, 6*, 368–373.
Klerman, G. L., & Weissman, M. M. (1989). Increasing rates of depression. *Journal of the American Medical Association, 261*, 2229–2235.
Klerman, G. L., & Weissman, M. M. (1992). The course, morbidity, and costs of depression. *Archives of General Psychiatry, 49*, 831–834.
Kohen, D. (2004). Diabetes mellitus and schizophrenia: Historical perspective. *The British Journal of Psychiatry, 184*, 64–66.
Koro, C. E., Fedder, D. O., L'Italien, G. J., Weiss, S. S., Magder, L. S., Kreyenbuhl, J., et al. (2002). Assessment of independent effect of olanzapine and risperidone on risk of diabetes among

patients with schizophrenia: Population based nested case-control study. *British Medical Journal, 325*(7358), 243–247.

Kreyenbuhl, J., Buchanan, R., Dickerson, F., & Dixon, L. (2010). The Schizophrenia Patient Outcomes Research Team (PORT): Updated treatment recommendations 2009. *Schizophrenia Bulletin, 36*(1), 94–103.

Kreyenbuhl, J., Dixon, L. B., McCarthy, J. F., Soliman, S., Ignacio, R. V., & Valenstein, M. (2008). Does adherence to medications for type 2 diabetes differ between individuals with vs without schizophrenia? *Schizophrenia Bulletin* (Advance online publication). doi:10.1093/schbul/sbn106.

Kroenke, K., Spitzer, R. L., & Williams, J. B. (2001). The PHQ-9: Validity of a brief depression severity measure. *International Journal of General Medicine, 16*(9), 606–613.

Kupka, R. W., Nolen, W. A., Post, R. M., McElroy, S. L., Altshuler, L. L., Denicoff, K. D., et al. (2002). High rate of autoimmune thyroiditis in bipolar disorder: Lack of association with lithium exposure. *Biological Psychiatry, 51*(4), 305–311.

Larkin, M. E., Capasso, V. A., Chen, C., Mahoney, E. K., Hazard, B., Cagliero, E., et al. (2008). Measuring psychological insulin resistance: Barriers to insulin use. *The Diabetes Educator, 34*(3), 511–517.

Lasser, K., Boyd, J., Woolhandler, S., Himmelstein, D., McCormick, D., & Bor, D. (2000). Smoking and mental illness: A population-based prevalence study. *Journal of the American Medical Association, 284*(20), 2606–2610.

Lee, P., Greenfield, J., & Campbell, L. (2009). Managing young people with type 1 diabetes in a 'rave' new world: Metabolic complications of substance abuse in type 1 diabetes. *Diabetic Medicine, 26*(4), 328–333.

Li, C., Barker, L., Ford, E. S., Zhang, X., Strine, T. W., & Mokdad, A. H. (2008). Diabetes and anxiety in US adults: Findings from the 2006 behavioral risk factor surveillance system. *Diabetic Medicine, 25*(7), 878–881.

Li, C., Ford, E., Zhao, G., Balluz, L., Berry, J., & Mokdad, A. (2010). Undertreatment of mental health problems in adults with diagnosed diabetes and serious psychological distress: The Behavioral Risk Factor Surveillance System, 2007. *Diabetes Care, 33*(5), 1061–1064.

Li, C., Ford, E. S., Zhao, G., Strine, T. W., Dhingra, S., Barker, L., et al. (2009). Association between diagnosed diabetes and serious psychological distress among U.S. adults: The Behavioral Risk Factor Surveillance System, 2007. *International Journal of Public Health, 54*, S43–S51.

Lin, E. H., Korff, M. V., Alonso, J., Angermeyer, M. C., Anthony, J., Bromet, E., et al. (2008). Mental disorders among persons with diabetes – Results from the World Mental Health Surveys. *Journal of Psychosomatic Research, 65*, 571–580.

Livingstone, C., & Rampes, H. (2006). Lithium: A review of its metabolic adverse effects. *Psychopharmacology, 20*, 347–355.

Llorente, M. D., & Uruita, V. (2006). Diabetes, psychiatric disorders, and the metabolic effects of antipsychotic medications. *Clinical Diabetes, 24*(1), 18–24.

Loh, C., Meyer, J., & Leckband, S. (2008). Accuracy of body image perception and preferred weight loss strategies in schizophrenia: A controlled pilot study. *Acta Psychiatrica Scandinavica, 117*(2), 127–132.

Lucksted, A., McGuire, C., Postrado, L., Kreyenbuhl, J., & Dixon, L. (2004). Specifying cigarette smoking and quitting among people with serious mental illness. *The American Journal on Addictions, 13*(2), 128–138.

Ludman, E., Katon, W., Russo, J., Simon, G., Von Korff, M., Lin, E., et al. (2006). Panic episodes among patients with diabetes. *General Hospital Psychiatry, 28*(6), 475–481.

Lustman, P. J., Anderson, R. J., Freedland, K. E., de Groot, M., Carney, R. M., & Clouse, R. E. (2000). Depression and poor glycemic control: A meta-analytic review of the literature. *Diabetes Care, 23*, 934–942.

Lustman, P., Clouse, R., Griffith, L., & Carney, R. (1997). Screening for depression in diabetes using the Beck Depression Inventory. *Psychosomatic Medicine, 59*(1), 24–31.

Lustman, P. J., Griffith, L. S., Clouse, R. E., Freedland, K. E., Eisen, S. A., Rubin, E. H., Carne, R. M., & McGill, J. B. (1995). Effects of alprazolam on glucose regulation in diabetes. Results of double-blind, placebo-controlled trial. *Diabetes Care, 18*(8), 1133–1139.
Lustman, P. J., Williams, M. M., Sayuk, G. S., Nix, B. D., & Clouse, R. E. (2007). Factors influencing glycemic control in type 2 diabetes during acute- and maintenance-phase treatment of major depressive disorder with bupropion. *Diabetes Care, 30*, 459–466.
MacGillivray, S., Arroll, B., Hatcher, S., Ogston, S., Reid, I., Sullivan, F., et al. (2003). Efficacy and tolerability of selective serotonin reuptake inhibitors compared with tricyclic antidepressants in depression treated in primary care: Systematic review and meta-analysis. *British Medical Journal, 326*, 1014–1020.
Mannucci, E., Tesi, F., Ricca, V., Pierazzuoli, E., Barciulli, E., Moretti, S., et al. (2002). Eating behavior in obese patients with and without type 2 diabetes mellitus. *Obesity (Silver Spring), 26*(6), 848–853.
Marder, S., Essock, S., Miller, A., Buchanan, R., Davis, J., Kane, J., et al. (2002). The Mount Sinai Conference on the pharmacotherapy of schizophrenia. *Schizophrenia Bulletin, 28*(1), 5–16.
Markowitz, S., Gonzalez, J., Wilkinson, J., & Safren, S. (2011). Treating depression in diabetes: Emerging findings. *Psychosomatics, 52*(1), 1–18.
McClave, A., Dube, S., Strine, T., Kroenke, K., Caraballo, R., & Mokdad, A. (2009). Associations between smoking cessation and anxiety and depression among U.S. adults. *Addictive Behaviors, 34*(6–7), 491–497.
McCreadie, R. G. (2003). Diet, smoking and cardiovascular risk in people with schizophrenia. *The British Journal of Psychiatry, 183*, 534–539.
McEvoy, J., & Allen, T. (2003). Substance abuse (including nicotine) in schizophrenic patients. *Current Opinion in Psychiatry, 16*(2), 199–205.
McEvoy, J., Meyer, J., Goff, D., Nasrallah, H., Davis, S., Sullivan, L., et al. (2005). Prevalence of the metabolic syndrome in patients with schizophrenia: Baseline results from the Clinical Antipsychotic Trials of Intervention Effectiveness (CATIE) schizophrenia trial and comparison with national estimates from NHANES III. *Schizophrenia Research, 80*(1), 19–32.
McGinnis, R. A., McGrady, A., Cox, S. A., & Grower-Dowling, K. A. (2005). Biofeedback-assisted relaxation in type 2 diabetes. *Diabetes Care, 28*, 2145–2149.
McGuffin, P., Rijsdijk, F., Andrew, M., Sham, P., Katz, R., & Cardno, A. (2003). The heritability of bipolar affective disorder and the genetic relationship to unipolar depression. *Archives of General Psychiatry, 60*, 497–502.
McIntyre, R. S., Konarski, J. Z., Misener, V. L., & Kennedy, S. H. (2005). Bipolar disorder and diabetes mellitus: Epidemiology, etiology, and treatment implications. *Annals of Clinical Psychiatry, 17*(2), 83–93.
McKibbin, C., Patterson, T., Norman, G., Patrick, K., Jin, H., Roesch, S., et al. (2006). A lifestyle intervention for older schizophrenia patients with diabetes mellitus: A randomized controlled trial. *Schizophrenia Research, 86*(1–3), 36–44.
Mezuk, B., Eaton, W. W., Albrecht, S., & Golden, S. H. (2008). Depression and type 2 diabetes over the lifespan: A meta-analysis. *Diabetes Care, 31*(12), 383–390.
Miller, M., & Pumariega, A. (2001). Culture and eating disorders: A historical and cross-cultural review. *Psychiatry, 64*(2), 93–110.
Miranda, J., Chung, J. Y., Green, B. L., Krupnick, J., Siddique, J., Revicki, D. A., et al. (2003). Treating depression in predominantly low-income young minority women: A randomized controlled trial. *Journal of the American Medical Association, 290*, 57–65.
Mitsonis, C., Dimopoulous, N., & Psarra, V. (2009). Clinical implications of anxiety in diabetes: A critical review of the evidence base. *European Psychiatry, 24*(1), 526.
Mollema, E. D., Snoek, F. J., Ader, H. J., Heine, R. J., & van der Ploeg, H. M. (2001). Insulin-treated diabetes patients with fear of self-injecting or fear of self-testing: Psychological comorbidity and general well-being. *Journal of Psychosomatic Research, 51*(5), 665–672.
Mollema, E. D., Snoek, F. J., Heine, R. J., & van der Ploeg, H. M. (2001). Phobia of self-injecting and self-testing in insulin-treated diabetes patients: Opportunities for screening. *Diabetic Medicine, 18*(8), 671–674.

Morse, S. A., Ciechanowski, P. S., Katon, W. J., & Hirsch, I. B. (2006). Isn't this just bedtime snacking? The potential adverse effects of night-eating symptoms on treatment adherence and outcomes in patients with diabetes. *Diabetes Care, 29*(8), 1800–1804.

Mueser, K., & Gingerich, S. (2006). *The complete family guide to schizophrenia*. New York, NY: Guilford.

Mueser, K., & McGurk, S. (2004). Schizophrenia. *The Lancet, 363*(9426), 2063–2072.

Musselman, D., Betan, E., Larsen, H., & Phillips, L. (2003). Relationship of depression to diabetes types 1 and 2: Epidemiology, biology, and treatment. *Biological Psychiatry, 54*(3), 317–329.

Myers, V. H., Boyer, B. A., Herbert, J. D., Barakat, L. P., & Scheiner, G. (2007). Fear of hypoglycemia and self reported posttraumatic stress in adults with diabetes type I treated by intensive regimens. *Journal of Clinical Psychology in Medical Settings, 14*(1), 11–21.

Nair, R., Lawler, L., & Miller, M. (2007). Chronic pancreatitis. *American Family Physician, 76*(11), 1679–1688.

Neumark-Sztainer, D., Patterson, J., Mellin, A., Ackard, D. M., Utter, J., Story, M., et al. (2002). Weight control practices and disordered eating behaviors among adolescent females and males with type 1 diabetes: Associations with sociodemographics, weight concerns, familial factors, and metabolic outcomes. *Diabetes Care, 25*(8), 1289–1296.

Newman, S., Steed, L., & Mulligan, K. (2004). Self-management interventions for chronic illness. *The Lancet, 364*, 1523–1537.

Nielsen, S., Emborg, C., & Molbak, A.-G. (2002). Mortality in concurrent type 1 diabetes and anorexia nervosa. *Diabetes Care, 25*, 309–312.

Norris, S. L., Engelgau, M. M., & Venkat Narayan, K. M. (2001). Self-management training in type 2 diabetes. *Diabetes Care, 24*, 561–578.

Norris, S., Zhang, X., Avenell, A., Gregg, E., Bowman, B., & Serdula, M. (2004). Long-term effectiveness of lifestyle and behavioral weight loss interventions in adults with type 2 diabetes: A meta-analysis. *The American Journal of Medicine, 117*, 762–774.

O'Kane, M. J., Bunting, B., Copeland, M., & Coates, V. E. (2008). Efficacy of self monitoring of blood glucose in patients with newly diagnosed type 2 diabetes (ESMON study): Randomised controlled trial. *British Medical Journal, 336*, 1177–1180.

Okada, S., Ichiki, K., Tanokuchi, S., Ishii, K., Hamada, H., & Ota, Z. (1994). Effect of an anxiolytic on lipid profile in non-insulin-dependent diabetes mellitus. *The Journal of International Medical Research, 22*(6), 338–342.

Osborn, C. Y., Trott, H. W., Buchowski, M. S., Patel, K. A., Kirby, L. D., Hargreaves, M. K., et al. (2010). Racial disparities in the treatment of depression in low-income persons with diabetes. *Diabetes Care, 5*, 1050–1054.

Papelbaum, M., Appolinario, J. C., Moreira Rde, O., Ellinger, V. C., Kupfer, R., & Coutinho, W. F. (2005). Prevalence of eating disorders and psychiatric comorbidity in a clinical sample of type 2 diabetes mellitus patients. *Revista Brasileira de Psiquiatria, 27*(2), 135–138.

Parks, J., Svendsen, D., Singer, P., Foti, M., & Mauer, B. (2006). *Morbidity and mortality in people with serious mental illness*. National Association of State Mental Health Program Directors. Retrieved November 11, 2009 from http://www.nasmhpd.org.

Peet, M. (2004). Diet, diabetes and schizophrenia: Review and hypothesis. *The British Journal of Psychiatry. Supplement, 47*, 102–105.

Pendlebury, J., & Holt, R. (2008). Supporting the lifestyle modification and treatment of type 2 diabetes for people with severe mental illness. *European Diabetes Nursing, 5*(2), 58–63.

Pennix, B. W., Guralnik, J. M., Lerrucci, L., Simonsick, E. M., Deeg, D. J., & Wallace, R. B. (1998). Depressive symptoms and physical decline in community-dwelling older persons. *Journal of the American Medical Association, 279*, 1720–1726.

Pennix, B. W., Leveille, S., Ferrucci, L., van Eijk, J. T., & Guralnik, J. M. (1999). Exploring the effects of depression of physical disability: Longitudinal evidence established populations for epidemiologic studies of the elderly. *American Journal of Public Health, 89*, 1346–1352.

Petrak, F., Herpertz, S., Albus, C., Hirsch, A., Kulzer, B., & Kruse, J. (2005). Psychosocial factors and diabetes mellitus: Evidence-based treatment guidelines. *Current Diabetes Reviews, 1*(3), 255–270.

Peveler, R. C., Bryden, K. S., Neil, H. A., Fairburn, C. G., Mayou, R. A., Dunger, D. B., et al. (2005). The relationship of disordered eating habits and attitudes to clinical outcomes in young adult females with type 1 diabetes. *Diabetes Care, 28*(1), 84–88.

Peyrot, M., McMurry, J. F., & Kruger, D. F. (1999). A biosocial model of glycemic control in diabetes: Stress, coping, and regimen influence. *Journal of Health and Social Behavior, 40*, 141–158.

Peyrot, M., & Rubin, R. (1997). Levels and risks of depression and anxiety symptomatology among diabetic adults. *Diabetes Care, 20*(4), 585–590.

Philip, N., Carpenter, L., Tyrka, A., & Price, L. (2008). Augmentation of antidepressants with atypical antipsychotics: A review of the current literature. *Journal of Psychiatric Practice, 14*(1), 34–44.

Phillips, P., & Johnson, S. (2001). How does drug and alcohol misuse develop among people with psychotic illness? A literature review. *Social Psychiatry and Psychiatric Epidemiology, 36*(6), 269–276.

Piette, J. D., Heisler, M., Ganoczy, D., McCarthy, J. F., & Valenstein, M. (2007). Differential medication adherence among patients with schizophrenia and comorbid diabetes and hypertension. *Psychiatric Services, 58*(2), 207–212.

Polivy, J., & Herman, C. (1985). Dieting and bingeing: A casual analysis. *The American Psychologist, 40*(2), 193–201.

Polonsky, W. (2002). Emotional and quality-of-life aspects of diabetes management. *Current Diabetes Reports, 2*(2), 153–159.

Polonsky, W. H., Davis, C. L., Jacobson, A. M., & Anderson, B. J. (1992). Correlates of hypoglycemic fear in type I and type II diabetes mellitus. *Health Psychology, 11*(3), 199–202.

Polonsky, W. H., Fisher, L., Earles, J., Dudl, R. J., Lees, J., Mullan, J. T., et al. (2005). Assessing psychosocial stress in diabetes. *Diabetes Care, 28*, 626–631.

Pramming, S., Thorsteinsson, B., Bendtson, I., & Binder, C. (1991). Symptomatic hypoglycaemia in 411 type 1 diabetic patients. *Diabetic Medicine, 8*(3), 217–222.

Pratt, L., Dey, A., & Cohen, A. (2007). Characteristics of adults with serious psychological distress as measured by the K6 scale: United States, 2001-04. *Advance Data, 382*, 1–18.

Purcell, S., Wray, N., Stone, J., Visscher, P., O'Donovan, M., Sullivan, P., et al. (2009). Common polygenic variation contributes to risk of schizophrenia and bipolar disorder. *Nature, 460*(7256), 748–752.

Radloff, L. S. (1977). The CES–D Scale: A self report depression scale for research in the general population. *Applied Psychological Measurement, 1*, 385–401.

Ravert, R. (2009). Alcohol management strategies of college students with diabetes. *Patient Education and Counseling, 77*(1), 97–102.

Regenold, W. T., Thapar, R. K., Marano, C., Gavirneni, S., & Kondapavuluru, P. V. (2002). Increased prevalence of type 2 diabetes mellitus among psychiatric in patients with bipolar I affective and schizoaffective disorders independent of psychotropic drug use. *Journal of Affective Disorders, 70*(1), 19–26.

Riggs, P., Levin, F., Green, A. I., & Vocci, F. (2008). Comorbid psychiatric and substance abuse disorders: Recent treatment research. *Substance Abuse, 29*(3), 51–63.

Risérus, U., & Ingelsson, E. (2007). Alcohol intake, insulin resistance, and abdominal obesity in elderly men. *Obesity (Silver Spring), 15*(7), 1766–1773.

Rodin, G., Craven, J., Littlefield, C., & Murray, M. (1991). Eating disorders and intentional insulin undertreatment in adolescent females with diabetes. *Psychosomatics, 32*(2), 171–176.

Rodin, G., & Daneman, D. (1992). Eating disorders and IDDM. A problematic association. *Diabetes Care, 15*(10), 1402–1412.

Rodin, G., Olmsted, M. P., Rydall, A. C., Maharaj, S. I., Colton, P. A., Jones, J. M., et al. (2002). Eating disorders in young women with type 1 diabetes mellitus. *Journal of Psychosomatic Research, 53*(4), 943–949.

Rosenzweig, S., Reibel, D., Greeson, J., Jasser, S., & McMearty, K. (2007). Mindfulness-based stress reduction is associated with improved glycemic control in type 2 diabetes mellitus: A pilot study. *Alternative Therapies in Health and Medicine, 13*, 36–37.

Rouillon, F., & Sorbara, F. (2005). Schizophrenia and diabetes: Epidemiological data. *European Psychiatry, 20*(Suppl 4), 345–348.

Rubin, R. (2005). Adherence to pharmacologic therapy in patients with type 2 diabetes mellitus. *The American Journal of Medicine, 118*(Suppl 5A), 27–34.

Rubin, R. R., & Peyrot, M. (2001). Psychological issues and treatments for people with diabetes. *Journal of Clinical Psychology, 57*(4), 457–478.

Rubin, R., Peyrot, M., & Saudek, C. (1993). The effect of a comprehensive diabetes education program incorporating coping skills training on emotional wellbeing and diabetes self-efficacy. *The Diabetes Educator, 19*(3), 210–214.

Russell, L. B., Suh, D. C., & Safford, M. A. (2005). Time requirements for diabetes self-management: Too much for many? *The Journal of Family Practice, 54*, 52–56.

Ruzickova, M., Slaney, C., Garnham, J., & Alda, M. (2003). Clinical features of bipolar disorder with and without comorbid diabetes mellitus. *Canadian Journal of Psychiatry, 48*(7), 458–461.

Ryan, M., Gallanagh, J., Livingstone, M. B., Gaillard, C., & Ritz, P. (2008). The prevalence of abnormal eating behaviour in a representative sample of the French diabetic population. *Diabetes & Metabolism, 34*(6 Pt 1), 581–586.

Rydall, A. C., Rodin, G. M., Olmsted, M. P., & Devenyi, R. G. (1997). Disordered eating behavior and microvascular complications in young women with insulin-dependent diabetes mellitus. *The New England Journal of Medicine, 336*(26), 1849–1854.

Safren, S., Gonzalez, J., & Soroudi, N. (2008a). *CBT for depression and adherence in individuals with chronic illness: Client workbook (treatments that work)*. New York, NY: Oxford University Press.

Safren, S., Gonzalez, J., & Soroudi, N. (2008b). *CBT for depression and adherence in individuals with chronic illness: Therapist guide (treatments that work)*. New York, NY: Oxford University Press.

Safren, S. A., O'Cleirigh, C., Tan, J., Raminani, S., Reilly, L. C., Otto, M. W., et al. (2009). A randomized controlled trial of cognitive behavioral therapy for adherence and depression (CBT-AD) in HIV-infected individuals. *Health Psychology, 28*(1), 1–10.

Saydah, S. H., Fradkin, J., & Cowie, C. C. (2004). Poor control of risk factors for vascular disease among adults with previously diagnosed diabetes. *Journal of the American Medical Association, 291*(3), 335–342.

Schenck, C. H. (2006). A study of circadian eating and sleeping patterns in night eating syndrome (NES) points the way to future studies on NES and sleep-related eating disorder. *Sleep Medicine, 7*(8), 653–656.

Schraufnagel, T. J., Wagner, A. W., Miranda, J., & Roy-Byrne, P. P. (2006). Treating minority patients with depression and anxiety: What does the evidence tell us? *General Hospital Psychiatry, 28*, 27–36.

Sclar, D. A., Robinson, L. M., Skaer, T. L., & Galin, R. S. (1998). Trends in the prescribing of antidepressant pharmacotherapy: Office-based visits, 1990-1995. *Clinical Therapeutics, 20*, 871–884.

Sernyak, M. J., Leslie, D. L., Alarcon, R. D., Losonczy, M. F., & Rosenheck, R. (2002). Association of diabetes mellitus with use of atypical neuroleptics in the treatment of schizophrenia. *The American Journal of Psychiatry, 159*(4), 561–566.

Seymour, H., Gilman, D., & Quin, J. (1996). Severe ketoacidosis complicated by 'ecstasy' ingestion and prolonged exercise. *Diabetic Medicine, 13*(10), 908–909.

Shaw, J., Sicree, R., & Zimmet, P. (2010). Global estimates of the prevalence of diabetes for 2010 and 2030. *Diabetes Research and Clinical Practice, 87*(1), 4–14.

Sheldon, B. H., & Quin, J. D. (2005). Diabetes and illicit drug use. *Practical Diabetes International, 22*(6), 222–224.

Smith, M., Hopkins, D., Peveler, R. C., Holt, R., Woodward, M., & Ismail, K. (2008). First-v. second-generation antipsychotics and risk for diabetes in schizophrenia: Systematic review and meta-analysis. *The British Journal of Psychiatry, 192*, 406–411.

Snoek, F. J., Mollema, E. D., Heine, R. J., Bouter, L. M., & van der Ploeg, H. M. (1997). Development and validation of the Diabetes Fear of Injecting and Self-Testing Questionnaire (D-FISQ): First findings. *Diabetic Medicine, 14*, 871–876.

Snoek, F. J., & Skinner, T. C. (2002). Psychological counselling in problematic diabetes: Does it help? *Diabetic Medicine, 19*(4), 265–273.

Soo, H., & Lam, S. (2009). Stress management training in diabetes mellitus. *Journal of Health Psychology, 14*, 933–943.

Soroudi, N., Perez, G., Gonzalez, J., Greer, J., Pollack, M., Otto, M., et al. (2008). CBT for medication adherence and depression (CBT-AD) in HIV-infected patients receiving methadone maintenance therapy. *Cognitive and Behavioral Practice, 15*, 93–106.

Spangler, J., Summerson, J., Bell, R., & Konen, J. (2001). Smoking status and psychosocial variables in type 1 diabetes mellitus. *Addictive Behaviors, 26*(1), 21–29.

Spencer, M. S., Kieffer, E. C., Sinco, B. R., Palmisano, G., Guzman, J., James, S., et al. (2006). Diabetes specific emotional distress among African Americans and Hispanics with type 2 diabetes. *Journal of Health Care for the Poor and Underserved, 17*, 88–105.

Spitzer, R. L., Kroenke, K., Linzer, M., Hahn, S. R., Williams, J. B., deGruy, F. V., III, et al. (1995). Health-related quality of life in primary care patients with mental disorders. Results from the PRIME-MD 1000 Study. *Journal of the American Medical Association, 274*, 1511–1517.

Spitzer, R. L., Kroenke, K., Williams, J. B., & Lowe, B. (2006). A brief measure for assessing generalized anxiety disorder: The GAD-7. *Archives of Internal Medicine, 166*(10), 1092–1097.

Steel, J. M., Young, R. J., Lloyd, G. G., & Clarke, B. F. (1987). Clinically apparent eating disorders in young diabetic women: Associations with painful neuropathy and other complications. *British Medical Journal, 294*(6576), 859–862.

Stewart, W. F., Ricci, J. A., Chee, E., Hahn, S. R., & Morganstein, D. (2003). Cost of lost productive work time among US workers with depression. *Journal of the American Medical Association, 289*, 3135–3144.

Substance Abuse and Mental Health Services Administration. (2009). *Results from the 2008 national survey on drug use and health: National findings*. Rockville, MD: Office of Applied Studies (NSDUH Series H-36, HHS Publication No. SMA 09-4434).

Sultan, S., Epel, E., Sachon, C., Vaillant, G., & Hartemann-Heurtier, A. (2008). A longitudinal study of coping, anxiety and glycemic control in adults with type 1 diabetes. *Psychology & Health, 23*(1), 73–90.

Surwit, R. S., Van Tilburg, M. A., Zucker, N., McCaskill, C. C., Parekh, P., Feinglos, M. N., et al. (2002). Stress management improves long-term glycemic control in type 2 diabetes. *Diabetes Care, 25*(1), 30–34.

Takii, M., Uchigata, Y., Tokunaga, S., Amemiya, N., Kinukawa, N., Nozaki, T., et al. (2008). The duration of severe insulin omission is the factor most closely associated with the microvascular complications of type 1 diabetic females with clinical eating disorders. *The International Journal of Eating Disorders, 41*(3), 259–264.

Thakore, J. H. (2005). Metabolic syndrome and schizophrenia. *The British Journal of Psychiatry, 186*, 455–456.

Thase, M., Haight, B., Richard, N., Rockett, C., Mitton, M., Modell, J., et al. (2005). Remission rates following antidepressant therapy with bupropion or selective serotonin reuptake inhibitors: A meta-analysis of original data from 7 randomized controlled trials. *The Journal of Clinical Psychiatry, 66*(8), 974–981.

Thomas, P., Raymondet, P., Charbonnel, B., & Vaiva, G. (2005). Are there specific care requirements for patients with schizophrenia and diabetes or with a risk of diabetes? *European Psychiatry, 20*, 358–363.

Tierney, S., Deaton, C., & Whitehead, J. (2009). Caring for people with type 1 diabetes mellitus engaging in disturbed eating or weight control: A qualitative study of practitioners' attitudes and practices. *Journal of Clinical Nursing, 18*(3), 384–390.

Tuncay, T., Musabak, I., Gok, D. E., & Kutlu, M. (2008). The relationship between anxiety, coping strategies and characteristics of patients with diabetes. *Health and Quality of Life Outcomes, 6*(79). doi:10.1186/1477-7525-6-79.

U. S. Department of Health and Human Services (2010). Healthy people 2020: The road ahead. Retrieved on January 3rd, 2011 from http://www.health.gov/healthypeople/url/.

Vileikyte, L., Leventhal, H., Gonzalez, J. S., Peyrot, M., Rubin, R. R., Ulbrecht, J. S., et al. (2005). Diabetic peripheral neuropathy and depressive symptoms: The association revisited. *Diabetes Care, 28*(10), 2378–2383.

Vileikyte, L., Peyrot, M., Gonzalez, J. S., Rubin, R. R., Garrow, A. P., Stickings, D., et al. (2009). Predictors of depressive symptoms in persons with diabetic peripheral neuropathy: A longitudinal study. *Diabetologia, 52*(7), 1265–1273.

Wang, P., Sachs, G., Zarate, C., Marangell, L., Calabrese, J., Goldberg, J., et al. (2006). Overweight and obesity in bipolar disorders. *Journal of Psychiatric Research, 40*(8), 762–764.

Weinberger, A., & George, T. (2009). Nicotine and tobacco use in patients with schizophrenia. In J. Meyer & H. Nasrallah (Eds.), *Medical illness and schizophrenia* (2nd ed., pp. 223–243). Arlington, VA: American Psychiatric Publishing.

Weinger, K. (2007). Psychosocial issues and self-care. *The American Journal of Nursing, 107*(6), 34–38.

Weinger, K., & Jacobson, A. M. (2001). Psychosocial and quality of life correlates of glycemic control during intensive treatment of type 1 diabetes. *Patient Education and Counseling, 42*, 123–131.

Weinger, K., & Lee, J. (2006). Psychosocial and psychiatric challenges of diabetes mellitus. *The Nursing Clinics of North America, 41*(4), 667–680.

Weiss, A. P., Henderson, D. C., Weilburg, J. B., Goff, D. C., Meigs, J. B., Cagliero, E., et al. (2006). Treatment of cardiac risk factors among patients with schizophrenia and diabetes. *Psychiatric Services, 57*(8), 1145–1152.

Whitebird, R. R., Kreitzer, M. J., & O'Connor, P. J. (2009). Mindfulness-based stress reduction and diabetes. *Diabetes Spectrum, 22*(4), 226–230.

Wild, D., von Maltzahn, R., Brohan, E., Christensen, T., Clauson, P., & Gonder-Frederick, L. (2007). A critical review of the literature on fear of hypoglycemia in diabetes: Implications for diabetes management and patient education. *Patient Education and Counseling, 68*, 10–15.

Willi, C., Bodenmann, P., Ghali, W., Faris, P., & Cornuz, J. (2007). Active smoking and the risk of type 2 diabetes: A systematic review and meta-analysis. *Journal of the American Medical Association, 298*(22), 2654–2664.

Wu, R. R., Zhao, J. P., Jin, H., Shao, P., Fang, M. S., Guo, X. F., et al. (2008). Lifestyle intervention and metformin for treatment of antipsychotic-induced weight gain: A randomized controlled trial. *Journal of the American Medical Association, 299*, 185–193.

Yi, J. P., Yi, J. C., Vitaliano, P. P., & Weinger, K. (2008). How does anger coping style affect glycemic control in diabetes patients? *International Journal of Behavioral Medicine, 15*(3), 167–172.

Young, E. A., Abelson, J. L., & Cameron, O. G. (2004). Effect of comorbid anxiety disorders on the hypothalamic–pituitary–adrenal axis response to a social stressor in major depression. *Biological Psychiatry, 56*, 113–120.

Zambanini, A., Newson, R. B., Maisey, M., & Feher, M. D. (1999). Injection related anxiety in insulin-treated diabetes. *Diabetes Research and Clinical Practice, 46*(3), 239–246.

Zhang, X., Norris, S. L., Gregg, E. W., Cheng, Y. J., Beckles, G., & Kahn, H. S. (2005). Depressive symptoms and mortality among persons with and without diabetes. *American Journal of Epidemiology, 161*, 652–660.

Ziedonis, D. M., & George, T. P. (1997). Schizophrenia and nicotine use: Report of a pilot smoking cessation program and review of neurobiological and clinical issues. *Schizophrenia Bulletin, 23*(2), 247–254.

Ziedonis, D., Williams, J. M., & Smelson, D. (2003). Serious mental illness and tobacco addiction: A model program to address this common but neglected issue. *The American Journal of the Medical Sciences, 326*(4), 223–230.

Zigmond, A. S., & Snaith, R. P. (1983). The Hospital Anxiety and Depression Scale. *Acta Psychiatrica Scandinavica, 67*, 361–370.

Chapter 3
Psychological Co-morbidities of Cardiovascular Disease

Matthew C. Whited, Amanda L. Wheat, Bradley M. Appelhans, and Sherry Pagoto

3.1 Introduction: Cardiovascular Disease

Cardiovascular disease (CVD) is very broadly defined by the ICD-10 as any disorder involving the circulatory system (World Health Organization, 2007). The most prominently investigated forms of CVD in the context of psychological co-morbidities include myocardial infarction (MI), coronary heart disease (CHD; also referred to as heart disease, coronary artery disease, or cardiac disease), and stroke. In this chapter, CVD will refer to diseases that are classified in the ICD-10 as ischemic heart diseases, cerebrovascular diseases, and heart failure, which is listed under "other forms of heart disease." These CVDs are chosen for review in this chapter because they have been extensively investigated and discussed in the context of co-morbid psychological illness. These diseases are also chronic in nature, developing over the life span, which has greater implications for psychological co-morbidities than congenital structural abnormalities.

3.2 Mood Disorders and CVD

Mood disorders including major depressive disorder (MDD), dysthymic disorder, and bipolar disorders I and II have been shown to have associations with CVD. In MDD, periods of depressed mood and/or anhedonia with accompanying symptoms are present for 2 weeks or longer. In dysthymic disorder, subthreshold depressive symptoms persist for a period of at least 2 years. The bipolar disorders are characterized by manic and/or hypomanic episodes that often alternate with major depressive episodes.

M.C. Whited (✉)
Department of Medicine, Division of Preventive and Behavioral Medicine, University of Massachusetts Medical School, 55 Lake Avenue North S7-746, Worcester, MA 01655, USA
e-mail: Matthew.Whited@umassmed.edu

S. Pagoto (ed.), *Psychological Co-morbidities of Physical Illness: A Behavioral Medicine Perspective*, DOI 10.1007/978-1-4419-0029-6_3,

3.2.1 Major Depressive Disorder

3.2.1.1 Prevalence of Co-occurring MDD and CVD

MDD is the most prevalent mental illness in the US with a 12-month point-prevalence of 6.7% (Kessler, Chiu, Demler, & Walters, 2005). Persons with MDD are 60–80% more likely to develop CVD than persons without MDD (Sowden & Huffman, 2009). In two meta-analyses, one of 10 prospective community studies (Wulsin & Singal, 2003) and another of 11 prospective cohort studies (Rugulies, 2002), persons with MDD were found to have a 64% greater chance of developing coronary artery disease than those without. In studies that used diagnostic interviews for MDD, the probability of developing CVD was higher than in studies using self-reported depressive symptom measures (Rugulies, 2002; Sowden & Huffman, 2009).

Not only are people with MDD at greater risk for CVD, but the prevalence of MDD among patients with CVD (15–20%) is substantially higher than in the general population (Kent & Shapiro, 2009), and depression is a risk factor for mortality and additional cardiovascular events (e.g., MI) in depressed CVD patients. In a prospective study of 457 patients with MI or unstable angina, depression was demonstrated to be an independent risk factor for mortality (Kronish, Rieckmann, Schwartz, Schwartz, & Davidson, 2009). The association was not entirely accounted for by depression's association with other CVD-related prognostic factors such as age, serum cardiac enzymes, systolic blood pressure, and ST segment deviation. Similarly, two meta-analyses of 20 and 22 prospective studies of patients with coronary heart disease (Barth, Schumacher, & Herrmann-Lingen, 2004) and MI (van Melle et al., 2004) reported that depression is a risk factor for mortality. Similar associations have been observed in heart failure. A meta-analysis of 36 studies demonstrated a point-prevalence of depression in heart failure patients of 21.5% and higher rates of death and secondary cardiovascular events in depressed compared to nondepressed patients (Rutledge, Reis, Linke, Greenberg, & Mills, 2006). Prevalence of depression in heart failure varies from 11 to 42% with higher rates observed at higher levels of disease severity (Rutledge et al.).

3.2.1.2 Pathophysiology of Depression and CVD

A fairly substantial literature has demonstrated that depression is prospectively associated with increased risk for CVD, and depression co-morbid with CVD is associated with poorer medical prognosis, even after controlling for CVD severity (Frasure-Smith & Lesperance, 2010). Although the associations are robust, no evidence has definitively established a causal relationship between depression and CVD. Potential mechanisms of the association between depression and CVD have been identified over the past several decades of research and include behavioral factors, altered autonomic balance, increased platelet aggregation, inflammation, genetic determinants, and in the case of stroke, brain lesions. It is unlikely that a single mechanism accounts entirely for the relationship between depression and CVD, and the relative contribution of these factors is a subject of ongoing research (Fang & Cheng, 2009; Frasure-Smith & Lesperance, 2010).

Lifestyle Factors

Depression is associated with several lifestyle risk factors for CVD, which may account for their association. Depressed persons are more likely to be sedentary and have a poor diet, which can lead to obesity and high cholesterol (Williams & Steptoe, 2007), both of which increase risk for CVD. For a thorough discussion of the association between obesity and depression, see Chap. 1, Sect. 1.2.1. Recently, several studies have investigated the associations between overall diet quality and depression (Jacka et al., 2010; Kuczmarski et al., 2010). In a population-based study of 1,046 Australian women, diet quality was related to the severity of psychological distress and odds of a depressive or anxiety disorder (Jacka et al.). Data from the Healthy Aging in Neighborhoods of Diversity Across the Life Span Study showed that both depression diagnosis and depressive symptom severity were associated with worse diet quality in an urban population (Kuczmarski et al.). Further research is required to determine the direction of the association between depression and diet quality and the extent to which worse diet quality mediates the association between depression and CVD.

Depressed persons are more likely to smoke, a significant CVD risk factor (Skala, Freedland, & Carney, 2006), and are less likely to quit (Anda et al., 1990). In a nationally representative sample, 37% of MDD patients were current smokers and 59% had been a smoker at some point in their life (Ziedonis et al., 2008). In a secondary analysis of a placebo-controlled randomized trial of buproprion therapy for smoking cessation among 245 smokers hospitalized with CVD, moderate-to-severe self-reported depressive symptoms during hospitalization resulted in a greater likelihood of resuming smoking by 4 weeks after discharge. Patients with minimal or mild depressive symptoms were more likely to remain abstinent across 1-year follow-up than moderate-to-severely depressed patients (Thorndike et al., 2008).

Depression is also associated with lower rates of adherence to medication regimens, especially preventive medication regimens (Ibishi et al., 2009; Williams & Steptoe, 2007). A systematic review of eight studies demonstrated a strong relationship between elevated depressive symptoms and poor adherence to antihypertensive medications (Eze-Nliam, Thombs, Lima, Smith, & Ziegelstein, 2010). Depressive symptoms have also been shown to predict worse adherence to daily aspirin. In a study of 165 CHD patients, patients who were persistently depressed as compared to nondepressed or remitted patients had worse adherence to daily aspirin over 3 months (Rieckmann, Gerin, et al., 2006; Rieckmann, Kronish, et al., 2006). A secondary analysis demonstrated that improvement in depressive symptoms over 1 month was associated with improved adherence (Rieckmann, Gerin, et al., 2006; Rieckmann, Kronish, et al., 2006). Another study of 492 patients with MI or unstable angina demonstrated poorer adherence for persistently depressed persons across multiple domains including exercise, quitting smoking, medications adherence, and attending cardiac rehabilitation (Kronish et al., 2006). All of these depression-related behavioral risk factors may be important intervention targets for CVD prevention and treatment in patients with depression.

Autonomic Nervous System Imbalance

Autonomic imbalance has been discussed as playing a role in the association between CVD and depression. The autonomic nervous system is divided into the sympathetic and parasympathetic branches, which act in a generally antagonistic fashion to modulate energy expenditure to match current environmental demands (Thayer & Lane, 2007). Autonomic imbalance occurs when one branch dominates the other. Some studies suggest that autonomic imbalance in the regulation of cardiac function (e.g., heart rate, contractile force) over time may promote the development of CVD (Thayer & Lane). In both CVD and depression, increases in sympathetic nervous system activity and decreases in parasympathetic nervous system activity are evident (Grippo, 2009; McConnell, Jacka, Williams, Dodd, & Berk, 2005; Williams & Steptoe, 2007). Heart rate variability (HRV) is a measure of cardiac autonomic imbalance and refers to beat-to-beat fluctuations in heart rate that occur during respiration (Bansal, Khan, & Salhan, 2009; Berntson et al., 1997). Low HRV is associated with depression, CVD (Agelink, Boz, Ullrich, & Andrich, 2002; Carney & Freedland, 2009; Koschke et al., 2009; Stein & Kleiger, 1999; Thayer & Lane, 2007), and mortality after MI (Bigger, Fleiss, Rolnitzky, & Steinman, 1993). Low HRV also partially mediates the relationship between depression and survival following acute MI (Carney et al., 2005). Some antidepressant medications including tricyclic antidepressants (TCAs) (Kemp et al., 2010; Licht et al., 2008; Van Zyl, Hasegawa, & Nagata, 2008), some selective serotonin reuptake inhibitors (SSRIs) (Bar et al., 2004; Koschke et al., 2009; Licht, De Geus, Van Dyck, & Penninx, 2010; Licht et al., 2008), and serotonin and norepinephrine reuptake inhibitors (SNRIs) (Bar et al., 2004; Koschke et al., 2009) have also been shown to suppress HRV. The relationships between depression, autonomic imbalance, and CVD point to autonomic imbalance as a potential mechanism in the relationship between depression and CVD. Further research is required to elucidate whether autonomic imbalance is a causal mechanism and to determine what other factors link depression, autonomic imbalance, and CVD.

Increased Platelet Activation

Platelets in plasma are responsible for blood clotting and become activated when chemical signals bind to their surface, resulting in a change of platelet shape and secretion of chemicals that facilitate the formation of clots (Bruce & Musselman, 2005; Scott, 2004). These clots are important in wound healing, but heightened platelet activation can stimulate plaque growth in the arteries which restricts blood flow and damages the tissue fed by occluded arteries (i.e., atherosclerosis), ultimately increasing risk for CVD (Scott). A review concluded that findings across studies have consistently shown that persons with depression display greater platelet activity than comparable control groups (Bruce & Musselman, 2005). A study of patients who had suffered a MI revealed greater platelet activation in depressed vs. nondepressed patients (Kuijpers, Hamulyak, Strik, Wellens, & Honig, 2002). Persons with depression also have a greater density of serotonin receptors on the surface of their platelets, which may result in greater platelet activation (McConnell et al., 2005). Platelet serotonin receptor density appears to be a modifiable condition, as evidenced by reduced receptor density resulting from SSRI treatment (McConnell et al.). Studies have demonstrated reduced platelet activation in patients with ischemic heart disease (Pollock, Laghrissi-Thode, & Wagner, 2000) and coronary artery disease (Serebruany, O'Connor, & Gurbel, 2001) who were treated with SSRIs. Though this evidence suggests that SSRIs may be an effective treatment for depressed persons with CVD, intervention research reviewed in Section "Pharmacological Treatments" is inconclusive on this issue.

Inflammation

Increased inflammation throughout the body plays a key role in the pathogenesis of atherosclerosis, and ultimately CVD (Scott, 2004). Arterial walls become damaged by an exaggerated inflammatory response, which subsequently expedites plaque formation and progression of the atherosclerotic process. Inflammatory markers are elevated in persons with depression, regardless of CVD status, and evidence suggests that the relationship between inflammation and depression is bidirectional (McConnell et al., 2005; Williams & Steptoe, 2007). On the one hand, treatment with a proinflammatory cytokine has been shown to increase depressive symptoms (Kop & Gottdiener, 2005), and heightened inflammation following stroke has been pointed to as a potential cause of poststroke depression (Fang & Cheng, 2009). On the other hand, a prospective longitudinal study of 263 healthy men and women demonstrated that baseline depressive symptoms predicted increasing inflammation over time (Stewart, Rand, Muldoon, & Kamarck, 2009). In a sample of 1,017 coronary artery disease patients, inflammation was a weak mediator and did not survive analyses that accounted for behavioral mediators such as physical activity, smoking, and medication adherence (Whooley et al., 2008). Inflammation appears to mediate the relationship between depression and CVD; however, it is a weak predictor compared to other factors.

Common Genetic Factors

Little research has examined the extent to which genetic predictors are responsible for the association between CVD and depression. One study using a population of male twins demonstrated that a genetic correlation of $r=0.42$ exists between lifetime depression and CVD (defined as angina, MI, CHD, or heart surgery) (Scherrer et al., 2003). Interestingly, the genetic correlation of CVD with hypertension was lower ($r=0.32$) than the correlation between depression and CVD ($r=0.42$). Specific genetic markers connecting depression and CVD have yet to be identified.

Brain Lesions in Stroke

Stroke results in brain damage either due to a lack of blood flow (i.e., ischemic stroke) or a burst blood vessel (i.e., hemorrhagic stroke). The location of brain lesions may affect the likelihood of poststroke depression. In a review, Fang and Cheng (2009) conclude that left hemisphere lesions seem to be related to depression directly following stroke, but the literature appears to be mixed, with other studies demonstrating an association between poststroke depression and right hemisphere lesion, and some showing no association (Fang & Cheng). A systematic review by Bhogal, Teasell, Foley, and Speechley (2004) demonstrated methodological differences between studies that led to conflicting conclusions on lesion location and poststroke depression. In hospitalized patient samples, poststroke depression was related to left hemisphere lesions, whereas community samples found depression to be related to right hemisphere lesions. This association may be explained by the timing of depression assessment, as depression assessed within 28 days of a stroke was associated with left hemisphere lesions, and assessing depression 1–4 months after stroke was associated with right hemisphere lesions (Bhogal, Teasell, et al.). Lesion location is an important area for future investigation, because few definitive conclusions exist. Santos et al. (2009) propose an alternate theory, stating that accumulation of macro- and microvascular lesions in the neural circuits responsible for mood regulation result in symptoms of depression following stroke, a phenomenon referred to as vascular depression. Though evidence for stroke-induced tissue damage is mixed at best, it remains a viable area of future inquiry.

Towards a Comprehensive Model

The association between depression and CVD is likely multifactorial in nature (Frasure-Smith & Lesperance, 2010). For example, autonomic imbalance is related to inflammation (McConnell et al., 2005) and sympathetic hyperarousal is related to overabundance of platelet receptors. Grippo (2009) outlines a more integrative model based on findings from both human and animal research that proposes several common mechanisms of CVD and depression. They propose that physiological reactions to environmental stressors results in disruptions in neurohormonal, immune, and autonomic processes (e.g., inflammation, autonomic imbalance, poor hormonal and immune regulation) and that neurotransmitters and neuropeptides such as oxytocin and serotonin play a role as links between these processes and behavior. Future research is needed of the interrelationships between the factors involved in the association between depression and CVD.

3.2.1.3 Clinical Care of Patients with Depression CVD

Assessment

Depressive symptoms are common following a CVD event, but symptoms do not meet criteria for MDD unless they are present for 2 or more weeks and cause significant distress or impairment (Carney & Freedland, 2008). In addition, somatic symptoms of depression such as fatigue and difficulty sleeping can be caused by CVD or, for inpatients, the hospital environment. A diagnostic interview, although time-consuming, is ideal to make a valid diagnosis of MDD, but not feasible in most clinical settings. Brief screening instruments can assess depressive symptoms easily and quickly, and as a result, at multiple points in care. Tracking the course of depressive symptoms is important because MDD can develop late in the course of treatment, and persistent MDD is a poor prognostic indicator.

Several brief screening instruments can be helpful to identify patients in need of more extensive assessment and treatment for depression. Supporting the use of screening instruments over purely clinical judgment is one study that showed that practitioner's judgment of which patients should be assessed for MDD missed 75% of patients who had elevated scores on the Beck Depression Inventory-I (Ziegelstein et al., 2005). A commonly used screening instrument is the Patient Health Questionnaire (PHQ), which exists in both 2 and 9 question formats (available at http://phqscreeners.com/ in many languages). The PHQ is recommended for screening in CVD patients by the NHLBI (Davidson et al., 2006) and it is recommended in several reviews (Carney & Freedland, 2008; Pozuelo et al., 2009). In a sample of patients with CHD, the PHQ-9 had a sensitivity of 54% and a specificity of 90% (McManus, Pipkin, & Whooley, 2005). Other instruments that have been found to effectively screen for MDD in persons with CVD include the Beck Depression Inventory-II (BDI-II), the Hamilton Rating Scale for Depression (HRSD), the Center for Epidemiologic Studies Depression Scale (CES-D), and the Hospital Anxiety and Depression Scale (HADS). The HADS especially has been extensively studied in medical populations including CVD patients (Berg, Lonnqvist, Palomaki, & Kaste, 2009; Sagen et al., 2009). The HADS should also be considered in patients where anxiety is a concern, as it assesses for both anxiety and depression.

Some debate exists as to whether screening and treatment for depression are necessary in CVD care settings. Thombs et al. (2008) suggested that screening for depression in a CVD care setting is not cost-effective at this time because the healthcare infrastructure does not support adequate depression assessment and treatment after the initial screening. They point out the lack of evidence that depression screening provides greater access to mental health care, results in reduced depressive symptoms, or improves cardiovascular morbidity and mortality. A reply to this contention by Carney, Freedland, and Jaffe (2009) points out that the American Heart Association recommends depression screening in CVD patients and that being aware of the presence of depression also guides clinical decision-making much in the same way that assessing other associated risk factors would, such as age. A positive screen for depression should, at least, alert the provider that the patient may have a poorer prognosis and require closer monitoring for adherence to their medical treatment. In addition, despite the fact that depression treatment may not impact cardiovascular mortality, many evidence-based treatments exist to improve depressive symptoms (Joynt & O'Connor, 2005), which can significantly impact quality of life even if it does not contribute to duration of life.

Treatment

Several randomized trials testing treatments for depression in persons with CVD have been conducted; however, no definitive conclusions have been made on the optimal depression treatment. Both pharmacological and psychotherapy interventions have been tested with varying efficacy. In addition to depression, trials typically include CVD morbidity and mortality as primary endpoints.

Pharmacological Treatments

SSRIs are the most commonly prescribed antidepressant medication, but safety in CVD patients has not been extensively tested (Carney & Freedland, 2008). Several observational studies have shown a relationship between antidepressant use and CVD events and death (Cohen, Gibson, & Alderman, 2000; Hippisley-Cox et al., 2001; Krantz et al., 2009; Smoller et al., 2009); however, randomized trials of antidepressants in CVD populations have not revealed a negative impact on CVD risk, events, or death. The most recent systematic review of cardiovascular adverse events in randomized trials for SSRIs reported the literature to be inconclusive due to a low number of thoroughly reported, serious, adverse events in published trials and a lack of large-scale randomized trials of CVD patients (Swenson, Doucette, & Fergusson, 2006). In the Sertraline Antidepressant Heart Attack Randomized Trial (SADHART), 369 patients with MDD who were recently hospitalized for MI or unstable angina were treated for 24 weeks with either sertraline or placebo (Glassman et al., 2002). Sertraline improved depression but did not adversely affect cardiac functioning; in fact, fewer severe cardiac events were observed in the sertraline condition, although the difference was not statistically significant and the study was not powered to detect group differences in cardiac events. In a subanalysis of SADHART data, people with more severe depression (i.e., history of depressive episodes, severe episodes) responded more favorably to sertraline treatment than to placebo. Persons with depression diagnoses following CVD hospitalization displayed a greater placebo response than patients who had MDD prior to hospitalization (Glassman, Bigger, Gaffney, Shapiro, & Swenson, 2006). Findings are consistent with a meta-analysis of antidepressant medication efficacy which showed antidepressant medication is consistently effective in severe MDD, but less so in mild-to-moderate MDD (Fournier et al., 2010).

A second study, SADHART-CHF, randomized participants with heart failure to 12 weeks of sertraline or placebo (O'Connor et al., 2010). All participants received nurse-facilitated support in the form of four telephone and two in-person meetings.

Unlike SADHART, results showed no effect of sertraline on depression or CVD improvement. SADHART and SADHART-CHF may show different results due to the unexpectedly large placebo response in SADHART-CHF, possibly due to the nursing support in both conditions.

In the CREATE trial, 284 depressed patients with coronary artery disease were randomized to citalopram or placebo (Lesperance et al., 2007). Participants also underwent a second randomization to receive 12 weeks of interpersonal therapy (IPT) or no psychotherapy. All participants received clinical management, which involved weekly 20–25 min sessions in which information was provided about depression and participants were encouraged to adhere to the medication/placebo and study protocol. Findings demonstrated that citalopram was superior to placebo in reducing depressive symptoms. Secondary analyses determined that persons with recurrent depression benefitted from citalopram relative to placebo, but persons experiencing their first episode of depression did not benefit from citalopram relative to placebo. No interaction between the efficacy of medication and psychotherapy was found.

Both the SADHART and CREATE studies found that SSRIs are most effective for persons with more severe or recurrent depression. Authors of the CREATE study strongly suggest that clinical management sessions accompany SSRI treatment so treatment providers can be responsive to medication-related adverse events and facilitate an optimal balance between depression symptoms reduction and medication side effects (Lesperance et al., 2007).

TCAs and monoamine oxidase inhibitors (MAOIs) have adverse cardiac effects and should not be used as a first-line treatment for CVD patients (Carney & Freedland, 2008). The Myocardial Infarction and Depression – Intervention Trial (MIND-IT) (van Melle et al.) randomized 331 post-MI patients to receive either mirtazapine, an SNRI, or usual care. Both the antidepressant treatment and usual care conditions received an SSRI if their depressive symptoms did not improve after 8 weeks. Findings revealed that mirtazapine was not effective in improving depressive symptoms or cardiovascular mortality at 18 months.

Reviews of treatment of poststroke depression support the use of antidepressants which in some cases have been shown to improve cognitive symptoms (Hackett, Anderson, House, & Xia, 2008; Zavoreo, Basic-Kes, Bosnar-Puretic, & Demarin, 2009). The use of antidepressants may not impact stroke risk, however, as data from the Framingham Heart Study suggest (Salaycik et al., 2007), although this study of 4,120 community-dwelling participants only saw an increased risk of stroke conferred by depressive symptoms in persons under 65 years old. Additional research on the treatment of poststroke depression is warranted to identify effective treatments, although the combination of psychotherapy and pharmacotherapy may be effective, as discussed below.

Psychotherapy

Both cognitive behavior therapy (CBT) and problem solving therapy (PST) have been tested in CVD populations with efficacy on depressive symptoms, with mixed outcomes on CVD-related endpoints. The Enhancing Recovery in Coronary Heart Disease (ENRICHD) trial randomized 2,481 patients with a recent MI and MDD, minor depression, and/or low perceived social support to CBT or usual care conditions (Berkman et al., 2003). Minor depression was defined as having 2–4 symptoms of depression, with one being either depressed mood or a loss of interest or pleasure. Low perceived social support was identified via a cut-off score on a social support measure developed for the ENRICHD study. CBT in the ENRICHD trial involved teaching patients to alter their cognitive appraisal of situations and thoughts that cause them to feel depressed. It also included training in social skills with emphasis on developing a social network, when relevant. Patients who did not respond to psychotherapy or who presented with more severe depression were considered for pharmacotherapy with sertraline. The treatment group improved in measures of social support and depressive symptoms, relative to the control group, but no effect on myocardial event-free survival was observed, which was the primary outcome of the study. A subanalysis of the ENRICHD study, however, demonstrated that persons who did not respond to treatment were more likely to have a myocardial event than persons who responded to treatment (de Jonge et al., 2007). Also worthy of note is a study that demonstrated a decreased risk of recurrent CVD following MI for patients who received CBT, but this study was not specific to patients with depression, and the primary target of CBT treatment was stress management (Gulliksson et al., 2011).

PST, also tested for the treatment of MDD among persons with CVD, teaches patients to systematically evaluate and take planned action to solve life problems, in addition to engaging in planned enjoyable activities. Davidson et al. utilized PST to treat 157 persistently depressed patients with acute coronary syndrome (ACS) (Davidson et al., 2010). Participants in this study were first observed for 3 months after diagnosis with ACS to ensure that their depression was persistent and not an acute reaction to ACS. Participants were then randomized to usual care or enhanced care conditions. Enhanced care participants were given a choice of initial treatment of PST or an antidepressant medication. The majority (75%) chose PST. Participants whose depressive symptoms did not improve with their original choice were offered the opportunity to switch to the other treatment, intensify their current treatment, or add the other treatment to current treatment. By the end of the study, 48% of enhanced care patients were taking an antidepressant compared to 30% in the usual care group, and 81% of the enhanced care group had received PST. Enhanced care was associated with improvement in depressive symptoms. This treatment was also associated with a lower number of adverse cardiac events, though the total number of events in this study was small and the study was not designed to determine the effect of depression treatment on CVD. This is the only randomized clinical trial to show a statistically significant reduction in cardiovascular events associated with psychotherapy, although the design did not allow for separation of psychotherapy effects from medication effects.

Other psychotherapies have not been found to be useful in the treatment of depression in CVD patients. The CREATE study (discussed in Section Pharmacological Treatments) utilized IPT, which focuses on addressing interpersonal conflicts, life transitions, grief and loss, and social isolation (Lesperance et al., 2007). In this study, participants were randomized to receive 12 weeks of IPT plus clinical management or clinical management alone. Half of participants were taking citalopram and half were taking a placebo. Results of this study demonstrated that IPT combined with clinical management did not result in lower depressive symptoms or fewer adverse cardiac events in comparison to clinical management alone. The efficacy of IPT did not differ based on medication status.

A recent Cochrane Review concluded that no adequately controlled studies demonstrated an effect of psychotherapy on poststroke depression (Hackett et al., 2008). Only four studies met the inclusion criteria for this review (Lincoln & Flannaghan, 2003; Towle, Lincoln, & Mayfield, 1989; Watkins et al., 2007; Zhao, Zhou, Su, Xiao, & Guo, 2004) because they utilized an adequate usual care comparison arm and provided outcome data regarding depressive symptoms. Therapies included in the review were PST, CBT, motivational interviewing, and psychological support. None of these therapies were effective in reducing depression in stroke patients. A more recent study of poststroke depression demonstrated the efficacy of antidepressant medication plus a brief behavioral activation-style intervention based on the "Seattle Protocols (Teri, Logsdon, & McCurry, 2005)" originally designed for persons with Alzheimer's disease (Mitchell et al., 2009). Patients ($n=101$) were randomized to receive the behavioral intervention plus usual care (which included antidepressant medication) or usual care alone. In both the usual care and behavioral intervention groups, 77% of participants were taking an antidepressant. The behavioral intervention resulted in improved depression scores beyond that conferred by usual care. The positive results of this study indicate that further research on the treatment of poststroke depression is warranted.

Although the psychotherapy trial literature has mixed outcomes on depression in CVD populations, different psychotherapies may operate via different processes and several effective depression therapies have not yet been tested in CVD populations. For example, behavioral activation and mindfulness-based cognitive therapy (Dimidjian & Davis, 2009) are efficacious in the treatment of depression and may have some relevance and applicability to the CVD population. The Seattle Protocols behavioral intervention discussed above heavily utilizes behavioral activation strategies. Behavioral activation has also been found effective in populations with other medical co-morbidities (e.g., cancer, obesity, nicotine dependence, HIV) (Daughters et al., 2008; Hopko, Lejuez, & Hopko, 2008; Hopko, Lejuez, LePage, Hopko, & McNeil, 2003) and mindfulness-based cognitive therapy has a strong stress reduction component which could be particularly relevant to CVD patients. Further research is needed to determine the optimal psychotherapy for depression in the context of CVD.

3.2.2 *Dysthymic Disorder*

Dysthymia has rarely been studied in the context of CVD. To the extent that depressive symptoms are central to both dysthymia and major depression, the pathophysiology linking them to CVD would seem to be similar; however, this assumption should be made with caution pending further investigation. In a population-based sample, MDD was more strongly associated with risk for stroke than dysthymia, but dysthymia was more strongly associated with risk for CHD than depression (Baune, Adrian, Arolt, & Berger, 2006). Rafanelli Milaneschi, Roncuzzi, and Pancaldi (2010) found that a retrospective diagnosis of dysthymia prior to the onset of heart disease predicted a second episode of heart disease 2.5 years later, whereas MDD did not. Dysthymia involves a persistent pattern of negative mood that can last several years, which could conceivably take a different toll on cardiovascular health than MDD which tends to be episodic, even if more severe in symptoms. The duration and severity of depression symptoms on CVD risk is an area for further study.

3.2.3 Bipolar Disorder

3.2.3.1 Prevalence

Persons with bipolar disorder are two to almost five times more likely to have CVD than the general population, with 1.5–2.5 times higher risk for CVD mortality (Baune, Adrian, et al., 2006; Garcia-Portilla et al., 2009). They also develop CVD 10–14 years earlier than their mentally healthy counterparts (Baune, Adrian, et al., 2006; Garcia-Portilla et al., 2009; Goldstein, Fagiolini, Houck, & Kupfer, 2009). A longitudinal study of a clinical sample found a greater risk for CVD mortality with bipolar I compared to bipolar II disorder, the former of which is characterized by manic episodes and the latter by hypomanic episodes (Fiedorowicz et al., 2009). The degree of mania in this study independently predicted CVD and may explain the difference in CVD risk between the two diagnoses.

3.2.3.2 Pathophysiology of Bipolar Disorder and CVD

The pathophysiology of bipolar disorder and CVD is not well studied, although some research suggests that unique mechanisms are involved beyond those associated with depression. Patients with bipolar disorder tend to have circadian rhythm disturbances, high rates of obesity, and cognitive and executive dysfunction, all of which are potentially related to CVD risk (Soreca, Frank, & Kupfer, 2009). Metabolic syndrome, which is strongly related to CVD, is also more prevalent in persons with bipolar disorder relative to the general population, with a combined prevalence ratio from multiple studies of 1.6 (Murray, Weiner, Prabhakar, & Fiedorowicz, 2009). Poor access to care, behavioral risk factors, and psychotropic medication have also been discussed as potential mechanisms of the relationship between bipolar disorder and CVD (Murray et al.).

Access to Care and Lifestyle Factors

Data from the National Health Interview Survey, a large nationally representative sample of noninstitutionalized individuals, demonstrate that individuals with bipolar disorder tend to have poorer access to medical care (Bradford et al., 2008). Patients with bipolar disorder were less likely than the general population to have a relationship with a primary care provider, which could result in reduced access to CVD preventive care (e.g., lipid screening and management). This is especially a concern because persons with bipolar disorder have poorer health behaviors than people without chronic mental illness. In a cross-sectional study of United States veterans, patients with bipolar disorder reported low rates of exercise and poor eating habits, such as meal skipping, than those without a severe mental illness (Kilbourne et al., 2007). In this same study, bipolar patients were less likely to discuss diet and exercise with their physician than those without a severe mental illness. Persons with bipolar disorder have higher rates of smoking than the general population (Diaz, James, et al., 2009; Diaz, Meary, et al., 2009).

Psychotropic Medication

Psychotropic medications for bipolar disorder may contribute to the development of CVD given that atypical antipsychotic medications, mood stabilizers, and anticonvulsants have metabolic and weight gain side effects. Chapter 1 (see Sects. 1.5.2.1 and "Psychopharmacology") contains a review of the effects of the antipsychotics, mood stabilizers, and anticonvulsants on weight. Section 3.4.2.1 of this chapter reviews the effects of antipsychotic medications on CVD risk factors. Some anticonvulsants have also been shown to increase CVD risk. A cross-sectional study of 77 patients with bipolar disorder and 119 healthy controls revealed that patients with bipolar disorder who were treated with valproic acid had poorer lipid profiles (e.g., higher LDL cholesterol, triglycerides, and total cholesterol) than untreated patients with bipolar disorder and healthy controls (Chang et al., 2010). In a prospective 12-month study of 53 children taking anticonvulsants, lipid levels increased after 3 months of treatment and remained high at 1-year follow-up for patients treated with carbamazepine, but not valproic acid (Yilmaz, Dosan, Gurgoze, & Gungor, 2001). Another study of women with epilepsy revealed that those on valproic acid were more obese and had higher rates of metabolic syndrome than those on carbamazepine, lamotrigne, and topiramate, with the latter two having the lowest rates of obesity and metabolic syndrome (Kim & Lee, 2007). Very few studies have examined CVD risk of anticonvulsants in samples with bipolar disorder, although existing literature in samples with epilepsy would suggest that CVD risk monitoring during treatment of bipolar is certainly indicated.

3.2.3.3 Clinical Care of Bipolar Patients with CVD

Assessment

Pharmacological treatment is paramount for the control of symptoms in bipolar disorder. Medications such as lithium, anticonvulsant mood stabilizers, and atypical antipsychotics are effective, but can have CVD-related side effects such as weight gain. In 2004, the American Diabetes Association, American Psychiatric Association, American Association of Clinical Endocrinologists, and the North American Association for the Study of Obesity (now named the Obesity Society) held a Consensus Development Conference to put forth a clinical guideline that recommends baseline screening of weight, waist circumference, blood pressure, plasma glucose, and fasting lipids for all patients who are prescribed atypical antipsychotics (American Diabetes Association, American Psychiatric Association, American Association of Clinical Endocrinologists, & North American Association for the Study of Obesity, 2004). Unfortunately, individuals with serious mental illnesses often do not receive CVD risk screening and treatment (Morrato et al., 2009; Murray et al., 2009). An article by Ketter details a protocol for monitoring CVD-related side effects of medications, depressive and manic symptoms, medication adherence, safety and tolerability, and medical co-morbidities in patients with bipolar disorder (Ketter, 2010). For the monitoring of symptom severity, the PHQ-9 is suggested for depressive symptoms and the Mood Disorders Questionnaire for the monitoring of manic symptoms (Hirschfeld et al., 2000).

Treatment Issues

Despite the potential side effects of medications used to treat bipolar disorder, medication treatment is associated with better mortality rates. A study of 220 patients with bipolar disorder followed for 34–38 years indicated that the patients who received treatment for bipolar disorder, despite having more severe impairment, lived longer and had a 2.5 times lower suicide rate than untreated patients with bipolar disorder (Angst, Stassen, Clayton, & Angst, 2002). Collaborative care between medicine and psychiatry is essential in bipolar disorder in order to effectively address both psychiatric symptoms and CVD risk factors. Kilbourne and colleagues tested a medical care model for the treatment of bipolar disorder in a sample of 58 older veterans with a CVD-related risk factor such as hypertension or diabetes. Treatment involved self-management sessions that addressed bipolar disorder and CVD preventive care followed by contact with a care manager who liaised between the patient and their care providers. All primary care and mental health providers also participated in a seminar series that focused on CVD risk in patients with bipolar disorder. This program has shown good patient satisfaction and attendance rates, while adding feasible additional cost to patient care; hiring additional staff is not required and care managers were not taxed with an overwhelming case load (Kilbourne, Post, Nossek, Drill, et al., 2008; Kilbourne, Post, Nossek, Sonel, et al., 2008). The program also enhanced physical health-related quality of life in patients who received treatment, as compared to a treatment as usual group (Kilbourne, Post, Nossek, Drill, et al.; Kilbourne, Post, Nossek, Sonel, et al.). Though this model is one template for collaborative care, additional research is needed on models of integrated and/or collaborative care to determine cost-effective approaches to managing both the mental and physical health of people with severe mental illness.

3.3 Anxiety Disorders and CVD

3.3.1 Prevalence

Several studies support a significant association between CVD and anxiety disorders. In a population study utilizing data from the Behavioral Risk Factor Surveillance System study, 16.1% of individuals with CVD had a lifetime history of anxiety disorder, compared to 10% of those without CVD (Fan, Strine, Jiles, & Mokdad, 2008). The lifetime prevalence of any anxiety disorder is 17.8% for individuals with CHD history (Sherbourne, Jackson, & Meredith, 1996), and a cross-sectional study of 2,315 patients with a depressive or anxiety disorder demonstrated that persons with an anxiety disorder were about three times more likely to have CHD (Vogelzangs et al., 2010). In this study, the relationship between depressive disorders and CHD was largely accounted for by co-morbid anxiety. Not only do people with CVD have higher rates of anxiety disorders, but people with anxiety disorders also have a higher prevalence of CVD. In a population-based study, 4.5% of individuals diagnosed with a lifetime anxiety disorder had CVD compared to 3.1% of those with no lifetime anxiety disorder (Goodwin, Davidson, & Keyes, 2009). The strongest evidence for links to CVD exist for generalized anxiety disorder (GAD), panic disorder, and posttraumatic stress disorder (PTSD).

3.3.1.1 Generalized Anxiety Disorder

In the general population, prevalence of GAD is 3.1% (Kessler et al., 2005), and it is 3.7% in primary care patients (Olfson et al., 1997). Among primary care patients with CHD or hypertension, the prevalence of GAD is much higher, ranging between 10.4 and 12.4% (Sherbourne, Jackson, et al., 1996). In a study examining a small sample of outpatients in a cardiology clinic, 24% of patients met criteria for GAD (Bankier, Januzzi, & Littman, 2004). In addition to higher rates of GAD in CVD patients, evidence exists for higher rates of CVD in GAD patients. In a population-based sample, 6.1% of persons with a history of GAD had CVD, while only 3.2% of individuals with no history of GAD had CVD (Goodwin, Davidson, et al., 2009). Also, in a sample of 1,015 patients with stable CHD, having a diagnosis of GAD conferred a 74% greater risk of a cardiovascular event over a 7–9-year follow-up period (Martens et al., 2010).

3.3.1.2 Panic Disorder

In the general population, prevalence of panic disorder is 2.7% (Kessler et al., 2005) and it is 3% in primary care patients (Olfson et al., 1997). Within CHD patients and cardiac outpatients, one review reported prevalence rates of panic disorder between 10 and 50% (Fleet, Lavoie, & Beitman, 2000). However, authors of the review acknowledge that rates may have been inflated due to liberally or poorly defined CHD status. Diagnosis of panic disorder in CHD patients may also be inflated due to overlapping symptoms (e.g., chest pain) (Potokar & Nutt, 2000). The prevalence of CVD is also heightened in people with panic disorder. A population-based study reported that 5.5% of persons with panic disorder had either current or prior CVD, compared to 3.3% of the total sample (Goodwin, Davidson, et al., 2009). A retrospective longitudinal study of veterans found that patients with panic disorder were at increased risk for incident MI as compared to mentally healthy patients (Scherrer et al., 2010). There is also evidence that panic disorder confers risk for stroke. A study using Taiwan's national health insurance database revealed a 2.4 times greater risk for stroke across a 3-year follow-up period among patients with panic disorder compared to age- and sex-matched controls (Chen, Hu, Lee, & Lin, 2010). A review of the literature on the effect of depression, anxiety, and anger on CVD risk reported a significant prospective risk of CVD development in patients with panic disorder (Suls & Bunde, 2005).

3.3.1.3 Posttraumatic Stress Disorder

The prevalence of PTSD over a 1-year period in the general population is 3.5% (Kessler et al., 2005) and about 2% in primary care patients (Olfson et al., 1997). Much higher rates have been observed in samples with CVD. For example, a study of 100 CHD outpatients reported that 29% met criteria for PTSD (Bankier, Januzzi, et al., 2004). Not all studies have shown a significant relationship between PTSD and CVD though, as evidenced in a review of this literature (Qureshi, Pyne, Magruder, Schulz, & Kunik, 2009). Two studies not included in that review found that male veterans (Kubzansky, Koenen, Spiro, Vokonas, & Sparrow, 2007) and community-dwelling females (Kubzansky, Koenen, Jones, & Eaton, 2009) with elevated PTSD symptoms were at increased risk for CHD. Male veterans with greater PTSD symptoms were 12–35% more likely to have CHD compared to male veterans with fewer PTSD symptoms (Kubzansky et al., 2007). Women with higher PTSD symptoms had 3.46 greater odds of negative CHD outcomes than the general population (Kubzansky et al., 2009). Among a population sample that was 52% female, patients with PTSD were at an increased likelihood of CVD (odds ratio: 2.4–3.4) as compared to persons without PTSD (Spitzer et al., 2009). This study used a clinical interview to assess PTSD and confirms the results of the investigation with veterans discussed above, extending the association between PTSD and CVD to clinically relevant PTSD and to the general population. A systematic review of 80 articles revealed evidence suggesting associations between PTSD and CVD-related morbidity and mortality, but some inconsistencies in findings necessitate additional investigation regarding the risk for CVD conferred by PTSD (Dedert, Calhoun, Watkins, Sherwood, & Beckham, 2010). These authors specifically recommend that future research may be strengthened through investigation of the relationship between PTSD and metabolic abnormalities using longitudinal designs, more diverse samples, utilizing diagnostic interviews to diagnose PTSD, and evaluating mediators and moderators such as co-morbid psychological conditions and socio-economic status.

Cardiovascular events can be life-threatening, painful, and traumatic, so much so that they can trigger PTSD in some patients. A review of PTSD following cardiac events reported that 22% of patients developed PTSD following an MI and 19–38% of sudden cardiac arrest survivors subsequently developed PTSD (Spindler & Pedersen, 2005). A study of 951 post-MI patients revealed that patients who were younger and had greater symptoms of helplessness and fear of dying were at higher risk of developing PTSD (Guler et al., 2009). PTSD resulting from MI also appears to persist over time. One study followed MI patients for an average of 21 months after their initial diagnosis of PTSD and found that two thirds of MI patients still met criteria for PTSD 21 months after their initial diagnosis (Abbas et al., 2009). Avoidance and hyperarousal were the most persistent symptoms. The relationship between PTSD and CVD is bidirectional, with CVD events precipitating PTSD in some cases and PTSD symptoms contributing to CVD risk in others.

3.3.1.4 Anxiety Symptoms

Much of the literature linking anxiety and CVD focuses on anxiety symptoms rather than anxiety disorders. A recent review examined the literature on a variety of CVD-related outcomes (e.g., documented MI, cardiac mortality) in relation to anxiety, panic, and worry to determine whether anxiety symptoms are related to the progression of (i.e., "prognostic studies") and onset of (i.e., "prospective studies") disease over time (Suls & Bunde, 2005). The majority of prospective studies reviewed support a link between anxiety symptoms and the onset of CVD, and those that did not support the association were less methodologically sound. Overall, prospective evidence indicated that anxiety symptoms conferred a 2–7-fold increased risk for cardiac morbidity or mortality over a range of follow-up periods between 2 and 35 years. Of 17 prognostic studies examining the association between progression of CVD and anxiety symptoms, only four studies provided evidence for such a positive relationship. Follow-up periods for these studies ranged from 4 months to 10 years. Although anxiety symptoms appear to increase risk for CVD onset, evidence is not as strong for the role of anxiety symptom severity in the progression or exacerbation of CVD. A study of 49,321 Swedish men (18–20 year old) provides strong evidence for the role of anxiety in CVD onset, because low age of the sample reduces the influence of confounding subclinical CVD (Janszky, Ahnve, Lundberg, & Hemmingsson, 2010). In this study, participants underwent a diagnostic interview and were categorized based on the presence of clinically significant anxiety symptoms (an interview diagnosis of any anxiety disorder) and were monitored for onset of CHD for 37 years. Anxiety was found to be a significant predictor of CHD onset and MI and was a much stronger predictor than depression.

A meta-analysis of 12 papers investigating the influence of anxiety on CVD post-MI revealed a 36% increased risk of adverse cardiovascular events and outcomes when anxiety was treated as a dichotomous variable based on self-report measures (Roest, Martens, Denollet, & de Jonge, 2010). Specifically, anxiety was associated with increased risk for new cardiac events, as well as all-cause and cardiovascular mortality. Interestingly, three studies, all using the HADS, revealed a protective effect of anxiety symptoms on cardiac and/or all-cause mortality (Herrmann, Brand-Driehorst, Buss, & Rüger, 2000; Mykletun et al., 2007; Meyer, Buss, & Herrmann-Lingen, 2010). One of those studies revealed that anxiety was protective for mortality in patients with less severe CVD, but predicted worse mortality in patients with more severe CVD, as measured by reduced left ventricular function (Meyer, Buss, & Herrmann-Lingen, 2010). They concluded that the prognostic value of anxiety symptoms appears to depend on disease severity. Further research is still needed to determine why anxiety is protective in some cases and destructive in others.

3.3.2 Pathophysiology of Anxiety and CVD

The majority of the literature examining the mechanisms for the association between anxiety and CVD focuses on anxiety in general rather than specific disorders; however, physiological, behavioral, and pharmacological mechanisms have been proposed.

3.3.2.1 Physiological Mechanisms

Cardiovascular Reactivity and Autonomic Imbalance

Cardiovascular reactivity, or the responsiveness of the cardiovascular system to stress, affects processes that lead to the development of CVD and may help to explain why heightened anxiety is linked to CVD (Rozanski & Kubzansky, 2005). The exaggerated physiological stress response observed in persons with heightened anxiety may cause increased wear and tear on the cardiovascular system, thus contributing to the development of CVD. In addition to cardiovascular reactivity, autonomic imbalance has been implicated in the association between anxiety and CVD. Autonomic imbalance is characterized by low HRV and poor baroreceptor sensitivity. HRV refers to naturally occurring beat-to-beat changes in heart rate, with low variability being a sign of autonomic imbalance (Malik et al., 1996). Baroreceptor sensitivity refers to how sensitive the baroreceptors are to changes in blood pressure. Poor baroreceptor sensitivity is also a sign of autonomic imbalance. Each of these indicators of autonomic imbalance is associated with heightened

CHD risk, cardiac events, and atherosclerosis. Low HRV and baroreflex dysfunction also have been linked to elevated phobic anxiety, panic, and general anxiety symptoms (White, 2008) which may explain the link between anxiety disorders and CVD.

CVD Risk Factors

Individuals with anxiety disorders and elevated anxiety symptoms appear to have higher cholesterol and blood pressure, even when controlling for confounding lifestyle factors (White, 2008). Cholesterol levels have been shown to be elevated up to three times more often in individuals with anxiety disorders compared to controls, and that association held even when accounting for avoidance of exercise due to anxiety and differences in diet (Peter, Goebel, Müller, & Hand, 1999). Associations between anxiety and hypertension have also been evidenced by examining presence of hypertension in psychiatric samples (Markovitz, Matthews, Wing, Kuller, & Meilahn, 1991) as well as examining longitudinal evidence for development of hypertension in samples that were normotensive at baseline (Wells, Golding, & Burnam, 1989). Still unknown are the mechanisms by which anxiety is related to elevated lipids and blood pressure.

3.3.2.2 Behavioral Risk Factors

People with anxiety disorders exhibit higher rates of behavioral risk factors for CVD than their counterparts without anxiety disorders which may explain their elevated risk for CVD (Bonnet et al., 2005; Roy-Byrne et al., 2008; White, 2008). In general, individuals with anxiety disorders tend to have worse diets, poor sleep, higher rates of drug use, poor medication adherence, and higher rates of both obesity (White) and smoking (Roy-Byrne, Davidson, et al., 2008) compared to individuals without anxiety disorders. Among a large sample of adults attending an outpatient clinic specializing in CVD, anxiety was linked to poor diet, physical inactivity, and smoking (Bonnet et al., 2005). Alcohol consumption has also been associated with both elevated anxiety and CVD risk (Roy-Byrne, Davidson, et al., 2008; Strine et al., 2008). Anxiety may also interfere with health behaviors following a CVD event. One study showed that greater anxiety was associated with worse exercise adherence in post-MI patients (Ljubic, Deane, Zecchin, & Denniss, 2006).

Finally, insomnia may play a role in the link between anxiety and CVD. One study examined the moderating effects of insomnia on the anxiety and CVD relationship in a large sample of community-dwelling women (Olafiranye et al., 2010). The association between anxiety and CVD symptoms was reduced by threefold when insomnia was accounted for statistically. The authors speculated that sleep may play a role in the co-morbidity because stress is related to sleep disturbance, and both sleep disturbance and stress are related to sympathetic hyperarousal which increases CVD risk. Additional examination of sleep as a factor in the association between anxiety disorders and CVD is merited.

3.3.2.3 Pharmacology

Anxiolytics and antidepressant medication are often used in the treatment of anxiety disorders, but may have implications for CVD risk. The Women's Ischemia Syndrome Evaluation study, a large longitudinal study of ischemic heart disease in women with CHD, found that antidepressant medication was associated with cardiovascular events over 6 years, whereas anxiolytic use was not associated with those events (Krantz et al., 2009). The combination of anxiolytics and antidepressants was associated with heightened risk for cardiovascular events (i.e., hazards ratio of 3.98) after controlling for both anxiety and depression symptom severity. A cross-sectional investigation of community-dwelling older adults found that benzodiazepine use was associated with higher rates of CHD, congestive heart failure, and hypertension, although severity of symptoms was not controlled in this investigation (Gleason et al., 1998). These findings suggest the possibility of increased CVD risk when anxiolytics are used in combination with antidepressants and/or in older adult populations. However, additional studies are needed to draw firm conclusions. An exhaustive discussion of antidepressants and CVD risk can be found in Section Pharmacological Treatments.

3.3.3 Clinical Care of Patients with Co-morbid Anxiety and CVD

3.3.3.1 Assessment

Given that the prevalence of anxiety disorders in CVD populations is elevated, combined with fact that anxiety is associated with factors that worsen CVD (e.g., smoking, cardiovascular reactivity), screening for anxiety disorders in CVD populations may aid in clinical care. Assessment may be particularly warranted for individuals with a known personal or familial history of anxiety or mood disorders, or those who may be experiencing significant distress due to psychosocial circumstances or recent trauma. Several measures can be used to assess anxiety disorders and symptoms in CVD patients. To formally diagnose an anxiety disorder, diagnostic interviews that address DSM-IV (American Psychiatric Association, 2000) criteria are ideal, although infeasible in many settings that have limited time for assessment and/or do not employ mental health professionals. The HADS is a 14-item questionnaire of anxiety symptoms designed specifically for use with medically ill patients, and cutoffs indicate possible or probable presence of an anxiety disorder (Sigmond & Snaith, 1983). The HADS requires approximately 2–5 min to complete (Aina & Susman, 2006) and has demonstrated validity, reliability, sensitivity, and specificity across hospital, primary care, psychiatry, and general samples (Bjelland, Dahl, Haug, & Neckelmann, 2002; Herrmann, 1997). One study of cardiac patients found that the HADS performed well compared to structured clinical interview in identifying individuals with anxiety disorders (Harter, Woll, Wunsch,

Bengel, & Reuter, 2006). Also, the HADS may be helpful in predicting who may need treatment referrals. For example, a study of 104 stroke patients revealed that patients assessed within 2 weeks of a stroke who had a HADS anxiety score of 8 or greater displayed clinically significant anxiety (i.e., at least one diagnosed anxiety disorder) at 4-month follow-up (Sagen et al., 2010). The HADS may be preferable to the State-Trait Anxiety Inventory (Spielberger, Gorsuch, & Lushene, 1970) and the Beck Anxiety Inventory (Beck, Epstein, Brown, & Steer, 1988), the most widely used instruments to measure anxiety in the general population because neither has been validated in samples of individuals with CVD. Both of the latter measures include items on somatic anxiety symptoms (e.g., heart palpitations and dizziness) which are often indistinguishable from somatic symptoms resulting from CVD.

An important assessment issue in CVD patients is differentiating between cardiac chest pain and panic attacks, which can also be characterized by chest pain. Evidence for panic disorder includes presence of agoraphobia, feelings of impending doom prior to the chest pain, younger age (given that cardiac chest pain and tachycardia are less likely to occur in younger patients), and pain location over the heart as opposed to beneath the sternum as in cardiac chest pain (Potokar & Nutt, 2000). When the patient reports that pain radiates to the left arm or shoulder, cardiac chest pain may be more likely. Because panic disorder and cardiac chest pain can coexist, a cardiovascular event should not be discounted in the presence of suspected panic. A cardiac event could trigger a panic attack, especially among people with preexisting panic disorder. Due to the increased risk of acute coronary syndrome in persons with panic disorder, treatment providers should treat panic disorder not only as a differential diagnosis, but also as an indicator of the potential for a patient to experience a future cardiovascular event (Soh & Lee, 2010).

3.3.3.2 Treatment of Anxiety Disorders in the Context of CVD

Both pharmacotherapy and psychotherapy are used in the treatment of anxiety disorders. However, very little research has tested these treatments in the context of CVD.

Pharmacotherapy

SSRIs are the most widely used drugs for anxiety disorders (Gulliksson, Burell, et al., 2011). Some, albeit limited, evidence exists for their safety and efficacy in CVD patient populations; however, more research is needed to make definitive conclusions (Davies, Jackson, Potokar, & Nutt, 2004; Sowden & Huffman, 2009). Benzodiazepines are also widely prescribed for the treatment of anxiety disorders, but research exploring cardiovascular effects in patients with anxiety disorders is lacking. A review of benzodiazepine treatment of chest pain revealed they are efficacious in reducing chest pain, and some evidence exists for additional CVD-related benefits such as reduced risk for reinfarction following MI and decreased nitroglyceride use (Huffman

& Stern, 2003). Further research is needed regarding the efficacy of benzodiazepines on anxiety symptoms in individuals with CVD and co-occurring anxiety. Selective norepinephrine reuptake inhibitors and anticonvulsants have been shown effective in treating anxiety disorders (Dell'Osso, Buoli, Baldwin, & Altamura, 2010; Hoffman & Mathew, 2008; Zwanzger, Diemer, & Jabs, 2009), but research on their effectiveness and safety in patients with CVD is lacking. Beta-blockers, primarily used for the treatment of hypertension, are sometimes used off-label to treat anxiety disorders, although efficacy data have been mixed (Bastien, 2010). Some promise may exist specifically for patients developing PTSD following a cardiac event or surgery, given one study's findings that use of beta-blockers following cardiac surgery resulted in fewer traumatic memories and stress symptoms 6 months following surgery (Schelling, 2007).

Psychotherapy

CBT and exposure therapy are evidence-based treatments for most anxiety disorders (Chambless & Ollendick, 2001; Deacon & Abramowitz, 2004; McIntosh et al., 2004; Norton & Price, 2007). CBT targets both the distorted thought patterns (e.g., overestimation of threat) and behavioral components (e.g., avoidance of feared places or situations) that maintain anxiety disorders. Therapeutic strategies include restructuring distorted thoughts and exposing clients to feared stimuli either imaginally or in vivo, among other techniques. Exposure therapy typically involves intense administration of the latter therapeutic component, and it is typically used when there is a discrete feared stimulus or situation to which the client can be exposed and for which related anxiety may be reduced (e.g., heights, germs), as in the case of specific phobias, PTSD, and obsessive compulsive disorder. Trials of CBT and other psychotherapies for anxiety disorders that co-occur with CVD are needed to determine efficacy for anxiety and CVD outcomes. One small study examined the use of CBT in 39 cardiac rehabilitation patients whose scores on the HADS indicated probable depression and/or anxiety (Hambridge, Turner, & Baker, 2009). At posttreatment and at 1- and 6-month follow-up, moderate-to-strong effect sizes were found reflecting significant change in anxiety. At the 6-month follow-up, HADS anxiety scores fell below clinical cutoffs. These results are encouraging, but more investigations with larger samples are warranted to determine the efficacy and effectiveness of CBT for anxiety in individuals with co-morbid CVD. Further, the optimal timing of psychotherapy for anxiety disorders in the context of CVD may also be an important clinical issue, particularly in the case of PTSD. Studies examining the effect of anxiety disorder treatments in CVD populations on CVD events and mortality are needed.

Clinical Considerations

Clinicians should consider that stigma may be attached to an anxiety disorder diagnosis in CVD patients (Janeway, 2009). They should be prepared to mitigate such stigmatization by communicating that having problems with anxiety does not reduce the legitimacy of the patient's medical issues. Janeway provides a useful clinical algorithm to use with CVD patients with anxiety disorders that suggests when to refer patients to a mental health provider, how to reduce stigma associated with anxiety disorders, and how to provide adequately integrated care.

3.3.4 Conclusion

In sum, anxiety disorders are somewhat more prevalent in the CVD population than in the general population. Anxiety disorders might increase risk for CVD via both physiological and behavioral processes. On the other hand, a traumatic CVD event can trigger anxiety, including PTSD (Hari et al., 2010). Such symptoms may even develop as late as 1 year following the event, which supports ongoing assessment. Although many evidence-based treatments for anxiety disorders exist, little examination of these interventions has occurred in CVD populations. When treating a psychological disorder in the context of a serious medical co-morbidity such as CVD, consultation with the entire medical team will help to insure that the treatment decision is the safest and most effective option.

3.4 Psychotic Disorders

3.4.1 Prevalence

The psychotic disorders (e.g., schizophrenia, schizoaffective disorder, and psychotic depression) are generally characterized by a constellation of symptoms including hallucinations, delusions, disordered thinking, social withdrawal, and cognitive deficits. Patients experience great difficulty with social, occupational, and independent functioning and typically require pharmacologic intervention to address disabling symptoms. Individuals with psychotic disorders are disproportionately affected by CVD. The prevalence of CVD has been reported at 27% in a population-based cohort of adults with schizophrenia compared to 17% in non-schizophrenic controls (Bresee, Majumdar, Patten, & Johnson, 2010). The CATIE study, the largest prospective randomized trial of antipsychotic medications to date, revealed that at baseline estimated 10-year CHD risk of 689 participants with schizophrenia was greater than matched controls from the general population for males (9.4 vs. 7.0%) and females (6.3 vs. 4.2%) (Goff et al., 2005). Further, about 40% of CATIE participants met criteria for the metabolic syndrome (McEvoy et al., 2005), a constellation of symptoms that increase risk for CVD, whereas in the general population it is estimated to be at 24% (Ford, Giles, & Dietz, 2002). Heart failure also is more prevalent among adults with schizophrenia compared to controls (8 vs. 4%), as is stroke (9 vs. 4%) (Bresee et al., 2010). The gap in CVD prevalence rates between people with and without schizophrenia is widest at younger ages, and female sex does not appear to confer protection against CVD among younger adults with schizophrenia as it does in the general population (Bresee et al.). CVD-related hospital admittance and emergency room visits are elevated as well; they are 43% higher among people with schizophrenia than the general population (Callaghan, Boire, Lazo, McKenzie, & Cohn, 2009). In addition to CVD in general, rate of sudden cardiac death is three times higher in people with schizophrenia compared to the general population (Koponen, Jokelainen, Keinanen-Kiukaanniemi, Kumpusalo, & Vanhala, 2008). Mortality rates in general among people with schizophrenia are twice that of the general population (Capasso, Lineberry, Bostwick, Decker, & Sauver, 2008), and CVD is responsible for 50% of the excess death (De Hert et al., 2006). CVD is the leading cause of premature mortality in adults with schizophrenia. Seventy-five percent of people with schizophrenia will die of CVD and about 25 years earlier than the average US adult (Hennekens, 2007).

3.4.2 Pathophysiology

CVD among persons with schizophrenia has been attributed to myriad factors including antipsychotic medications, autonomic dysfunction associated with disease itself, and lifestyle factors, including smoking, dietary intake, and sedentary lifestyles.

3.4.2.1 Antipsychotic Medication

Atypical antipsychotic medications can cause weight gain and other metabolic disturbances that increase risk for CVD. A thorough discussion of weight gain-related side effects of atypical antipsychotic medications can be found in Chap. 1, Sect. 1.5.2.1. Weight gain contributes to other CVD risk factors, such as elevated lipids, C-reactive protein (Carrizo et al., 2008), and insulin resistance (Newcomer, 2009). However, atypical antipsychotics have been shown to also have direct effects on certain CVD risk factors including lipids, glucose metabolism, and QT interval prolongation.

The impact of atypical antipsychotic medications on blood lipids is well documented (Diaz, James, et al., 2009; Diaz, Meary, et al., 2009; Meyer & Koro, 2004), but the magnitude and direction of effects vary significantly by medication. Triglycerides, a form of fat in the blood that is linked to MI, stroke, and CVD, appear to be most affected by antipsychotic medications (Meyer et al., 2008). In the CATIE study, 3-month changes in nonfasting triglycerides varied by medication, with *elevations* observed with quetiapine and olanzipine, *reductions* observed with risperidone and perphenizine, and *no effect* observed with ziprasidone. In terms of blood cholesterol, the CATIE study revealed that olanzipine and quetipine were associated with increased 10-year CHD risk from baseline, whereas perphenizine, risperidone, and ziprasidone were associated with decreased risk from baseline (Daumit et al., 2008). Differences were attributable to decreases in total cholesterol in participants treated with risperidone and ziprasidone and increases in high density lipoprotein cholesterol in participants treated with perphenazine and ziprasidone.

In addition to lipids, atypical antipsychotics have been shown to increase risk for hyperglycemia, possibly via glucose metabolism interference, thereby contributing to risk for metabolic syndrome and type 2 diabetes. A meta-analysis revealed that increased risk for hyperglycemia was evident for clozapine- and olanzipine-treated groups relative to BMI-matched groups treated with other antipsychotic medications or healthy controls (Newcomer & Haupt, 2006). Hypertension also has been cited as a side effect of atypical antipsychotic medications, but clozapine is the only medication for which a direct effect has been consistently observed (De Leon & Diaz, 2007). Finally, people with schizophrenia who are treated with antipsychotic medications have been shown to have prolonged QT interval, a risk factor for sudden death (Blasco-Fontecilla, Baca-Garcia, & de Leon, 2010). One cross-sectional study reported results of electrocardiograms in 1,017 people with schizophrenia and showed first-generation antipsychotic medications, but not atypical antipsychotics, were associated with increased risk for QT interval prolongation (Ozeki et al., 2010). Overall, antipsychotic medications seem to have significant implications for CVD risk, but vary greatly in the extent to which they influence various CVD risk factors.

3.4.2.2 Autonomic Dysfunction

Although atypical antipsychotic medications have been implicated in heightened risk for CVD and sudden death, unmedicated individuals also have heightened risk for CVD and sudden death (Jindal, MacKenzie, Baker, & Yeragani, 2005), which suggests that either schizophrenia itself, lifestyle factors, or some combination contribute to that risk. Autonomic dysfunction as reflected by low HRV, reduced baroreflex sensitivity, and reduced QT variability have been observed during acute psychosis in unmedicated samples, and each increases risk for cardiac arrhythmias, which can precipitate a cardiac event or sudden death (Bar, Boettger, et al., 2007; Bar, Koschke, et al., 2007). Degree of severity of psychotic symptoms correlates with QT variability, making patients in acute psychosis at particularly heightened risk for sudden death (Bar, Boettger, et al., 2007; Bar, Koschke, et al., 2007). The known association between acute psychosis and autonomic dysfunction has treatment implications given that some antipsychotic medications also contribute to autonomic dysfunction, as discussed above. Electrocardiograms may be indicated to assess changes in electrical activity of the heart as a result of antipsychotic treatment in schizophrenia.

3.4.2.3 Lifestyle Factors

The prevalence rates of lifestyle factors associated with increased risk for CVD, including smoking, obesity, unhealthy diet, and sedentary lifestyles, also are elevated in people with schizophrenia. For example, three quarters of people with schizophrenia smoke, compared to about one quarter of adults in the general US population (Hennekens, Hennekens, Hollar, & Casey, 2005). Obesity also affects people with schizophrenia disproportionately with rates of 42% (Bell, Farmer, Ries, & Srebnik, 2009) compared to 34% in the general US population (Flegal, Carroll, & Ogden, 2010). The dietary quality in persons with schizophrenia is also lower than controls. In one study, dietary patterns of 30 hospitalized patients with schizophrenia were compared to 30 healthy age- and sex-matched controls, and findings revealed that dietary scores were lower for patients than controls among women, but not men (Amani, 2007). Women with schizophrenia had higher intake of cream and carbonated beverages and lower intake of fruits, vegetables, nuts, dairy, and chicken compared to controls. Men with schizophrenia were heavier than controls and had higher intake of cream and hydrogenated fat, and lower intake of nuts. Another study compared 74 general practice patients with severe mental illness (i.e., schizophrenia, schizoaffective disorder, or other psychotic disorder) to 148 people without such diagnoses on fat and fiber intake as well as other lifestyle factors, controlling for socioeconomic status and medication use (Osborn, Nazareth, & King, 2007). People with severe mental illness had higher saturated fat intake and lower fiber intake than controls. They also were less likely to exercise and more likely to smoke.

People with schizophrenia have also been shown to be less physically active in general than controls, although very few studies have addressed this question, and data are mixed depending on measures used. In one study, physical activity levels of community-dwelling adults with schizophrenia were compared to sex- and age-matched controls (Lindamer et al., 2008). Results from self-report measures showed that adults with schizophrenia engaged in less than half the time in physical activity and expended less than half the calories as controls. However, differences in expenditure were not observed via accelerometry data. Another study, also using self-reported physical activity, compared 185 outpatients with severe mental illness (i.e., schizophrenia or schizoaffective disorder) to an age-, gender-, and race-matched sample from National Health and Nutrition Examination Survey-III (NHANES) on the proportion of people who are inactive, active but less than recommended levels, and active and at recommended levels (Daumit et al., 2005). Results revealed that people with severe mental illness had higher rates of inactivity (25.7 vs. 17.5%) and higher rates of less than recommended levels of activity (45.2 vs. 35.7%), but no differences in rates of recommended levels of activity (38.9 vs. 38.9%). Among the severely mentally ill patients, education was the strongest predictor of meeting the recommended level of activity and number of social contacts in the last month was the stronger predictor of inactivity.

3.4.3 Screening and Interventions to Reduce CVD Risk in Schizophrenia

3.4.3.1 Screening for CVD Risk Factors

In 2004, the American Diabetes Association, American Psychiatric Association, American Association of Clinical Endocrinologists, and the North American Association for the Study of Obesity (now named the Obesity Society) held a Consensus Development Conference to put forth a clinical guideline that recommends baseline screening of weight, waist circumference, blood pressure, plasma glucose, and fasting lipids for all patients who are prescribed atypical antipsychotics (American Diabetes Association et al., 2004). Unfortunately, two recent studies showed that the Consensus guidelines had a minimal effect on screening rates. In a retrospective cohort analysis of a large managed care database, screening rates of glucose increased from 17.3 to only 21.8% over 2 years and from 8.4 to only 10.5% for lipids (Haupt et al., 2009). A second retrospective cohort study of a managed care database showed that the rates of increase in screening rates for lipid and glucose were no different pre- and postguidelines (Morrato et al., 2009). More work is clearly needed to promote widespread adoption of screening guidelines.

3.4.3.2 Managing CVD Risk in People with Schizophrenia

Reducing CVD risk in people with schizophrenia may involve a number of approaches including antipsychotic medication switching, weight loss/lifestyle interventions, smoking cessation, and CVD preventive care. Medication switching and weight loss interventions are discussed in Chap. 1, Sect. 1.5.3.2 in this book, and smoking cessation interventions in people with schizophrenia are discussed in Chap. 5. Briefly, behavioral weight loss interventions involving dietary and physical activity counselling have a modest but significant impact on both preventing and reducing medication-induced weight gain (see Chap. 1). In addition to impact on weight, some randomized trials also reported improvements in cardiovascular risk factors such as triglycerides (Chen, Chen, & Huang, 2009; Lindenmayer et al., 2009; McKibbin et al., 2006; Wu et al., 2007), fasting glucose (Lindenmayer et al., 2009), insulin resistance (Wu et al., 2007), cholesterol (Kwon et al., 2006), blood pressure (Brar et al., 2005), and metabolic syndrome (Lindenmayer et al., 2009). For smoking, nicotine replacement therapies and bupropion have been shown to increase cessation rates in people with schizophrenia (see Chap. 5).

CVD Preventive Care

In addition to antipsychotic medication management and lifestyle interventions, people with schizophrenia should be assisted in securing routine primary care, where comprehensive CVD preventive care typically occurs. CVD preventive care includes screening, referral, and pharmacological management of risk factors. However, access to care appears to be a challenge for people with schizophrenia (Bradford et al., 2008). They are more likely to need medical care and not receive it, more likely to delay medical care due to cost, and less likely to receive a needed prescription than people without mental illness (Bradford et al.). Reduced access might not be the only contributor to inadequate CVD preventive care. A recent study revealed that even when patients with schizophrenia attended the same number of physician visits as their peers, they were still less likely to receive treatment for CVD (Vahia et al., 2008). In the CATIE trial, only 11% of participants with dyslipidemia were taking statins at baseline (Nasrallah et al., 2006). In a study of people with type 2 diabetes (Kreyenbuhl et al., 2006), only 20% of people with schizophrenia were in statin treatment compared to 48% of people who had no mental illness, even though the schizophrenia group had more CVD risk factors. A third study using a database of primary care medical records in the UK found that patients with CVD and schizophrenia were significantly less likely to receive cholesterol screening and treatment than people with CVD and no mental illness (Hippisley-Cox, Parker, Coupland, & Vinogradova, 2007). These findings point to barriers to care that occur during or after the healthcare visit. One reason suggested is that symptoms experienced by people with schizophrenia may affect the care they receive (Felker, Yazel, & Short, 1996). The severity of psychotic symptoms has been associated with less adequate treatment (Vahia et al., 2008). Such symptoms affect the patient's insight and ability to communicate, as well as both treatment delivery and receipt. Physicians report discomfort treating patients with florid symptoms, which could affect the quality of the encounter (Vahia et al.). Uncontrolled psychiatric symptoms might also overshadow other healthcare concerns. In addition, the patient may not have the skills to navigate the healthcare system (Felker, Yazel, et al., 1996). People with severe mental illness often have difficulty keeping appointments, tolerating waiting rooms, following up on referrals, and communicating with healthcare professionals (McConnell, Inderbitzin, & Pollard, 1992). Finally, physicians report that clinical assessment can be more challenging with patients with schizophrenia. Psychotropic medication regimens with complicated side effect profiles along with numerous psychiatric complaints and symptoms present challenging differential diagnostic issues (Felker, Yazel, et al., 1996).

The elevated prevalence of CVD in this population combined with reduced rates of care makes CVD prevention in schizophrenia an urgent area for research. One study revealed that having a schizophrenia diagnosis predicted 1-year post-MI mortality and the association was attributable to the level of care received post-MI (Druss, Bradford, Rosenheck, Radford, & Krumholz, 2001), which suggests that reduced care may account for increased CVD death in people with schizophrenia. The literature is lacking in intervention studies for improving CVD screening and treatment rates. Vahia et al. (2008) recommend that health education interventions that teach patients about preventive care and that motivate them to ask for the care they need may improve care receipt among people with schizophrenia. Collaborative care models that bring preventive care into the psychiatry setting may also be a promising approach.

3.4.4 Summary

People with schizophrenia are disproportionately affected by CVD and CVD mortality. Multiple factors account for their increased risk, including psychotropic medications, cardiac changes associated with psychotic symptoms, lifestyle factors, and inadequate screening and preventive care. Very little research has addressed CVD risk reduction approaches in this population. Some data suggest that behavioral weight loss interventions and pharmacological smoking cessation interventions are effective, although it remains unclear if these treatments are widely accessible to this patient population. Comprehensive care models are needed that address both the mental and physical health needs of people with schizophrenia.

References

Abbas, C. C., Schmid, J. P., Guler, E., Wiedemar, L., Begre, S., Saner, H., et al. (2009). Trajectory of posttraumatic stress disorder caused by myocardial infarction: A two-year follow-up study. *International Journal of Psychiatry in Medicine, 39*(4), 359–376.

Agelink, M. W., Boz, C., Ullrich, H., & Andrich, J. (2002). Relationship between major depression and heart rate variability. Clinical consequences and implications for antidepressive treatment. *Psychiatry Research, 113*(1–2), 139–149.

Aina, Y., & Susman, J. L. (2006). Understanding comorbidity with depression and anxiety disorders. *Journal of the American Osteopathic Association, 106*(Suppl 2), S9–S14.

Amani, R. (2007). Is dietary pattern of schizophrenia patients different from healthy subjects? *BMC Psychiatry, 7*, 15.

American Diabetes Association, American Psychiatric Association, American Association of Clinical Endocrinologists & North American Association for the Study of Obesity. (2004). Consensus development conference on antipsychotic drugs and obesity and diabetes. *Diabetes Care, 27*(2), 596–601.

American Psychiatric Association. (2000). *Diagnostic and statistical manual of mental disorders*. Washington: American Psychiatric Association.

Anda, R. F., Williamson, D. F., Escobedo, L. G., Mast, E. E., Giovino, G. A., & Remington, P. L. (1990). Depression and the dynamics of smoking – A national perspective. *Journal of the American Medical Association, 264*(12), 1541–1545.

Angst, F., Stassen, H. H., Clayton, P. J., & Angst, J. (2002). Mortality of patients with mood disorders: Follow-up over 34–38 years. *Journal of Affective Disorders, 68*(2–3), 167–181.

Bankier, B., Januzzi, J. L., & Littman, A. B. (2004). The high prevalence of multiple psychiatric disorders in stable outpatients with coronary heart disease. *Psychosomatic Medicine, 66*(5), 645–650.

Bansal, B., Khan, M., & Salhan, A. K. (2009). A review of measurement and analysis of heart rate variability. *International conference on computer and automation engineering*, 8–10 March, pp. 243–246.

Bar, K. J., Boettger, M. K., Koschke, M., Schulz, S., Chokka, P., Yeragani, V. K., et al. (2007). Non-linear complexity measures of heart rate variability in acute schizophrenia. *Clinical Neurophysiology, 118*(9), 2009–2015.

Bar, K. J., Greiner, W., Jochum, T., Friedrich, M., Wagner, G., & Sauer, H. (2004). The influence of major depression and its treatment on heart rate variability and pupillary light reflex parameters. *Journal of Affective Disorders, 82*(2), 245–252.

Bar, K. J., Koschke, M., Boettger, M. K., Berger, S., Kabisch, A., Sauer, H., et al. (2007). Acute psychosis leads to increased QT variability in patients suffering from schizophrenia. *Schizophrenia Research, 95*(1–3), 115–123.

Barth, J., Schumacher, M., & Herrmann-Lingen, C. (2004). Depression as a risk factor for mortality in patients with coronary heart disease: A meta-analysis. *Psychosomatic Medicine, 66*(6), 802–813.

Bastien, D. L. (2010). Pharmacological treatment of combat-induced PTSD: A literature review. *British Journal of Nursing (Mark Allen Publishing), 19*(5), 318–321.

Baune, B. T., Adrian, I., Arolt, V., & Berger, K. (2006). Associations between major depression, bipolar disorders, dysthymia and cardiovascular diseases in the general adult population. *Psychotherapy and Psychosomatics, 75*(5), 319–326.

Beck, A. T., Epstein, N., Brown, G., & Steer, R. A. (1988). An inventory for measuring clinical anxiety: Psychometric properties. *Journal of Consulting and Clinical Psychology, 56*(6), 893–897.

Bell, R. C., Farmer, S., Ries, R., & Srebnik, D. (2009). Metabolic risk factors among medicaid outpatients with schizophrenia receiving second-generation antipsychotics. *Psychiatric Services, 60*(12), 1686–1689.

Berg, A., Lonnqvist, J., Palomaki, H., & Kaste, M. (2009). Assessment of depression after stroke a comparison of different screening instruments. *Stroke, 40*(2), 523–529.

Berkman, L. F., Blumenthal, J., Burg, M., Carney, R. M., Catellier, D., Cowan, M. J., et al. (2003). Effects of treating depression and low-perceived social support on clinical events after myocardial infarction – The enhancing recovery in coronary heart disease patients (ENRICHD) randomized trial. *Journal of the American Medical Association, 289*(23), 3106–3116.

Berntson, G. G., Bigger, J. T., Eckberg, D. L., Grossman, P., Kaufmann, P. G., Malik, M., et al. (1997). Heart rate variability: Origins, methods, and interpretive caveats. *Psychophysiology, 34*(6), 623–648.

Bhogal, S. K., Teasell, R., Foley, N., & Speechley, M. (2004). Lesion location and poststroke depression – Systematic review of the methodological limitations in the literature. *Stroke, 35*(3), 794–802.

Bigger, J. T., Fleiss, J. L., Rolnitzky, L. M., & Steinman, R. C. (1993). The ability of several short-term measures of RR variability to predict mortality after myocardial-infarction. *Circulation, 88*(3), 927–934.

Bjelland, I., Dahl, A. A., Haug, T. T., & Neckelmann, D. (2002). The validity of the hospital anxiety and depression scale – An updated literature review. *Journal of Psychosomatic Research, 52*(2), 69–77.

Blasco-Fontecilla, H., Baca-Garcia, E., & de Leon, J. (2010). Do atypical antipsychotic drugs reduce the risk of ischemic heart disease and mortality? Possible role of 5-HT2A receptor blockade. *Schizophrenia Research, 119*(1–3), 160–163.

Bonnet, F., Irving, K., Terra, J. L., Nony, P., Berthezene, F., & Moulin, P. (2005). Anxiety and depression are associated with unhealthy lifestyle in patients at risk of cardiovascular disease. *Atherosclerosis, 178*(2), 339–344.

Bradford, D. W., Kim, M. M., Braxton, L. E., Marx, C. E., Butterfield, M., & Elbogen, E. B. (2008). Access to medical care among persons with psychotic and major affective disorders. *Psychiatric Services, 59*(8), 847–852.

Brar, J. S., Ganguli, R., Pandina, G., Turkoz, I., Berry, S., & Mahmoud, R. (2005). Effects of behavioral therapy on weight loss in overweight and obese patients with schizophrenia or schizoaffective disorder. *The Journal of Clinical Psychiatry, 66*(2), 205–212.

Bresee, L. C., Majumdar, S. R., Patten, S. B., & Johnson, J. A. (2010). Prevalence of cardiovascular risk factors and disease in people with schizophrenia: A population-based study. *Schizophrenia Research, 117*(1), 75–82.

Bruce, E. C., & Musselman, D. L. (2005). Depression, alterations in platelet function, and ischemic heart disease. *Psychosomatic Medicine, 67*, S34–S36.

Callaghan, R. C., Boire, M. D., Lazo, R. G., McKenzie, K., & Cohn, T. (2009). Schizophrenia and the incidence of cardiovascular morbidity: A population-based longitudinal study in Ontario, Canada. *Schizophrenia Research, 115*(2–3), 325–332.

Capasso, R. M., Lineberry, T. W., Bostwick, J. M., Decker, P. A., & Sauver, J. S. (2008). Mortality in schizophrenia and schizoaffective disorder: An Olmsted county, Minnesota cohort: 1950–2005. *Schizophrenia Research, 98*(1–3), 287–294.

Carney, R. M., Blumenthal, J. A., Freedland, K. E., Stein, P. K., Howells, W. B., Berkman, L. F., et al. (2005). Low heart rate variability and the effect of depression on post-myocardial infarction mortality. *Archives of Internal Medicine, 165*(13), 1486–1491.

Carney, R. M., & Freedland, K. E. (2008). Depression in patients with coronary heart disease. *The American Journal of Medicine, 121*(11 Suppl 2), S20–S27.

Carney, R. M., & Freedland, K. E. (2009). Depression and heart rate variability in patients with coronary heart disease. *Cleveland Clinic Journal of Medicine, 76*(Suppl 2), S13–S17.

Carney, R. M., Freedland, K. E., & Jaffe, A. S. (2009). Depression screening in patients with heart disease. *Journal of the American Medical Association, 301*(13), 1337.

Carrizo, E., Fernandez, V., Quintero, J., Connell, L., Rodriguez, Z., Mosquera, M., et al. (2008). Coagulation and inflammation markers during atypical or typical antipsychotic treatment in schizophrenia patients and drug-free first-degree relatives. *Schizophrenia Research, 103*(1–3), 83–93.

Chambless, D. L., & Ollendick, T. H. (2001). Empirically supported psychological interventions: Controversies and evidence. *Annual Review of Psychology, 52*, 685–716.

Chang, H. H., Yang, Y. K., Gean, P. W., Huang, H. C., Chen, P. S., & Lu, R. B. (2010). The role of valproate in metabolic disturbances in bipolar disorder patients. *Journal of Affective Disorders, 124*(3), 319–323.

Chen, C. K., Chen, Y. C., & Huang, Y. S. (2009). Effects of a 10-week weight control program on obese patients with schizophrenia or schizoaffective disorder: A 12-month follow up. *Psychiatry and Clinical Neurosciences, 63*(1), 17–22.

Chen, Y. H., Hu, C. J., Lee, H. C., & Lin, H. C. (2010). An Increased risk of stroke among panic disorder patients: A 3-year follow-up study. *Canadian Journal of Psychiatry-Revue Canadienne De Psychiatrie, 55*(1), 43–49.

Cohen, H. W., Gibson, G., & Alderman, M. H. (2000). Excess risk of myocardial infarction in patients treated with antidepressant medications: Association with use of tricyclic agents. *The American Journal of Medicine, 108*(1), 2–8.

Daughters, S. B., Braun, A. R., Sargeant, M. N., Reynolds, E. K., Hopko, D. R., Blanco, C., et al. (2008). Effectiveness of a brief behavioral treatment for inner-city illicit drug users with elevated depressive symptoms: The life enhancement treatment for substance use (LETS Act!). *The Journal of Clinical Psychiatry, 69*(1), 122–129.

Daumit, G. L., Goff, D. C., Meyer, J. M., Davis, V. G., Nasrallah, H. A., McEvoy, J. P., et al. (2008). Antipsychotic effects on estimated 10-year coronary heart disease risk in the CATIE schizophrenia study. *Schizophrenia Research, 105*(1–3), 175–187.

Daumit, G. L., Goldberg, R. W., Anthony, C., Dickerson, F., Brown, C. H., Kreyenbuhl, J., et al. (2005). Physical activity patterns in adults with severe mental illness. *The Journal of Nervous and Mental Disease, 193*(10), 641–646.

Davidson, K. W., Kupfer, D. J., Bigger, J. T., Califf, R. M., Carney, R. M., Coyne, J. C., et al. (2006). Assessment and treatment of depression in patients with cardiovascular disease: National Heart, Lung, and Blood Institute working group report. *Psychosomatic Medicine, 68*(5), 615–650.

Davidson, K. W., Rieckmann, N., Clemow, L., Schwartz, J. E., Shimbo, D., Medina, V., et al. (2010). Enhanced depression care for patients with acute coronary syndrome and persistent depressive symptoms coronary psychosocial evaluation studies randomized controlled trial. *Archives of Internal Medicine, 170*(7), 600–608.

Davies, S. J. C., Jackson, P. R., Potokar, J., & Nutt, D. J. (2004). Treatment of anxiety and depressive disorders in patients with cardiovascular disease. *British Medical Journal, 328*(7445), 939–943.

De Hert, M., Kalnicka, D., van Winkel, R., Wampers, M., Hanssens, L., Van Eyck, D., et al. (2006). Treatment with rosuvastatin for severe dyslipidemia in patients with schizophrenia and schizoaffective disorder. *The Journal of Clinical Psychiatry, 67*(12), 1889–1896.

de Jonge, P., Honig, A., van Melle, J. P., Schene, A. H., Kuyper, A. M. G., Tulner, D., et al. (2007). Nonresponse to treatment for depression following myocardial infarction: Association with subsequent cardiac events. *The American Journal of Psychiatry, 164*(9), 1371–1378.

De Leon, J., & Diaz, F. J. (2007). Planning for the optimal design of studies to personalize antipsychotic prescriptions in the post-CATIE era: The clinical and pharmacoepidemiological data suggest that pursuing the pharmacogenetics of metabolic syndrome complications (hypertension, diabetes mellitus and hyperlipidemia) may be a reasonable strategy. *Schizophrenia Research, 96*(1–3), 185–197.

Deacon, B. J., & Abramowitz, J. S. (2004). Cognitive and behavioral treatments for anxiety disorders: A review of meta-analytic findings. *Journal of Clinical Psychology, 60*(4), 429–441.

Dedert, E., Calhoun, P., Watkins, L., Sherwood, A., & Beckham, J. (2010). Posttraumatic stress disorder, cardiovascular, and metabolic disease: A review of the evidence. *Annals of Behavioral Medicine, 39*(1), 61–78.

Dell'Osso, B., Buoli, M., Baldwin, D. S., & Altamura, A. C. (2010). Serotonin norepinephrine reuptake inhibitors (SNRIs) in anxiety disorders: A comprehensive review of their clinical efficacy. *Human Psychopharmacology-Clinical and Experimental, 25*(1), 17–29.

Diaz, F. J., James, D., Botts, S., Maw, L., Susce, M. T., & de Leon, J. (2009). Tobacco smoking behaviors in bipolar disorder: A comparison of the general population, schizophrenia, and major depression. *Bipolar Disorders, 11*(2), 154–165.

Diaz, F. J., Meary, A., Arranz, M. J., Ruano, G., Windemuth, A., & de Leon, J. (2009). Acetyl-coenzyme A carboxylase alpha gene variations may be associated with the direct effects of some antipsychotics on triglyceride levels. *Schizophrenia Research, 115*(2–3), 136–140.

Dimidjian, S., & Davis, K. J. (2009). Newer variations of cognitive-behavioral therapy: Behavioral activation and mindfulness-based cognitive therapy. *Current Psychiatry Reports, 11*, 453–458.

Druss, B. G., Bradford, W. D., Rosenheck, R. A., Radford, M. J., & Krumholz, H. M. (2001). Quality of medical care and excess mortality in older patients with mental disorders. *Archives of General Psychiatry, 58*(6), 565–572.

Eze-Nliam, C. M., Thombs, B. D., Lima, B. B., Smith, C. G., & Ziegelstein, R. C. (2010). The association of depression with adherence to antihypertensive medications: A systematic review. *Journal of Hypertension, 28*(9), 1785–1795.

Fan, A. Z., Strine, T. W., Jiles, R., & Mokdad, A. H. (2008). Depression and anxiety associated with cardiovascular disease among persons aged 45 years and older in 38 states of the United States. *Preventive Medicine, 46*(5), 445–450.

Fang, J., & Cheng, Q. (2009). Etiological mechanisms of post-stroke depression: A review. *Neurological Research, 31*(9), 904–909.

Felker, B., Yazel, J. J., & Short, D. (1996). Mortality and medical comorbidity among psychiatric patients: A review. *Psychiatric Services, 47*(12), 1356–1363.

Fiedorowicz, J. G., Solomon, D. A., Endicott, J., Leon, A. C., Li, C. S., Rice, J. P., et al. (2009). Manic/hypomanic symptom burden and cardiovascular mortality in bipolar disorder. *Psychosomatic Medicine, 71*(6), 598–606.

Fleet, R., Lavoie, K., & Beitman, B. D. (2000). Is panic disorder associated with coronary artery disease? A critical review of the literature. *Journal of Psychosomatic Research, 48*(4–5), 347–356.

Flegal, K. M., Carroll, M. D., & Ogden, C. L. (2010). Prevalence and trends in obesity among US Adults, 1999–2008. *Journal of the American Medical Association, 303*(3), 235–241.

Ford, E. S., Giles, W. H., & Dietz, W. H. (2002). Prevalence of the metabolic syndrome among US adults: Findings from the third national Health and Nutrition Examination Survey. *Journal of the American Medical Association, 287*, 356–359.

Fournier, J. C., DeRubeis, R. J., Hollon, S. D., Dimidjian, S., Amsterdam, J. D., Shelton, R. C., et al. (2010). Antidepressant drug effects and depression severity a patient-level meta-analysis. *Journal of the American Medical Association, 303*(1), 47–53.

Frasure-Smith, N., & Lesperance, F. (2010). Depression and cardiac risk: Present status and future directions. *Heart, 96*(3), 173–176.

Garcia-Portilla, M. P., Saiz, P. A., Bascaran, M. T., Martinez, S., Benabarre, A., Sierra, P., et al. (2009). Cardiovascular risk in patients with bipolar disorder. *Journal of Affective Disorders, 115*(3), 302–308.

Glassman, A. H., Bigger, J. T., Gaffney, M., Shapiro, P. A., & Swenson, J. R. (2006). Onset of major depression associated with acute coronary syndromes – Relationship of onset, major depressive disorder history, and episode severity to sertraline benefit. *Archives of General Psychiatry, 63*(3), 283–288.

Glassman, A. H., O'Connor, C. M., Califf, R. M., Swedberg, K., Schwartz, P., Bigger, J. T., et al. (2002). Sertraline treatment of major depression in patients with acute MI or unstable angina. *Journal of the American Medical Association, 288*(6), 701–709.

Gleason, P. P., Schulz, R., Smith, N. L., Newsom, J. T., Kroboth, P., Kroboth, F. J., et al. (1998). Correlates and prevalence of benzodiazepine use in community-dwelling elderly. *Journal of General Internal Medicine, 13*(4), 243–250.

Goff, D. C., Sullivan, L. M., McEvoy, J. P., Meyer, J. M., Nasrallah, H. A., Daumit, G. L., et al. (2005). A comparison of ten-year cardiac risk estimates in schizophrenia patients from the CATIE study and matched controls. *Schizophrenia Research, 80*(1), 45–53.

Goldstein, B. I., Fagiolini, A., Houck, P., & Kupfer, D. J. (2009). Cardiovascular disease and hypertension among adults with bipolar I disorder in the United States. *Bipolar Disorders, 11*(6), 657–662.

Goodwin, R. D., Davidson, K. W., & Keyes, K. (2009). Mental disorders and cardiovascular disease among adults in the United States. *Journal of Psychiatric Research, 43*(3), 239–246.

Grippo, A. J. (2009). Mechanisms underlying altered mood and cardiovascular dysfunction: The value of neurobiological and behavioral research with animal models. *Neuroscience and Biobehavioral Reviews, 33*(2), 171–180.

Guler, E., Schmid, J. P., Wiedemar, L., Saner, H., Schnyder, U., & von Kanel, R. (2009). Clinical diagnosis of posttraumatic stress disorder after myocardial infarction. *Clinical Cardiology, 32*(3), 125–129.

Gulliksson, M., Burell, G., Vessby, B., Lundin, L., Toss, H., & Svardsudd, K. (2011). Randomized controlled trial of cognitive behavioral therapy vs standard treatment to prevent recurrent cardiovascular events in patients with coronary heart disease: Secondary Prevention in Uppsala Primary Health Care Project (SUPRIM). *Archives of Internal Medicine, 171*(2), 134–140.

Hackett, M. L., Anderson, C. S., House, A., & Xia, J. (2008). Interventions for treating depression after stroke. *Cochrane Database of Systematic Reviews,* (4), CD003437.

Hambridge, J. A., Turner, A., & Baker, A. L. (2009). BraveHeart begins: Pilot results of group cognitive behaviour therapy for depression and anxiety in cardiac patients. *The Australian and New Zealand Journal of Psychiatry, 43*(12), 1171–1177.

Hari, R., Begre, S., Schmid, J. P., Saner, H., Gander, M. L., & von Kanel, R. (2010). Change over time in posttraumatic stress caused by myocardial infarction and predicting variables. *Journal of Psychosomatic Research, 69*(2), 143–150.

Harter, M., Woll, S., Wunsch, A., Bengel, J., & Reuter, K. (2006). Screening for mental disorders in cancer, cardiovascular, and musculoskeletal diseases. *Social Psychiatry and Psychiatric Epidemiology, 41*, 56–62.

Haupt, D. W., Rosenblatt, L. C., Kim, E., Baker, R. A., Whitehead, R., & Newcomer, J. W. (2009). Prevalence and predictors of lipid and glucose monitoring in commercially insured patients treated with second-generation antipsychotic agents. *The American Journal of Psychiatry, 166*(3), 345–353.

Hennekens, C. H. (2007). Increasing global burden of cardiovascular disease in general populations and patients with schizophrenia. *The Journal of Clinical Psychiatry, 68*(Suppl 4), 4–7.

Hennekens, C. H., Hennekens, A. R., Hollar, D., & Casey, D. E. (2005). Schizophrenia and increased risks of cardiovascular disease. *American Heart Journal, 150*(6), 1115–1121.

Herrmann, C. (1997). International experiences with the hospital anxiety and depression scale – A review of validation data and clinical results. *Journal of Psychosomatic Research, 42*, 17–41.

Herrmann, C., Brand-Driehorst, S., Buss, U., & Rüger, U. (2000). Effects of anxiety and depression on 5-year mortality in 5057 patients referred for exercise testing. *Journal of Psychosomatic Research, 48*(4–5), 455–462.

Hippisley-Cox, J., Parker, C., Coupland, C., & Vinogradova, Y. (2007). Inequalities in the primary care of patients with coronary heart disease and serious mental health problems: A cross-sectional study. *Heart, 93*(10), 1256–1262.

Hippisley-Cox, J., Pringle, M., Hammersley, V., Crown, N., Wynn, A., Meal, A., et al. (2001). Antidepressants as risk factor for ischaemic heart disease: Case-control study in primary care. *British Medical Journal, 323*(7314), 666–669.

Hirschfeld, R. M. A., Williams, J. B. W., Spitzer, R. L., Calabrese, J. R., Flynn, L., Keck, P. E., et al. (2000). Development and validation of a screening instrument for bipolar spectrum disorder: The mood disorder questionnaire. *The American Journal of Psychiatry, 157*(11), 1873–1875.

Hoffman, E. J., & Mathew, S. J. (2008). Anxiety disorders: A comprehensive review of pharmacotherapies. *The Mount Sinai Journal of Medicine, 75*(3), 248–262.

Hopko, D. R., Lejuez, C. W., & Hopko, S. D. (2008). Cognitive-behavior therapy for depressed cancer patients in a medical care setting. *Behavior Therapy, 39*, 126–136.

Hopko, D. R., Lejuez, C. W., LePage, J. P., Hopko, S. D., & McNeil, D. W. (2003). A brief behavioral activation treatment for depression: A randomized trial within an inpatient psychiatric hospital. *Behavior Modification, 27*, 458–469.

Huffman, J. C., & Stern, T. A. (2003). The use of benzodiazepines in the treatment of chest pain: A review of the literature. *The Journal of Emergency Medicine, 25*(4), 427–437.

Ibishi, N. F., Musliu, N. R., Kamberi, A., Qirko, S., Brokaj, S., Lezha, M., et al. (2009). Impact of depression and cardiovascular disease. *Psychiatric Annals, 39*(1), 22–25.

Jacka, F. N., Pasco, J. A., Mykletun, A., Williams, L. J., Hodge, A. M., O'Reilly, S. L., et al. (2010). Association of Western and traditional diets with depression and anxiety in women. *The American Journal of Psychiatry, 167*(3), 305–311.

Janeway, D. (2009). An Integrated approach to the diagnosis and treatment of anxiety within the practice of cardiology. *Cardiology in Review, 17*(1), 36–43.

Janszky, I., Ahnve, S., Lundberg, I., & Hemmingsson, T. (2010). Early-onset depression, anxiety, and risk of subsequent coronary heart disease: 37-year follow-up of 49,321 young Swedish men. *Journal of the American College of Cardiology, 56*(1), 31–37.

Jindal, R., MacKenzie, E. M., Baker, G. B., & Yeragani, V. K. (2005). Cardiac risk and schizophrenia. *Journal of Psychiatry & Neuroscience, 30*(6), 393–395.

Joynt, K. E., & O'Connor, C. M. (2005). Lessons from SADHART, ENRICHD, and other trials. *Psychosomatic Medicine, 67*, S63–S66.

Kemp, A. H., Quintana, D. S., Gray, M. A., Felmingham, K. L., Brown, K., & Gatt, J. M. (2010). Impact of depression and antidepressant treatment on heart rate variability: A review and meta-analysis. *Biological Psychiatry, 67*(11), 1067–1074.

Kent, L. K., & Shapiro, P. A. (2009). Depression and related psychological factors in heart disease. *Harvard Review of Psychiatry, 17*(6), 377–388.

Kessler, R. C., Chiu, W. T., Demler, O., & Walters, E. E. (2005). Prevalence, severity, and comorbidity of 12-month DSM-IV disorders in the National Comorbidity Survey Replication. *Archives of General Psychiatry, 62*(6), 617–627.

Ketter, T. A. (2010). Strategies for monitoring outcomes in patients with bipolar disorder. *The Primary Care Companion to the Journal of Clinical Psychiatry, 12*(Suppl 1), 10–16.

Kilbourne, A. M., Post, E. P., Nossek, A., Drill, L., Cooley, S., & Bauer, M. S. (2008). Improving medical and psychiatric outcomes among individuals with bipolar disorder: A randomized controlled trial. *Psychiatric Services, 59*(7), 760–768.

Kilbourne, A. M., Post, E. P., Nossek, A., Sonel, E., Drill, L. J., Cooley, S., et al. (2008). Service delivery in older patients with bipolar disorder: A review and development of a medical care model. *Bipolar Disorders, 10*(6), 672–683.

Kilbourne, A. M., Rofey, D. L., McCarthy, J. F., Post, E. P., Welsh, D., & Blow, F. C. (2007). Nutrition and exercise behavior among patients with bipolar disorder. *Bipolar Disorders, 9*(5), 443–452.

Kim, J. Y., & Lee, H. W. (2007). Metabolic and hormonal disturbances in women with epilepsy on antiepileptic drug monotherapy. *Epilepsia, 48*(7), 1366–1370.

Kop, W. J., & Gottdiener, J. S. (2005). The role of immune system parameters in the relationship between depression and coronary artery disease. *Psychosomatic Medicine, 67*, S37–S41.

Koponen, H., Jokelainen, J., Keinanen-Kiukaanniemi, S., Kumpusalo, E., & Vanhala, M. (2008). Metabolic syndrome predisposes to depressive symptoms: A population-based 7-year follow-up study. *The Journal of Clinical Psychiatry, 69*(2), 178–182.

Koschke, M., Boettger, M. K., Schulz, S., Berger, S., Terhaar, J., Voss, A., et al. (2009). Autonomy of autonomic dysfunction in major depression. *Psychosomatic Medicine, 71*(8), 852–860.

Krantz, D. S., Whittaker, K. S., Francis, J. L., Rutledge, T., Johnson, B. D., Barrow, G., et al. (2009). Psychotropic medication use and risk of adverse cardiovascular events in women with suspected coronary artery disease: Outcomes from the Women's Ischemia Syndrome Evaluation (WISE) study. *Heart, 95*(23), 1901–1906.

Kreyenbuhl, J., Dickerson, F. B., Medoff, D. R., Brown, C. H., Goldberg, R. W., Fang, L., et al. (2006). Extent and management of cardiovascular risk factors in patients with type 2 diabetes and serious mental illness. *The Journal of Nervous and Mental Disease, 194*(6), 404–410.

Kronish, I. M., Rieckmann, N., Halm, E. A., Shimbo, D., Vorchheimer, D., Haas, D. C., et al. (2006). Persistent depression affects adherence to secondary prevention behaviors after acute coronary syndromes. *Journal of General Internal Medicine, 21*(11), 1178–1183.

Kronish, I. M., Rieckmann, N., Schwartz, J. E., Schwartz, D. R., & Davidson, K. W. (2009). Is depression after an acute coronary syndrome simply a marker of known prognostic factors for mortality? *Psychosomatic Medicine, 71*(7), 697–703.

Kubzansky, L. D., Koenen, K. C., Jones, C., & Eaton, W. W. (2009). A prospective study of posttraumatic stress disorder symptoms and coronary heart disease in women. *Health Psychology, 28*(1), 125–130.

Kubzansky, L. D., Koenen, K. C., Spiro, A., Vokonas, P. S., & Sparrow, D. (2007). Prospective study of posttraumatic stress disorder symptoms and coronary heart disease in the normative aging study. *Archives of General Psychiatry, 64*, 110–116.

Kuczmarski, M. F., Sees, A. C., Hotchkiss, L., Cotugna, N., Evans, M. K., & Zonderman, A. B. (2010). Higher healthy eating index-2005 scores associated with reduced symptoms of depression in an urban population: Findings from the Healthy Aging in Neighborhoods of Diversity Across the Life Span (HANDLS) study. *Journal of the American Dietetic Association, 110*(3), 383–389.

Kuijpers, P., Hamulyak, K., Strik, J., Wellens, H. J. J., & Honig, A. (2002). Beta-thromboglobulin and platelet factor 4 levels in post-myocardial infarction patients with major depression. *Psychiatry Research, 109*(2), 207–210.

Kwon, J. S., Choi, J. S., Bahk, W. M., Yoon Kim, C., Hyung Kim, C., Chul Shin, Y., et al. (2006). Weight management program for treatment-emergent weight gain in olanzapine-treated patients with schizophrenia or schizoaffective disorder: A 12-week randomized controlled clinical trial. *The Journal of Clinical Psychiatry, 67*(4), 547–553.

Lesperance, F., Frasure-Smith, N., Koszycki, D., Laliberte, M. A., van Zyl, L. T., Baker, B., et al. (2007). Effects of citalopram and interpersonal psychotherapy on depression in patients with coronary artery disease – The Canadian Cardiac Randomized Evaluation of Antidepressant and Psychotherapy Efficacy (CREATE) trial. *Journal of the American Medical Association, 297*(4), 367–379.

Licht, C. M. M., De Geus, E. J. C., Van Dyck, R., & Penninx, B. W. J. H. (2010). Longitudinal evidence for unfavorable effects of antidepressants on heart rate variability. *Biological Psychiatry, 68*(9), 861–868.

Licht, C. M. M., de Geus, E. J. C., Zitman, F. G., Hoogendijk, W. J. G., van Dyck, R., & Penninx, B. W. J. H. (2008). Association between major depressive disorder and heart rate variability in the Netherlands Study of Depression and Anxiety (NESDA). *Archives of General Psychiatry, 65*(12), 1358–1367.

Lincoln, N. B., & Flannaghan, T. (2003). Cognitive behavioral psychotherapy for depression following stroke – A randomized controlled trial. *Stroke, 34*(1), 111–115.

Lindamer, L. A., McKibbin, C., Nonnan, G. J., Jordan, L., Harrison, K., Abeyesinhe, S., et al. (2008). Assessment of physical activity in middle-aged and older adults with schizophrenia. *Schizophrenia Research, 104*(1–3), 294–301.

Lindenmayer, J. P., Khan, A., Wance, D., Maccabee, N., Kaushik, S., & Kaushik, S. (2009). Outcome evaluation of a structured educational wellness program in patients with severe mental illness. *The Journal of Clinical Psychiatry, 70*(10), 1385–1396.

Ljubic, M. A., Deane, F. P., Zecchin, R. P., & Denniss, R. (2006). Motivation, psychological distress, and exercise adherence following myocardial infarction. *Australian Journal of Rehabilitation Counseling, 12*(1), 21–32.

Malik, M., Bigger, J. T., Camm, A. J., Kleiger, R. E., Malliani, A., Moss, A. J., et al. (1996). Heart rate variability: standards of measurement, physiological interpretation, and clinical use. *Circulation, 93*(5), 1043–1065.

Markovitz, J. H., Matthews, K. A., Wing, R. R., Kuller, L. H., & Meilahn, E. N. (1991). Psychological, biological and health behavior predictors of blood pressure changes in middle-aged women. *Journal of Hypertension, 9*(5), 399–406.

Martens, E. J., de Jonge, P., Na, B., Cohen, B. E., Lett, H., & Whooley, M. A. (2010). Scared to death? Generalized anxiety disorder and cardiovascular events in patients with stable coronary heart disease the heart and soul study. *Archives of General Psychiatry, 67*(7), 750–758.

McConnell, S., Jacka, F. N., Williams, L. J., Dodd, S., & Berk, M. (2005). The relationship between depression and cardiovascular disease. *International Journal of Psychiatry in Clinical Practice, 9*(3), 157–167.

McConnell, S. D., Inderbitzin, L. B., & Pollard, W. E. (1992). Primary health care in the CMHC: A role for the nurse practitioner. *Hospital and Community Psychiatry, 43*(7), 724–727.

McEvoy, J. P., Meyer, J. M., Goff, D. C., Nasrallah, H. A., Davis, S. M., Sullivan, L., et al. (2005). Prevalence of the metabolic syndrome in patients with schizophrenia: Baseline results from the Clinical Antipsychotic Trials of Intervention Effectiveness (CATIE) schizophrenia trial and comparison with national estimates from NHANES III. *Schizophrenia Research, 80*(1), 19–32.

McIntosh, A., Cohen, A., Turnbull, N., Esmonde, L., Dennis, P., Eatock, J., et al. (2004). *Clinical guidelines and evidence review for panic disorder and generalised anxiety disorder*. Sheffield: National Collaborating Centre for Primary Care.

McKibbin, C. L., Patterson, T. L., Norman, G., Patrick, K., Jin, H., Roesch, S., et al. (2006). A lifestyle intervention for older schizophrenia patients with diabetes mellitus: A randomized controlled trial. *Schizophrenia Research, 86*(1–3), 36–44.

McManus, D., Pipkin, S. S., & Whooley, M. A. (2005). Screening for depression in patients with coronary heart disease (data from the heart and soul study). *The American Journal of Cardiology, 96*(8), 1076–1081.

Meyer, J. M., Davis, V. G., Goff, D. C., McEvoy, J. P., Nasrallah, H. A., Davis, S. M., et al. (2008). Change in metabolic syndrome parameters with antipsychotic treatment in the CATIE Schizophrenia Trial: Prospective data from phase 1. *Schizophrenia Research, 101*(1–3), 273–286.

Meyer, J. M., & Koro, C. E. (2004). The effects of antipsychotic therapy on serum lipids: A comprehensive review. *Schizophrenia Research, 70*(1), 1–17.

Meyer, T., Buss, U., & Herrmann-Lingen, C. (2010). Role of cardiac disease severity in the predictive value of anxiety for all-cause mortality. *Psychosomatic Medicine, 72*(1), 9–15.

Mitchell, P. H., Veith, R. C., Becker, K. J., Buzaitis, A., Cain, K. C., Fruin, M., et al. (2009). Brief psychosocial-behavioral intervention with antidepressant reduces poststroke depression significantly more than usual care with antidepressant living well with stroke: Randomized, controlled trial. *Stroke, 40*(9), 3073–3078.

Morrato, E. H., Newcomer, J. W., Kamat, S., Baser, O., Harnett, J., & Cuffel, B. (2009). Metabolic screening after the American diabetes association's consensus statement on antipsychotic drugs and diabetes. *Diabetes Care, 32*(6), 1037–1042.

Murray, D. P., Weiner, M., Prabhakar, M., & Fiedorowicz, J. G. (2009). Mania and mortality: Why the excess cardiovascular risk in bipolar disorder? *Current Psychiatry Reports, 11*(6), 475–480.

Mykletun, A., Bjerkeset, O., Dewey, M., Prince, M., Overland, S., & Stewart, R. (2007). Anxiety, depression, and cause-specific mortality: The HUNT study. *Psychosomatic Medicine, 69*(4), 323–331.

Nasrallah, H. A., Meyer, J. M., Goff, D. C., McEvoy, J. P., Davis, S. M., Stroup, T. S., et al. (2006). Low rates of treatment for hypertension, dyslipidemia and diabetes in schizophrenia: Data from the CATIE schizophrenia trial sample at baseline. *Schizophrenia Research, 86*(1–3), 15–22.

Newcomer, J. W. (2009). Comparing the safety and efficacy of atypical antipsychotics in psychiatric patients with comorbid medical illnesses. *The Journal of Clinical Psychiatry, 70*, 30–36.

Newcomer, J. W., & Haupt, D. W. (2006). The metabolic effects of antipsychotic medications. *Canadian Journal of Psychiatry-Revue Canadienne De Psychiatrie, 51*(8), 480–491.

Norton, P. J., & Price, E. C. (2007). A meta-analytic review of adult cognitive-behavioral treatment outcome across the anxiety disorders. *The Journal of Nervous and Mental Disease, 195*(6), 521–531.

O'Connor, C. M., Jiang, W., Kuchibhatla, M., Silva, S. G., Cuffe, M. S., Callwood, D. D., et al. (2010). Safety and efficacy of sertraline for depression in patients with heart failure. *Journal of the American College of Cardiology, 56*(9), 692–699.

Olafiranye, O., Jean-Louis, G., Magai, C., Zizi, F., Brown, C. D., Dweck, M., et al. (2010). Anxiety and cardiovascular symptoms: The modulating role of insomnia. *Cardiology, 115*(2), 114–119.

Olfson, M., Fireman, B., Weissman, M., Leon, A. C., Sheehan, D. V., Kathol, R. G., et al. (1997). Mental disorders and disability among patients in a primary care group practice. *The American Journal of Psychiatry, 154*(12), 1734–1740.

Osborn, D. P., Nazareth, I., & King, M. B. (2007). Physical activity, dietary habits and coronary heart disease risk factor knowledge amongst people with severe mental illness: A cross sectional comparative study in primary care. *Social Psychiatry and Psychiatric Epidemiology, 42*(10), 787–793.

Ozeki, Y., Fujii, K., Kurimoto, N., Yamada, N., Okawa, M., Aoki, T., et al. (2010). QTc prolongation and antipsychotic medications in a sample of 1017 patients with schizophrenia. *Progress in Neuro-Psychopharmacology & Biological Psychiatry, 34*(2), 401–405.

Peter, H., Goebel, P., Müller, S., & Hand, I. (1999). Clinically relevant cholesterol elevation in anxiety disorders: A comparison with normal controls. *International Journal of Behavioral Medicine, 6*(1), 30–39.

Pollock, B. G., Laghrissi-Thode, F., & Wagner, W. R. (2000). Evaluation of platelet activation in depressed patients with ischemic heart disease after paroxetine or nortriptyline treatment. *Journal of Clinical Psychopharmacology, 20*(2), 137–140.

Potokar, J. P., & Nutt, D. J. (2000). Chest pain: Panic attack or heart attack? *International Journal of Clinical Practice, 54*(2), 110–114.

Pozuelo, L., Zhang, J. P., Franco, K., Tesar, G., Penn, M., & Jiang, W. (2009). Depression and heart disease: What do we know, and where are we headed? *Cleveland Clinic Journal of Medicine, 76*(1), 59–70.

Qureshi, S. U., Pyne, J. M., Magruder, K. M., Schulz, P. E., & Kunik, M. E. (2009). The link between post-traumatic stress disorder and physical comorbidities: A systematic review. *Psychiatry Quarterly, 80*, 87–97.

Rafanelli, C., Milaneschi, Y., Roncuzzi, R., & Pancaldi, L. G. (2010). Dysthymia before myocardial infarction as a cardiac risk factor at 2.5-year follow-up. *Psychosomatics, 51*(1), 8–13.

Rieckmann, N., Gerin, W., Kronish, I. M., Burg, M. M., Chaplin, W. F., Kong, G., et al. (2006). Course of depressive symptoms and medication adherence after acute coronary syndromes – An electronic medication monitoring study. *Journal of the American College of Cardiology, 48*(11), 2218–2222.

Rieckmann, N., Kronish, I. M., Haas, D., Gerin, W., Chaplin, W. F., Burg, M. M., et al. (2006). Persistent depressive symptoms lower aspirin adherence after acute coronary syndromes. *American Heart Journal, 152*(5), 922–927.

Roest, A. M., Martens, E. J., Denollet, J., & de Jonge, P. (2010). Prognostic association of anxiety post myocardial infarction with mortality and new cardiac events: A meta-analysis. *Psychosomatic Medicine, 72*(6), 563–569.

Roy-Byrne, P. P., Davidson, K. W., Kessler, R. C., Asmundson, G. J. G., Goodwin, R. D., Kubzansky, L., et al. (2008). Anxiety disorders and comorbid medical illness. *General Hospital Psychiatry, 30*(3), 208–225.
Rozanski, A., & Kubzansky, L. D. (2005). Psychologic functioning and physical health: A paradigm of flexibility. *Psychosomatic Medicine, 67*, S47–S53.
Rugulies, R. (2002). Depression as a predictor for coronary heart disease – A review and meta-analysis. *American Journal of Preventive Medicine, 23*(1), 51–61.
Rutledge, T., Reis, V. A., Linke, S. E., Greenberg, B. H., & Mills, P. J. (2006). Depression in heart failure – A meta-analytic review of prevalence, intervention effects, and associations with clinical outcomes. *Journal of the American College of Cardiology, 48*(8), 1527–1537.
Sagen, U., Finset, A., Moum, T., Morland, T., Vik, T. G., Nagy, T., et al. (2010). Early detection of patients at risk for anxiety, depression and apathy after stroke. *General Hospital Psychiatry, 32*(1), 80–85.
Sagen, U., Vik, T. G., Moum, T., Morland, T., Finset, A., & Dammen, T. (2009). Screening for anxiety and depression after stroke: Comparison of the Hospital Anxiety and Depression Scale and the Montgomery and Asberg Depression Rating Scale. *Journal of Psychosomatic Research, 67*(4), 325–332.
Salaycik, K. J., Kelly-Hayes, M., Beiser, A., Nguyen, A. H., Brady, S. M., Kase, C. S., et al. (2007). Depressive symptoms and risk of stroke – The Framingham study. *Stroke, 38*(1), 16–21.
Santos, M., Koevari, E., Gold, G., Bozikas, V. P., Hof, P. R., Bouras, C., et al. (2009). The neuroanatomical model of post-stroke depression: Towards a change of focus? *Journal of the Neurological Sciences, 283*(1–2, Sp. Iss. 1), 158–162.
Schelling, G. (2007). Post-traumatic stress disorder in somatic disease: Lessons from critically ill patients. In E. R. DeKloet & E. Vermetten (Eds.), *Stress hormones and post traumatic stress disorder: Basic studies and clinical perspectives* (pp. 229–237). Amsterdam: Elsevier.
Scherrer, J. F., Chrusciel, T., Zeringue, A., Garfield, L. D., Hauptman, P. J., Lustman, P. J., et al. (2010). Anxiety disorders increase risk for incident myocardial infarction in depressed and nondepressed veterans administration patients. *American Heart Journal, 159*(5), 772–779.
Scherrer, J. F., Xian, H., Bucholz, K. K., Eisen, S. A., Lyons, M. J., Goldberg, J., et al. (2003). A twin study of depression symptoms, hypertension, and heart disease in middle-aged men. *Psychosomatic Medicine, 65*(4), 548–557.
Scott, J. (2004). Pathophysiology and biochemistry of cardiovascular disease. *Current Opinion in Genetics and Development, 14*(3), 271–279.
Serebruany, V. L., O'Connor, C. M., & Gurbel, P. A. (2001). Effect of selective serotonin reuptake inhibitors on platelets in patients with coronary artery disease. *The American Journal of Cardiology, 87*(12), 1398–1400.
Sherbourne, C. D., Jackson, C. A., & Meredith, L. S. (1996). Prevalence of comorbid anxiety disorders in primary care outpatients. *Archives of Family Medicine, 5*(1), 27–34.
Sigmond, A. S., & Snaith, R. P. (1983). The hospital anxiety and depression scale. *Acta Psychiatrica Scandinavica, 67*(6), 361–370.
Skala, J. A., Freedland, K. E., & Carney, R. M. (2006). Coronary heart disease and depression: A review of recent mechanistic research. *Canadian Journal of Psychiatry-Revue Canadienne De Psychiatrie, 51*(12), 738–745.
Smoller, J. W., Allison, M., Cochrane, B. B., Curb, J. D., Perlis, R. H., Robinson, J. G., et al. (2009). Antidepressant use and risk of incident cardiovascular morbidity and mortality among postmenopausal women in the Women's Health Initiative study. *Archives of Internal Medicine, 169*(22), 2128–2139.
Soh, K. C., & Lee, C. (2010). Panic attack and its correlation with acute coronary syndrome – More than just a diagnosis of exclusion. *Annals of the Academy of Medicine, Singapore, 39*(3), 197–202.
Soreca, I., Frank, E., & Kupfer, D. J. (2009). The phenomenology of bipolar disorder: What drives the high rate of medical burden and determines long-term prognosis? *Depression and Anxiety, 26*(1), 73–82.

Sowden, G. L., & Huffman, J. C. (2009). The impact of mental illness on cardiac outcomes: A review for the cardiologist. *International Journal of Cardiology, 132*(1), 30–37.

Spielberger, C. D., Gorsuch, R. L., & Lushene, R. E. (1970). *Manual for the state-trait anxiety inventory*. Paolo Alto: Consulting Psychologists Press.

Spindler, H., & Pedersen, S. S. (2005). Posttraumatic stress disorder in the wake of heart disease: Prevalence, risk factors, and future research directions. *Psychosomatic Medicine, 67*(5), 715–723.

Spitzer, C., Barnow, S., Volzke, H., John, U., Freyberger, H. J., & Grabe, H. J. (2009). Trauma, posttraumatic stress disorder, and physical illness: Findings from the general population. *Psychosomatic Medicine, 71*(9), 1012–1017.

Stein, P. K., & Kleiger, R. E. (1999). Insights from the study of heart rate variability. *Annual Review of Medicine, 50*, 249–261.

Stewart, J. C., Rand, K. L., Muldoon, M. F., & Kamarck, T. W. (2009). A prospective evaluation of the directionality of the depression-inflammation relationship. *Brain, Behavior, and Immunity, 23*(7), 936–944.

Strine, T. W., Mokdad, A. H., Balluz, L. S., Gonzalez, O., Crider, R., Berry, J. T., et al. (2008). Depression and anxiety in the united states: Findings from the 2006 behavioral risk factor surveillance system. *Psychiatric Services, 59*(12), 1383–1390.

Suls, J., & Bunde, J. (2005). Anger, anxiety, and depression as risk factors for cardiovascular disease: The problems and implications of overlapping affective dispositions. *Psychological Bulletin, 131*(2), 260–300.

Swenson, J. R., Doucette, S., & Fergusson, D. (2006). Adverse cardiovascular events in antidepressant trials involving high-risk patients: A systematic review of randomized trials. *Canadian Journal of Psychiatry-Revue Canadienne De Psychiatrie, 51*(14), 923–929.

Teri, L., Logsdon, R. G., & McCurry, S. M. (2005). The Seattle protocols: Advances in behavioral treatment of Alzheimer's disease. In M. Grundman, H. Feldman, L. J. Fitten, B. Winblad, & E. Giacobini (Eds.), *Research and practice in Alzheimer's disease* (pp. 153–158). Paris: Serdi.

Thayer, J. F., & Lane, R. D. (2007). The role of vagal function in the risk for cardiovascular disease and mortality. *Biological Psychology, 74*(2), 224–242.

Thombs, B. D., de Jonge, P., Coyne, J. C., Whooley, M. A., Frasure-Smith, N., Mitchell, A. J., et al. (2008). Depression screening and patient outcomes in cardiovascular care a systematic review. *Journal of the American Medical Association, 300*(18), 2161–2171.

Thorndike, A. N., Regan, S., McKool, K., Pasternak, R. C., Swartz, S., Torres-Finnerty, N., et al. (2008). Depressive symptoms and smoking cessation after hospitalization for cardiovascular disease. *Archives of Internal Medicine, 168*(2), 186–191.

Towle, D., Lincoln, N. B., & Mayfield, L. M. (1989). Evaluation of social work on depression after stroke. *Clinical Rehabilitation, 3*(2), 89–96.

Vahia, I. V., Diwan, S., Bankole, A. O., Kehn, M., Nurhussein, M., Ramirez, P., et al. (2008). Adequacy of medical treatment among older persons with schizophrenia. *Psychiatric Services, 59*(8), 853–859.

van Melle, J. P., de Jonge, P., Spijkerman, T. A., Tijssen, J. G. P., Ormel, J., van Veldhuisen, D. J., et al. (2004). Prognostic association of depression following myocardial infarction with mortality and cardiovascular events: A meta-analysis. *Psychosomatic Medicine, 66*(6), 814–822.

Van Zyl, L. T., Hasegawa, T., & Nagata, K. (2008). Effects of antidepressant treatment on heart rate variability in major depression: A quantitative review. *BioPsychoSocial Medicine, 2*, 12.

Vogelzangs, N., Seldenrijk, A., Beekman, A. T. F., van Hout, H. P. J., de Jonge, P., & Penninx, B. (2010). Cardiovascular disease in persons with depressive and anxiety disorders. *Journal of Affective Disorders, 125*(1–3), 241–248.

Watkins, C. L., Auton, M. F., Deans, C. F., Dickinson, H. A., Jack, C. I. A., Lightbody, C. E., et al. (2007). Motivational interviewing early after acute stroke – A randomized, controlled trial. *Stroke, 38*(3), 1004–1009.

Wells, K. B., Golding, J. M., & Burnam, M. A. (1989). Affective, substance use, and anxiety disorders in persons with arthritis, diabetes, heart disease, high blood pressure, or chronic lung conditions. *General Hospital Psychiatry, 11*(5), 320–327.

White, K. S. (2008). Cardiovascular disease and anxiety. In M. J. Zvolensky & J. A. Smith (Eds.), *Anxiety in health behaviors and physical illness* (pp. 279–315). New York: Springer.

Whooley, M. A., de Jonge, P., Vittinghoff, E., Otte, C., Moos, R., Carney, R. M., et al. (2008). Depressive symptoms, health behaviors, and risk of cardiovascular events in patients with coronary heart disease. *Journal of the American Medical Association, 300*(20), 2379–2388.

Williams, E. D., & Steptoe, A. (2007). The role of depression in the etiology of acute coronary syndrome. *Current Psychiatry Reports, 9*(6), 486–492.

World Health Organization. (2007). International statistical classification of diseases and health-related problems: 10th revision, from http://apps.who.int/classifications/apps/icd/icd10online/. Retreived 2-1-11

Wu, M. K., Wang, C. K., Bai, Y. M., Huang, C. Y., & Lee, S. D. (2007). Outcomes of obese, clozapine-treated in patients with schizophrenia placed on a six-month diet and physical activity program. *Psychiatric Services, 58*(4), 544–550.

Wulsin, L. R., & Singal, B. M. (2003). Do depressive symptoms increase the risk for the onset of coronary disease? A systematic quantitative review. *Psychosomatic Medicine, 65*(2), 201–210.

Yilmaz, E., Dosan, Y., Gurgoze, M. K., & Gungor, S. (2001). Serum lipid changes during anticonvulsive treatment serum lipids in epileptic children. *Acta Neurologica Belgica, 101*(4), 217–220.

Zavoreo, I., Basic-Kes, V., Bosnar-Puretic, M., & Demarin, V. (2009). Post-stroke depression. *Acta Clinica Croatica, 48*(3), 329–333.

Zhao, H. W., Zhou, C. X., Su, X. L., Xiao, X. C., & Guo, Y. (2004). Effect of a mental intervention on post-stroke depression and rehabilitation of neurological function. *Chinese Journal of Clinical Rehabilitation, 8*(13), 2408–2409.

Ziedonis, D., Hitsman, B., Beckham, J., Zvolensky, M., Adler, L., Audrain-McGovern, J., et al. (2008). Tobacco use and cessation in psychiatric disorders: National Institute of Mental Health report. *Nicotine & Tobacco Research, 10*(12), 1691–1715.

Ziegelstein, R. C., Kim, S. Y., Kao, D., Fauerbach, J. A., Thombs, B. D., McCann, U., et al. (2005). Can doctors and nurses recognize depression in patients hospitalized with an acute myocardial infarction in the absence of formal screening? *Psychosomatic Medicine, 67*(3), 393–397.

Zwanzger, P., Diemer, J., & Jabs, B. (2009). Comparison of combined psycho- and pharmacotherapy with monotherapy in anxiety disorders: Controversial viewpoints and clinical perspectives. *Journal of Neural Transmission, 116*(6), 759–765.

Chapter 4
Psychological Co-morbidities of Cancer

Paul B. Jacobsen and Kristine A. Donovan

4.1 Introduction

4.1.1 Overview of Cancer

Approximately one out of every two American men and one out of every three American women will develop cancer at some point during their lifetime (American Cancer Society, 2009). The chances for these individuals to survive cancer vary considerably depending on the specific type diagnosed, the extent of disease at the time of initial diagnosis, and the responsiveness of the disease to treatment. Much of the early effort to combat cancer focused exclusively on testing new therapies to improve the quantity of patients' lives (i.e., survival). These efforts, combined with improvements in early detection, have yielded impressive gains for certain forms of the disease (American Cancer Society, 2009).

More recently, there has been growing recognition that comprehensive cancer care should also seek to preserve or restore the quality of patients' lives (Institute of Medicine, 2007). This recognition is due, in part, to the large body of evidence documenting the adverse impact of a cancer diagnosis on mental well-being and the adverse impact of cancer treatment (e.g., surgery, chemotherapy, and radiotherapy) on mental and physical well-being (Institute of Medicine, 2007). These problems are not confined to the period of active cancer treatment. The burgeoning field of cancer survivorship research has shown that mental and physical problems first arising during treatment can persist for months or years after treatment completion

P.B. Jacobsen (✉)
H. Lee Moffitt Cancer Center and Research Institute, Tampa, FL, USA
e-mail: Paul.Jacobsen@moffitt.org

S. Pagoto (ed.), *Psychological Co-morbidities of Physical Illness: A Behavioral Medicine Perspective*, DOI 10.1007/978-1-4419-0029-6_4,

(Institute of Medicine, 2006). In addition, research has shown that new problems affecting mental and physical well-being can arise long after treatment have been completed (Institute of Medicine, 2006).

4.1.2 Chapter Aim and Organization

The aim of this chapter is to summarize knowledge about common psychological problems (i.e., co-morbidities) related to cancer diagnosis and treatment in adults in a manner designed to be useful to researchers and clinicians. The primary focus is on depression and anxiety because a considerable body of research exists about the nature of these problems and their treatment. Sleep and sexual problems in people with cancer are also covered, but to a lesser extent given the limited research to date on these topics.

The general organization of the chapter is to first describe the etiology of each co-morbidity, noting in particular factors relatively specific to its occurrence in people with cancer. Next, procedures commonly used in oncology settings to assess each co-morbidity are described, followed by a summary of findings about its prevalence and course. We then provide an overview of research on the management of each co-morbidity that includes examples of evidence-supported interventions. Finally, we consider future directions for addressing psychological co-morbidities in people with cancer.

4.2 Depression

4.2.1 Prevalence and Course

Estimates of the prevalence of depression in people with cancer vary widely. For example, one review reported prevalence rates for depression in cancer patients ranging from 1 to 42% (Pirl, 2004). This variability may be attributed, in part, to differences across studies in the methods used to estimate prevalence. In some studies, prevalence was estimated using cut-off scores applied to continuous measures of depressive symptomatology, while in other studies it was estimated using interviews based on DSM-IV criteria. Variability may also reflect the heterogeneous nature of the samples studied. Considerable differences are evident across the various study samples in such clinical characteristics as the types of cancers represented, participants' hospital status (inpatient or outpatient), the cancer treatments they received, and their disease stage.

Two published reviews have provided comparisons of prevalence rates for depression obtained using different assessment methods. The first review included studies of cancer patients published between 1966 and 2001 (Pirl, 2004). Among 11 studies that used DSM criteria, the majority of studies report rates between 10 and

25% for major depressive disorder; of the remaining studies, 25% reported rates below this range and 17% reported rates above this range. Among 14 studies that used the HADS to identify depression, the majority of studies report rates between 7 and 21% for probable cases; of the remaining studies, 14% reported rates below this range and 14% reported rates above this range. These comparisons must be interpreted with caution since there is no overlap among studies using each method. The other review is limited to studies of depression in people with breast cancer published between 1987 and 2007 (Fann et al., 2008). Among the 36 studies examined, estimates of rates of depression based on screening instruments mostly ranged between 15 and 30%. These rates were noted to be generally higher and more variable than those based on structured interviews, most of which ranged between 5 and 15%.

Studies of the prevalence of depression in cancer patients based on diagnostic criteria have typically been cross-sectional in design. Consequently, they do not yield information about changes in depression prevalence over time. In one of the few studies to address this issue, patients who underwent curative resection for nonsmall cell lung cancer at a major cancer treatment center in Japan were assessed for depression using the SCID at one, three, and 12 months after surgery (Akechi, Okamura, Nishiwaki, & Uchitomi, 2001). The prevalence of major depression at these time points was 4.7, 2.8, and 1.4%, respectively. Information about the course of depression indicates that, among patients with major depression at 1 month postsurgery, 10% were still depressed at 12 months postsurgery. Among patients without major depression at 1 month postsurgery, 1% developed depression by 12 months postsurgery. These data appear to indicate that major depression was relatively uncommon in the sample studied and did not increase in prevalence over the year following surgical resection. However, the authors note that the 12-month figure may be an underestimate of depression due to selective attrition and to psychiatric consultations being provided as part of routine care.

To summarize, the evidence currently available allows few conclusions to be drawn regarding the prevalence and course of depression in people with cancer. Limitations of the existing evidence base include relatively few studies reporting depression prevalence rates based on established diagnostic criteria and even fewer studies in which patients have been evaluated longitudinally using diagnostic criteria. Additional limitations include marked differences in the clinical characteristics of the samples studied, which makes it difficult to compare findings across studies, and the widespread use of convenience sampling as opposed to population-based sampling, which raises questions about the representativeness of the samples studied. With these limitations in mind, it is not surprising that precise estimates of the prevalence of depression in cancer patients are not available. Findings from two reviews suggest that rates of current major depression based on structured interviews typically fall between 5 and 25%. To provide context for these figures, a nationally (U.S.) representative study estimated that 6.7% of adults met criteria for major depressive disorder at some point in the previous 12 months (Kessler, Chiu, Demler, & Walters, 2005). Accordingly, the prevalence of major depressive disorder in cancer patients can be estimated to be between one and four times that observed in the general population.

4.2.2 Etiology

There are many possible sources of depression in people with cancer. For some individuals, the presence of depressive symptomatology simply reflects the continued presence of problems that predate their cancer diagnosis. For many individuals with no preexisting problems, symptoms of depression can occur as a psychological response to the diagnosis of a severe and potentially life-threatening illness. Concerns about how the disease may disrupt life plans, diminish quality of life, and fail to respond to treatment are common among those diagnosed with cancer and have the potential to elicit a wide range of emotional reactions.

Depression has also been observed to present in cancer patients as part of a "symptom cluster," which has been defined as two or more concurrent symptoms related to each other (Kim, McGuire, Tulman, & Barsevick, 2005). Fatigue, pain, and sleep problems are among the symptoms most frequently found to co-occur with depression in people with cancer (Barsevick, 2007). The reasons for this clustering are an active area of investigation. One possible explanation is that symptoms such as pain and fatigue contribute to depressive symptomatology because they are experienced as unpleasant and interfere with daily functioning (Barsevick, 2007). Another possible explanation is that the symptom co-occurrence reflects a common underlying biological mechanism. For example, it has been hypothesized that fatigue and depression in cancer patients may both represent "sickness behaviors" attributable to treatment-induced cytokine dysregulation (Cleeland et al., 2000). Support for this hypothesis comes from research that has evaluated side effects associated with the use of supraphysiologic doses of interferon-alpha as a cancer treatment. Interferon-alpha is a cytokine that is released early during viral infection which has both antiviral and antiproliferative properties. Administration of interferon-alpha has been found to produce symptoms that overlap with major depression, such as depressed mood, anhedonia, fatigue, anorexia, impaired concentration, and sleep disturbance (Capuron et al., 2002). Indeed, studies suggest that approximately 30–45% of patients treated with interferon-alpha will develop symptoms consistent with the presence of a major depressive disorder during the course of therapy (Musselman et al., 2001). Although interferon-alpha is perhaps the most striking example, other drugs used in the treatment of cancer (e.g., corticosteroids) can also result in depressive symptoms via biological mechanisms.

An additional mechanism by which depression may occur in people with cancer is through the direct biological effects of the disease. Evidence of this mechanism consists primarily of research that has examined links between depression and pancreatic cancer. A number of studies have shown that, among newly or recently diagnosed patients, symptoms of mood disturbance are more common for pancreatic cancer than for other types of cancer (Fras & Pearson, 1967; Holland et al., 1986). Beyond this, retrospective studies suggest that symptoms of depression often predate the diagnosis of pancreatic cancer by many months (Fras & Pearson, 1967; Joffe, Rubinow, Demicoff, Maher, & Sindelar, 1986). Additional evidence comes from a population-based longitudinal study of the relationship between depression and pancreatic cancer in the general population (Carney, Jones, Woolson, Noyes, &

Doebbeling, 2003). Findings based on insurance claims data confirmed that depression more commonly preceded pancreatic cancer than it did other gastrointestinal malignancies as well as all other cancers. Although the possibility that depression causes pancreatic cancer cannot be ruled out, attention has focused on biological mechanisms by which pancreatic cancer may result in depressive symptoms. One theory with empirical support is that pancreatic tumors secrete serotonin in sufficient quantities to deplete central nervous system stores of serotonin, thereby resulting in depression (Brown & Parakevas, 1982). Another theory under study is that pancreatic tumor cells secrete antibodies that either block central nervous system receptors for serotonin or reduce the synaptic availability of serotonin (Jacobsson, 1971).

Depression has been identified as a factor that may affect survival after cancer diagnosis through biological or behavioral pathways (Spiegel & Giese-Davis, 2003). Evidence for its impact includes the finding, based on a meta-analysis of 68 prospective studies, of a pooled relative risk ratio of 1.18 ($p < 0.001$) for the relationship of depression with cancer mortality (Pinquart & Duberstein, 2010). Drawing conclusions about the prognostic importance of depression from observational studies is complicated, however, by the difficulty of controlling for relevant confounding variables. Randomized controlled trials of interventions to address depression and related psychological symptoms have the potential to address this methodological challenge and provide more definitive evidence. Positive findings for the impact on mortality from at least two such trials (Andersen et al., 2008; Spiegel, Bloom, Kramer, & Gottheil, 1989) have been used to argue that psychological interventions can enhance the survival of cancer patients. This conclusion has been disputed by others (Coyne, Stefanek, & Palmer, 2007; Stefanek, Palmer, Thombs, & Coyne, 2009) who cite numerous studies that found no significant effects for psychological interventions on cancer survival and can identify important methodological limitations in those studies that have reported effects on survival. Accordingly, the question of whether depression affects cancer survival cannot be answered conclusively at this time.

4.2.3 Assessment

Depression in people with cancer has been assessed using a single symptom approach, a multisymptom approach, and a clinical syndrome approach (Jacobsen, Donovan, Swaine, & Watson, 2006). The single symptom approach refers to assessment methods that generally focus on measuring depressed mood as a continuous variable (e.g., visual analog scales assessing severity of depressed mood) or as a categorical variable (e.g., clinical interview questions assessing presence/absence of anxious or depressed mood). The advantages of these methods over other methods are their brevity and the absence of item content (e.g., loss of appetite) that might reflect disease symptoms or treatment side effects rather than the presence of emotional difficulties. Their disadvantages include the potential for single-item measures to yield unreliable findings, the limited information they yield about depression, and the challenge of identifying clinically significant problems based solely on information about mood.

The multisymptom approach refers to assessment methods that focus on measuring constellations of depressive symptoms. Common multisymptom approaches to measuring depression in cancer patients include self-report scales such as Center for Epidemiologic Studies Depression Scale (CES-D) (Radloff, 1977) and the Depression Subscale of the Hospital Anxiety and Depression Scale (HADS-D) (Zigmond & Snaith, 1983), the Beck Depression Inventory-II (BDI-II) (Beck, Steer, & Brown, 1996), and the Patient Health Questionnaire-9 (PHQ-9) (Kroenke, Spitzer, & Williams, 2001). The advantages of these methods over other methods are their established reliability and validity and the ability to compare scores across a variety of medical and nonmedical populations. Disadvantages include the presence of some measures (e.g., BDI-II and PHQ-9) of item content (e.g., loss of appetite) that might reflect disease symptoms or treatment side effects rather than the presence of emotional difficulties. Other measures (e.g., CES-D and HADS-D) have little or no item content overlapping with disease symptoms or treatment side effects, but, as a consequence, do not include somatic symptoms generally considered to be key features of depression. Another disadvantage of many of these measures is the lack of well-validated cut-off scores for identifying clinically significant depression in cancer patients. The PHQ-9 does possess a cut-off score that has been shown to be a sensitive and specific indicator of the presence/absence of major depressive disorder in a variety of populations (Kroenke et al., 2001). Published evidence of the utility of this cut-off score with cancer patients is not yet available.

The clinical syndrome approach refers to assessment methods used to detect the presence of a mood disorder (e.g., major depressive disorder). This approach typically involves the application of criteria identified in the fourth edition of the American Psychiatric Association's *Diagnostic and Statistical Manual of Mental Disorders (DSM-IV)* (American Psychiatric Association, 1994). In research studies, the application of these criteria is typically conducted using interview schedules, such as the Structured Clinical Interview for DSM-IV Disorders (SCID) (First, Gibbons, & Spitzer, 1996). The advantage of these methods over other methods is their utility in identifying the presence of clinically significant forms of depression. Disadvantages include the extensive training required to conduct diagnostic interviews, the presence of criteria (e.g., fatigue) that might reflect disease symptoms or treatment side effects rather than the presence of emotional difficulties, and the relatively high threshold that presence of a mood disorder poses for identifying individuals who may be experiencing emotional difficulties.

4.3 Anxiety

4.3.1 Prevalence and Course

According to recent reviews, between 25 and 48% of cancer patients report significant anxiety symptoms (Miovic & Block, 2007), while prevalence rates for diagnosable anxiety disorders range from 10 to 30% (Roy-Byrne et al., 2008). Commonly reported anxiety disorders in cancer patients include specific phobias, panic disorder with and without agoraphobia, generalized anxiety disorder (GAD), acute stress disorder (ASD), and posttraumatic stress disorder (PTSD). Prevalence rates of symptoms as well as diagnosable anxiety disorders vary because of differences across studies in the clinical characteristics of the samples, including cancer type and stage, treatment modalities, and time since diagnosis, and differences in the assessment methodologies used to estimate prevalence (Harter et al., 2001; Roy-Byrne et al., 2008). Some studies have estimated prevalence based on cut-off scores on continuous multisymptom measures of anxiety. For example, Dahl et al. (2005) used the HADS to identify anxiety in long-term survivors of testicular cancer. Nineteen percent of survivors scored at or above the HADS cut-off for clinically significant anxiety. Other studies have estimated prevalence based on published diagnostic criteria for clinically significant anxiety disorders. For example, Harter et al. (2001) reported a 12-month prevalence rate of 20.5% for anxiety disorders in total in a sample of cancer patients who were interviewed using the Composite International Diagnostic Interview, a standardized clinical interview using DSM-IV criteria. While the overall prevalence rates for anxiety generally were similar, 12-month prevalence rates for specific disorders were: specific phobia 12%, panic disorder with or without agoraphobia 5.5%, social phobia 2%, PTSD 1.5%, and GAD 1%. The differences in prevalence rates for anxiety symptoms versus specific anxiety disorders reflect the different approaches to assessment. This is further illustrated in a study by Stark et al. (2002) of a sample of adults with cancer. Based on scores on the HADS, the prevalence rate for significant anxiety was 48%. Eighteen percent of these patients met International Classification of Disorders, tenth Revision (ICD-10) criteria for an anxiety disorder using a semistructured clinical interview administered subsequently. Prevalence rates for specific disorders were: specific phobia 14%, panic disorder 9%, and GAD 8%. According to the researchers, the most common reasons for failure to fulfill ICD-10 criteria were that anxiety was not disruptive enough to be considered abnormal and that patients had too few anxiety symptoms.

Information about the course of specific anxiety disorders over time is limited as most studies of the prevalence of anxiety in cancer patients based on diagnostic criteria have been cross-sectional. Kangas, Henry, and Bryant (2005) conducted one of the few prospective studies of ASD and PTSD in the first year after a cancer diagnosis. Participants were adults with head and neck or lung cancer. In the initial month following their cancer diagnosis, 23% met criteria for ASD. Forty percent of patients with a diagnosis of ASD at 1 month met criteria for PTSD at 12 months. No patients who did not meet criteria for ASD at 1 month met criteria for PTSD at 12 months. With respect to other anxiety disorders, at 6 months, 33% of the sample met criteria for an anxiety disorder, excluding PTSD. At 12 months, 20% met criteria for an anxiety disorder including PTSD; 40% of these patients had a chronic course of anxiety since diagnosis. Although this study was limited by a high rate of attrition over the course of the study, its findings are generally consistent with cross-sectional prevalence studies. Findings also suggest that trauma-related distress generally subsides within the year following a cancer diagnosis.

In summary, previous research suggests that up to nearly one half of cancer patients experience significant anxiety and that prevalence rates for anxiety disorders based on diagnostic criteria range from 10 to 30%; this is for all anxiety disorders combined. Prevalence rates for specific disorders based on diagnostic criteria are predictably less and vary based on the disorder. By comparison, a recent nationally representative study (Kessler et al., 2005) estimated that 18% of adults in the general population met criteria for an anxiety disorder at some point in the previous 12 months. In this study, rates for specific disorders ranged from 2.7% for panic disorder to 8.7% for specific phobia (Kessler et al., 2005). Taken together, these data suggest that anxiety symptoms and diagnosable anxiety disorders are more prevalent in cancer patients compared to the general population. It is difficult to draw more definitive conclusions from the existing evidence base, however. This is because most studies of anxiety in cancer patients have not relied on diagnostic criteria to assess anxiety, but have relied instead on multisymptom reports of anxiety that paint a more general picture of anxiety. As well, the clinical characteristics of the samples studied have varied considerably making it difficult to provide precise estimates of anxiety disorders in cancer patients.

4.3.2 Etiology

Anxiety is a predictable response to the diagnosis of a life-threatening illness. For some people, cancer serves to reawaken or exacerbate symptoms of an anxiety disorder that predates the diagnosis. For others, anxiety symptoms are a psychological reaction to cancer and its treatment. Typical symptoms and signs of anxiety include somatic symptoms (e.g., heart palpitations and sweating), behavioral symptoms (e.g., restlessness and agitation), and cognitive symptoms (e.g., anxious thoughts in the form of apprehension and worry (Miller & Massie, 2006; Stark & House, 2000; Stark et al., 2002)). While these symptoms may be relatively common, symptoms that cause significant distress and interfere with functioning may suggest pathological anxiety and meet standard clinical criteria for an anxiety disorder. Reactive anxiety or adjustment disorder with anxious mood is an excessive response to an identifiable stressful event that begins relatively soon after the event. GAD is characterized by more anxious symptoms and symptoms must persist for a longer period of time. The anxiety seen in both reactive anxiety and GAD is typically free-floating (i.e., occurring without a particular trigger or in a particular pattern), pervasive, and difficult to control (Kerrihard, Breitbart, Dent, & Strout, 1999; Stark et al., 2002). Phobias reflect extreme anxiety that occurs in relation to a clearly defined situation or object and persistent anxiety in anticipation of these stimuli. In panic disorder, fear and intense discomfort occur suddenly and unpredictably. The anxiety seen in panic disorder and phobias typically builds in a crescendo pattern (Miller & Massie, 2006; Stark et al., 2002). PTSD is a reaction to a traumatic event, defined as a threat to life or serious injury. The disorder is characterized by symptoms organized into three clusters: reexperiencing, avoidance, and arousal (American Psychiatric Association, 1994; Kerrihard et al., 1999).

Cancer represents a threat to social roles, interpersonal relationships, future health, and life plans. Anxiety is generally high soon after the onset of cancer-related symptoms and during evaluation and diagnosis (Fallowfield, Hall, Maguire, Baum, & A'Hern, 1994). Anxiety also increases with progression of disease; research suggests that more advanced disease is associated with higher levels of anxiety (Miovic & Block, 2007; Roth & Massie, 2007; Stark & House, 2000). Cancer treatment is often associated with increases in anxious symptomatology. In general, high levels of anxiety occur prior to surgery and generally diminish after surgery (Tjemsland, Soreide, & Malt, 1998). Chemotherapy and radiotherapy are also associated with increased anxiety (Miller & Massie, 2006; Stark & House, 2000). The toxicity associated with chemotherapy and the worsening side effects as radiotherapy progresses may each represent a threat, although research suggests that not receiving treatment may produce more anxiety (Stark & House, 2000). The end of treatment may also serve to increase anxiety as patients may feel more vulnerable without the close monitoring and routine of scheduled treatment.

While anxiety may occur as a psychological reaction to cancer, anxiety also may be caused or exacerbated by medications used to treat cancer or other conditions that arise as a result of cancer and its treatment, including pain and endocrine and metabolic changes (Miller & Massie, 2006; Roy-Byrne et al., 2008). Uncontrolled acute pain is often associated with high levels of anxiety. Corticosteroids often cause anxiety symptoms such as restlessness and agitation. Prednisone is frequently used to reduce nausea and vomiting with chemotherapy or as a component of standard treatment regimens. High doses or rapid tapering of this medication may result in symptoms of anxiety (Kerrihard et al., 1999). Similarly, psychostimulants used to treat fatigue and other symptoms can cause irritability and tremulousness (Miller & Massie, 2006). In addition, abnormal metabolic states, such as hypoglycemia and hypoxia, may induce restlessness, agitation, and high levels of anxiety (Kerrihard et al., 1999; Miller & Massie, 2006).

4.3.3 Assessment

Anxiety in people with cancer has also been assessed using various approaches focusing on a single symptom, multiple symptoms, and the presence of a clinical syndrome. The single symptom approach generally focuses on measuring anxious mood as a continuous variable (e.g., visual analog scales assessing severity of anxious mood) or as a categorical variable (clinical interview questions assessing presence/absence of anxious mood). As with depression, there are advantages and disadvantages to this approach. Single-item measures, while focused and brief, provide limited information and cannot determine whether a clinical syndrome is present. The multisymptom assessment approach to anxiety focuses on measuring constellations of anxious symptoms, including, for example, shakiness, numbness or tingling, nervousness, and fear. Self-report scales representative of this approach are the State-Trait Anxiety Inventory (STAI) (Spielberger, 1983), the Anxiety Subscale of the Hospital Anxiety and Depression Scale (HADS-A) (Zigmond & Snaith, 1983), and the Beck Anxiety Inventory (BAI) (Beck & Steer, 1990). Perhaps the greatest advantage of this approach over other methods of assessing anxiety is the well-established psychometric properties of these commonly used measures. The greatest disadvantages are perhaps the lack of well-validated cut-off scores for identifying clinically significant anxiety and the inability of these measures to adequately distinguish among the various types of anxiety disorders (e.g., GAD vs. specific phobia). Finally, the clinical syndrome approach to assessing anxiety, like that for assessing depression, typically involves applying the criteria set forth in the DSM-IV (American Psychiatric Association, 1994) and the use of interview schedules. The advantages and disadvantages of this approach for assessing anxiety mirror those for assessing depression using this approach. The clinical syndrome approach enables one to more accurately gauge the presence of clinically significant anxiety and to distinguish among types of anxiety disorders. However, it includes criteria (e.g. heart palpitations) that might reflect disease symptoms or treatment-related side effects rather than emotional difficulties. Further, the threshold for presence of an anxiety disorder based on diagnostic criteria is relatively high. A cancer patient who does not meet criteria for an anxiety disorder may nevertheless be experiencing emotional difficulties worthy of clinical attention.

4.4 Management of Depression and Anxiety in Cancer Patients

4.4.1 Systematic Reviews and Meta-Analyses of Intervention Research

In this section, we attempt to summarize major conclusions from all existing systematic reviews and meta-analyses of the effects of psychosocial and pharmacological interventions on depression and anxiety in adults with cancer. Relevant publications were identified through several methods including electronic searches of major databases (e.g., MEDLINE, PsycINFO, Cochrane Systematic Reviews) and inspection of the reference lists of identified publications. Seventeen publications were identified that reached conclusions about the efficacy of psychosocial interventions for depression or anxiety (see Table 4.1). Five publications were identified that reached conclusions about the efficacy of pharmacological interventions for depression or anxiety (see Table 4.2).

4.4.1.1 Depression

Sixteen of the publications identified reached conclusions about the efficacy of psychosocial interventions for depression in cancer patients. Ten of the 16 publications reached positive conclusions. Seven of the ten publications yielding positive

Table 4.1 Systematic reviews and meta-analyses of psychosocial interventions for anxiety or depression in adults with cancer

Reference	Psychosocial intervention focus	Studies reviewed	Findings	Conclusions
Devine and Westlake (1995)	Psychoeducational care	Randomized and nonrandomized studies of cancer patients	Positive results for anxiety reported in 95% of studies; $d=0.56$, 95% CI=0.42–0.70 Positive results for depression reported in 92% of studies; $d=0.54$, 95% CI=0.43–0.65	Many types of psychoeducational care show beneficial effects on anxiety and depression
Lovejoy et al. (2000)	Cognitive-behavioral interventions	Randomized and nonrandomized studies of cancer patients	Knowledge base for management of cancer-related depression with cognitive-behavioral therapy is in the beginning phases of development	Several studies suggest that simple, brief therapy (6 sessions or less) provides effective relief in milder cases of cancer-related depression
Bottomley (1998)	Pharmacological and psychosocial interventions	Randomized and nonrandomized studies	Positive results for depression with individual and group interventions	A number of psychological approaches to the treatment of depression demonstrate positive effects
Sellick and Crooks (1999)	Individual psychosocial counseling interventions	Randomized studies of cancer patients	Magnitude of treatment effects for depression in the 10 studies reviewed was classified as: large (5), moderate (2), low (2), and none (1)	There is sufficient evidence to credit a counseling intervention with a positive effect on depression for both statistical and clinical significance
Sheard and Maguire (1999)	Psychosocial interventions	Randomized studies of cancer patients	Anxiety: $d=0.42$, 95% CI=0.08–0.74; $d=0.36$ based on criteria for developing a robust estimate Depression: $d=0.36$, 95% CI=0.06–0.66; $d=0.19$ with positive outliers removed	Preventative psychological interventions may have a moderate clinical effect on anxiety but not depression
Luebbert et al. (2001)	Relaxation training	Randomized studies of nonsurgical cancer patients	Anxiety: $d=0.45$, 95% CI=0.23–0.67 Depression: $d=0.54$, 95% CI=0.30–0.78	Relaxation training has a significant (small) effect on anxiety and a significant (medium) effect on depression

(continued)

Table 4.1 (continued)

Reference	Psychosocial intervention focus	Studies reviewed	Findings	Conclusions
Redd et al. (2001)	Behavioral interventions for cancer treatment side effects	Randomized and nonrandomized studies	4 of 5 randomized studies and 13 of 14 nonrandomized studies demonstrated beneficial effects of behavioral intervention on anxiety	Multimodal behavioral intervention can ameliorate anxiety associated with invasive medical treatments
Barsevick et al. (2002)	Psychoeducational interventions	Randomized and nonrandomized studies of cancer patients	Positive results for depression reported in 63% of studies reviewed	Psychoeducational interventions are effective in reducing depression. In particular, behavioral therapy, counseling/psychotherapy, and either of these combined with education are beneficial
Newell et al. (2002)	Psychosocial interventions	Randomized studies of cancer patients of fair or better quality	Recommendations for anxiety tentatively against 8 strategies, neither for nor against 7 strategies, and tentatively for 1 strategy	Music therapy can be tentatively recommended for reducing anxiety and several other strategies warrant further exploration
			Recommendations for depression were tentatively against 7 strategies, neither for nor against 6 strategies, and tentatively for 0 strategies	No-intervention strategy can be recommended for reducing depression, but several warrant further exploration
Uitterhoeve et al. (2004)	Psychological interventions	Randomized studies of patients with advanced cancer	1 of 10 studies reviewed showed a significant intervention effect for anxiety 6 of 10 studies reviewed showed a significant intervention effect for depression	The main benefit of psychological interventions in advanced cancer is an improvement of depression and feelings of sadness

Zabalegui et al. (2005)	Support groups	Randomized studies of cancer patients	Anxiety: $d=0.71$, 95% CI=0.38–1.04 Depression: $d=0.63$, 95% CI=0.28–0.98	Participation in a support group is associated with improvements in depression and anxiety
Jacobsen et al. (2002)	Psychosocial interventions	Randomized studies of cancer patients	36% of analyses yielded significant results for anxiety favoring the intervention condition 41% of analyses yielded significant results for depression favoring the intervention condition	Numerous evidence-based recommendations can be made for the use of psychological interventions in the management of anxiety and depression
Osborn et al. (2006)	Psychosocial interventions	Randomized studies of cancer patients with posttreatment follow-up evaluations	Anxiety: $g=1.99$, 95% CI=0.69–3.31 (cognitive-behavioral therapy); $g=-0.02$; 95% CI=−0.36–0.31 (psychoeducation) Depression: $g=1.21$, 95% CI=0.22–2.19 (cognitive-behavioral therapy; $g=-0.06$, 95% CI=−0.24–0.13 (psychoeducation))	Cognitive-behavioral therapy is effective for the short-term (<8 months) management of anxiety and depression in cancer survivors
Williams and Dale (2006)	Psychosocial interventions	Randomized studies of cancer patients with depression/depressive symptoms	3 of 4 studies showed a benefit of psychological intervention in treating depression; 7 of 10 trials showed a benefit of cognitive-behavioral therapy in reducing depressive symptoms	There is limited trial data on the efficacy of psychotherapeutic interventions in treating depression. Cognitive-behavioral therapy appears effective in reducing depressive symptoms
Rodin et al. (2007)	Psychosocial interventions	Randomized and nonrandomized studies of cancer patients with depression/depressive symptoms	2 of 4 studies showed a benefit of psychological intervention in reducing depressive symptoms	The evidence for nonpharmacological treatment of depression in cancer is mixed

(continued)

Table 4.1 (continued)

Reference	Psychosocial intervention focus	Studies reviewed	Findings	Conclusions
Akechi et al. (2008)	Psychosocial interventions	Randomized studies of patients with incurable cancer	Depression: $d=0.44$, 95% CI=0.08–0.80	Psychological interventions are useful in treating depressive states in advanced cancer patients; no evidence supports effectiveness in patients with clinically diagnosed depression
Hersch et al. (2009)	Psychosocial interventions	Randomized and nonrandomized studies of gynecological cancer patients	3 of 4 randomized studies showed that counseling reduced anxiety or depression; 3 of 7 randomized studies of cognitive-behavior therapy reduced anxiety or depression	Evidence was mixed regarding intervention effects. Symptoms of anxiety and depression seemed to be amenable to counseling

Table 4.2 Systematic reviews and meta-analyses of pharmacological interventions for anxiety or depression in adults with cancer

Reference	Pharmacological intervention focus	Studies reviewed	Number of studies reviewed	Conclusions
Ly, Chidgey, Addington-Hall, and Hotopf (2002)	Medications evaluated for effects on depression	Randomized studies of palliative care patients (at least 50% with cancer)	3	There are too few adequate studies to draw clear conclusions about management of depression in this setting
Pirl (2004)	Medications evaluated for effects on depression	Randomized studies of cancer patients	13	There appeared to be some efficacy data for selective serotonin reuptake inhibitors, tricyclic antidepressants, and minanserin (an atypical antidepressant)
Jacobsen et al. (2002)	Medications evaluated for effects on anxiety or depression	Randomized studies of cancer patients	12	Evidence for efficacy against depression is strongest for paroxetene and mianserin. Evidence for efficacy against anxiety is strongest for lorazepam
Williams and Dale (2006)	Medications evaluated for effects on depression	Randomized studies of cancer patients with depression/depressive symptoms	6	There is some evidence that antidepressants are effective in reducing depression/depressive symptoms in cancer patients. The small number of trials argues against drawing definitive conclusions about which antidepressants are most effective or well tolerated
Rodin et al. (2007)	Medications evaluated for effects on depression	Randomized and nonrandomized studies of cancer patients with depression/depressive symptoms	7	The limited evidence available suggests that cancer patients may benefit from pharmacological treatments for depression. Many newer antidepressants have not been systematically evaluated with cancer patients

conclusions were systematic reviews. The supporting evidence presented by Bottomley (1998) and Lovejoy, Tabor, Matteis, and Lillis (2000) consisted primarily of summaries of clinical trials that yielded positive findings for psychosocial interventions. Sellick and Crooks (1999) based their positive recommendation on evidence that intervention effects were large or moderate in seven of ten RCTs reviewed. Barsevick, Sweeney, Haney, and Chung (2002) reported that 30 of 48 randomized and nonrandomized studies identified (63%) yielded evidence supporting the benefits of psychosocial intervention. Among the many interventions evaluated in these studies, the evidence was viewed as sufficient to specifically recommend behavioral therapy, counseling/psychotherapy, and either of these approaches combined with education. Jacobsen et al. (2006) identified 47 RCTs of psychosocial interventions in which depression was measured as an outcome. Of the 102 outcome analyses reported in these studies, 42 (41%) yielded significant results favoring the intervention condition. Finally, Uitterhoeve et al. (2004) focused on RCTs conducted with patients with advanced cancer. Based on results showing a significant intervention effect for depression in six of ten studies, the authors concluded that a main benefit of psychosocial intervention in this patient population is improvement of depression and feelings of sadness.

The other publications reached positive conclusions based on the results of meta-analyses demonstrating significant effect sizes for psychosocial interventions. Luebbert, Dahme, and Hasenbring (2001) reported a significant effect of medium size ($d=0.54$) for relaxation training with cancer patients not undergoing surgery based on six studies. Devine and Westlake (1995) reported a significant effect of medium size ($d=0.54$) for psychosocial intervention based on 40 studies. Additional analyses limited to interventions tested in four or more studies yielded significant effect sizes (range = 0.40–0.66) for each of the following: education, counseling, relaxation training, and combinations of the preceding strategies. Zabalegui, Sanchez, Sanchez, and Juando (2005) reported a significant effect of medium size ($d=0.71$) for group psychosocial interventions based on 13 studies. Finally, Osborn, Demoncada, and Feuerstein (2006) reported a significant effect of large size ($g=1.21$) for cognitive-behavioral therapy in the posttreatment period based on five studies. The same publication reported a nonsignificant effect for educational intervention ($d=-0.06$) based on two studies.

In contrast, six of the 16 publications did not reach positive conclusions about the efficacy of psychosocial interventions in the management of depression. Newell, Sanson-Fisher, and Savolainen (2002) evaluated the results of 15 RCTs of psychosocial interventions judged to be of fair or better quality in which depression was measured as an outcome. Using criteria described previously, none of the 13 strategies evaluated merited a tentative recommendation. However, several therapies (e.g., cognitive-behavioral therapy and guided imagery) were judged to warrant further exploration based on patterns of significant results deemed inconsistent. Sheard and Maguire (1999) conducted a meta-analysis that yielded a significant effect of small size ($d=0.36$) for psychosocial interventions based on 20 studies. Results showed, however, that exclusion of three studies with very large positive effects reduced the effect size to a magnitude ($d=0.19$) considered by the authors to be clinically weak to negligible. The latter finding led to a conclusion that psychosocial interventions did not have a clinically significant effect on depression in cancer patients. Williams and Dale (2006) conducted a systematic review that distinguished studies based on whether the outcome was a reduction in clinically significant depression (a categorical measure) or in depressive symptomatology (a continuous measure). With regard to the former, the benefits of psychosocial intervention were evident in three of four RCTs. With regard to the latter, the benefits were evident in seven of ten RCTs of cognitive-behavioral therapy (the most frequently studied psychosocial intervention). These two results led to mixed conclusions. Although the authors concluded that more research was needed to determine the efficacy of psychosocial interventions in treating depression (i.e., limiting clinically significant levels of depression), they also noted that cognitive-behavioral therapy appeared to be effective in reducing depressive symptoms. Rodin et al. (2007) limited their systematic review to studies in which clinically significant depression was an eligibility criterion for participants. Based on findings showing that two of four studies demonstrated greater improvement in patients who received a psychosocial intervention, the authors concluded that the evidence for nonpharmacological treatment of depression in cancer is mixed. Akechi, Okuyama, Onishi, Morita, and Furukawa (2008) limited their meta-analysis to randomized studies of patients with incurable cancer. They observed a significant effect of small size ($d=0.44$) for psychosocial interventions based on six studies, but noted that none of these studies were of patients with clinically diagnosed depression. These findings led to the conclusion that psychosocial interventions were useful in treating depressive states in patients with advanced cancer; however, no evidence supports the effectiveness of these interventions in treating clinically diagnosed depression. In the final report, Hersch, Juraskova, Price, and Mullan (2009) limited their systematic review to studies of psychosocial interventions with gynecological cancer patients. Based on a review of 22 studies, they concluded that evidence was mixed regarding interventions. Results were strongest for counseling, which was found to be effective in two randomized trials determined to be of good quality.

Four of the publications identified reported information about the efficacy of pharmacological interventions for depression in cancer patients. All four publications were systematic reviews. Two publications concluded there was some evidence for the efficacy of pharmacological interventions (Bottomley, 1998; Williams & Dale, 2006) and one publication concluded that the evidence was limited (Rodin et al., 2007). The fourth publication identified specific medications for which the evidence was strongest (Jacobsen et al., 2006). However, one review cautioned against drawing definitive conclusions about which antidepressant medications are most effective or well tolerated given the limited number of trials conducted (Williams & Dale, 2006) and another review noted that many newer antidepressant medications have yet to be systematically evaluated with cancer patients (Rodin et al., 2007).

4.4.1.2 Anxiety

Ten publications identified offered conclusions about the efficacy of psychosocial interventions for anxiety in cancer patients. Seven of the ten publications reached positive conclusions. Redd, Montgomery, and DuHamel (2001) conducted a systematic review of studies of behavioral interventions for cancer patients undergoing treatment (primarily chemotherapy). Recommendations for the use of behavioral interventions were based on findings showing that four of five RCTs and 14 of 15 nonrandomized studies yielded significant results favoring the behavioral intervention condition. Jacobsen et al. (2006) conducted a systematic review of RCTs of psychosocial interventions in which anxiety was measured as an outcome. Among the 54 RCTs identified, 49 of 135 outcome analyses (36%) yielded significant results favoring the intervention condition. The other four publications reached positive conclusions based on the results of meta-analyses demonstrating significant effect sizes for psychosocial interventions. Luebbert et al. (2001) reported a significant effect of small size ($d=0.45$) for relaxation training with cancer patients not undergoing surgery based on eight studies. Devine and Westlake (1995) reported a significant effect of medium size ($d=0.56$) for psychosocial interventions based on 55 studies. Additional analyses limited to interventions tested in five or more studies yielded significant effect sizes (range=0.46–0.74) for all the subcategories examined including educational interventions and relaxation training interventions. Sheard and Maguire (1999) reported a significant effect of small size ($d=0.42$) for psychosocial intervention based on 19 studies. Exclusion of nonrandomized trials and trials that did not meet other criteria for quality yielded a similar-sized effect ($d=0.36$). Zabalegui et al. (2005) reported a significant effect of medium size ($d=0.71$) for group interventions based on outcomes reported in 11 studies. Finally, Osborn et al. (2006) reported a significant effect of large size ($g=1.99$) for cognitive-behavioral therapy in the post-treatment period based on four studies. The same publication reported a nonsignificant effect for educational intervention ($d=-0.02$) based on one study.

In contrast, three of the ten publications did not reach positive conclusions about the efficacy of psychosocial interventions in the management of anxiety. Both publications were systematic reviews. Hersch et al. (2009) limited their systematic review to studies of psychosocial interventions with gynecological cancer patients. Based on a review of 22 studies, they concluded that evidence was mixed regarding interventions. Results were strongest for counseling, which was found to be effective in two randomized trials determined to be of good quality. Uitterhoeve et al. (2004) focused on psychosocial interventions for patients with advanced cancer. No recommendations were offered about use of psychosocial interventions for management of anxiety in this patient population based on evidence that only one of ten RCTs showed a significant intervention effect. Newell et al. (2002) evaluated the results of 25 RCTs of psychosocial interventions judged to be of fair or better quality in which anxiety was measured as an outcome. For a strategy to earn at least a tentative recommendation, at least 75% of the trials evaluating the strategy had to yield statistically significant results. Based on this criterion, only one of 16 strategies evaluated merited a tentative recommendation. Specifically, music therapy earned this recognition based on evidence that the only trial conducted of this therapy with anxiety as an outcome yielded positive results. Several additional therapies (e.g., cognitive-behavioral therapy, communication skills training, and guided imagery) were judged to warrant further exploration based on patterns of significant results deemed inconsistent.

Only one publication reported information about the efficacy of pharmacological interventions for anxiety in cancer patients. Based on a systematic review of the literature, Jacobsen et al. (2006) observed that evidence was strongest for the efficacy of lorazepam. It should be noted, however, that only eight trials of pharmacological interventions were identified in which anxiety was measured as an outcome and only three of these trials evaluated lorazepam.

4.4.2 Limitations of Existing Intervention Research

With regard to pharmacological interventions, there seems to be general agreement that additional research is needed in order to be able to formulate specific evidence-based recommendations about use of medications to treat anxiety and depression in cancer patients. With regard to psychosocial interventions, differences in the scope of the reviews, the methods used to summarize findings across studies, and the manner in which recommendations were reached seriously limit the conclusions that can be drawn from these publications. Although the majority of publications reached favorable conclusions about the efficacy of psychosocial interventions against anxiety and depression in adults with cancer, nearly all identified weaknesses in the research base that have important implications for clinical practice. These weaknesses can be distilled down to four major areas of concern.

First, there are notable gaps in the literature regarding the benefits of psychosocial interventions for patients with certain demographic, disease, and treatment characteristics. With regard to demographic characteristics, one review found that eligibility was limited to men in only 5% of studies (Jacobsen et al., 2006). Similarly, there is little evidence regarding the efficacy of psychosocial interventions with members of ethnic and racial minority groups (Moyer, Sohl, Knapp-Oliver, & Schneider, 2009). With regard to disease characteristics, there are limitations in the evidence base related to disease type and disease status. Most studies are based on samples with several different types of cancer and, except for breast cancer, very few studies are limited to a single form of cancer (Jacobsen et al., 2006). The significance of this issue lies in the possibility that the sources of anxiety and depression and the psychosocial interventions needed to treat them may vary considerably across different cancers. A similar situation exists with regard to disease status. One review found that 73% of studies did not focus on a specific disease stage and, of those that did, only 9% focused on patients with stage IV or metastatic disease (Jacobsen et al., 2006). Although research suggests that psychosocial interventions are effective against depression in patients with advanced disease (Uitterhoeve et al., 2004), the issue merits additional study based on evidence suggesting that several forms of psychosocial distress worsen with advancing disease (Fallowfield et al., 2001). With regard to treatment status, one review found that only 8% of studies were found to be limited to patients not currently receiving treatment (Jacobsen et al., 2006). Although research suggests that cognitive-behavioral therapy is effective in relieving anxiety and depression in the posttreatment period (Osborn et al., 2006), too few studies have been conducted to adequately evaluate any other form of psychosocial intervention.

The presence of inconsistent findings is a second notable limitation of the evidence base. One of the more negative evaluations of psychosocial interventions comes from a review that evaluated whether at least 75% of the trials evaluating a specific strategy yielded statistically significant positive results (Newell et al., 2002). As noted previously, only one strategy met this criterion for anxiety and none met it for depression (Newell et al., 2002). This lack of consistency can be attributed, in part, to differences across studies evaluating the same intervention strategy in the demographic, disease, and treatment characteristics of the samples recruited, the number and timing of the outcome assessments performed, and the outcome measures used. In addition, there may be considerable variation across studies in the number and content of sessions for interventions that share the same name (e.g., relaxation training). Adoption of common outcome measures and common terminology to describe the format and content of interventions is needed to promote greater standardization of methodology across studies.

The quality of the studies is a third area of concern. Inadequate reporting of study methodology appears to be a major problem (Moyer et al., 2009). One review found that only 3% of trials provided sufficient information to permit evaluation of ten indicators of study quality (Newell et al., 2002). However, problems are also evident when study methodology is adequately described. For example, the majority of studies conducted in the 1990s failed to account for patients lost to follow-up in the outcome analyses performed (Newell et al., 2002). The widespread adoption by major journals of standardized descriptions of clinical trials procedures, such as the Consolidated Standards of Reporting Trials (CONSORT) criteria (Moher, Schulz, & Altman, 2001), should have a positive influence on the quality of future studies.

The general lack of research on patients experiencing clinically significant levels of anxiety and depression is a fourth area of concern. One review found that only 5% of studies limited eligibility to patients experiencing some degree of anxiety, depression, or psychosocial distress (Jacobsen et al., 2006). Based on the reported prevalence of anxiety and depression in oncology settings (Kessler et al., 2005; Pirl, 2004), the average patient in most intervention studies was likely to be experiencing low levels of anxiety and depression at the time they were recruited. In addition to limiting the statistical power to detect intervention effects, the lack of eligibility criteria based on current anxiety or depression raises questions about whether the findings are generalizable to patients experiencing clinically significant symptomatology. In the one review limited to studies of patients experiencing elevated levels of depression (Rodin et al., 2007), evidence from the four studies identified was mixed regarding the efficacy of psychosocial interventions in treating depression, suggesting the need for additional research on this topic. By evaluating psychosocial interventions with patients experiencing moderate-to-severe symptoms of anxiety and depression, future research is likely to yield findings of greater relevance to clinical practice.

4.4.3 Evidence-Based Recommendations for Management of Depression and Anxiety

The systematic reviews and meta-analyses described previously provide abundant information about the efficacy of psychosocial interventions in managing anxiety and depression in adults with cancer. The challenge is to translate this abundance of information into evidence-based recommendations that are relevant to clinical practice.

In 2003, the National Breast Cancer Centre and the National Cancer Control Initiative in Australia published the first edition of "Clinical Practice Guidelines for the Psychosocial Care of Adults with Cancer" (National Breast Cancer Centre and National Cancer Control Initiative, 2003). These guidelines, based on available research evidence, are presented in the form of a series of recommendations accompanied by identification of the levels and sources of research support. Included in the document is a table summarizing recommendations for the psychosocial care of cancer patients that are based on systematic review of all relevant RCTs (Level I evidence) or on at least one properly designed RCT (Level II evidence). Those recommendations that relate primarily to the management of anxiety and depression appear in adapted form in Table 4.3. With regard to psychosocial interventions, the guidelines indicate that cognitive-behavioral and psychoeducational interventions are among several interventions effective in the treatment of anxiety and depression. An assumption underlying these guidelines is that evidence collected from other populations is generalizable to cancer patients. Specifically, some of the evidence cited in support of these recommendations includes systematic reviews and randomized trials conducted on populations other than cancer patients.

An approach we developed previously that may be useful is to summarize the literature in terms of the number of RCTs that demonstrated efficacy in managing anxiety or depression based on intervention type and patient disease or treatment status (Jacobsen et al., 2006). An adapted version of this summary appears in the following list. Specifically, the list includes RCTs published between 1980 and 2003 for which significant ($p<0.05$) effects were obtained for an intervention relative to a control condition. This listing is comprised only of studies retrieved as part of the review that could be classified according to intervention type and the disease or treatment status of the participants.

Evidence-based recommendations for the use of psychological interventions:

Relaxation techniques, alone or combined with education/skills training, are effective in preventing or relieving:

- Anxiety (Arakawa, 1997; Bindemann, Soukop, & Kaye, 1991) and depression (Arakawa, 1997; Bindemann et al., 1991; Edgar, Rosberger, & Collet, 2001) in newly diagnosed patients.
- Anxiety (Liossi & White, 2001) and depression (Liossi & White, 2001) in patients in the terminal phase of illness.
- Anxiety (Burish, Carey, Krozely, & Greco, 1987; Burish & Lyles, 1981; Carey & Burish, 1987; Jacobsen et al., 2002; Mantovani et al., 1996; Morrow, 1986) and

Table 4.3 National Breast Cancer Centre and National Cancer Control Initiative Recommendations Relevant to Management of Anxiety and Depression Supported by Level I or Level II Evidence

Recommendation	Evidence level
Providing question prompt sheets to patients with cancer during an initial consultation promotes patient questions, reduces anxiety, improves recall, and shortens the consultation	II
Providing patients with information about the procedure they are about to undergo reduces emotional distress and improves psychological and physical recovery	I
Providing patients with practical details about the procedure (procedural information), a booklet, and/or a videotape decreases anxiety and psychological distress	II
Providing patients with information about what they are likely to experience before, during, and after a procedure (sensory information) decreases anxiety	I
Providing patients with psychological support before undergoing surgery reduces psychological distress	I
Cognitive-behavioral, psychoeducational, and crisis interventions, as well as combinations of education and behavioral or nonbehavioral interventions and antianxiety medications, are effective in the treatment of anxiety	I
Cognitive-behavioral, psychoeducational, and supportive interventions, as well as combinations of education and behavioral or nonbehavioral interventions and cognitive-behavioral interventions and antidepressants, are effective in the treatment of depression	I
Supportive psychotherapy, in combination with antidepressants, such as selective serotonin reuptake inhibitors is effective for the management of posttraumatic stress disorder	I
Depression can be managed by incorporating a combination of supportive psychotherapy, cognitive and behavioral techniques, and pharmacotherapy	I
There is no evidence that any particular antidepressant is superior to another in the management of depression in people with cancer	I

Note: Adapted from National Breast Cancer Centre and National Cancer Control Initiative (2003)

depression (Burish et al., 1987; Burish & Lyles, 1981; Jacobsen et al., 2002; Mantovani et al., 1996) in patients undergoing chemotherapy.

- Anxiety (Decker, Cline-Elsen, & Gallagher, 1992; Evans & Connis, 1995) and depression (Decker et al., 1992; Evans & Connis, 1995; Pruitt et al., 1993) in patients undergoing radiotherapy.
- Anxiety (Cheung, Molassiotis, & Chang, 2003; Petersen & Quinlivan, 2002) and depression (Fawzy et al., 1990; Petersen & Quinlivan, 2002) in patients undergoing surgery.
- Anxiety (Elsesser, van Berkel, & Sartory, 1994) and depression (Simpson, Carlson, & Trew 2001) following completion of active treatment.

Psychoeducation is effective in preventing or relieving:

- Anxiety (McQuellon et al., 1998; Wells, McQuellon, Hinkle, & Cruz, 1995) and depression (McQuellon et al., 1998) in newly diagnosed patients.

- Anxiety (Ali & Khalil, 1989) and depression (McArdle et al., 1996) in patients undergoing surgery.
- Anxiety (Jacobs, Ross, Walker, & Stockdale, 1983) and depression (Rawl et al., 2002) in patients undergoing chemotherapy.

Supportive and supportive-expressive therapies are effective in preventing or relieving:

- Anxiety (Goodwin et al., 2001; Spiegel, Bloom, & Yalom, 1981) and depression (Edelman, Bell, & Kidman, 1999; Goodwin et al., 2001) in patients with metastatic disease.
- Anxiety (Mantovani et al., 1996) and depression (Mantovani et al., 1996) in patients undergoing chemotherapy.
- Anxiety (Evans & Connis, 1995) and depression (Evans & Connis, 1995) in patients undergoing radiotherapy.
- Depression (Watson, Denton, Baum, & Greer, 1988) in patients undergoing surgery.

Couples counseling is effective in preventing or relieving:

- Depression (Christensen, 1983) in patients undergoing surgery.

Cognitive-behavioral therapy is effective in preventing or relieving:

- Depression (Edelman et al., 1999) in patients with metastatic disease.
- Anxiety (Moynihan, Bliss, Davidson, Burchell, & Horwich, 1998) in patients undergoing surgery.

Cognitive therapy is effective in preventing or relieving:

- Depression (Marchioro et al., 1996) in patients undergoing chemotherapy.

This list can serve several useful purposes. First, it can be used to identify specific applications of psychosocial interventions for which there is empirical support. That is, treatment providers and patients can readily determine when in the disease course or at what point in the treatment process a specific intervention has been shown to be effective in preventing or relieving anxiety or depression. Second, inspection of the number of unique citations next to each listing provides information about the extent of the evidence for the identified use of a specific intervention strategy. Finally, the citations themselves identify specific studies that provide information about the content and delivery of the intervention strategy and the methodology used to evaluate it.

4.4.4 Examples of Evidence-Supported Interventions

In this section, we provide examples of interventions effective in preventing or reducing depression or anxiety in people with cancer. We were guided by three considerations in selecting examples. First and foremost, the intervention had to have been found superior to a control condition in a published RCT. Second, we sought to spotlight interventions with good potential for dissemination. Specifically, we sought to identify interventions that possessed features suggesting they would be generally acceptable to patients and relatively easy to implement in terms of the professional time and resources required. Finally, we sought to identify interventions that addressed common indications for preventing or reducing depression or anxiety in people with cancer.

4.4.4.1 Cognitive Therapy for Depression in Patients with Metastatic Cancer

Savard et al. (2006) adapted a form of cognitive therapy developed for treatment of depression in the general population (Beck, Rush, Shaw, & Emery, 1979) to meet the needs of patients with metastatic cancer. The goal of this therapy is to foster an optimistic but realistic attitude in patients toward their situation as opposed to an overly negative attitude (e.g., only thinking of death) or overly positive attitude (e.g., hoping only to be cured). The intervention consists of 8 weekly 60–90 min sessions followed by three booster sessions at 3-week intervals. The sessions focus primarily on helping patients to modify dysfunctional or irrational thoughts about their cancer and other important situations in their lives.

The efficacy of this intervention was evaluated against a wait-list control condition using an RCT design. Participants were women with metastatic breast cancer who met criteria for having clinically significant depressive symptomatology. Patient-reported outcomes were assessed before and after the initial intervention period and 3- and 6-months after intervention in all participants who received cognitive therapy. Results indicated that patients in the cognitive therapy condition demonstrated significantly ($p<0.01$) less depression postintervention than patients in the wait-list condition on a standardized multisymptom clinician rating measure. Additional analyses indicated that a further significant ($p<0.01$) reduction in depression occurred during the 6-month follow-up period among patients receiving cognitive therapy.

As noted previously, psychosocial distress tends to be greater in cancer patients with more advanced disease. Accordingly, there is likely to be considerable need for psychosocial interventions effective against depression in patients with metastatic disease. Previous research has documented the benefit of weekly supportive-expressive group psychotherapy conducted over the course of a year in preventing or relieving depression in women with metastatic breast cancer who were not selected on the basis of preexisting psychosocial distress (Goodwin et al., 2001). The cognitive therapy evaluated by Savard et al. (2006) has the advantages of being much shorter in duration and of having been tested in a sample of patients with preexisting depressive symptomatology.

4.4.4.2 Group Cognitive-Behavioral Therapy for Cancer Survivors

Simpson et al. (2001) developed a group cognitive-behavioral intervention for women who had completed treatment for early-stage breast cancer. The intervention consists of 6 weekly 90-min sessions led by a psychiatrist, with two breast cancer survivors serving as lay coleaders. Building on a similar program developed by Cunningham and Tocco (1989), the topics addressed during these meetings are: progressive muscle relaxation; inner relaxation (self-hypnosis); other stress management techniques; mental imagery; goal setting; and planning and achieving change.

The investigators evaluated the efficacy of this intervention in an RCT in which it was compared to a no-intervention control condition. Study participants were women who had completed treatment for stage 0, I, or II breast cancer no more than 2 years previously. Individuals with mood or anxiety disorders were not excluded and comprised approximately 20% of the study sample. Patient-reported outcomes were assessed prior to randomization, immediately following intervention, and one and 2 years later. Findings indicated that patients who received the group cognitive-behavioral intervention reported significantly ($p<0.05$) less depression on a standardized multisymptom self-report measure immediately postintervention and at the 2-year follow-up than patients who did not receive the intervention. As part of the same study, the investigators also examined participants' total billings to their Canadian provincial healthcare plan in the postintervention follow-up period. These were calculated to be 23.5% lower in the intervention condition than in the control condition.

This brief intervention demonstrated long-lasting effects on depression in the posttreatment period in a sample that included a considerable number of women with preexisting problems with depression and anxiety. Evidence from the study suggests that addressing psychosocial distress in this patient population can also yield savings in healthcare costs. Given the limited resources required for implementation and the potential cost savings that may result, this intervention would appear to have considerable potential to be adopted as a program routinely offered to patients finishing treatment for early-stage breast cancer to promote positive adjustment to cancer survivorship.

4.4.4.3 Collaborative Depression Care for Cancer Patients

Strong et al. (2008) evaluated the use of a collaborative care model approach (Katon et al., 1995) adapted for oncology settings to identify and treat depressed cancer patients. The intervention consists of up to ten sessions with a cancer nurse who provides education about depression and its treatment (including antidepressant medication), and problem-solving therapy to overcome feelings of helplessness. In addition, the nurse consults with each patient's oncologist and primary care physician about management of depression.

The efficacy of this intervention was evaluated against a usual care condition using a RCT design. Patients being treated for cancer at a regional center, who were found to have major depressive disorder through screening, were assigned to usual care or usual care plus a collaborative care intervention. Findings showed significantly lower scores on a measure of depressive symptomatology 3 months postrandomization for patients who received the collaborative care intervention relative to usual care controls. These differences are reflected in the percentages of usual care patients (45%) vs. collaborative care patients (68%) whose major depressive disorder had remitted in the 3-month period. The beneficial effects of collaborative care observed at 3 months were still evident at 6- and 12-month follow-up assessments. As part of the same study, the investigators also calculated the costs of delivering the depression management intervention versus provision of usual care only. Incremental cost of the intervention was $668 over 6 months.

This study provides strong evidence that an integrated model of care delivery, which includes routine screening and care delivered according to a standardized protocol, can improve the management of depression in cancer patients beyond usual care. It is noteworthy that the intervention incorporated a form of psychotherapy (i.e., problem-solving therapy) found previously to be effective against depressive symptomatology in a randomized controlled trial with cancer patients (Nezu, Nezu, Felgoise, McClure, & Houts, 2003). Thus, the study provides an excellent example of how a research-tested psychosocial intervention can be incorporated into a broader intervention strategy designed for dissemination into clinical practice. The next phase in the development of this collaborative care model would be to identify strategies to facilitate its dissemination to professionals working with cancer patients and to promote its implementation in oncology settings.

4.4.4.4 Cognitive-behavioral Stress Management for Cancer Patients

Antoni et al. (2009) tested the effects of a cognitive-behavioral stress management intervention for women undergoing treatment for breast cancer using an RCT design. The intervention consisted of 10 weekly group-based sessions focused on teaching stress reduction techniques. Group facilitations encouraged emotional expression and skill building in anxiety reduction via muscle relaxation and relaxing imagery. Sessions included didactic content, in-session experiential exercises, and out-of-sessions assignments.

In the RCT, women with stage I–III breast cancer who had undergone surgery but had not yet begun adjuvant treatment were randomized to the intervention condition or a one-day psychoeducational control group. Patient-reported outcomes and clinician ratings of anxiety were assessed prior to randomization, 6 months after randomization (3 months after the intervention), and approximately 1 year after randomization. Women who participated in the intervention demonstrated significantly ($p<0.05$) lower cancer-related anxiety and interviewer-rated general anxiety symptoms; this effect persisted across the 12-month follow-up period.

Much of the existing intervention literature has focused on depression, particularly in breast cancer patients. This relatively brief but intensive intervention demonstrated long-lasting effects on anxiety in women with nonmetastatic breast cancer.

4.5 Sleep Problems

4.5.1 Prevalence and Course

Previous research suggests that sleep problems affect between 30 and 50% of cancer patients (Savard & Morin, 2001). This range of prevalence estimates reflects differences in the methods used to assess sleep problems across studies as well as differences in the patient populations that were recruited.

A recently published study that used a standardized interview to diagnose the presence of an insomnia syndrome provides more precise information to date about the prevalence and course of clinically significant insomnia in people with cancer (Savard, Villa, Ivers, Simard, & Morin, 2009). In the study, investigators sought to recruit all patients scheduled to receive curative surgery for a first diagnosis of non-metastatic cancer at two major treatment centers. Individuals who agreed to participate were administered the Insomnia Interview Schedule prior to surgery and 2 months later. Findings indicated that 28.5% of patients met diagnostic criteria for an insomnia syndrome prior to surgery, with 56.3% of these patients reporting problems that were greater than 6 months in duration. An additional 31% of patients reported insomnia symptoms that did not meet the diagnostic criteria and the remaining 40.5% of patients were classified as good sleepers. At follow-up, the prevalence of an insomnia syndrome declined to a nonsignificant extent to 26.2%. The percentage of patients who were experiencing insomnia symptoms that did not meet diagnostic criteria declined significantly to 22%, while the percentage classified as good sleepers increased significantly to 52%. With regard to incidence, remission, and persistence, findings indicated that 18.6% of good sleepers prior to surgery developed insomnia symptoms or an insomnia syndrome. Among patients with insomnia (either symptoms or syndrome), 32% became good sleepers and 68% remained insomniacs. The authors note that the 28.5 and 22% prevalence rates for clinically significant insomnia before and after surgery are substantially higher than the rate of 9.5% found in the general population using similar criteria (Morin, LeBlanc, Daley, Gregoire, & Merette, 2006). Future reports based on this patient cohort are expected to describe the course of insomnia for up to 18 months following surgery.

4.5.2 Etiology

Similar to depression and anxiety, there are many possible sources of sleep problems in people with cancer. In discussing the etiology of these problems, it is important to recognize the existence of different types of sleep and arousal disorders. According to the American Academy of Sleep Medicine classification system (American Academy of Sleep Medicine, 2005), the major types include insomnia (i.e., difficulty falling or staying asleep), sleep-related breathing disorders, hypersomnia, circadian rhythm sleep disorders, parasomnias, and sleep-related movement disorders.

Most research on the etiology of sleep problems in cancer patients has focused on insomnia. The psychological distress frequently experienced by cancer patients represents a major potential source of sleep problems given the well-documented relationships between distress responses and insomnia. The presence of other symptoms that can disturb sleep, such as nocturnal hot flashes, have also been shown to contribute to insomnia in people with cancer (Savard et al., 2004). In many instances, insomnia presents in cancer patients as part of a symptom cluster that may also include fatigue, pain, and depression. As described previously, this clustering may be attributable to a common underlying biological mechanism, such as cytokine dysregulation induced by cancer treatment. Cancer and its treatment can also result in breathing problems that interfere with sleep. Breathing-related sleep problems are particularly common in patients with tumors in the head and neck region that affect the airway (Nesse et al., 2006).

4.5.3 Assessment

Sleep problems can be assessed using objective methods (e.g., polysomnography) as well as subjective self-report methods. Although examples of studies using objective methods can be identified (Parker et al., 2008), most research on sleep problems in cancer patients has relied on self-report methods. The Pittsburgh Sleep Quality Index (PSQI) (Buysse, Reynolds, Monk, Berman, & Kupfer, 1989) is among the more commonly used self-report measures. The 19-item version yields seven component scores: sleep quality, sleep latency, sleep duration, sleep efficiency, sleep disturbances, use of sleeping medication, and daytime dysfunction. At least two studies have evaluated the psychometric characteristics of the PSQI with cancer patients and reported favorable results (Beck, Schwartz, Towsley, Dudley, & Barsevick, 2004; Carpenter & Andrykowski, 1998). Another self-report measure used in oncology settings is the Insomnia Severity Index (Morin, 1993). This 7-item measure provides a global index of the severity of insomnia and has been shown to be an effective method of screening for clinically significant insomnia in cancer patients (Savard, Savard, Simard, & Ivers, 2005). Additionally, the semistructured Insomnia Interview Schedule (Morin, 1993) has been used with cancer patients to assess the presence of insomnia according to DSM-IV criteria and ICSD criteria.

4.5.4 Management of Sleep Problems in Cancer Patients

4.5.4.1 Summary of Research Literature

A recent state of the science review of sleep-wake disturbances in adults with cancer by Berger (2009) summarized research into the management of sleep problems. The review noted that no intervention studies have tested the effects of prescription sleep drugs in patients with cancer. Accordingly, use of these medications in oncology settings is guided primarily by evidence demonstrating their efficacy in other populations.

In contrast to the lack of pharmacologic research, the review identified 18 new studies of nonpharmacologic interventions for people with cancer published since 2005 in which sleep was a primary or secondary outcome. Based on the findings from these studies and 20 additional studies published before 2005, several classes of interventions have been evaluated with regard to the weight of evidence supporting their use as part of the Oncology Nursing Society's Putting Evidence into Practice (PEP) initiative. The categorization scheme provides specific definitions for ratings that can range from "recommended for practice" (e.g., effectiveness demonstrated by strong evidence from rigorously conducted studies) to "not recommended for practice" (e.g., lack of effectiveness or harmfulness demonstrated by strong evidence from rigorously conducted studies). At present, exercise interventions, and education and information interventions are rated as "effectiveness not established" based primarily on the limited number of rigorous studies conducted. Complementary therapies are also rated as "efficacy not established" based on the limited number of rigorous studies conducted and the varied nature of the interventions tested. In contrast, cognitive-behavioral therapy is rated as "likely to be effective" based on evidence from several relatively large randomized clinical trials that yielded positive results for sleep outcomes.

4.5.4.2 Example of Evidence-Supported Intervention

In this section, we provide an example of an intervention effective for sleep problems in people with cancer. This example was selected from among several interventions that have been shown to be superior to a control condition in a published RCT and possess good potential for dissemination.

Berger et al. (2008) developed an intervention for insomnia in cancer patients that featured four components commonly found in empirically supported behavioral therapy approaches for insomnia. These components are: modified stimulus control, modified sleep restriction, relaxation therapy, and sleep hygiene counseling. The intervention was delivered by nurses who developed individualized therapy plans drawing from these components based on patients' responses to standardized questionnaires assessing sleep difficulties. The intervention was first delivered to patients 2 days before they started chemotherapy treatment. Revisions to the therapy plan were made during contacts that occurred two days prior to each later treatment. In addition, reinforcement of the therapy plan was provided during contacts that occurred seven days after each plan revision.

The efficacy of this intervention was evaluated in a RCT against a time and attention control condition that focused on healthy eating. Participants were women with nonmetastatic breast cancer scheduled to begin chemotherapy. Sleep was assessed using self-report measures (PSQI and sleep diaries) and objective measures (wrist actigraphy) before the start of treatment, at the first four treatments, and 30 days after the last treatment. Findings indicated that sleep quality as measured by the PSQI improved significantly over time in the intervention group, but not the control group. In addition, diary data and actigraphy data showed that patients in the intervention group experienced significantly fewer nighttime awakenings. As part of a follow-up study (Berger et al., 2009), participants in the intervention group met again with nurses to revise the therapy plan 60 and 90 days after the last treatment. Reassessment of all study participants 90 days after the last treatment demonstrated that the intervention group continued to experience significantly better sleep quality relative to the control group. An assessment conducted 1 year following the baseline assessment yielded similar results that approached statistical significance ($p=0.052$).

Given the high likelihood that patients undergoing chemotherapy will experience sleep disturbance (Palesh et al., 2009), an argument can be made for intervening prophylactically with all patients before the start of treatment. In addition to its demonstrated short-term and long-term efficacy, the intervention tested in the study by Berger et al. (2008) has three features that are notable strengths for dissemination purposes. First, it has the potential to be delivered by nurses as part of routine clinical care of chemotherapy patients. Second, it can be individualized to address only those factors relevant to the patient's sleep problems. Third, there are frequent opportunities to revise the plan. The last feature is particularly important since it provides flexibility to address new or worsening sleep problems that are not unlikely to occur over the course of repeated chemotherapy treatments.

4.6 Sexual Problems

4.6.1 Prevalence and Course

The most common sexual problems after cancer treatment are erectile dysfunction (ED) in men, pain with sexual activity in women, and loss of sexual desire in men and women (Schover, 2005). Other sexual problems that may occur include ejaculatory disorders, including retrograde ejaculation and alterations in ejaculation in men (Havenga, Maas, DeRuiter, Welvaart, & Trimbos, 2000). Changes in genital arousal and lubrication are often the root cause of pain in sexual activity in women. Relatively nonspecific sexual problems such as a decrease in sexual satisfaction or body image concerns also have been identified in both men and women following treatment for cancer. Prevalence rates of sexual problems vary widely by cancer type and by type of sexual problem. For example, studies have demonstrated that between 30 and 63% of women treated for cervical cancer experience sexual problems (Jensen et al., 2003, 2004), while between 30 and 100% of women treated for breast cancer may report sexual problems (Sadovsky et al., 2010). An 85% rate of ED has been reported in men after prostate cancer (Schover et al., 2002). Reviews of sexual problems with testicular cancer have demonstrated rates of ejaculatory disorders as high as 50% (Jonker-Pool et al., 2001; Nazareth, Lewin, & King, 2001).

Prevalence rates also vary based on the treatment modalities used to treat the disease. For example, ED rates of 30–40% have been reported for prostate cancer patients treated with external-beam radiotherapy (Sadovsky et al., 2010), while the rate of ED may be as high as 100% after radical prostatectomy (Burnett et al., 2007). The wide range of prevalence rates is also attributable to the heterogeneity of methodologies used to assess and define sexual problems, the timing of assessments (including whether patients' sexual functioning was assessed prior to the start of treatment), and the differences across studies in the demographic and clinical characteristics of the individuals studied.

4.6.2 Etiology

Sexual problems in individuals with cancer are typically the result of the physical and psychological effects of cancer and cancer treatment (Schover & Jensen, 1988). Surgical treatment may remove reproductive organs or damage the physiological systems involved in the sexual response. Chemotherapy often causes side effects such as weight changes, hair loss, fatigue, ovarian failure in premenopausal women, and hypogonadism in men. These effects may directly impair the sexual response or indirectly affect an individual's ability and motivation to engage in sexual activity. Radiation may cause fatigue and tissue damage that in the short term adversely affects body image in both men and women. Radiation to the pelvis may cause fatigue and bowel and bladder changes that affect an individual's capacity for intimacy. In men, sexual problems after pelvic radiation may result from damage to pelvic nerves and blood vessels involved in erection and from slowing of testosterone production. Alterations in vaginal anatomy and decreased vaginal lubrication secondary to pelvic radiation often cause sexual problems in women. As well, radiation to the whole pelvis is likely to result in ovarian failure in premenopausal women. Androgen deprivation therapy may result in profound sexual problems in men, while hormone manipulation therapy in women may exacerbate women's menopausal symptoms. Finally, supportive medications such as opioids for pain control, antidepressants, antianxiety medications, and antiemetics may cause sexual problems in men and women.

4.6.3 Assessment

The assessment of sexual problems in cancer patients should include a physical exam with laboratory tests of fasting glucose, cholesterol, lipids, and hormonal profile to identify or confirm a specific cause or to evaluate the role of potential co-morbid conditions in the development and maintenance of sexual problems (Hatzichristou et al., 2004, 2010). There are also a number of specialized diagnostic tests and procedures available (e.g., pudendal arteriogram in women and nocturnal penile tumescence and rigidity in men); however, these tests typically have little impact on how sexual problems are managed. Thus, to date, the assessment of sexual problems in cancer patients has consisted predominantly of patient's self-report of sexual problems.

A recent review of sexual function measures used with cancer patients (Jeffery et al., 2009) noted that few measures have both undergone extensive psychometric testing and been used widely in research and clinical settings with cancer patients. Two measures designed to assess sexual functioning in men meet these criteria. The International Index of Erectile Function (IIEF) (Rosen et al., 1997) is a 15-item self-report measure. Scores are calculated for five domains: erectile function, orgasmic function, sexual desire, intercourse satisfaction, and overall satisfaction. The psychometric properties of the IIEF have been well established and the instrument has been used to evaluate sexual function in men with a variety of cancers, including bladder, colon, prostate, testicular, and rectal cancer (Jeffery et al., 2009). The University of California-Los Angeles (UCLA) Prostate Cancer Index (PCI) (Litwin et al., 1998) and its longer version, the Expanded Prostate Index Composite (EPIC) (Wei, Dunn, Litwin, Sandler, & Sanda, 2000), have been widely used to assess sexual problems in prostate cancer patients. The UCLA PCI is a 20-item measure that was originally designed to be used with the Rand 36-item Health Survey to assess quality of life in men with prostate cancer. Both the PCI and the 26- and 50-item versions of EPIC include items about urinary and bowel function in addition to items about sexual functioning and sexual bother. In women, the most widely used and psychometrically sound measure is the Female Sexual Function Index (FSFI) (Rosen et al., 2000; Wiegel, Meston, & Rosen, 2005), a 19-item self-report measure designed to assess the multidimensional nature of female sexual function. Scores are calculated for six domains: desire, arousal, lubrication, orgasmic capacity, dyspareunia, and sexual satisfaction. A total scale score is obtained by adding the six domain scores. The reliability and validity of the FSFI are well established and the measure has been shown to discriminate between clinical and nonclinical populations. It has been used to evaluate sexual function in women with a variety of cancers, including bladder, breast, cervix, colon, gynecologic, rectal, and vulvar cancer (Jeffery et al., 2009).

4.6.4 Management of Sexual Problems in Cancer Patients

4.6.4.1 Summary of Research Literature

A number of therapies are currently available to address sexual problems in men with cancer. Testosterone replacement therapy is often effective in increasing sexual desire and may improve erectile function in men with clinically low levels of serum testosterone. Oral therapy with phosphodiesterase type 5 (PDE5) inhibiting drugs is considered first-line treatment for erectile dysfunction. Standard second-line therapies for erectile dysfunction include intracavernosal injections with prostaglandin

E_1 alone or in combination with papaverine and phentolamine. Side effects include pain at the injection site, penile fibrosis, and corporal plaque, and many patients switch to oral medications or discontinue injections because of these side effects or because they find injections cumbersome and inconvenient (Zippe, Nandipati, Agarwal, & Raina, 2006). Intraurethral prostaglandin E_1 delivered with the medicated urethral system for erection (MUSE®) represents an alternative for those not willing to consider injections; research indicates that compliance is higher with MUSE® than with injections but that its efficacy is lower. Vacuum constriction devices are one of the oldest treatments available for erectile dysfunction. Side effects with these devices are rare, and the device represents a one-time cost that is relatively inexpensive compared to other available therapies. However, the lack of spontaneity with their use as well as their labor-intensive nature make this a less appealing option for many men. Finally, implanted silicone rods or inflatable penile implants are used when there is a clearly identified medical cause for erectile dysfunction and erections are not likely to improve. Cancer survivors who have had nerve-sparing surgical procedures are encouraged to wait at least 1 year before considering a penile prosthesis because surgery to implant the prosthesis destroys one's own capacity for erection.

Available treatment options for sexual problems in women with cancer are relatively fewer in number. Water- or silicone-based vaginal lubricants and vaginal moisturizers are routinely recommended to combat vaginal dryness. When these are not sufficient to alleviate dyspareunia, low-dose vaginal estrogen preparations may be considered (North American Menopause Society, 2007). Pelvic floor muscle training and vaginal dilators are recommended as a prophylactic measure after pelvic radiotherapy to prevent vaginal stenosis (Denton & Maher, 2003). Evidence for the effectiveness of these therapies among cancer survivors, however, is limited (Miles et al., 2007). With respect to vaginal dilation in particular, there is a lack of consistency in patient education regarding this therapy (White & Faithfull, 2006) and compliance rates for vaginal dilation are universally low (Robinson, Faris, & Scott, 1999; Jeffries, Robinson, Craighead, & Keats, 2006). In general, there are limited efficacy and safety data for testosterone therapy for low desire associated with ovarian failure, and it is not recommended (Ganz & Greendale, 2007; Schover, 2008).

Research strongly suggests that sexual problems are multifactorial in nature and factors such as an individual's age, emotional well-being, partner relationship quality, and sexual health history may play a role in the development and maintenance of sexual problems after cancer (Ganz et al., 2000; Northouse, Mood, Templin, Mellon, & George, 2000; Schmidt, Bestmann, Kuchler, & Kremer, 2005). Thus, efforts to manage sexual problems in cancer patients should begin with a comprehensive assessment. It is important to identify the specific nature of the sexual problem as well as factors that may be perpetuating the problem. Relatively simple sexual problems can often be dealt with by providing information and suggestions for behavior change. More complex and severe problems will require more intensive intervention and efforts that combine medical and psychological therapies are likely to be most effective.

4.6.4.2 Example of Evidence-Supported Intervention

In this section, we provide an example of an intervention found to be effective in improving sexual adjustment and body image in women after cancer. The example was selected because the intervention was evaluated in an RCT and because the intervention itself was a couple-based intervention. Although a recent systematic review of randomized controlled interventions for sexual problems in women after cancer (Scott & Kayser, 2009) noted the difficulty in recruiting men (either as patients or partners) to psychosocial oncology intervention studies, the review concluded that the strongest effects were seen for couple-focused interventions. Including partners in interventions for sexual problems in women acknowledges the multiplicity of factors that may contribute to the development and maintenance of sexual problems and the important role that a partner often plays in effectively addressing sexual problems.

Scott and Halford (2004) developed a couple-based intervention referred to as CanCOPE that focused on helping couples in which the women has been diagnosed with cancer cope with cancer and support each other. The intervention involves five 2-h sessions before surgery, after surgery, 1 week later, 5 weeks later, and at 6 months follow-up. All of the sessions took place at the couple's home. Two 30-min telephone calls at 1 and 3 months postsurgery serve to review client progress. Both partners receive educational material, coping skills training, and supportive counseling. Couples are also taught supportive communication and partner support and received sexual counseling. In a test of the CanCOPE intervention, women with early-stage breast or gynecologic cancer were randomly assigned to this intervention, individual coping training, or a medical education control. The individual coping intervention was delivered in the patient's home, and with the exception of the 5-week postsurgery session, followed the same schedule as the CanCOPE intervention. The intervention consisted of the provision of medical information and coping education and supportive counseling. The medical education intervention provided high-quality education on all aspects of medical care, but with no specific psychological intervention. Women in this condition received five brief telephone calls conducted prior to surgery, 1 and 2 weeks postsurgery, and 6 and 9 months postsurgery. Relative to the individual coping and medication education conditions, the CanCOPE intervention significantly increased couple-coping supportive communication, reduced women's psychological distress and avoidance of intrusive negative thoughts, and improved women's sexual self-schema, sexual intimacy with their partners, and perceptions of their partner's acceptance of their body. Although the CanCOPE intervention did not have a differential effect on women's sexual dysfunction, the researchers hypothesized that this was due to a floor effect; women in the study reported rates of sexual dysfunction comparable to healthy women.

Although the intervention in the Scott and Halford (2004) possesses limited potential for dissemination, its effectiveness highlights several important components for consideration in future intervention studies (Scott & Kayser, 2009). These are the provision of education for both partners about the women's diagnosis and treatment, the promotion of couples' mutual coping and support processes, and the provision of specific therapies to address sexual problems.

4.7 Future Directions

The number and variety of studies reviewed in this chapter attest to the depth and breadth of research on psychological co-morbidities of cancer. Nevertheless, important gaps exist in the literature. As noted previously, there is a dearth of research focusing on men and on ethnic and racial minority groups. In addition, few studies have focused on the characterization and management of psychological co-morbidities in patients with advanced disease and patients who have completed treatment. Another important gap is the relative lack of systematic research on biological risk factors for psychological co-morbidities in cancer patients. Along these lines, research examining the potential interactive effects of genetic polymorphisms with treatment exposure would appear to have promise (Ahles et al., 2003; Collado-Hidalgo, Bower, Ganz, Irwin & Cole, 2008).

Three additional recommendations are offered that go beyond addressing existing gaps to reconsidering the current approach to the management of psychological co-morbidities of cancer. All three recommendations reflect the need for research more relevant to clinical practice. First, studies of psychological interventions should be informed by the growing body of research demonstrating that cancer patients tend to experience symptoms in clusters rather than in isolation (Miaskowski, Dodd, & Lee, 2004). Depression, for example, frequently co-occurs with pain, fatigue, and sleep problems in cancer patients (Gaston-Johansson et al., 2000; Donovan & Jacobsen, 2007). Recognizing this pattern, several RCTs have been designed specifically to test whether psychological interventions are effective against symptom clusters of this type (Williams, 2007). Second, psychological interventions need to be evaluated in combination with other approaches used to manage psychological co-morbidities. Specifically, RCTs are needed that explicitly test whether the combination of pharmacotherapy and psychotherapy is better than either approach alone in managing anxiety, depression, and sleep problems. RCTs should also be conducted to test whether certain personal, disease, or treatment characteristics predict whether a patient is likely to benefit more from psychotherapy or medication. Third, research is needed that evaluates the entire clinical pathway through which a patient might receive an intervention for a psychological co-morbidity. For example, NCCN Clinical Practice Guidelines recommend that patients be screened routinely for distress and that patients found to have moderate to severe distress receive care that includes psychotherapy (Anonymous, 1999). Whether or not this strategy (routine screening followed by referral to psychosocial professionals only for distressed patients) results in better management of psychological co-morbidities than other strategies (e.g., preventive interventions offered to all patients) has yet to be adequately evaluated.

References

Ahles, T. A., Saykin, A. J., Noll, W. W., Furstenberg, C. T., Guerin, S., Cole, B., et al. (2003). The relationship of APOE genotype to neuropsychological performance in long-term cancer survivors treated with standard dose chemotherapy. *Psycho-Oncol, 12*, 612–619.

Akechi, T., Okamura, H., Nishiwaki, Y., & Uchitomi, Y. (2001). Psychiatric disorders and associated and predictive factors in patients with unresectable nonsmall cell lung carcinoma. *Cancer, 92*, 2609–2622.

Akechi T., Okuyama T., Onishi J., Morita T., & Furukawa, T. A. (2008). Psychotherapy for depression among incurable cancer patients. *Cochrane Database Syst Rev* 2, CD005537.

Ali, N. S., & Khalil, H. Z. (1989). Effect of psychoeducational intervention on anxiety among Egyptian bladder cancer patients. *Cancer Nurs, 12*, 236–242.

American Academy of Sleep Medicine. (2005). *International classification of sleep disorders: Diagnostic and coding manual* (2nd ed.). Westchester: American Academy of Sleep Medicine.

American Cancer Society. (2009). *Cancer facts and figures 2009*. Atlanta: American Cancer Society.

American Psychiatric Association. (1994). *Diagnostic and statistical manual of mental disorders* (4th ed.). Washington: American Psychiatric Association.

Andersen, B. L., Yang, H., Farrar, W. B., Golden-Kruetz, D. M., Emery, C. F., Thornton, L. M., et al. (2008). Psychological intervention improves survival for breast cancer patients. *Cancer, 113*, 450–458.

Anonymous. (1999). NCCN practice guidelines for the management of psychosocial distress. *Oncol, 13*, 113–147.

Antoni, M. H., Lechner, S., Diaz, A., Vargas, S., Holley, H., Phillips, K., et al. (2009). Cognitive behavioral stress management effects on psychosocial and physiological adaptation in women undergoing treatment for breast cancer. *Brain Behav Immun, 23*, 580–591.

Arakawa, S. (1997). Relaxation to reduce nausea, vomiting, and anxiety induced by chemotherapy in Japanese patients. *Cancer Nurs, 20*, 342–349.

Barsevick, A. M. (2007). The concept of symptom cluster. *Semin Oncol Nurs, 23*, 89–98.

Barsevick, A. M., Sweeney, C., Haney, E., & Chung, E. (2002). A systematic qualitative analysis of psychoeducational interventions for depression in patients with cancer. *Oncol Nurs Forum, 29*, 73–84.

Beck, A. T., Rush, A. J., Shaw, B. F., & Emery, G. (1979). *Cognitive therapy of depression*. New York: Guilford Press.

Beck, S. L., Schwartz, A. L., Towsley, G., Dudley, W., & Barsevick, A. M. (2004). Psychometric evaluation of the Pittsburgh sleep quality index in cancer patients. *J Pain Symptom Manage, 27*, 140–148.

Beck, A. T., & Steer, R. A. (1990). *Manual for the Beck Anxiety Inventory*. San Antonio: Psychological Corporation.

Beck, A. T., Steer, R. A., & Brown, G. K. (1996). *BDI-II Beck Depression Inventory – Second edition manual*. San Antonio: Psychological Corporation.

Berger, A. M. (2009). Update on the state of the science: Sleep-wake disturbances in adult patients with cancer. *Oncol Nurs Forum, 36*, 165–177.

Berger, A. M., Kuhn, B. R., Farr, L. A., Lynch, J. C., Agrawal, S., Chamberlain, J., et al. (2008). Behavioral therapy intervention trial to improve sleep quality and cancer-related fatigue. *Psycho-Oncol, 16*, 634–646.

Berger, A. M., Kuhn, B. R., Farr, L. A., Von Essen, S. G., Chamberlain, J., Lynch, J. C., et al. (2009). One-year outcomes of a behavioral therapy intervention trial on sleep quality and cancer-related fatigue. *J Clin Onc, 27*, 6033–6040.

Bindemann, S., Soukop, M., & Kaye, S. B. (1991). Randomised controlled study of relaxation training. *Eur J Cancer, 27*, 170–174.

Bottomley, A. (1998). Depression in cancer patients: A literature review. *Eur J Cancer Care, 7*, 181–191.

Brown, J. H., & Parakevas, F. (1982). Cancer and depression. Cancer presenting with depressive illness: an autoimmune disease? *Br J Psychiatry, 141*, 227–232.

Burish, T. G., Carey, M. P., Krozely, M. G., & Greco, F. A. (1987). Conditioned side effects induced by cancer chemotherapy: Prevention through behavioral treatment. *J Consult Clin Psychol, 55*, 42–48.

Burish, T. G., & Lyles, J. N. (1981). Effectiveness of relaxation training in reducing adverse reactions to cancer chemotherapy. *J Behav Med, 4*, 65–78.

Burnett, A. L., Aus, G., Canby-Hagino, E. D., Cookson, M. S., D'Amico, A. V., Dmochowski, R. R., et al. (2007). Erectile function outcome reporting after clinically localized prostate cancer treatment. *J Urol, 178*, 597–601.

Buysse, D. J., Reynolds, C. F., Monk, T. H., Berman, S. R., & Kupfer, D. J. (1989). The Pittsburgh Sleep Quality Index: A new instrument for psychiatric practice and research. *J Psychiatr Res, 28*, 193–213.

Capuron, L., Gumnick, J. F., Musselman, D. L., Lawson, D. H., Reemsnyder, A., Nemeroff, C. B., et al. (2002). Neurobehavioral effects of interferon-alpha in cancer patients: Phenomenology and paroxetine responsiveness of symptom dimensions. *Neuropsychopharmacol, 26*, 643–652.

Carey, M. P., & Burish, T. G. (1987). Providing relaxation training to cancer chemotherapy patients: A comparison of three delivery techniques. *J Consult Clin Psychol, 55*, 732–737.

Carney, C. P., Jones, L., Woolson, R. F., Noyes, R., & Doebbeling, B. N. (2003). Relationship between depression and pancreatic cancer in the general population. *Psychosom Med, 65*, 884–888.

Carpenter, J. S., & Andrykowski, M. A. (1998). *Psychometric evaluation of the Pittsburgh Sleep Quality Index J Psychosom Res, 45*, 5–13.

Cheung, Y. L., Molassiotis, A., & Chang, A. M. (2003). The effect of progressive muscle relaxation training on anxiety and quality of life after stoma surgery in colorectal cancer patients. *Psycho-Oncol, 12*, 254–266.

Christensen, D. N. (1983). Postmastectomy couple counseling: An outcome study of a structured treatment protocol. *J Sex Marital Ther, 9*, 266–275.

Cleeland, C. S., Mendoza, T. R., Wang, X. S., Chou, C., Harle, M. T., Morrissey, M., et al. (2000). Assessing symptom distress in cancer patients: The M. D. Anderson Symptom Inventory. *Cancer, 89*, 1634–1646.

Collado-Hidalgo, A., Bower, J. E., Ganz, P. A., Irwin, M. R., & Cole, S. W. (2008). Cytokine gene polymorphisms and fatigue in breast cancer survivors: Early findings. *Brain Behav Immun, 22*, 1197–1200.

Coyne, J. C., Stefanek, M., & Palmer, S. C. (2007). Psychotherapy and survival in cancer: The conflict between hope and evidence. *Psychol Bull, 133*, 367–394.

Cunningham, A. J., & Tocco, E. K. (1989). A randomized trial of group psychoeducational therapy for cancer patients. *Patient Care Counsel, 14*, 101–114.

Dahl, A. A., Haaland, C. F., Mykletun, A., Bremnes, R., Dahl, O., Klepp, O., et al. (2005). Study of anxiety disorder and depression in long-term survivors of testicular cancer. *J Clin Oncol, 23*, 2389–2395.

Decker, T. W., Cline-Elsen, J., & Gallagher, M. (1992). Relaxation therapy as an adjunct in radiation oncology. *J Clin Psychol, 48*, 388–393.

Denton, A. S. & Maher, E. J. (2003). Interventions for the physical aspects of sexual dysfunction in women following pelvic radiotherapy. *Cochrane Database Syst Rev*, CD003750.

Devine, E. C., & Westlake, S. K. (1995). The effects of psychoeducational care provided to adults with cancer: Meta-analysis of 116 studies. *Oncol Nurs Forum, 22*, 1369–1381.

Donovan, K. A., & Jacobsen, P. B. (2007). Fatigue, depression, and insomnia: Evidence for a symptom cluster. *Sem Onc Nurs, 23*, 127–135.

Edelman, S., Bell, D. R., & Kidman, A. D. (1999). A group cognitive behaviour therapy programme with metastatic breast cancer patients. *Psycho-Oncol, 8*(4), 295–305.

Edgar, L., Rosberger, Z., & Collet, J. P. (2001). Lessons learned: Outcomes and methodology of a coping skills intervention trial comparing individual and group formats for patients with cancer. *Int J Psychiatry Med, 31*, 289–304.

Elsesser, K., van Berkel, M., & Sartory, G. (1994). The effects of anxiety management training on psychological variables and immune parameters in cancer patients: A pilot study. *Beh Cog Psychoth, 22*, 13–23.

Evans, R. L., & Connis, R. T. (1995). Comparison of brief group therapies for depressed cancer patients receiving radiation treatment. *Public Health Rep, 110*, 306–311.

Fallowfield, L. J., Hall, A., Maguire, P., Baum, M., & A'Hern, R. P. (1994). Psychological effects of being offered choice of surgery for breast cancer. *BMJ, 309*, 448.
Fallowfield, L. J., Ratcliffe, D., Jenkins, V., & Saul, J. (2001). Psychiatric morbidity and its recognition by doctors in patients with cancer. *Br J Cancer, 84*, 1011–1015.
Fann, J. R., Thomas-Rich, A. M., Katon, W. J., Cowley, D., Pepping, M., McGregor, B. A., et al. (2008). Major depression after breast cancer: a review of epidemiology and treatment. *Gen Hosp Psychiatry, 30*, 112–126.
Fawzy, F. I., Cousins, N., Fawzy, N. W., Kemeny, M. E., Elashoff, R., & Morton, D. (1990). A structured psychiatric intervention for cancer patients. I. Changes over time in methods of coping and affective disturbance. *Arch Gen Psychiatry, 47*, 720–725.
First, M. B., Gibbons, M. & Spitzer, R. L. (1996). Users guide for the structured clinical interview for DSM-IV Axis I disorders: Research version. In (Ed.). New York: Biometrics Research.
Fras, I. L., & Pearson, J. S. (1967). Comparison of psychiatric symptoms in carcinoma of the pancreas with those in some other intra-abdominal neoplasms. *Am J Psychiatry, 123*, 1553–1562.
Ganz, P. A., & Greendale, G. A. (2007). Female sexual desire–beyond testosterone. *J Natl Cancer Inst, 99*, 659–661.
Ganz, P. A., Greendale, G. A., Petersen, L., Zibecchi, L., Kahn, B., & Belin, T. R. (2000). Managing menopausal symptoms in breast cancer survivors: results of a randomized controlled trial. *J Natl Cancer Inst, 92*, 1054–1064.
Gaston-Johansson, F., Fall-Dickson, J. M., Nanda, J., Ohly, K. V., Stillman, S., Krumm, S., et al. (2000). The effectiveness of the comprehensive coping strategy program on clinical outcomes in breast cancer autologous bone marrow transplantation. *Cancer Nurs, 23*, 277–285.
Goodwin, P. J., Leszcz, M., Ennis, M., Koopmans, J., Vincent, L., Guther, H., et al. (2001). The effect of group psychosocial support on survival in metastatic breast cancer. *N Engl J Med, 345*, 1719–1726.
Harter, M., Reuter, K., Aschenbrenner, A., Schretzmann, B., Marschner, N., Hasenburg, A., et al. (2001). Psychiatric disorders and associated factors in cancer: results of an interview study with patients in inpatient, rehabilitation and outpatient treatment. *Eur J Cancer, 37*, 1385–1393.
Hatzichristou, D., Rosen, R. C., Broderick, G., Clayton, A., Cuzin, B., Derogatis, L., et al. (2004). Clinical evaluation and management strategy for sexual dysfunction in men and women. *J Sex Med, 1*, 49–57.
Hatzichristou, D., Rosen, R. C., Derogatis, L. R., Low, W. Y., Meuleman, E. J., Sadovsky, R., et al. (2010). Recommendations for the clinical evaluation of men and women with sexual dysfunction. *J Sex Med, 7*, 337–348.
Havenga, K., Maas, C. P., DeRuiter, M. C., Welvaart, K., & Trimbos, J. B. (2000). Avoiding long-term disturbance to bladder and sexual function in pelvic surgery, particularly with rectal cancer. *Semin Surg Oncol, 18*, 235–243.
Hersch, J., Juraskova, I., Price, M., & Mullan, B. (2009). Psychosocial interventions and quality of life in gynaecological cancer patients: a systematic review. *Psycho-Oncol, 18*, 795–810.
Holland, J. D., Korzun, A. H., Tross, S., Silberfarb, P., Perry, M., Comis, R., et al. (1986). Comparative psychological disturbance in patients with pancreatic and gastric cancer. *Am J Psychiatry, 143*, 982–986.
Institute of Medicine. (2006). *From cancer patient to cancer survivor: Lost in transition*. Washington: National Academies Press.
Institute of Medicine. (2007). *Cancer care for the whole patient: Meeting psychosocial health needs*. Washington: National Academies Press.
Jacobs, C., Ross, R. D., Walker, I. M., & Stockdale, F. E. (1983). Behavior of cancer patients: A randomized study of the effects of education and peer support groups. *Am J Clin Oncol, 6*, 347–353.
Jacobsen, P. B., Donovan, K. A., Swaine, Z. N. & Watson, I. S. (2006). Management of anxiety and depression in adult cancer patients: Toward an evidence-based approach. In A. E. Chang, P. A. Ganz, D. F. Hayes, T. J. Kinsella, et al. (Ed.), *Oncology: An evidence-based approach* (1552–1579). New York: Springer.

Jacobsen, P. B., Meade, C. D., Stein, K. D., Chirikos, T. N., Small, B. J., & Ruckdeschel, J. C. (2002). Efficacy and costs of two forms of stress management training for cancer patients undergoing chemotherapy. *J Clin Oncol, 20*, 2851–2862.

Jacobsson, L. O. (1971). Initial mental disorders in carcinoma of pancreas and stomach. *Acta Psychiatric Scand, 220*, 120–127.

Jeffery, D. D., Tzeng, J. P., Keefe, F. J., Porter, L. S., Hahn, E. A., Flynn, K. E., et al. (2009). Initial report of the cancer Patient-Reported Outcomes Measurement Information System (PROMIS) sexual function committee: review of sexual function measures and domains used in oncology. *Cancer, 115*, 1142–1153.

Jeffries, S. A., Robinson, J. W., Craighead, P. S., & Keats, M. R. (2006). An effective group psychoeducational intervention for improving compliance with vaginal dilation: a randomized controlled trial. *Int J Radiat Oncol Biol Phys, 65*, 404–411.

Jensen, P. T., Groenvold, M., Klee, M. C., Thranov, I., Petersen, M. A., & Machin, D. (2003). Longitudinal study of sexual function and vaginal changes after radiotherapy for cervical cancer. *Int J Radiat Oncol Biol Phys, 56*, 937–949.

Jensen, P. T., Groenvold, M., Klee, M. C., Thranov, I., Petersen, M. A., & Machin, D. (2004). Early-stage cervical carcinoma, radical hysterectomy, and sexual function. A longitudinal study. *Cancer, 100*, 97–106.

Joffe, R., Rubinow, D., Demicoff, K., Maher, M., & Sindelar, W. F. (1986). Depression and carcinoma of the pancreas. *Gen Hosp Psychiatry, 8*, 241–245.

Jonker-Pool, G., Van de Wiel, H. B., Hoekstra, H. J., Sleijfer, D. T., Van Driel, M. F., Van Basten, J. P., et al. (2001). Sexual functioning after treatment for testicular cancer–review and meta-analysis of 36 empirical studies between 1975–2000. *Arch Sex Behav, 30*, 55–74.

Kangas, M., Henry, J., & Bryant, R. (2005). The Course of Psychological Disorder in the 1st Year After Cancer Diagnosis. *J Consult Clin Psychol, 73*, 763–768.

Katon, W., Von Korff, M., Lin, E., Walker, E., Simon, G. E., Bush, T., et al. (1995). Collaborative management to achieve treatment guidelines. Impact on depression in primary care. *JAMA, 273*, 1026–1031.

Kerrihard, T., Breitbart, W., Dent, R., & Strout, D. (1999). Anxiety in patients with cancer and human immunodeficiency virus. *Semin Clin Neuropsychiatry, 4*, 114–132.

Kessler, R. C., Chiu, W. T., Demler, O., & Walters, E. E. (2005). Prevalence, severity, and comorbidity of 12-month DSM-IV disorders in the national comorbidity survey replication. *Arch Gen Psychiatry, 62*(617–627).

Kim, H., McGuire, D. B., Tulman, L., & Barsevick, A. M. (2005). Symptom clusters: concept analysis and clinical implications for cancer nursing. *Cancer Nurs, 28*, 270–282.

Kroenke, K., Spitzer, R. L., & Williams, J. B. W. (2001). The PHQ-9: Validity of a brief depression severity measure. *J Gen Intern Med, 16*, 606–613.

Liossi, C., & White, P. (2001). Efficacy of clinical hypnosis in the enhancement of quality of life of terminally ill cancer patients. *Cont Hypn, 18*, 145–160.

Litwin, M. S., Hays, R. D., Fink, A., Ganz, P. A., Leake, B., & Brook, R. H. (1998). The UCLA Prostate Cancer Index: Development, reliability, and validity of a health-related quality of life measure. *Med Care, 36*, 1002–1012.

Lovejoy, N. C., Tabor, D., Matteis, M., & Lillis, P. (2000). Cancer-related depression: Part I – neurologic alterations and cognitive-behavioral therapy. *Oncol Nurs Forum, 27*, 667–678.

Luebbert, K., Dahme, B., & Hasenbring, M. (2001). The effectiveness of relaxation training in reducing treatment-related symptoms and improving emotional adjustment in acute non-surgical cancer treatment: A meta-analytic review. *Psychooncology, 10*, 490–502.

Ly, K. L., Chidgey, J., Addington-Hall, J., & Hotopf, M. (2002). Depression in palliative care: A systematic review. Part 2. Treatment. *Palliat Med, 16*, 279–284.

Mantovani, G., Astara, G., Lampis, B., Bianchi, A., Curreli, L., Orru, W., et al. (1996). Evaluation by multidimensional instruments of health-related quality of life of elderly cancer patients undergoing three different "psychosocial" treatment approaches. A randomized clinical trial. *Support Care Cancer, 4*, 129–140.

Marchioro, G., Azzarello, G., Checchin, F., Perale, M., Segati, R., Sampognaro, E., et al. (1996). The impact of a psychological intervention on quality of life in non-metastatic breast cancer. *Eur J Cancer, 32A*, 1612–1615.

McArdle, J. M., George, W. D., McArdle, C. S., Smith, D. C., Moodie, A. R., Hughson, A. V., et al. (1996). Psychological support for patients undergoing breast cancer surgery: A randomised study. *BMJ, 312*, 813–816.

McQuellon, R. P., Wells, M., Hoffman, S., Craven, B., Russell, G., Cruz, J., et al. (1998). Reducing distress in cancer patients with an orientation program. *Psycho-Oncol, 7*(3), 207–217.

Miaskowski, C., Dodd, M., & Lee, K. (2004). Symptom clusters: The new frontier in symptom management research. *J Natl Cancer Inst Monogr, 32*, 17–21.

Miles, C. L., Candy, B., Jones, L., Williams, R., Tookman, A. & King, M. (2007). Interventions for sexual dysfunction following treatments for cancer. *Cochrane Database Syst Rev*, CD005540.

Miller, K., & Massie, M. J. (2006). Depression and anxiety. *Cancer J, 12*, 388–397.

Miovic, M., & Block, S. (2007). Psychiatric disorders in advanced cancer. *Cancer, 110*, 1665–1676.

Moher, D., Schulz, K. F., & Altman, D. G. (2001). The CONSORT statement: revised recommendations for improving the quality of reports of parallel-group randomized trials. *Ann Intern Med, 134*, 657–662.

Morin, C. M. (1993). *Insomnia: Psychological assessment and management*. New York: Guilford Press.

Morin, C. M., LeBlanc, M., Daley, M., Gregoire, J. P., & Merette, C. (2006). Epidemiology of insomnia: Prevalence, self-help treatments, consultations, and determinants of help-seeking behaviors. *Sleep Med, 7*, 123–130.

Morrow, G. R. (1986). Effect of the cognitive hierarchy in the systematic desensitization treatment of anticipatory nausea in cancer patients: A component comparison with relaxation only, counseling, and no treatment. *Cog Ther Res, 10*, 421–446.

Moyer, A., Sohl, S. J., Knapp-Oliver, S. K., & Schneider, S. (2009). Characteristics and methodological quality of 25 years of research investigating psychosocial interventions for cancer patients. *Cancer Treat Rev, 35*, 475–484.

Moynihan, C., Bliss, J. M., Davidson, J., Burchell, L., & Horwich, A. (1998). Evaluation of adjuvant psychological therapy in patients with testicular cancer: Randomised controlled trial. *BMJ, 316*, 429–435.

Musselman, D. L., Lawson, D. H., Gumnick, J. F., Manatunga, A. K., Penna, S., Goodkin, R. S., et al. (2001). Paroxetine for the prevention of depression induced by high-dose interferon alfa. *N Engl J Med, 344*, 961–966.

National Breast Cancer Centre and National Cancer Control Initiative. (2003). *Clinical Practice Guidelines for the Psychosocial Care of Adults with Cancer*. Camperdown, Australia: National Breast Cancer Centre.

Nazareth, I., Lewin, J., & King, M. (2001). Sexual dysfunction after treatment for testicular cancer: a systematic review. *J Psychosom Res, 51*, 735–743.

Nesse, W., Hoekema, A., Stegenga, B., van der Hoeven, J. H., de Bont, L. G., & Roodenburg, J. L. (2006). Prevalence of obstructive sleep apnoea following head and neck cancer treatment: A cross sectional study. *Oral Oncol, 42*, 107–113.

Newell, S. A., Sanson-Fisher, R. W., & Savolainen, N. J. (2002). Systematic review of psychological therapies for cancer patients: Overview and recommendations for future research. *J Natl Cancer Inst, 94*, 558–584.

Nezu, A. M., Nezu, C. M., Felgoise, S. H., McClure, K. S., & Houts, P. S. (2003). Project genesis: Assessing the efficacy of problem-solving therapy for distressed adult cancer patients. *J Consult Clin Psychol, 71*, 1036–1048.

North American Menopause Society. (2007). The role of local vaginal estrogen for treatment of vaginal atrophy in post menopausal women: 2007 position statement of the North American Menopause Society. *Menopause, 14*, 355–369.

Northouse, L. L., Mood, D., Templin, T., Mellon, S., & George, T. (2000). Couples' patterns of adjustment to colon cancer. *Soc Sci Med, 50*, 271–284.

Osborn, R. L., Demoncada, A. C., & Feuerstein, M. (2006). Psychosocial interventions for depression, anxiety, and quality of life in cancer survivors: Meta-analyses. *Int J Psychiatry Med, 36*, 13–34.

Palesh, O. G., Roscoe, J. A., Mustian, K. M., Roth, T., Savard, J., Ancoli-Israel, S., et al. (2009). Prevalence, demographics, and psychological associations of sleep disruption in patients with cancer: University of Rochester Cancer Center-Community Clinical Oncology Program. *J Clin Oncol, 28*, 292–298.

Parker, K. P., Bliwise, D. L., Ribeiro, M., Jain, S. R., Vena, C. I., Kohles-Baker, M., et al. (2008). Sleep/wake patterns of individuals with advanced cancer measured by ambulatory polysomnography. *J Clin Oncol, 26*, 2464–2472.

Petersen, R. W., & Quinlivan, J. A. (2002). Preventing anxiety and depression in gynaecological cancer: A randomised controlled trial. *BJOG, 109*, 386–394.

Pinquart, M., & Duberstein, P. R. (2010). Depression and cancer mortality: A meta-analysis. *Psychol Med., 40*(11), 1797–810.

Pirl, W. F. (2004). Evidence report on the occurrence, assessment, and treatmentof depression in cancer patients. *J Natl Cancer Inst Monogr, 32*, 32–39.

Pruitt, B. T., Waligora-Serafin, B., McMahon, T., Byrd, G., Besselman, L., Kelly, G. M., et al. (1993). An educational intervention for newly-diagnosed cancer patients undergoing radiotherapy. *Psycho-Oncol, 2*, 55–62.

Radloff, L. S. (1977). The CES-D Scale: A self-report depression scale for research in the general population. *Appl Psychol Meas, 1*, 385–401.

Rawl, S. M., Given, B. A., Given, C. W., Champion, V. L., Kozachik, S. L., Barton, D., et al. (2002). Intervention to improve psychological functioning for newly diagnosed patients with cancer. *Oncol Nurs Forum, 29*, 967–975.

Redd, W. H., Montgomery, G. H., & DuHamel, K. N. (2001). Behavioral intervention for cancer treatment side effects. *J Natl Cancer Inst, 93*, 810–823.

Robinson, J. W., Faris, P. D., & Scott, C. B. (1999). Psychoeducational group increases vaginal dilation for younger women and reduces sexual fears for women of all ages with gynecological carcinoma treated with radiotherapy. *Int J Radiat Oncol Biol Phys, 44*, 497–506.

Rodin, G., Lloyd, N., Katz, M., Green, E., Mackay, J. A., & Wong, R. K. S. (2007). The treatment of depression in cancer patients: a systematic review. *Support Care Cancer, 15*, 123–136.

Rosen, R., Brown, C., Heiman, J., Leiblum, S., Meston, C., Shabsigh, R., et al. (2000). The Female Sexual Function Index (FSFI): a multidimensional self-report instrument for the assessment of female sexual function. *J Sex Marital Ther, 26*, 191–208.

Rosen, R. C., Riley, A., Wagner, G., Osterloh, I. H., Kirkpatrick, J., & Mishra, A. (1997). The international index of erectile function (IIEF): a multidimensional scale for assessment of erectile dysfunction. *Urology, 49*, 822–830.

Roth, A. J., & Massie, M. J. (2007). Anxiety and its management in advanced cancer. *Curr Opin Support Palliat Care, 1*, 50–56.

Roy-Byrne, P. P., Davidson, K. W., Kessler, R. C., Asmundson, G. J., Goodwin, R. D., Kubzansky, L., et al. (2008). Anxiety disorders and comorbid medical illness. *Gen Hosp Psychiatry, 30*, 208–225.

Sadovsky, R., Basson, R., Krychman, M., Morales, A. M., Schover, L., Wang, R., et al. (2010). Cancer and sexual problems. *J Sex Med, 7*, 349–373.

Savard, J., Davidson, J., Ivers, H., Quesnel, C., Rioux, D., Dupere, V., et al. (2004). The association between nocturnal hot flashes and sleep in breast cancer survivors. *J Pain Symptom Manage, 27*, 513–522.

Savard, J., & Morin, C. M. (2001). Insomnia in the context of cancer: A review of a neglected problem. *J Clin Oncol, 19*, 895–908.

Savard, M., Savard, J., Simard, S., & Ivers, H. (2005). Empirical validation of the insomnia severity index in cancer patients. *Psycho-Oncol, 14*, 429–441.

Savard, J., Simard, S., Giguere, I., Ivers, H., Morin, C. M., Maunsell, E., et al. (2006). Randomized clinical trial on cognitive therapy for depression in women with metastatic breast cancer: Psychological and immunological effects. *Palliat Support Care, 4*, 219–237.

Savard, J., Villa, J., Ivers, H., Simard, S., & Morin, C. M. (2009). Prevalence, natural course, and risk factors of insomnia comorbid with cancer over a 2-month period. *J Clin Oncol, 27*, 5233–5239.

Schmidt, C. E., Bestmann, B., Kuchler, T., & Kremer, B. (2005). Factors influencing sexual function in patients with rectal cancer. *Int J Impot Res, 17*, 231–238.

Schover, L. R. (2005). Sexuality and fertility after cancer. *Hematology Am Soc Hematol Educ Program*, 523–7.

Schover, L. R. (2008). Androgen therapy for loss of desire in women: is the benefit worth the breast cancer risk? *Fertil Steril, 90*, 129–140.

Schover, L. R., Fouladi, R. T., Warneke, C. L., Neese, L., Klein, E. A., Zippe, C., et al. (2002). Defining sexual outcomes after treatment for localized prostate carcinoma. *Cancer, 95*, 1773–1785.

Schover, L. R., & Jensen, S. B. (1988). *Sexuality and chronic illness: A comprehensive approach.* New York: Guilford Press.

Scott, J. L., & Halford, W. K. (2004). United we stand? The effects of a couple-coping intervention on adjustment to early stage breast or gynecological cancer. *J Consul Clin Psychol, 72*, 1122–1135.

Scott, J. L., & Kayser, K. (2009). A review of couple-based interventions for enhancing women's sexual adjustment and body image after cancer. *Cancer J, 15*, 48–56.

Sellick, S. M., & Crooks, D. L. (1999). Depression and cancer: An appraisal of the literature for prevalence, detection, and practice guideline development for psychological interventions. *Psychooncology, 8*, 315–333.

Sheard, T., & Maguire, P. (1999). The effect of psychological interventions on anxiety and depression in cancer patients: Results of two meta-analyses. *Br J Cancer, 80*, 1770–1780.

Simpson, J. S., Carlson, L. E., & Trew, M. E. (2001). Effect of group therapy for breast cancer on healthcare utilization. *Cancer Pract, 9*, 19–26.

Spiegel, D., Bloom, J. R., Kramer, H. C., & Gottheil, E. (1989). Effect of psychosocial treatment on survival of patients with metastatic breast cancer. *Lancet, 2*, 888–891.

Spiegel, D., Bloom, J. R., & Yalom, I. (1981). Group support for patients with metastatic cancer. A randomized outcome study. *Arch Gen Psychiatry, 38*, 527–533.

Spiegel, D., & Giese-Davis, J. (2003). Depression and cancer: Mechanisms and disease progression. *Biol Psychiatry, 54*, 269–282.

Spielberger, C. D. (1983). Manual for the state-trait anxiety inventory. In (Ed.). Palo Alto: Consulting Psychologists Press.

Stark, D. P. H., & House, A. (2000). Anxiety in cancer patients. *Br J Cancer, 83*, 1261–1267.

Stark, D., Kiely, M., Smith, A., Velikova, G., House, A., & Selby, P. (2002). Anxiety disorders in cancer patients: their nature, associations, and relation to quality of life. *J Clin Oncol, 20*, 3137–3148.

Stefanek, M. E., Palmer, S. C., Thombs, B. D., & Coyne, J. C. (2009). Finding what is not there. *Cancer, 115*, 5612–5616.

Strong, V., Waters, R., Hibberd, C., et al. (2008). Management of depression for people with cancer (SMaRt oncology 1): a randomised trial. *Lancet, 372*(9632), 40–48.

Tjemsland, L., Soreide, J. A., & Malt, U. F. (1998). Posttraumatic stress symptoms in operable breast cancer III: Status one year after surgery. *Breast Cancer Res Treat, 47*, 141–151.

Uitterhoeve, R. J., Vernooy, M., Litjens, M., Potting, K., Bensing, J., De Mulder, P., et al. (2004). Psychosocial interventions for patients with advanced cancer – a systematic review of the literature. *Br J Cancer, 91*, 1050–1062.

Watson, M., Denton, S., Baum, M., & Greer, S. (1988). Counselling breast cancer patients: A specialist nurse service. *Counsel Psychol Quart, 1*, 25–34.

Wei, J. T., Dunn, R. L., Litwin, M. S., Sandler, H. M., & Sanda, M. G. (2000). Development and validation of the expanded prostate cancer index composite (EPIC) for comprehensive assessment of health-related quality of life in men with prostate cancer. *Urology, 2000*(56), 899–905.

Wells, M. E., McQuellon, R. P., Hinkle, J. S., & Cruz, J. M. (1995). Reducing anxiety in newly diagnosed cancer patients: A pilot program. *Cancer Pract, 3*, 100–104.

White, I. D., & Faithfull, S. (2006). Vaginal dilation associated with pelvic radiotherapy: a UK survey of current practice. *Int J Gynecol Cancer, 16*, 1140–1146.

Wiegel, M., Meston, C., & Rosen, R. (2005). The female sexual function index (FSFI): cross-validation and development of clinical cutoff scores. *J Sex Marital Ther, 31*, 1–20.

Williams, L. A. (2007). Clinical management of symptom clusters. *Sem Onc Nurs, 23*, 113–120.

Williams, S., & Dale, J. (2006). The effectiveness of treatment for depression/depressive symptoms in adults with cancer: a systematic review. *Br J Cancer, 94*, 372–390.

Zabalegui, A., Sanchez, S., Sanchez, P. D., & Juando, C. (2005). Nursing and cancer support groups. *J Adv Nurs, 51*, 369–381.

Zigmond, A. S., & Snaith, R. P. (1983). The hospital anxiety and depression scale. *Acta Psychiatr Scand, 67*(6), 361–370.

Zippe, C., Nandipati, K., Agarwal, A., & Raina, R. (2006). Sexual dysfunction after pelvic surgery. *Int J Impot Res, 18*, 1–18.

Chapter 5
Tobacco Addiction and Psychological Co-morbidities

Douglas Ziedonis, David Kalman, Monika Kolodziej, Chris W. Johnson, and Sun Kim

5.1 Introduction

Nicotine dependence is a psychiatric disorder characterized by a recurrent, periodic compulsion to use tobacco due to neurophysiological, psychological, and social factors (American Psychiatric Association, 2000; DiFranza et al., 2010). Nicotine dependence has behavioral and physiological characteristics that are similar to those of other addictions, but also unique aspects that require special attention because of its ubiquity on a global scale, its staggering effects on rates of morbidity and mortality, and its high prevalence of psychological co-morbidities, including psychiatric disorders. About 50% of all smokers are estimated to die from medical diseases caused by or worsened by their smoking accounting for about 450,000 deaths in the United States and more than five million deaths worldwide (U.S. Centers for Disease Control and Prevention, 2002; World Health Organization, 2009).

Compared to the general population, individuals with psychiatric disorders are much more likely to smoke cigarettes (Kleber et al., 2006). Epidemiological surveys show that at least 44% of all the cigarettes consumed in the United States are by individuals with a psychiatric disorder (Lasser et al., 2000). Rates are even higher among clinical populations, typically exceeding 50–75% (Kleber et al., 2006; Rustin, 1998; Williams et al., 2005). These individuals are also more likely to be nicotine-dependent, experience greater difficulty with tobacco use cessation, and have other problems associated with difficulty quitting including lack of social support, living with another smoker, and depressed mood ((Kleber et al., 2006). This chapter will focus on the psychiatric disorders most often associated with nicotine dependence, underlying biobehavioral mechanisms of co-morbidity, cultural factors, and treatment approaches.

D. Ziedonis (✉)
Department of Psychiatry, University of Massachusetts Medical School, 55 Lake Avenue North, Rm S7-850, Worcester, MA 01655, USA
e-mail: douglas.ziedonis@umassmemorial.org

S. Pagoto (ed.), *Psychological Co-morbidities of Physical Illness: A Behavioral Medicine Perspective*, DOI 10.1007/978-1-4419-0029-6_5,

5.2 Epidemiology

According to the Centers for Disease Control and Prevention, 20.4% of people in the United States are currently classified as smokers (Heyman, Barnes, & Schiller, 2009). Using data from a national community-based survey, Grant, Hasin, Chou, Stinson, and Dawson (2004) suggest that 12.8% of adults in the United States meet DSM-IV criteria for nicotine dependence and the majority of these smokers (55% of the smokers) have a co-morbid DSM-IV psychiatric disorder. This study found lower overall rates of nicotine dependence than other studies, perhaps because the sample only included adults and was based on DSM criteria versus just regular tobacco use or periodic compulsion to use. Rates of DSM-IV defined nicotine dependence among individuals with a psychiatric disorder are reported as follows: 34.5% with an alcohol use disorder, 52.4% with any drug use disorder, 29.2% with any mood disorder, 25.3% with any anxiety disorder, and 27.3% with any personality disorder (see Table 2 in Grant et al., 2004).

Smokers with a psychiatric disorder are also more likely to be heavier smokers than smokers without a psychiatric disorder (Beckham et al., 1997; Olincy, Young, & Freedman, 1997; Ziedonis, Kosten, Glazer, & Frances, 1994). Rates of heavy smoking (typically defined as 25–30 or more cigarettes per day) are often between 30 and 40% in clinical psychiatric populations, compared to about 10% in the general population (De Leon & Diaz, 2005). There appears to be a direct relationship between greater psychiatric illness severity and the likelihood of being a heavy smoker (Vanable, Carey, Carey & Maisto, 2003). Unfortunately, smokers with a psychiatric disorder are also less likely to quit than their counterparts without a psychiatric disorder. In a population-based study, lifetime quit rates were between 20 and 30% for smokers with a psychiatric diagnosis compared to 43% for smokers without a mental illness (Lasser et al., 2000). While data are limited, lifetime quit rates rarely exceed 20% in clinical samples (De Leon & Diaz, 2005). Taken together, this information suggests that persons with a psychiatric disorder are more likely to become smokers, are more likely to be heavy smokers, and are less likely to quit.

Rates of tobacco-caused medical co-morbidities and mortality are also significantly higher in smokers with versus without psychiatric disorders (Boscarino, 2006; Brown & Barraclough, 2000; Carney, Freedland, Miller, & Jaffe, 2002; Grant et al., 2004). Smoking significantly increases risk of negative health events and, in the case of co-morbid tobacco and alcohol use disorder, the adverse effect on health is synergistic. At the highest level of joint consumption of tobacco and alcohol, for example, Castellsaguè et al. (1999) found that compared to men who neither smoked nor drank, the odds ratio for esophageal cancer was 6.84 for men who never drank but smoked heavily, 14.13 for men who drank heavily but never smoked, and 50.85 for men who both drank and smoked heavily (see also Zheng et al., 1990). In addition, a 20-year retrospective study found that alcoholic smokers in alcohol dependence treatment were more likely to die from the effects of tobacco (all causes) than alcohol (Hurt et al., 1996). As noted earlier, 50% of all smokers die from a smoking-related disease.

5.3 Biobehavioral Mechanisms of Co-morbidity

Tobacco use and addiction commonly begin during adolescence due to a variety of biopsycho-social factors, including peer group, initial response to smoking cigarettes, and rapidity of progression to compulsive use and association of difficulty with quitting. Many individuals become nicotine-dependent and then develop a psychiatric disorder and others develop psychological problems and then become nicotine-dependent. There are also strong cultural influences, especially throughout the world, that influence tobacco use by gender. There have been many attempts to explain the high association of mental illness and nicotine dependence; however, there is little evidence to support most of the attributions such as the self-medication theory. Nicotine dependence is clearly a powerful addiction with prominent features of compulsion to use and difficulty quitting. There is evidence that psychiatric patients have more difficulty quitting tobacco use (Kleber et al., 2006); however, there may be many factors to account for this. Some patients report that they smoke in an attempt to self-regulate or alleviate emotional distress (Zvolensky & Bernstein, 2005) or to manage dysphoria (Srinivasan & Thara, 2002). Some individuals are likely to have genetic susceptibility to nicotine dependence and a mental illness (Ziedonis et al., 2008). There is also a growing literature questioning whether tobacco use during adolescence may influence the development of some mental health problems and psychiatric disorders. For example, one study found that adolescents and young adults who were nicotine-dependent first were more likely to develop a depressive disorder; however, those who had a depressive disorder first did not have a higher risk to develop nicotine dependence (Wu & Anthony, 1999). These developmental pathways may also be bidirectional. For example, Koenen et al. (2005) report that PTSD increased the risk for nicotine dependence, and that nicotine dependence increased the risk for development of PTSD. Mental health and addiction treatment settings have historically been a place where the social acceptance and encouragement of tobacco use resulted in individuals becoming tobacco-dependent, including due to cigarettes being used as a behavioral tool to reinforce specific behaviors (Kleber et al., 2006).

5.3.1 Genetic and Neurobiological Factors of Co-morbidity

The underlying neurobiology of nicotine dependence has a genetic component and there are also epigenetic changes influenced by ongoing tobacco use (Gardner, Tapper, King, & Ziedonis, 2009). Twin studies have demonstrated that common genetic factors exert an important influence on the co-occurrence of tobacco dependence and other psychiatric disorders. Lyons et al. (2002) studied a sample of individuals with schizophrenia probands and their cotwins without schizophrenia and controls. Among cotwins of a proband with schizophrenia, the odds of being a regular smoker were 3.7 times greater than the odds of being a regular smoker among twins from pairs in which neither had schizophrenia. In their study of male twins,

True et al. (1999) found a substantial genetic correlation ($r=0.68$) between lifetime tobacco and alcohol dependence. Similarly, in a study of female twins, the relationship between lifetime tobacco dependence and lifetime major depression was higher in monozygotic vs. dizygotic twins (Kendler et al., 1999; see also McCaffery, Papandonatos, Stanton, Lloyd-Richardson, & Niaura, 2008). In a twin study of the association between tobacco dependence and PTSD, shared genetic factors accounted for 63% of the relationship (Koenen et al., 2005). The influence of common genetic factors in the co-occurrence of tobacco dependence and other anxiety disorders is weaker (Sullivan & Kendler, 1999).

New discoveries are identifying likely neurobiological mechanisms that mediate genetic risk for the co-morbidity between tobacco dependence and other psychiatric disorders. Most work in this area has focused on the neurobiological mechanisms that mediate genetic risk for the co-morbidity between tobacco and alcohol dependence (see review in Kalman, Kim, DiGirolamo, Smelson, & Ziedonis, 2010). Ehringer et al. (2007) found an association between polymorphisms in a gene that codes for sensitivity to the biobehavioral effects of both alcohol and nicotine. Polymorphisms in neurobiological systems implicated in the development of addictive behaviors, including the dopaminergic, gamma-aminobutyric acid, and opioid systems, may also account for individual differences in sensitivity to alcohol and nicotine (Agrawal et al., 2008; Connor et al., 2007; Ray et al., 2006).

Freedman et al. (1997) found evidence for an abnormality in a type of nicotinic receptor (called the alpha 7 receptor) in patients with schizophrenia that was associated with auditory processing deficiencies (see also Adler, Hoffer, Wiser, & Freedman, 1993). The auditory processing deficiency in schizophrenia is also associated with an abnormality in inhibition of the P50 brainwave (Adler, Hoffer, Griffith, Waldo, & Freedman, 1992). Interestingly, the P50 defect is reversed by nicotine, and the abnormalities in both the P50 and the gene that codes for the alpha 7 nicotinic receptor are linked to the same chromosome (Freedman et al., 2001). Stimulation of dopaminergic activity by nicotine in the prefrontal and frontal cortex may temporarily "correct" abnormalities in metabolic activity in these areas of the brain, abnormalities that are associated with auditory processing as well as negative symptoms associated in schizophrenia (Dalack, Healy, & Meador-Woodruff, 1998). Although there may be temporary enhancements due to nicotine, there is an attenuation and tolerance that develops. The difficulty of nicotine withdrawal for these individuals compared to the general population is a substantial clinical issue and has likely resulted in retaining the high rates of co-morbidity.

No studies to date have investigated neurobiological mechanisms mediating the genetic risk for the co-morbidity between tobacco dependence and depression or any anxiety disorder, although multiple potential genetic pathways are almost certainly involved. Li, Volkow, Baler, and Egli (2007) suggest that these genetic pathways are likely to involve "multiple genes that interact with one another and with the environment in ways that are strongly influenced by developmental processes" (p. 2). We currently possess only a rudimentary understanding of these pathways and their effect on the neurobiological substrates that mediate smoking behavior. The interplay between nicotine dependence and psychological disorders can be further elucidated, however, by an understanding of the physiological effects of certain chemicals in tobacco smoke and how these effects often interact with co-morbid psychiatric disorders.

5.3.2 *Cultural Considerations in Nicotine Dependence and Psychological Co-morbidities*

Rates of nicotine dependence and psychiatric co-morbidities vary in different cultures and countries and this is likely due to both genetic and social factors. For example, the rate of tobacco addiction in China among individuals with schizophrenia varies greatly by gender. Men with schizophrenia have high rates of tobacco addiction (75%) and women have low rates (5–10%). These rates differ from the United States where there is no gender difference for tobacco addiction among individuals with schizophrenia; however, the findings in China mirror the general population in China suggesting social factors may be more powerful than biological ones in regard to onset of use.

In the United States, the initiation of smoking, smoking prevalence, patterns of tobacco use, and factors associated with smoking behavior and behavioral change are not consistent across all ethnic and cultural population subgroups. A much higher percentage of African Americans, for example, smoke mentholated cigarettes than do White Americans (80 vs. 20%, respectively; Kabat, Morabia, & Wynder, 1991). Interestingly, non-Hispanic White individuals with schizophrenia also have high rates of mentholated cigarette use compared to controls (Williams et al., 2007). African Americans in the general population smoke an average of ten fewer cigarettes per day than White Americans (Hahn, Folsom, Sprafka, & Norsted, 1990).

There is even substantial evidence for racial differences in the metabolism of nicotine and cotinine, a metabolite of nicotine (see Benowitz, Hukkanen, & Jacob, 2009 for review of nicotine kinetics and metabolism). In addition to influencing the development and maintenance of dependence, these differences in nicotine metabolism directly influence the dose of nicotine replacement therapy in smoking cessation treatment. Ethnopharmacologically, differences in the metabolism of medications may contribute to differences in tobacco use and treatment outcomes. Human cytochrome P450 1A2 (CYP1A2), for example, has been shown to exhibit considerable interindividual variability stemming from genetic, epigenetic, and environmental factors (Zhou, 2009). CYP1A2 is responsible for the metabolism of many medications, including some psychiatric medications, and is induced by polycyclic aromatic hydrocarbons found in tobacco smoke (Zevin & Benowitz, 1999). Berg, Mason, Boettcher, Hatsukami, and Murphy (2010) found significantly different levels of excreted glucuronide conjugates (a marker of nicotine and cotinine metabolism) in African American and European American smokers. There is limited research to date on nicotine dependence among ethnic groups and psychiatric co-morbidity; however, there are some consistencies of high rates of mental illness and tobacco addiction in different countries (Kleber et al., 2006).

5.3.2.1 Culture of Mental Health and Addiction Treatment Settings

An important factor within tobacco addiction and its treatment is the culture of mental health and addiction settings. Use of tobacco within these settings has often been accepted without hesitation or even actively reinforced, such as with the use of cigarettes or cigarette breaks as a reward for good behavior. Numerous myths regarding the perceived therapeutic benefit of tobacco use, the potential "issues" created by its treatment, and an assumed inability of patients to quit continue to pervade such settings. Treatment for nicotine dependence can be provided concurrently with treatment for other addictions and/or mental health problems (e.g., Prochaska, Hall, & Tsoh, 2008; see also Williams & Ziedonis, 2004). Addiction and mental health treatment programs are beginning to treat tobacco addiction, and more individuals entering such programs are willing to engage in tobacco addiction treatment (Friend & Pagano, 2005; Kleber et al., 2006).

5.4 Smoking and Symptoms of Psychiatric Disorders

Tobacco use can alter symptoms of psychiatric disorders through nicotine's effect on the brain and also by altering psychiatric medication blood levels. Tobacco use is also associated with poly-drug addiction among psychiatric patients. The associations between smoking and symptoms of specific disorders are outlined below.

5.4.1 Schizophrenia

Individuals with schizophrenia are more likely to be heavy smokers and there have been reports of smokers having higher rates of positive symptoms and lower rates of negative symptoms (Kleber et al., 2006; Ziedonis et al., 1994); however, Barnes et al. (2006) did not find any differences in positive or negative symptoms between nonsmoker and smoker groups with schizophrenia (see also Aguilar, Gurpegui, Diaz, & de Leon, 2005). Smith, Meyers, and Miller (2001) conducted the only experimental investigation of the acute effects of smoking and nicotine on positive and negative symptoms. Participants smoked a cigarette containing nicotine in one session and a nicotine-free cigarette in a second session. A reduction in negative symptoms was observed in both sessions, though no effect on positive symptoms was observed. This suggests that the effect on negative symptoms was due to the act of smoking, not to the nicotine content of the cigarette. Barr, Pizzagalli, Culhane, Goff, and Evins (2008) found stronger association between smoking motives to increase alertness and calmness among smokers with schizophrenia than smokers without schizophrenia. Forchuk et al. (2002) found that in their sample of smokers with schizophrenia, 37% said that smoking provided "no benefit" to them.

5.4.2 Anxiety Disorders

The effect of smoking and nicotine on anxiety symptoms has been studied among persons with posttraumatic stress disorder (PTSD) and those with panic disorder. Among smokers with PTSD, smoking was described as a way to cope with affective reactions to trauma-related stimuli (2005, Beckham et al., 1997; Feldner, Babson, & Zvolensky, 2007; McClernon et al., 2004); however, there is limited evidence to suggest that this is an effective coping strategy and clearly increased morbidity and mortality would negate this as a recommended clinical strategy. In the only experimental study conducted to date, smokers with and without PTSD smoked either a regular or nicotine-free cigarette following exposure to a trauma script (Beckham et al., 2007). Among smokers with PTSD, smoking either the nicotine-free or regular cigarette decreased negative affect and PTSD symptoms, but a greater decrease was observed for the regular cigarette. Smokers with panic disorder are more likely to report smoking to decrease negative affect (Zvolensky & Bernstein, 2005). At the same time, daily smoking is associated with greater risk of current panic attacks (Breslau & Klein, 1999; Goodwin & Hamilton, 2002). While these latter studies are correlational, they are consistent with the effect of nicotine on the sympathetic nervous system and suggest that smoking may worsen certain anxiety symptoms. No research has investigated the effect of smoking on anxiety in smokers with a generalized anxiety disorder. Overall, these studies point to the difficulty with attribution studies, highlighting the need to investigate the association between cigarette smoking and anxiety symptoms through systemic, laboratory investigations.

5.4.3 Mood Disorders

There is mixed evidence suggesting nicotine can enhance mood. The mechanism may be through positive reinforcement mechanisms and/or the ability to reverse negative mood due to nicotine withdrawal. Mechanisms for direct mood-enhancing effect (Kalman, 2002, and Picciotto, Addy, Mineur, & Brunzell, 2008 reviews) have been postulated due to its effect on nACHRs in the nervous system. Heightening cholinergic activity and/or sensitivity contributes to the development and exacerbation of symptoms of depression. Overactivation of nAChRs by endogenous acetylcholine could potentially be part of this complex mechanism (Picciotto & Zoli, 2008). Although acute doses of nicotine activate nAChRs and, by extension, endogenous acetylcholine, chronic doses effectively desensitize nAChRs which limits the endogenous acetylcholine to have an effect on these receptors which is similar to some antidepressants (see Shytle et al., 2002, for a detailed review).

Acute nicotine administration results in dopamine release in a brain region (e.g., the mesolimbic pathway) believed to mediate positive reinforcement (Brody et al., 2004; Leshnar & Koob, 1999). Individual differences that are due to genetic variation in relevant neurobiological systems (e.g., the dopaminergic and acetylcholine systems) may also be important in determining the mood-enhancing effects of acute doses of nicotine. Even with some mood-enhancing aspects, the need to treat withdrawal symptoms of craving and mood irritability is a powerful factor in relapse on ongoing tobacco use. This mechanism is clear.

In addition, recent studies have demonstrated the importance of nonpharmacological factors in the effect of smoking on mood (e.g., Perkins, Ciccocioppo, Conklin, & Milanak, 2008). The smoking ritual alone, independent of nicotine, relieved negative affect during a negative mood induction. Interestingly, reduction in negative affect was observed even in participants who were informed prior to the mood induction that they would be smoking a nicotine-free cigarette. In other words, the results were not due to placebo effects (i.e., expecting but not receiving nicotine while smoking). As the authors conclude, the smoking ritual itself, particularly the sensory effects of smoke inhalation, had a much greater influence on mood than actual or expected nicotine intake.

In addition to investigating the association between smoking and depressive symptoms, researchers have examined the associations between other mood symptoms, especially in relation to bipolar and schizoaffective disorders. In a cross-sectional study, bipolar disorder in tobacco users is associated with rapid cycling, more frequent depressive and manic mood episodes, and greater mood episode severity compared to nonsmokers (Waxmonsky et al., 2005). Findings from a recent prospective study of smoking on outcomes in bipolar and schizoaffective disorder show that individuals with these conditions who were smokers had poorer mental health outcomes during a 24-month period than those who were nonsmokers (Dodd et al., 2010). Based on these findings, the authors suggest a number of complex interactions between smoking and mood and/or psychotic symptoms as well as medications. These include decreased metabolism of psychotropic medications, changes in multiple neurotransmitter systems, and lower social acceptance of persons who smoke. Lower social acceptance may, in turn, result in lower social support and more severe mental health problems (Dodd et al., 2010). The mood-enhancing effects of nicotine observed in laboratory or cross-sectional studies may not persist when one examines the debilitating effects of nicotine over time.

5.4.4 Substance Use Disorders

Nicotine dependence is common among individuals with other substance use disorders and this addiction is often the last to be addressed. Ongoing tobacco use can be a cue and trigger for these individuals to relapse to other drugs. Among smokers with substance use disorders, only a minority (20%) believe that smoking helps them to cope with urges to drink or use other drugs (Monti, Rohsenow, Colby, & Abrams, 1995). In smokers seeking smoking cessation treatment, fewer than 10% reported that smoking is an important strategy for coping with urges to drink (Kalman, Rohsenow, Colby, Hayes, & Monti, 2001; Kalman, Herz, Monti, Kahler, Mooney, Rodrigues, & O'Conner, in press). In addition, in an experimental study, smoking deprivation did not increase urge to drink during exposure to alcohol cues (Cooney, Litt, & Cooney, 2002). Data have shown that individuals who are addicted to opiates are most likely to be heavy smokers (Stark & Campbell, 1993). Despite the documented problems associated with co-occurring opiate and nicotine addiction, traditional addiction treatment programs, including methadone maintenance programs, typically have not included tobacco addiction in the treatment plans or program. Overall, only a limited number of studies have addressed co-occurring nicotine and other substance use problems.

5.5 Tobacco Cessation Treatment

This section provides an overview of nicotine dependence treatment considerations for persons with psychiatric disorders, including medication and behavioral therapies, treatment outcomes, and the association between quit attempts and return of psychiatric symptoms. Organizational change strategies for health treatment settings are discussed. This section also includes treatment recommendations for smokers not ready to quit (lower motivated) and those ready to quit (higher motivated) who will benefit from behavioral interventions and medications.

5.5.1 Broad Treatment Considerations

There are numerous evidence-based nicotine dependence treatment options available, including medications, behavioral therapies, and phone/internet-based programs (Kleber et al., 2006; Ziedonis, Kalman, Johnson, & Mistler, in press). Creating a tailored individualized nicotine dependence treatment plan for smokers with psychological co-morbidities includes consideration of the severity of nicotine dependence, motivation to quit, preferences for treatment options, potential interactions with their psychiatric medications, past treatment attempts, social support, and co-morbid medical disorders. The 2008 Public Health Service Clinical Practice Guideline for Treating Tobacco Use and Dependence recommends that individuals presenting with a co-morbid psychiatric disorders be offered tobacco dependence treatment and clinicians must overcome any hesitation to provide treatment (Fiore et al., 2008). The American Psychiatric Association (APA) encourages psychiatrists to assess the smoking status of all of their patients and to assist them in quitting (Kleber et al., 2006). While recognizing that in some cases there is limited study of interventions tailored to specific co-morbid disorders, the APA guidelines recommend the use of traditional evidence-based behavioral therapies with motivational enhancement tools and nicotine dependence treatment medications, including nicotine replacement therapies (NRT) (gum, patch, inhaler, spray, or lozenge). Other evidence-based medications (bupropion and varenicline) are also helpful for this population; however, they require a prescription and careful monitoring.

Evidence suggests that smokers with psychiatric disorders are becoming more interested in smoking cessation treatment (Morris et al., 2006), although some continue to place a high value on smoking (Spring, Pingitore, & McChargue, 2003). In a study of 322 smokers in treatment for depression, 79% expressed an intention to quit, including 24% who reported that they were planning to quit in the next month. Many of these individuals had also made a quit attempt in the past year (Prochaska, Delluchi, & Hall, 2004; see also Acton, Prochaska, Kaplan, Small, & Hall, 2001). Orleans and Hutchinson (1993) found that 46% of substance-dependent persons in treatment reported making a quit attempt in the past year. In a survey of 108 substance-dependent inpatients, Irving, Seidner, Burling, Thomas, and Brenner (1994) found that 49% were "very certain" that they wanted to quit and 28% were "somewhat certain;" only 12% said that they did not want to quit.

5.5.2 *Specific Interventions*

Interventions should be tailored to the clinical needs of patients by taking into consideration severity of nicotine dependence (number of cigarettes per day and how soon they smoke their first cigarette after waking in the morning), symptoms of nicotine withdrawal symptoms (craving, affective, physical), psychiatric symptom stability, desire to quit, confidence in their ability to quit, history of quit attempts, and environmental factors such as the presence of other smokers in the person's life. Tobacco cessation treatment in individuals with co-morbid psychiatric conditions should generally follow established clinical guidelines, and while research to date provides limited guidance, many may require extended and more intensive treatment.

Tobacco cessation treatments for persons with psychiatric disorders consist of medication and behavioral therapy interventions, provided alone or in combination (el-Guebaly, Cathcart, Currie, Brown, & Gloster, 2002; Evins et al., 2008; Kleber et al., 2006; Sonne et al., 2010). Factors that influence the use of one intervention method over another include the interaction of co-morbid conditions over time, patient preference, cost (e.g., access to low-cost medications), interactions of medications, and availability (such as that of self-help groups in a geographical area). Types of medication and behavioral interventions are outlined below, followed by a brief review of treatment outcome studies for smokers with psychiatric disorders.

5.5.2.1 Medication Treatment

There are seven FDA approved medications, including five nicotine-based medications, known as NRT and two nonnicotine-based medications. The NRT medications include nicotine gum, lozenges, transdermal patches, nasal spray, and oral inhaler. Three of the NRT medications are available over-the-counter (OTC), including the nicotine patch, gum, and lozenge. The two nonnicotine smoking cessation medications are bupropion and varenicline. Each of the seven medications has recommended dosages based on FDA studies; however, clinical practice and postmarketing studies support the consideration of using higher dosages of nicotine replacement, multiple medications (multiple NRTs and bupropion and NRT), and longer time periods remaining on the medication (Kleber et al., 2006).

There is rich empirical support that medications significantly increase quit rates, including among smokers with co-morbid psychological symptoms or disorders. Given that persons with psychiatric disorders appear to have more severe tobacco withdrawal symptoms than those without co-morbid psychiatric disorders, the use of medications is especially important for this group. The nicotine patch is often a preferred NRT platform for people with psychiatric co-morbidities because of its high compliance rate and ease of use, and the off-label use of multiple NRTs is used in clinical practice. Each of the NRTs has particular dosages, advantages and precautions, side effects, costs, and patient education issues. The nicotine gum, lozenge, and oral inhaler are all absorbed in the oral mucosa and the absorption into the body is affected if the person consumes acidic beverages within 15 min of using the medication. The gum and lozenge are available in 2 and 4 mg dosages and may cause hiccups, nausea, and heartburn as a side effect. The NRTs are relatively safe, although the patch can have side effects of skin reaction/rash where the patch is applied, vivid dreams, or sleep disturbances if worn during the night. Because of the rapid absorption of nicotine nasal spray, there is a risk of possible dependence. The nicotine nasal spray is the fastest NRT medication method to get nicotine to the brain (about 5 min) compared to a cigarette (about 12 s). Due to the relatively more rapid pace to have an effect, some have postulated and found that this treatment might have some advantages clinically for the heavy smokers with schizophrenia and schizoaffective disorder due to the patients' perception that the medication was being delivered quicker and more potently and to its direct role in alleviating withdrawal distress (Williams, Ziedonis, & Foulds, 2004). Patients are advised not to continue to use tobacco when they are on the NRT medications; however, clinical practice may allow a very small amount of use for a short period of time. This is more likely a symptom of not getting enough NRT or perhaps not being ready to quit.

Bupropion, a nonnicotine medication also used to treat depression, can be integrated with NRT treatment. This medication is prescribed and should not be used for patients with a seizure disorder, on a MAO Inhibitor medication, with electrolyte abnormalities, or eating disorder. Common side effects are insomnia, dry mouth, headache, rash, or agitation. Varenicline is a partial agonist at the nicotine receptor and is usually a solo treatment for nicotine dependence treatment. The common side effect of nausea can be bothersome; however, there are more serious neuropsychiatric symptoms that can occur during withdrawal and with ongoing smoking, including suicidal ideation and behavior, agitation, and depressed mood. There may be a worsening of psychiatric symptoms for patients with preexisting psychiatric illness; however, this is being used in clinical practice with careful monitoring and studies of this medication with smokers with schizophrenia are currently just being done. Families and caregivers can be helpful in monitoring for symptoms. Overall, all of the 7 FDA approved medications can be helpful in treatment for smokers with psychological co-morbidities. There is a need to tailor to patient preference, monitor the medication treatment closely, and consider the interaction with psychiatric medications.

A very important clinical issue is to be aware that many psychiatric medication blood levels can be affected by smoking status. Tobacco smoke (the tar not the nicotine) effects the P450 CYP 1A2 isoenzyme and the medications that are metabolized in this part of the liver, including antidepressants (amitriptyline, nortriptyline, trazadone, fluvoxamine, clomipramine, and imipramine), antipschotics (haloperidol, olanzapine, clozapine, chlorpromazine, and fluphenazine), and other medications (apirin, codeince, propanolol, theophyline, etc.). Smoking lowers the medication blood levels, and quitting raises the medication blood levels. Of note, caffeine is also metabolized in this part of the liver and smoking cessation can result in a doubling of the blood level of caffeine.

5.5.2.2 Behavioral Therapy Approaches

Behavioral therapy approaches for smoking cessation typically begin with the assessment of the person's motivation to quit and are tailored according to whether motivation is low or high. Behavioral strategies include motivational enhancement therapy, cognitive-behavioral therapy, and 12-step facilitation (Nicotine Anonymous). These treatments can be provided via individual and group counseling, family-based interventions, and peer-support through groups such as Nic-A or specialized support by peer specialists (Schroeder & Morris, 2010).

Klesges, Klesges, Myers, Klem, and Isbell (1990) have demonstrated the benefit of using an initial motivational enhancement intervention for individuals with co-morbid psychological conditions, with the intervention often serving to bolster an individual's confidence in the ability to quit, commitment, and readiness to change. The efficacy of motivational enhancement interventions has been demonstrated in clinical populations of people with alcohol use disorders and community-based samples of smokers (Miller & Rollnick, 2002; Prochaska, Velicer, Fava, Rossi, & Tsoh, 2001). Only four studies of a motivational enhancement intervention have been conducted among smokers with another psychiatric disorder, however. In a study of smokers with schizophrenia, a greater proportion of participants receiving a one-session motivational intervention vs. psychoeducational counseling and advice-only conditions sought treatment for their tobacco dependence within 1 month of the intervention (Steinberg, Ziedonis, Krejci, & Brandon, 2004). The motivational enhancement intervention consisted of personalized feedback (e.g., medical and financial consequences of smoking) designed to create a discrepancy between the participant's smoking behavior and future goals (e.g., to be healthy and responsible with money). A motivational enhancement intervention was not effective in two studies with alcoholic smokers (Bobo, McIlvain, Lando, Walker, & Leed-Kelly, 1998; Rohsenow, Monti, Colby, & Martin, 2002), however. Hall, Humfleet, Reus, Munoz, and Cullen (2004) have found some benefit in providing specialized staged-care intervention for smokers with current depression.

Kalman, Kahler, Garvey, and Monti (2006) reported that quit rates among smokers in recovery from alcohol dependence were related to number of months of alcohol abstinence at the time of the smoking quit attempt. The quit rate among smokers with more than a year of alcohol abstinence was 29%; the rate was 7% among smokers with fewer than 12 months. In a meta-analysis of eight clinical trials of concurrent smoking and alcohol treatment, the mean quit rate at follow-up for both intervention and control conditions was 7% (see Table 1 in Prochaska et al., 2004, for a description of each study). Notably, the highest quit rate (18%) was achieved in a trial where the treatment provided was especially intensive (Burling, Burling, & Latini, 2001).

McFall et al. (2005) randomly assigned 66 smokers with PTSD to either integrated care or usual care. Integrated care was provided by a participant's mental health treatment provider and was designed to capitalize on the treatment relationship while usual care was provided by a tobacco dependence specialist. Quit rates at a 6-month follow-up were 21 and 10%, respectively, in the integrated care and usual care conditions. Similar quit rates were observed for integrated care in an observational study of smoking cessation treatment (McFall et al., 2005). McFall and colleagues are currently conducting a large-scale trial of integrated vs. usual care for smokers with PTSD (personal communication, September 26, 2009).

Three randomized clinical trials have been conducted among smokers with schizophrenia. In the first study, George et al. (2002) randomly assigned 32 smokers to bupropion or placebo. End of treatment quit rates were 47 and 15%, respectively, in the bupropion and placebo conditions; at 6-month follow-up, they were 22 and 8%, respectively. In the second study, Evins et al. (2005) randomly assigned 53 smokers to bupropion or placebo. At the end of treatment, quit rates were 16 and 0%, respectively. In the third study, George et al. (2000) randomly assigned 45 smokers to either standard behavioral counseling or tailored counseling, which included social skills training. Quit rates did not differ between groups at the end of treatment (standard and integrated care: 35%) or 6-month follow-up (standard care: 18%; integrated care: 11%). Interestingly, however, 17% of smokers taking an atypical antipsychotic vs. 7% taking a typical antipsychotic were smoking abstinent. George et al. (2002) observed a similar effect of type of antipsychotic medication on quit rates. Evins et al. (2005) observed an effect on smoking reduction. Interestingly, Evins et al. (2005) and George et al. (2002) both observed an effect of bupropion on negative symptoms (see also Evins et al., 2001). While speculative, the effects of atypical antipsychotics and perhaps bupropion on negative symptoms associated with hypofrontality may improve quit rates by reducing the need to use nicotine to achieve these effects.

Only one study has been conducted among smokers with current major depression (Hall et al., 2004, see above). In addition, a number of studies have investigated the efficacy of smoking cessation treatment on smokers with a past history of depressive illness. Mixed results have been found for the use of a mood management vs. a standard care intervention (Hall et al., 1996; Hall, Munoz, & Reus, 1994) and generally suggest that these smokers may benefit more from increased therapeutic contact than any specific therapeutic content (e.g., treatment focused on teaching mood management skills, Hall et al., 1998). Hughes (2007a, 2007b) identified seven clinical trials that investigated the effect of a quit attempt on the emergence of major depression among smokers with a past history of depression. Rates ranged from 3 to 5% (four studies) to 24% (one study); within each study, these smokers were more likely to develop major depression following a quit attempt compared to smokers without a past history.

While more research with larger samples and more frequent assessments during the postquit phase are needed before firm conclusions can be reached, the limited evidence to date suggests that close monitoring of smokers with histories of depression is warranted during smoking cessation treatment (see Hughes, 2007a, 2007b). However, clinicians and patients should understand that depressed mood is not uncommon among smokers following a quit attempt and that it often resolves within 1–4 weeks. In other words, while careful monitoring of smokers with histories of major depression is advised, negative affect following cessation should not be considered an inevitable precursor to the emergence of a major depressive episode (Hughes, 2007a, 2007b).

5.6 Quit Attempts and Clinical Symptoms

Several studies have investigated the effect of quit attempts on clinical symptoms in psychiatric populations. In a meta-analysis of 12 clinical trials of concurrent tobacco and alcohol and other drug (AOD) treatment, Prochaska et al. (2004) found that participants in the concurrent intervention vs. alcohol treatment only condition were significantly more likely to be abstinent from AODs. In the largest study of tobacco treatment for smokers with co-morbid alcohol dependence ($n=499$), Joseph, Willenbring, Nugent, and Nelson (2004) found that the alcohol abstinence rate for participants in the concurrent alcohol and tobacco treatment condition was modestly but significantly lower than that for participants who received smoking cessation treatment 6 months after beginning alcohol treatment; alcohol abstinence at follow-up in the concurrent and "delayed" conditions were 67 and 74%, respectively. Kalman et al. (2001) and Kalman et al. (in press) found that few (<10%) of these smokers report that quitting smoking has a negative effect on their ability to cope with urges to drink and Rohsenow, Colby, Martin, and Monti (2005) found that smoking to cope with urges to drink does not predict relapse to alcohol following a quit attempt. Taken together, the evidence suggests and supports concurrent treatment, although treatment providers will want to closely monitor their patients' alcohol status,

McFall and colleagues report that smoking cessation treatment did not have an adverse effect on PTSD symptoms for either those who successfully quit or those who were unable to quit (McFall et al., 2005, 2006). There is also little evidence that quitting smoking has an adverse effect on the symptoms of schizophrenia. Evins et al. (2005) did not find any evidence of clinical worsening as a result of smoking cessation attempts on negative or positive symptoms. Instead, an improvement was observed in negative symptoms in both the bupropion and placebo groups, though the improvement over baseline was not statistically significant. George et al. (2002) reported a statistically significant improvement in negative symptoms among participants in the bupropion group, but study samples were too small to investigate differences according to smoking status.

5.6.1 Considerations Unique to Treatment and Co-morbid Psychological Disorders

The timing of tobacco cessation treatment is particularly difficult to ascertain among patients with psychiatric disorders. While the 2008 Public Health Service's Clinical Practice Guideline suggests that all tobacco users with co-morbid psychological disorders should be offered timely treatment for their nicotine dependence; it acknowledges that in some circumstances it may be advisable to wait until a psychological disorder is stabilized or less severe before beginning treatment (Fiore et al., 2008). As was mentioned in the previous section, for example, smoking cessation may elicit or exacerbate depressive symptoms in individuals with a prior history of affective disorder (Killen, Fortmann, Schatzberg, Hayward, & Varady, 2003). Most of the literature on nicotine-dependent individuals with a co-morbid substance use disorder, however, finds that tobacco cessation does not harm recovery from other substance dependency and may in some instances be associated with better outcome (e.g., Prochaska et al., 2004).

Treatment blending is relatively commonplace in tobacco addiction treatment, in part because changes adopted during the course of treatment are oftentimes general lifestyle changes towards healthier living. To this end, treatment programs have been developed that attempt to blend nicotine dependence treatment into broader, more comprehensive wellness paradigms. Learning About Healthy Living (LAHL – Williams et al., 2005) is one such program, and it is intended to facilitate nicotine dependence treatment in populations with co-morbid mental illness. Although there is emphasis on the treatment of tobacco addiction, LAHL includes sections on improving diet, managing stress, and increasing activity. A pilot study using LAHL in nine community treatment programs received positive feedback from both consumers and staff (Williams et al., 2009).

Individuals will often seek treatment for one condition, but be unmotivated for treatment of their nicotine dependence. This occurs more frequently as facilities begin to institute tobacco-free grounds for the well-being of their consumers and employees. The situation does not have to be a source of conflict, however. Instead, motivational enhancement techniques, in conjunction with the use of a carbon monoxide monitor, if available, can be used to create a "teachable moment," wherein the clinician gently inquires about any concerns the patient has had about smoking while also allowing him/her to express unhappiness with the policy. The opportunity for a teachable moment may be especially ripe if the consumer's placement in the facility is related to his/her tobacco use (e.g., cardiovascular problems, emphysema, etc.).

Another important consideration in concurrent treatment of nicotine dependence and psychiatric disorders is the interaction between tobacco smoke and psychiatric medications (see review by Desai, Seabolt, & Jann, 2001). Polycyclic aromatic hydrocarbons present in cigarette smoke increase metabolic clearance of many medications through their actions on liver enzymes. Compared to nonsmokers, smokers are likely to require higher doses of some antidepressants (e.g., imipramine, clomipramine, fluvoxamine, trazadone), antipsychotics (both typical and atypical), and anxiolytics (particularly alprazolam). Among persons with schizophrenia, one study found that the dosage of antipsychotic medication was 17% greater in smokers than nonsmokers (Ziedonis et al., 1994). In addition, limited evidence suggests that the activation of dopaminergic pathways by nicotine may increase the risk of tardive dyskenesia among smokers who take antipsychotic medication (Kirch, Alho, & Wyatt, 1988). Individual difference variables (e.g., age, ethnicity, and gender), as well as the concurrent use of AODs with abuse liability, are likely to influence the effect of smoking on the disposition of medications. As such, dose adjustments are often needed following smoking cessation.

5.6.2 Effectiveness of Treatment Methods in Ethnic Population Subgroups

Studies have been conducted with respect to the efficacy of nicotine dependence treatment in different ethnic populations (see Okuyemi, Sanderson, Cho, & Ahluwalia, 2004); however, few that consider nicotine dependence, psychiatric disorder, and ethnicity. Kim, Ziedonis, and Chen (2007) reviewed the literature concerning tobacco use and dependence in Asian Americans. With respect to psychological co-morbidity, high levels of stress or anxiety have been associated with higher rates of smoking among Korean American men (Lew et al., 2001), and depression is associated with higher rates of smoking among Vietnamese American men (Wiecha, Lee, & Hodgkins, 1998). Some studies have found an association between alcohol use and cigarette smoking among Asian American populations (Yu, Chen, Kim, & Abdulrahim, 2002; Juon, Kim, Han, Ryu, & Han, 2003; Kim et al., 2000), while some have not (Thridandam, Fong, Jang, Louie, & Forst, 1998). Kim et al. (2007) suggest that this may be the result of cultural differences among population subgroups, but that it might also stem from methodological differences between studies (e.g., some studied alcohol use and others studied alcohol dependence).

Six randomized studies among Latinos demonstrate enhanced short-term abstinence from tobacco with smoking cessation interventions and three studies that demonstrate significant long-term abstinence rates (Okuyemi et al., 2004). More recently, Borrelli, McQuaid, Novak, Hammond, and Becker (2010) have demonstrated the utility of a culturally sensitive, theory-driven model of tobacco cessation treatment among Latino caregivers of children with asthma. Interestingly, higher rates of abstinence from tobacco have been associated with longer periods of acculturation into American culture among Latino men living in the United States, although this relationship has not been shown for Latino women (Castro et al., 2009).

As with Latino men, there is an inverse relationship between levels of acculturation among Asian American men and rates of smoking (i.e., higher levels of acculturation are associated with lower rates of smoking); however, a *positive* correlation between acculturation and rates of smoking is seen with Asian American women (i.e., higher levels of acculturation are associated with higher rates of smoking; Kim et al., 2007). Smoking cessation interventions targeted at Vietnamese males in California suggest that involving the family in treatment results in higher rates of abstinence than for interventions that do not include the family (Jenkins et al., 1997). Chen (2001) has shown a significant increase in tobacco abstinence among Southeast Asian men with a cessation intervention led by a nonclinical "lay" community member, and Ma et al. (2005) demonstrated the efficacy of a culturally sensitive treatment involving cognitive-behavioral therapy and the nicotine patch among Chinese and Korean Americans. Wu et al. (2009) recently conducted a larger randomized trial among Chinese Americans in New York City that showed a 67% abstinence rate at 6 months using culturally adapted motivational interviewing techniques and nicotine replacement therapy.

Very few studies have been conducted pertaining specifically to tobacco use among American Indians and Alaska Natives. There is a particular need for such studies given the extremely high rates of smoking among American Indians (40.8% according to Centers for Disease Control and Prevention, 2004). Further, Falk, Yi, and Hiller-Sturmhofel (2006) report that American Indians and Alaskan Natives are the most likely population subgroup to have co-morbid nicotine dependence and alcohol use disorder, and Dickerson, O'Malley, Canive, Thuras, and Westermeyer (2009) call attention to the unique context of nicotine dependence and psychiatric co-morbidities among American Indian populations.

In summary, studies of nicotine dependence treatment interventions in U.S. ethnic minority populations show that clinical interventions are successful more often than community-based interventions, and future studies should further assess psychological co-morbidity. There is a dearth of studies on the treatment of nicotine dependence and co-morbid conditions in minority populations (Lettlow, 2004).

5.6.3 Smoking Cessation in Mental Health and Addiction Treatment Settings

An underappreciated consideration in the concurrent treatment of nicotine dependence and co-morbid psychological disorders is the culture of the mental health and addiction treatment settings. Smoking is often overlooked in mental health programs due to a variety of barriers including the beliefs of treatment staff (e.g., smoking cessation will worsen symptoms, smoking is an important part of the "impoverished" lives of patients, patients are not interested in quitting smoking), lack of knowledge about the treatment of nicotine dependence, and a treatment culture amenable to smoking (e.g., "smoke-breaks" structured into the treatment day). Additionally, in substance use disorder programs, staff may believe that patients should avoid major life changes including smoking cessation during their first year of recovery and that stopping smoking may jeopardize drug/alcohol recovery. However, as already discussed, most mental health patients in treatment are concerned about their smoking, and the preponderance of evidence indicates that trying to quit does not interfere with other psychiatric symptoms.

Short staff trainings to address barriers to treating nicotine dependence have had little effect (Bobo, Anderson, & Bowman, 1997). Ziedonis and colleagues have developed a more intensive, manual-based approach, called "Addressing Tobacco through Organizational Change" (ATTOC), designed to facilitate and support the full integration of tobacco treatment into mental health or addiction treatment programs and agencies (Guydish et al., 2009; Williams et al., 2005; Ziedonis, Williams, & Smelson, 2003; Ziedonis, Guydish, Williams, Steinberg, & Foulds, 2006; Hoffman & Slade, 1993; Backer, 1995; Rogers, Feighery, Tencati, Butler, & Weiner, 1995). Key elements of the ATTOC model include developing strong support from key leaders, identifying a champion/cochampion, creating broad goals in patient, staff, and environment, creating a leadership group, and developing and implementing a change plan and communication plan. The strategic plan should clearly spell out the implementation process, including addressing sources of resistance, development of policies, and standard operating procedures that support the effort, and develop methods for monitoring this process.

The treatment program/agency develops the key patient, staff, and environment goals that might include (or not) a tobacco-free environment in which state-of-the-art treatment is provided. The model emphasizes the importance of *gradually* integrating tobacco treatment, however, and uses "transitional" goals to promote incremental change. The overarching goal of the model remains assisting these programs in the creation of a *self-sustaining treatment culture* wherein tobacco dependence is treated like any other drug dependence. While additional research is clearly needed, studies evaluating the model support its success (Sharp, Schwartz, Nightingale, & Novak, 2003; Guydish et al., 2009).

5.7 Conclusion

In conclusion, nicotine dependence is common among individuals with psychiatric disorders. This combination of disorders is associated with more difficult withdrawal syndromes and poorer smoking cessation outcomes. Treatment starts with a careful assessment and treatment planning, and is followed by integrating medication and behavioral therapy approaches. Although there is a need to conduct many more studies with this population, findings to date suggest use of all the current evidence-based approaches available for longer periods of time than would be used for persons without co-occurring psychiatric disorders. Monitoring psychiatric medication doses and side effects during early abstinence is important given the rise in blood levels that can occur with some medication. There is a need for a culture change in mental health and addiction treatment settings to address tobacco and provide treatment for all in need.

References

Acton, G. S., Prochaska, J. J., Kaplan, A. S., Small, T., & Hall, S. M. (2001). Depression and stages of change for smoking in psychiatric outpatients. *Addictive Behaviors, 26*, 621–631.

Adler, L. E., Hoffer, L. J., Griffith, J., Waldo, M. C., & Freedman, R. (1992). Normalization by nicotine of deficient auditory sensory gating in the relatives of schizophrenics. *Biological Psychiatry, 32*, 607–616.

Adler, L. E., Hoffer, L. D., Wiser, A., & Freedman, R. (1993). Normalization of auditory physiology by cigarette smoking in schizophrenic patients. *The American Journal of Psychiatry, 150*, 1856–1861.

Agrawal, A., Pergadia, M. L., Saccone, S. F., Hinrichs, A. L., Lessov-Schlaggar, C. N., Saccone, N. L., et al. (2008). Gamma-aminobutyric acid receptor genes and nicotine dependence: Evidence for association from a case-control study. *Addiction, 103*, 1027–1038.

Aguilar, M. C., Gurpegui, M., Diaz, F. J., & de Leon, J. (2005). Nicotine dependence and symptoms in schizophrenia: Naturalistic study of complex interactions. *The British Journal of Psychiatry, 186*, 215–221.

American Psychiatric Association. (2000). *Diagnostic and statistical manual of mental disorders: DSM-IV-TR* (4th ed.). Washington: American Psychiatric Association.

Backer, T. E. (1995). Assessing and enhancing readiness for change: Implications for technology transfer. In T. E. Backer, S. L. David, & G. Saucy (Eds.), *Reviewing the behavioral science knowledge base on technology transfer. NIDA Research Monograph 155*. Rockville: National Institute on Drug Abuse.

Barnes, M., Lawford, B. R., Burton, S. C., Heslop, K. R., Noble, E. P., Hausdorf, K., et al. (2006). Smoking and schizophrenia: Is symptom profile related to smoking and which antipsychotic medication is of benefit in reducing cigarette use? *The Australian and New Zealand Journal of Psychiatry, 40*, 575–580.

Barr, R. S., Pizzagalli, D. A., Culhane, M. A., Goff, D. C., & Evins, A. E. (2008). A single dose of nicotine enhances reward responsiveness in nonsmokers: Implications for development of dependence. *Biological Psychiatry, 63*, 1061–1065.

Beckham, J. C., Dennis, M. F., McClernon, F. J., Mozley, S. L., Collie, C. F., & Vrana, S. R. (2007). The effects of cigarette smoking on script-driven imagery in smokers with and without posttraumatic stress disorder. *Addictive Behaviors, 32*, 2900–2915.

Beckham, J. C., Feldman, M. E., Vrana, S. R., Mozley, S. L., Erkanli, A., Clancy, C. P., et al. (2005). Immediate antecedents of cigarette smoking in smokers with and without posttraumatic stress disorder: A preliminary study. *Experimental and Clinical Psychopharmacology, 13*, 219–228.

Beckham, J. C., Kirby, A. C., Feldman, M. E., Hertzberg, M. A., Moore, S. D., Crawford, A. L., et al. (1997). Prevalence and correlates of heavy smoking in Vietnam veterans with chronic posttraumatic stress disorder. *Addictive Behaviors, 22*, 637–647.

Benowitz, N. L., Hukkanen, J., & Jacob, P., III. (2009). Nicotine chemistry, metabolism, kinetics, and biomarkers. In J. E. Henningfield et al. (Eds.), *Nicotine psychopharmacology. Handbook of Experimental Pharmacology 192*. Berlin: Springer.

Berg, J. Z., Mason, J., Boettcher, A. J., Hatsukami, D. K., & Murphy, S. E. (2010). Nicotine metabolism in African Americans and European Americans: Variation in Glucuronidation by Ethnicity and UGT2B10 Haplotype. *The Journal of Pharmacology and Experimental Therapeutics, 332*, 202–209.

Bobo, J. K., Anderson, J. R., & Bowman, A. (1997). Training chemical dependency counselors to treat nicotine dependence. *Addictive Behaviors, 22*, 23–30.

Bobo, J. K., McIlvain, H. E., Lando, H. A., Walker, R. D., & Leed-Kelly, A. (1998). Effect of smoking cessation counseling on recovery from alcoholism: Findings from a randomized community intervention trial. *Addiction, 93*, 877–887.

Borrelli, B., McQuaid, E. L., Novak, S. P., Hammond, S. K., & Becker, B. (2010). Motivating Latino caregivers of children with asthma to quit smoking: a randomized trial. *Journal of Consulting and Clinical Psychology, 78*, 34–43.

Boscarino, J. A. (2006). Posttraumatic stress disorder and mortality among U.S. Army veterans 30 years after military service. *Annals of Epidemiology, 16*, 248–256.
Breslau, N., & Klein, D. F. (1999). Smoking and panic attacks: An epidemiologic investigation. *Archives of General Psychiatry, 56*, 1141–1147.
Brody, A. L., Mandelkern, M. A., Jarvik, M. E., Lee, G. S., Smith, E. C., Huang, J. C., et al. (2004). Differences between smokers and nonsmokers in regional gray matter volumes and densities. *Biological Psychiatry, 55*, 77–84.
Brown, S., & Barraclough, B. (2000). Causes of the excess mortality of schizophrenia. *The British Journal of Psychiatry, 177*, 212–217.
Burling, T. A., Burling, A. S., & Latini, D. (2001). A controlled smoking cessation trial for substance dependent inpatients. *Journal of Consulting and Clinical Psychology, 69*, 295–304.
Carney, R. M., Freedland, K. E., Miller, G. E., & Jaffe, A. S. (2002). Depression as a risk factor for cardiac mortality and morbidity: A review of potential mechanisms. *Journal of Psychosomatic Research, 53*, 897–902.
Castellsaguè, X., Muñoz, N., De Stefani, E., Victora, C. G., Castelletto, R., Rolón, P. A., et al. (1999). Independent and joint effects of tobacco smoking and alcohol drinking on the risk of esophageal cancer in men and women. *International Journal of Cancer, 82*, 657–664.
Castro, Y., Reitzel, L. R., Businelle, M. S., Kendzor, D. E., Mazas, C. A., Li, Y., et al. (2009). Acculturation differentially predicts smoking cessation among Latino men and women. *Cancer Epidemiology, Biomarkers & Prevention, 18*, 3468–3475.
Centers for Disease Control and Prevention. (2002). Annual smoking-attributable mortality, years of potential life lost, and economic costs – United States, 1995–1999. *Morbidity and Mortality Weekly Report, 51*, 300–303.
Centers for Disease Control and Prevention. (2004). Prevalence of cigarette use among 14 racial/ethnic populations: United States 1999–2001. *Morbidity and Mortality Weekly Report, 53*(3), 49–52.
Chen, M. S. (2001). The status of tobacco cessation research for Asian Americans and Pacific Islanders. *Asian American and Pacific Islander Journal of Health, 9*, 61–65.
Connor, J. P., Young, R. M., Lawford, B. R., Saunders, J. B., Ritchie, T. L., & Noble, E. P. (2007). Heavy nicotine and alcohol use in alcohol dependence is associated with D2 dopamine receptor (DRD2) polymorphism. *Addictive Behaviors, 32*, 310–319.
Cooney, N. L., Litt, M. D., & Cooney, J. L. (2002). In vivo assessment of the effects of smoking cessation in alcoholic smokers. *Alcoholism, Clinical and Experimental Research, 26*, 1952–1953.
Dalack, G. W., Healy, D. J., & Meador-Woodruff, J. H. (1998). Nicotine dependence in schizophrenia: Clinical phenomena and laboratory findings. *The American Journal of Psychiatry, 155*, 1490–1501.
De Leon, J., & Diaz, F. J. (2005). A meta-analysis of worldwide studies demonstrates an association between schizophrenia and tobacco smoking behaviors. *Schizophrenia Research, 76*, 135–157.
Desai, H. D., Seabolt, J., & Jann, M. W. (2001). Smoking in patients receiving psychotropic medications: A pharmacokinetic perspective. *CNS Drugs, 15*, 469–494.
Dickerson, D. L., O'Malley, S. S., Canive, J., Thuras, P., & Westermeyer, J. (2009). Nicotine dependence and psychiatric and substance use comorbidities in a sample of American Indian male veterans. *Drug and Alcohol Dependence, 99*(1–3), 169–175.
DiFranza, J., Ursprung, W. W., Lauzon, B., Bancej, C., Wellman, R. J., Ziedonis, D., et al. (2010). A systematic review of the diagnostic and statistical manual diagnostic criteria for nicotine dependence. *Addictive Behaviors (Epub 2009 Dec 21), 35*(5), 373–382.
Dodd, S., Brnabic, A. J., Berk, L., Fitzgerald, P. B., de Castella, A. R., Filia, S. (2010). A prospective study of the impact of smoking on outcomes in bipolar and schizoaffective disorder. *Comprehensive Psychiatry, 51*, 504–509.
Ehringer, M. A., Clegg, H. V., Collins, A. C., Corley, R. P., Crowley, T., Hewitt, J. K., et al. (2007). Association of the neuronal nicotinic receptor beta2 subunit gene (CHRNB2) with subjective responses to alcohol and nicotine. *American Journal of Medical Genetics. Part B, Neuropsychiatric Genetics, 144B*, 596–604.

el-Guebaly, N., Cathcart, J., Currie, S., Brown, D., & Gloster, S. (2002). Smoking cessation approaches for persons with mental illness or addictive disorders. *Psychiatric Services, 53*(9), 1166–1170.
Evins, E. A., Cather, C., Deckersbach, T., Freudenreich, O., Culhane, M. A., Olm-Shipman, C. M., et al. (2005). A double-blind placebo-controlled trial of bupropion sustained-release for smoking cessation in schizophrenia. *Journal of Clinical Psychopharmacology, 25*, 218–225.
Evins, A. E., Culhane, M. A., Alpert, J. E., Pava, J., Liese, B. S., Farabaugh, A., et al. (2008). A controlled trial of bupropion added to nicotine patch and behavioral therapy for smoking cessation in adults with unipolar depressive disorders. *Journal of Clinical Psychopharmacology, 28*, 660–668.
Evins, A., Mays, V., Cather, C., Rigotti, N., Tisdale, T., & Goff, D. (2001). A pilot trial of sustained release bupropion added to cognitive behavioral group therapy for smoking cessation in schizophrenia. *Nicotine & Tobacco Research, 3*, 391–396.
Falk, D. E., Yi, H. Y., & Hiller-Sturmhofel, S. (2006). An epidemiologic analysis of co-occurring alcohol and tobacco use and disorders: Findings from the National Epidemiologic Survey on alcohol and related conditions. *Alcohol Research & Health, 29*(3), 162–171.
Feldner, M. T., Babson, K. A., & Zvolensky, M. J. (2007). Smoking, traumatic event exposure, and posttraumatic stress: A critical review of the empirical literature. *Clinical Psychology Review, 27*, 14–45.
Fiore, M. C., Jaen, C. R., Baker, T. B., Bailey, W. C., Benowitz, N. L., Curry S. J., et al. (2008). *Treating tobacco use and dependence, 2008 Update. Clinical Practice Guideline*. Rockville: U.S. Department of Health and Human Services. Public Health Service.
Forchuk, C., Norman, R., Malla, A., Martin, M., McLean, T., Cheng, S., et al. (2002). Schizophrenia and the motivation for smoking. *Perspectives in Psychiatry, 38*, 41–46.
Freedman, R., Coon, H., Myles-Worsley, M., Orr-Urtreger, A., Olincy, A., Davis, A., et al. (1997). Linkage of a neurophysiological deficit in schizophrenia to a chromosome 15 locus. *Proceedings of the National Academy of Sciences, 94*, 587–592.
Freedman, R., Leonard, S., Olincy, A., Kaufmann, C. A., Malaspina, D., Cloninger, C. R., et al. (2001). Evidence for the multigenic inheritance of schizophrenia. *American Journal of Medical Genetics. Part B, Neuropsychiatric Genetics, 105*, 794–800.
Friend, K. B., & Pagano, M. E. (2005). Smoking cessation and alcohol consumption in individuals in treatment for alcohol use disorders. *Journal of Addictive Diseases, 24*, 61–75.
Gardner, P. D., Tapper, A. R., King, J. A., & Ziedonis, D. M. (2009). The neurobiology of nicotine addiction: Clinical and public policy implications. *Journal of Drug Issues, 39*, 1045–1067.
George, T. P., Vessicchio, J. C., Termaine, A., Bregartner, T. A., Feingold, A., Rounsaville, B. J., et al. (2002). A placebo controlled trial of bupropion for smoking cessation in schizophrenia. *Biological Psychiatry, 52*, 53–61.
George, T. P., Ziedonis, D. M., Feingold, A., Pepper, W. T., Satterburg, C. A., Winkel, J., et al. (2000). Nicotine transdermal patch and atypical antipsychotic medications for smoking cessation in schizophrenia. *The American Journal of Psychiatry, 157*, 1835–1842.
Goodwin, R. D., & Hamilton, S. P. (2002). The early-onset fearful panic attack as a predictor of severe psychopathology. *Psychiatry Research, 109*, 71–79.
Grant, B. F., Hasin, D. S., Chou, S. P., Stinson, F. S., & Dawson, D. A. (2004). Nicotine dependence and psychiatric disorders in the United States: Results from the national epidemiologic survey on alcohol and related conditions. *Archives of General Psychiatry, 61*, 1107–1115.
Guydish, J., Ziedonis, D., Tajima, B., Brigham, G., Zammarelli, L., & Levy, M. (2009). *Addressing nicotine dependence in drug treatment settings: Organizational change.* Poster session presented at the annual meeting of the College on Problems of Drug Dependence, Reno.
Hahn, L. P., Folsom, A. R., Sprafka, J. M., & Norsted, S. W. (1990). Cigarette smoking and cessation behaviors among urban blacks and whites. *Public Health Reports, 105*, 290–295.
Hall, S. M., Humfleet, G. L., Reus, V. I., Munoz, R. F., & Cullen, J. (2004). Extended nortriptyline and psychological treatment for cigarette smoking. *The American Journal of Psychiatry, 161*, 2100–2107.

Hall, S. M., Munoz, R. F., & Reus, V. I. (1994). Cognitive-behavioral intervention increases abstinence rates for depressive-history smokers. *Journal of Consulting and Clinical Psychology, 62*, 141–146.

Hall, S. M., Reus, V. I., Munoz, R. F., Sees, K. L., Humfleet, G., Hartz, E., et al. (1998). Nortriptyline and cognitive-behavioral therapy in the treatment of cigarette smoking. *Archives of General Psychiatry, 55*, 683–690.

Hall, S. M., Sees, K. L., Munoz, R. F., Reus, V. I., Duncan, C., Humfleet, G. L., et al. (1996). Mood management and nicotine gum in smoking treatment: A therapeutic contact and placebo controlled study. *Journal of Consulting and Clinical Psychology, 64*, 1003–1009.

Heyman, K. M., Barnes, P. M., & Schiller, J. S. (2009). *Early release of selected estimates based on data from the 2008 National Health Interview Survey*. Hyattsville: National Center for Health Statistics.

Hoffman, A. L., & Slade, J. (1993). Following the pioneers: Addressing tobacco in chemical dependency treatment. *Journal of Substance Abuse Treatment, 10*, 153–160.

Hughes, J. R. (2007a). Depression during tobacco abstinence. *Nicotine & Tobacco Research, 9*, 443–446.

Hughes, J. R. (2007b). Effects of abstinence from tobacco: Etiology, animal models, epidemiology, and significance: A subjective review. *Nicotine & Tobacco Research, 9*, 329–339.

Hurt, R. D., Offord, K. P., Croghan, I. T., Gomez-Dahl, L., Kotkke, T. E., Morse, R. M., et al. (1996). Mortality following inpatient addictions treatment: Role of tobacco use in a community-based cohort. *Journal of the American Medical Association, 275*, 1097–1103.

Irving, L. M., Seidner, A. L., Burling, T. A., Thomas, R. G., & Brenner, G. F. (1994). Drug and alcohol inpatients' attitudes about smoking cessation. *Journal of Substance Abuse, 6*, 267–278.

Jenkins, C. N., McPhee, S. J., Le, A., Pham, G. Q., Ha, N. T., & Stewart, S. (1997). The effectiveness of a media-led intervention to reduce smoking among Vietnamese-American men. *American Journal of Public Health, 87*(6), 1031–1034.

Joseph, A. M., Willenbring, M. L., Nugent, S. M., & Nelson, D. B. (2004). A randomized trial of concurrent versus delayed smoking intervention for patients in alcohol dependence treatment. *Journal of Studies on Alcohol, 65*, 681–691.

Juon, H. S., Kim, M., Han, H., Ryu, J. P., & Han, W. (2003). Acculturation and cigarette smoking among Korean American men. *Yonsei Medical Journal, 4*, 875–882.

Kabat, G. C., Morabia, A., & Wynder, E. L. (1991). Comparison of smoking habits of blacks and whites in a case-control study. *American Journal of Public Health, 81*(11), 1483–1486.

Kalman, D. (2002). The subjective effects of nicotine on humans: Methodological issues, a review of human laboratory studies and recommendations for future research. *Nicotine & Tobacco Research, 4*, 25–70.

Kalman, D., Kahler, C., Garvey, A. J., & Monti, P. M. (2006). High dose nicotine patch therapy for smokers with a past history of alcohol dependence: 36 week outcomes. *Journal of Substance Abuse Treatment, 30*, 213–217.

Kalman, D., Kim, S., DiGirolamo, G., Smelson, D., & Ziedonis, D. (2010). Addressing tobacco use disorder in smokers in early remission from alcohol dependence: The case for integrating smoking cessation services in substance use disorder treatment programs. *Clinical Psychology Review., 30*(1), 12–24.

Kalman, D. A., Morissette, S. B., & George, T. P. (2005). Co-morbidity of smoking in patients with psychiatric and substance use disorders. *The American Journal on Addictions, 14*, 106–123.

Kalman, D., Rohsenow, D., Colby, S., Hayes, K., & Monti, P. M. (2001). Concurrent vs. delayed smoking cessation treatment for alcoholics in early recovery: A pilot study. *Journal of Substance Abuse Treatment, 20*, 233–238.

Kendler, K. S., Neale, M. C., Sullivan, P., Corey, L. A., Gardner, C. O., & Prescott, C. A. (1999). A population-based twin study in women of smoking initiation and nicotine dependence. *Psychological Medicine, 29*, 299–308.

Killen, J. D., Fortmann, S. P., Schatzberg, A., Hayward, C., & Varady, A. (2003). Onset of major depression during treatment for nicotine dependence. *Addictive Behaviors, 28*, 461–470.

Kim, K. K., Yu, E. S. H., Chen, E. H., Kim, J., Brintnall, R., & Vance, S. (2000). Smoking behavior, knowledge, and beliefs among Korean Americans. *Cancer Practice, 8*, 223–230.

Kim, S. S., Ziedonis, D., & Chen, K. W. (2007). Tobacco use and dependence in Asian Americans: A review of the literature. *Nicotine & Tobacco Research, 9*, 169–184.

Kirch, D. G., Alho, A., & Wyatt, R. J. (1988). Hypothesis: A nicotine-dopamine interaction linking smoking with Parkinson's disease and tardive disease. *Cellular and Molecular Neurobiology, 8*, 285–291.

Kleber, H. D., Weiss, R. D., Anton, R. F., Rounsaville, B. J., George, T. P., Strain, E. C., et al. (2006). Greenfield, S.F., Ziedonis, D. M., Kosten, T. R., Hennessy, G., O'Brien, C. P., Connery, H.S. American Psychiatric Association Steering Committee on Practice Guidelines; McIntyre, J. S., Charles, S. C., Anzia, D. J., Nininger, J. E., Cook, I. A., Summergrad, P., Finnerty, M. T., Woods, S. M., Johnson, B. R., Yager, J., Pyles, R., Lurie, L., Cross, C. D., Walker, R. D., Peele, R., Barnovitz, M. A., Gray, S. H., Shemo, J. P., Saxena, S., Tonnu, T., Kunkle, R., Albert, A. B., Fochtmann, L. J., Hart, C., Regier, D. Treatment of patients with substance use disorders, second edition. *American Journal of Psychiatry, 163*, 5–82.

Klesges, R. C., Klesges, L. M., Myers, A. W., Klem, M. L., & Isbell, T. (1990). The effects of phenylpropanolamine on dietary intake, physical activity, and body weight after smoking cessation. *Clinical Pharmacology and Therapeutics, 47*, 747–754.

Koenen, K. C., Hitsman, B., Lyons, M. J., Niaura, R., McCaffery, J., Goldberg, J., et al. (2005). A twin registry study of the relationship between posttraumatic stress disorder and nicotine dependence in men. *Archives of General Psychiatry, 62*, 1258–1265.

Lasser, K., Boyd, J. W., Woolhandler, S., Himmelstein, D. U., McCormick, D., & Bor, D. H. (2000). Smoking and mental illness: A population-based prevalence study. *The Journal of the American Medical Association, 284*, 2606–2610.

Leshnar, A. I., & Koob, G. F. (1999). Drugs of abuse and the brain. *Proceedings of the Association of American Physicians, 111*, 99–108.

Lettlow, H. (2004). Commentary on Smoking Cessation in U.S. Ethnic Minority Populations. *VA in the Vanguard: Building on Success in Smoking Cessation. Proceeding of a Conference Held September 21, 2004*. San Francisco.

Lew, R., Moskowitz, J. M., Wismer, B. A., Min, K., Kang, S. H., Chen, A. M., et al. (2001). Correlates of cigarette smoking among Korean American adults in Alameda County, California. *Asian American and Pacific Islander Journal of Health, 19*, 50–60.

Li, T. K., Volkow, N. D., Baler, R. D., & Egli, M. (2007). The biological bases of nicotine and alcohol co-addiction. *Biological Psychiatry, 61*, 1–3.

Lyons, M. J., Bar, J. L., Kremen, W. S., Toomey, R., Eisen, S. A., Goldberg, J., et al. (2002). Nicotine and familial vulnerability to schizophrenia: A discordant twin study. *Journal of Abnormal Psychology, 111*, 687–693.

Ma, G. X., Fang, C., Shive, S., Su, X., Toubbeh, J. I., Miller, S., et al. (2005). A culturally enhanced smoking cessation study among Chinese and Korean smokers. *The International Journal of Health Education, 8*, 1–10.

McCaffery, J. M., Papandonatos, G. D., Stanton, C., Lloyd-Richardson, E. E., & Niaura, R. (2008). Depressive symptoms and cigarette smoking in twins from the National Longitudinal Study of Adolescent Health. *Health Psychology, 3*, S207–S215.

McClernon, F. J., Beckham, J. C., Mozley, S. L., Feldman, M. E., Vrana, S. R., & Rose, J. E. (2004). The effects of trauma recall on smoking topography in posttraumatic stress disorder and non-posttraumatic stress disorder trauma survivors. *Addictive Behaviors, 30*, 247–257.

McFall, M., Atkins, D. C., Yoshimoto, D., Thompson, C. E., Kanter, E., Malte, C. A., et al. (2006). Integrating tobacco cessation treatment into mental health care for patients with posttraumatic stress disorder. *The American Journal on Addictions, 15*, 336–344.

McFall, M., Saxon, A. J., Thompson, C. E., Yoshimoto, D., Malte, C., Straits-Troster, K., et al. (2005). Improving the rates of quitting smoking for veterans with posttraumatic stress disorder. *The American Journal of Psychiatry, 162*, 1311–1319.

Miller, W. R., & Rollnick, S. (2002). *Motivational interviewing: Preparing people for change*. New York: Guilford Press.

Monti, P. M., Rohsenow, D. J., Colby, S. M., & Abrams, D. B. (1995). Smoking among alcoholics during and after treatment: Implications for models, treatment strategies, and policy. In J. B. Fertig & J. P. Allen (Eds.), *Alcohol and tobacco: From basic science to clinical practice. NIAAA Research Monograph No. 30* (pp. 187–206). Bethesda: National Institutes on Health.
Morris, C. D., Giese, A. A., Turnbull, J. J., Dickinson, M., & Johnson-Nagel, N. (2006). Predictors of tobacco use among persons with mental illnesses in a statewide population. *Psychiatric Services, 57*, 1035–1038.
Okuyemi, K. S., Sanderson, C. L., Cho, W. S., & Ahluwalia, J. S. (2004). Smoking Cessation in U.S. Ethnic Minority Populations. *VA in the Vanguard: Building on Success in Smoking Cessation. Proceeding of a Conference Held September 21, 2004*. San Francisco.
Olincy, A., Young, D. A., & Freedman, R. (1997). Increased levels of the nicotine metabolite cotinine in schizophrenic smokers compared to other smokers. *Biological Psychiatry, 42*, 1–5.
Orleans, C. T., & Hutchinson, D. (1993). Tailoring nicotine addiction treatments for chemical dependency. *Journal of Substance Abuse Treatment, 9*, 197–208.
Perkins, K. A., Ciccocioppo, M., Conklin, C. A., & Milanak, M. E. (2008). Mood influences on acute smoking responses are independent of nicotine intake and dose expectancy. *Journal of Abnormal Psychology, 117*, 79–93.
Picciotto, M. R., Addy, N. A., Mineur, Y. S., & Brunzell, D. H. (2008). It is not "either/or": Activation and desensitization of nicotinic acetylcholine receptors both contribute to behaviors related to nicotine addiction and mood. *Progress in Neurobiology, 84*, 329–342.
Picciotto, M. R., & Zoli, M. (2008). Neuroprotection via nAChRs: The role of nAChRs in neurodegenerative disorders such as Alzheimer's and Parkinson's disease. *Frontiers in Bioscience, 13*, 492–504.
Prochaska, J. J., Delluchi, K., & Hall, S. M. (2004). A meta-analysis of smoking cessation interventions with individuals in substance abuse treatment or recovery. *Journal of Consulting and Clinical Psychology, 72*, 1144–1156.
Prochaska, J. J., Hall, S. M., Tsoh, J. Y., Eisendrath, S., Rossi, J. S., Redding, C. A., et al. (2008). Treating tobacco dependence in clinically depressed smokers: effect of smoking cessation on mental health functioning. *American Journal of Public Health, 98*(3), 446–448.
Prochaska, J. O., Velicer, W. F., Fava, J. L., Rossi, J. S., & Tsoh, J. Y. (2001). Evaluating a population-based recruitment approach and a stage-based expert system intervention for smoking cessation. *Addictive Behaviors, 26*, 583–602.
Ray, R., Jepson, C., Patterson, F., Strasser, A., Rukstalis, M., Perkins, K., et al. (2006). Association of OPRM1 A118G variant with the relative reinforcing value of nicotine. *Psychopharmacology, 188*, 355–363.
Rogers, T., Feighery, E. C., Tencati, E. M., Butler, J. L., & Weiner, L. (1995). Community mobilization to reduce point of purchase advertising of tobacco products. *Health Education Quarterly, 22*, 427–442.
Rohsenow, D. J., Colby, S. M., Martin, R. A., & Monti, P. M. (2005). Nicotine and other substance interaction expectancies questionnaire: Relationship of expectancies to substance use. *Addictive Behaviors, 30*, 629–641.
Rohsenow, D. J., Monti, P. M., Colby, S. M., & Martin, R. A. (2002). Brief interventions for smoking cessation in alcoholic smokers. *Alcoholism, Clinical and Experimental Research, 26*, 1950–1951.
Rustin, T. A. (1998). Incorporating nicotine dependence into addiction treatment. *Journal of Addictive Diseases, 17*, 83–108.
Schroeder, S. A., & Morris, C. D. (2010). Confronting a neglected epidemic: Tobacco cessation for persons with mental illnesses and substance abuse problems. *Annual Review of Public Health, 31*, 297–314.
Sharp, J., Schwartz, S., Nightingale, T., & Novak, S. (2003). Targeting nicotine addiction in a substance abuse program. *Science & Practice Perspectives, 2*, 33–40.
Shytle, R. D., Silver, A. A., Lukas, R. J., Newman, M. B., Sheehan, D. V., & Sanberg, P. R. (2002). Nicotinic acetylcholine receptors as targets for antidepressants. *Molecular Psychiatry, 7*, 525–535.

Smith, J. E., Meyers, R. J., & Miller, W. R. (2001). The community reinforcement approach to the treatment of substance use disorders. *Addiction, 10*(Suppl), 51–59.

Sonne, S. C., Nunes, E. V., Jiang, H., Tyson, C., Rotrosen, J., & Reid, M. S. (2010). The relationship between depression and smoking cessation outcomes in treatment-seeking substance abusers. *The American Journal on Addictions, 19*, 111–118.

Spring, B., Pingitore, R., & McChargue, D. E. (2003). Reward value of cigarette smoking for comparably heavy smoking schizophrenic, depressed, and nonpatient smokers. *The American Journal of Psychiatry, 160*, 316–322.

Srinivasan, T. N., & Thara, R. (2002). Smoking in Schizophrenia – all is not biological. *Schizophrenia Research, 56*(1–2), 67–74.

Stark, M. J., & Campbell, B. K. (1993). Drug use and cigarette smoking in applicants for drug abuse treatment. *Journal of Substance Abuse, 5*, 175–181.

Steinberg, M. L., Ziedonis, D. M., Krejci, J. A., & Brandon, T. H. (2004). Motivational interviewing with personalized feedback: A brief intervention for motivating smokers with schizophrenia to seek treatment for tobacco dependence. *Journal of Consulting and Clinical Psychology, 72*, 723–728.

Sullivan, P. F., & Kendler, K. S. (1999). The genetic epidemiology of smoking. *Nicotine & Tobacco Research, 1*, S69–S70.

Thridandam, M., Fong, W., Jang, M., Louie, L., & Forst, M. (1998). A tobacco and alcohol use profile of San Francisco's Chinese community. *Journal of Drug Education, 28*, 377–393.

True, W. R., Xian, H., Scherrer, J. F., Madden, P. A. F., Bucholz, K. K., Heath, A. C., et al. (1999). Common genetic vulnerability for nicotine and alcohol dependence in men. *Archives of General Psychiatry, 56*, 655–661.

Vanable, P. A., Carey, M. P., Carey, K. B., & Maisto, S. P. (2003). Smoking among psychiatric outpatients: Relationship to substance use, diagnosis, and illness severity. *Psychology of Addictive Behaviors, 17*, 259–265.

Waxmonsky, J. A., Thomas, M. R., Miklowitz, D. J., Allen, M. H., Wisniewski, S. R., Zhang, H.(2005). Prevalence and correlates of tobacco use in bipolar disorder: data from the first 2000 participants in the Systematic Treatment Enhancement Program. *General Hospital Psychiatry, 27*, 321–328.

Wiecha, J. M., Lee, V., & Hodgkins, J. H. (1998). Patterns of smoking, risk factors for smoking, and smoking cessation among Vietnamese men in Massachusetts (United States). *Tobacco Control, 7*, 27–34.

Williams, J. M., Foulds, J., Dwyer, M., Order-Connors, B., Springer, M., Gadde, P., et al. (2005). The integration of tobacco dependence treatment and tobacco-free standards into residential addictions treatment in New Jersey. *Journal of Substance Abuse Treatment, 28*(4), 331–340.

Williams, J. M., Gandhi, K. K., Steinberg, M. L., Foulds, J., Ziedonis, D. M., & Benowitz, N. L. (2007). Higher nicotine and carbon monoxide levels in menthol cigarette smokers with and without schizophrenia. *Nicotine & Tobacco Research, 9*(8), 873–881.

Williams, J. M., & Ziedonis, D. M. (2004). Addressing tobacco among individuals with a mental illness or an addiction. *Addictive Behaviors, 29*, 1067–1083.

Williams, J. M., Ziedonis, D. M., & Foulds, J. (2004). Case series of nicotine nasal spray in the combination treatment of tobacco dependence among patients with schizophrenia. *Psychiatric Services, 55*(9), 1064–1066.

Williams, J., Ziedonis, D. M., Vreeland, B., Speelman-Edwards, N., Zechner, M. R., Williams, M. T., et al. (2009). A wellness approach to addressing tobacco in mental health settings: Learning about healthy living. *American Journal of Psychiatric Rehabilitation., 12*(4), 352–369.

World Health Organization. (2009). *Who report on the global tobacco epidemic 2009: Implementing smoke-free environments*. Geneva: World Health Organization.

Wu, L. T., & Anthony, J. C. (1999). Tobacco smoking and depressed mood in late childhood and early adolescence. *American Journal of Public Health, 89*, 1837–1840.

Wu, D., Ma, G. X., Zhou, K., Zhou, D., Liu, A., & Poon, A. N. (2009). The effect of a culturally tailored smoking cessation for Chinese American smokers. *Nicotine & Tobacco Research, 11*(12), 1448–1457.

Yu, E. S., Chen, E. H., Kim, K. K., & Abdulrahim, S. (2002). Smoking among Chinese Americans: Behavior, knowledge, and beliefs. *American Journal of Public Health, 92*, 1007–1012.
Zevin, S., & Benowitz, N. L. (1999). Drug interactions with tobacco smoking. An update. *Clinical Pharmacokinetics., 36*, 425–438.
Zheng, T. Z., Boyle, P., Hu, H. F., Duan, J., Jiang, P. J., Ma, D. Q., et al. (1990). Tobacco smoking, alcohol consumption and risk of oral cancer: a case-control study in Beijing, People's Republic of China. *Cancer Causes & Control, 1*, 173–179.
Zhou, S.-F. (2009). Polymorphism of human cytochrome P450 2D6 and its clinical significance: Part I. *Clinical Pharmacokinetics, 48*, 689–723.
Ziedonis, D. M., Guydish, J., Williams, J., Steinberg, M., & Foulds, J. (2006). Barriers and solutions to addressing tobacco dependence in addiction treatment programs. *Alcohol Research & Health, 29*, 228–235.
Ziedonis, D. M., Hitsman, B., Beckham, J. C., Zvolensky, M., Adler, L. E., Audrain-McGovern, J., et al. (2008). Tobacco use and cessation in psychiatric disorders: National Institute of Mental Health Report. *Nicotine & Tobacco Research, 10*, 1691–1715.
Ziedonis, D. M., Kalman, D., Johnson, C.W., & Mistler, L. A. (in press). Nicotine dependence management. In Lowinson & Ruiz (Eds.), *Substance abuse: A comprehensive textbook* (5th ed.). Baltimore: Lippincott Williams & Wilkins.
Ziedonis, D. M., Kosten, T. R., Glazer, W. M., & Frances, R. J. (1994). Nicotine dependence and schizophrenia. *Hospital & Community Psychiatry, 45*, 204–206.
Ziedonis, D. M., Williams, J. M., & Smelson, D. (2003). Serious mental illness and tobacco addiction: A model program to address this common but neglected issue. *The American Journal of the Medical Sciences, 326*, 223–230.
Zvolensky, M. J., & Bernstein, A. (2005). Cigarette smoking and panic psychopathology. *Current Directions in Psychological Science, 14*, 301–305.

Chapter 6
Psychological Co-morbidities of HIV/AIDS

Christina Psaros, Jared Israel, Conall O'Cleirigh, C. Andres Bedoya, and Steven A. Safren

6.1 Introduction

Although great strides have been made in human immunodeficiency virus (HIV) prevention, detection, and treatment since HIV first emerged as a public health concern in the early 1980s, the number of people living with HIV in the United States (U.S.) remains staggeringly high and continues to increase. Current estimates by the Centers for Disease Control and Prevention (CDC) indicate that 1.1 million people in the United States were living with HIV infection at the end of 2006 and that 56,300 individuals were infected that year (CDC, 2009a). Since the inception of the epidemic, however, the face of HIV has changed. It was first considered a disease only affecting men who have sex with men (MSM) and intravenous drug users (IDU). While MSM are still infected with HIV at the highest rates domestically (50% of new infections in 2005), other at-risk groups have emerged. Women accounted for 26% of new infections in 2005 and are considered an at-risk group; women of color in particular are now disproportionately infected with HIV. Among all new diagnoses in women living in the U.S. in 2005, 64% occurred in African American women and 15% among Latina women (CDC, 2008a). While women of color are infected with HIV at high rates relative to their Caucasian counterparts, racial and ethnic disparities in transmission trends exist across both sexes. The rate of new infections in 2006 for African Americans was 7 times that of whites and represented 45% of all new infections (CDC, 2009b). The rate of new infections that year for Hispanics was 3 times that of Whites and represented 17% of all new infections (CDC, 2008b).

C. Psaros (✉)
Department of Psychiatry, Massachusetts General Hospital/Harvard Medical School, One Bowdoin Square, Boston, MA, USA
e-mail: cpsaros@partners.org

S. Pagoto (ed.), *Psychological Co-morbidities of Physical Illness: A Behavioral Medicine Perspective*, DOI 10.1007/978-1-4419-0029-6_6,

Advances in treatment, namely highly active antiretroviral therapy (HAART), have allowed most individuals to manage HIV as a chronic versus an acutely fatal illness. Antiretroviral therapy has both extended the life expectancy and resulted in overall improved quality of life for those living with HIV. However, managing HIV over the long term represents a substantial challenge for both HIV-positive individuals and those who provide health care for them. One such challenge is mental health. Numerous psychological co-morbidities are associated with HIV infection, including mood, anxiety, and substance use disorders, among others. Certain mood and anxiety disorders are more prevalent among HIV-positive individuals than they are in the general population (Beyer, Taylor, Gersing, & Krishnan, 2007; Pence, Miller, Whetten, Eron, & Gaynes, 2006) and can be associated with worse self-care behaviors and more advanced disease progression (e.g., DiMatteo, Lepper, & Croghan, 2000; Zorrilla, McKay, Luborsky, & Schmidt, 1996), making these disorders of particular importance to clinicians working with this population.

One self-care behavior of particular importance is adherence to HIV medications, or antiretroviral therapy. A large and growing body of literature has identified psychosocial barriers to medication adherence, including depression and anxiety, among HIV-positive individuals (for comprehensive reviews see Ammassari et al., 2002; Simoni, Frick, Pantalone, & Turner, 2003). To fully understand the significance of this problem, it is important to understand the goal of antiretroviral therapy, which is to suppress the viral load to undetectable levels. Although this goal may be achieved at variable levels of adherence, 95% or greater adherence is most frequently referenced as ideal, both to suppress viral replication and to minimize the development of drug resistance (Patterson et al., 2000). While newer regimens may require lower levels of adherence at least with respect to frequency of dosing (e.g., regimens dosed once daily versus twice daily), resistance to treatment can result from nonadherence. Because some medications (particularly those in the same class) share similar resistance profiles, cross-resistance can occur, eliminating the future use of drugs from an entire class (Panel on Antiretroviral Guidelines for Adults and Adolescents, 2011).

In addition to adherence to antiretroviral therapy, links between healthcare utilization and depression and anxiety have been observed among HIV-positive individuals. Some evidence suggests that anxiety and depressive symptoms may result in decreased adherence to regularly scheduled medical visits and provider recommendations. Furthermore, at least one study suggests HIV-positive individuals with depression tend to use higher levels of inpatient or emergency room care (Joyce, Chan, Orlando, & Burnam, 2005). Because of the chronicity and complexity of managing the disease, effective HIV care requires sustained and frequent contact with healthcare providers. In other words, retention in care over long periods of time is critical to successful HIV management, and symptoms of depression and/or anxiety may compromise patients' success at this.

The aforementioned factors underscore the need for accurate assessment and effective treatment of depression and anxiety in this population. Many symptoms of depression and anxiety overlap with symptoms of advanced HIV disease or its treatment (e.g., fatigue and concentration problems), which makes assessing depression and anxiety a complex task. Few psychotherapy interventions for the specific treatment of anxiety or depressive *disorders* have empirical support for use among HIV-positive individuals in particular, as patients with a diagnosable mood or anxiety disorder are often excluded from intervention studies. However, numerous studies have attempted to intervene on stress or other precursors to clinically significant affective dysregulation, with some success.

This chapter will explore some of the issues raised here. Research into the psychological co-morbidities of HIV-infected individuals has exploded in the past decade, and a great deal is currently known about depressive and anxiety disorders in this population; the chapter will focus most heavily on these areas. We first present an overview of the epidemiology and pathophysiology of depression in HIV, followed by a discussion of clinical considerations for assessment and treatment, including a review of existing evidence supporting the efficacy of psychotherapy interventions that target reductions in depressive symptoms. This will be followed by a similar review for anxiety disorders in HIV-positive individuals. Suggestions for clinicians who work with patients with HIV and one of these psychological co-morbidities will be provided.

While depression and anxiety disorders have received the most attention in the literature, other psychological co-morbidities affect HIV-positive individuals, including substance use disorders, psychotic disorders, sleep disorders, and pain disorders. Because the epidemiology, pathophysiology, treatment, and assessment of substance use disorders vary greatly based on the nature of the substance of abuse, the breadth and depth of reporting that would be required to provide a systematic review is beyond the scope of this chapter. However, information on the epidemiology of substance abuse in relation to anxiety and depression will be presented as appropriate. In addition, a very brief overview of data on the prevalence, pathophysiology, and possible clinical considerations for less prevalent Axis I disorders will be provided, including schizophrenia, sleep disorders, sexual disorders, and pain disorders. Finally, the chapter will conclude with a section on cultural considerations for the clinician working with HIV-positive individuals.

6.2 Depression and HIV

Individuals with HIV are disproportionately affected by mood disorders, especially major depression. Although prevalence studies of bipolar disorder in the HIV-positive individuals are generally lacking, one study found that in a sample of over 1,200 psychiatric outpatients diagnosed with bipolar disorder, 2.6% were HIV positive (Beyer et al., 2007), which is consistent with the general population prevalence, which is also 2.6% (Kessler, Chiu, Demler, & Walters, 2005). Because people with HIV do not appear to be disproportionately affected by bipolar disorder and the majority of research among HIV positive individuals is on unipolar depression, the following section will focus on unipolar depression. This section includes a review of data on the epidemiology and pathophysiology of HIV and depression, a discussion of the relationship of depression to self-care in HIV, and clinical considerations with respect to assessment and treatment of depression in this population.

6.2.1 Epidemiology

Depressive disorders affect from 20 to 37% of those with HIV (e.g., Atkinson & Grant, 1994; Bing et al., 2001; Cruess et al., 2003; Dew et al., 1997; Maj et al., 1994; Rabkin, 1996). A meta-analysis of 10 studies revealed a twofold increase in rates of depression in HIV-positive individuals compared with HIV-negative individuals (Ciesla & Roberts, 2001). The HIV Cost and Services Utilization Study (HCSUS), a nationally representative sample of 2,864 HIV-positive adults, revealed that 47% met criteria for any psychiatric disorder, 36% screened positive for major depression, and 26.5% for dysthymia using a diagnostic interview screener (Bing et al., 2001). These rates are between 4 and 8 times higher than those obtained from the National Household Survey on Drug Abuse (Substance Abuse and Mental Health Services Association, 2002) and 2–4 times higher than rates detected among the general population as assessed in the National Co-morbidity Survey (Kessler et al., 2005). Results from a study of 1,125 urban and rural dwelling patients receiving care from an HIV clinic in North Carolina were consistent with the HCSUS study, with 39% of clinic patients estimated to have had a mood and/or anxiety disorder in the past year based on a structured clinical interview (Pence et al., 2006). A number of large-scale studies conducted with both community and clinic-based samples that have utilized self-report screening instruments and symptom checklists (versus diagnostic interviews) have noted high rates of depressive symptomatology; the results of these studies suggest that 20–50% of HIV-positive individuals endorse recent significant depressive symptoms (Burak et al., 1993; Ickovics et al., 2001; Kilbourne, Justice, Rabeneck, Rodriguez-Barradas, & Weissman, 2001; Lyketsos et al., 1993; Lyketsos, Hutton, Fishman, Schwartz, & Treisman, 1996).

6.2.1.1 Epidemiology of Depression Among HIV-Positive Intravenous Drug Users

IDU is still a primary path of HIV infection, with over 6,600 cases (or about 12%) related to IDU occurring in the U.S. in 2006 (CDC, 2009b). Patients with HIV and a history of IDU may be at increased risk for depression (Knowlton et al., 2000).

Some studies have attempted to ascertain levels of depression among HIV-positive individuals attending drug treatment centers. For example, Turrina et al. (2001) found the prevalence of major depression among HIV-positive patients attending a methadone maintenance clinic was greater than 36%. In a study comparing the prevalence rates of depression among two cohorts of IDUs in Rhode Island, Brienza et al. (2000) reported significantly higher rates of major depression, as measured by structured clinical interview, in patients in methadone maintenance treatment (54%) than among patients enrolled in a needle exchange program (42%). While replication is needed, these findings suggest that certain HIV-positive IDUs may be more susceptible to depression that others.

6.2.2 HIV and the Pathophysiology of Depression

HIV-positive individuals may have preexisting mood disorders or may develop a new onset or recurrence of mood disorder after diagnosis and/or during treatment for HIV. In fact, some evidence suggests premorbid depression may be a risk factor for acquisition of sexually transmitted infections, such as HIV (e.g., Holden et al., 2008; Reisner et al., 2009; Williams & Latkin, 2005). An overview of a select number of these issues is provided below.

6.2.3 Depression and Risk for HIV Infection or Transmission

Depressed mood is a risk factor for engaging in health behaviors that directly impact one's susceptibility to contracting HIV, such as sexual risk behaviors and substance use (e.g., Davidson & Ritson, 1993; Dixit & Crum, 2000). These behaviors may not only result in behavioral vulnerabilities for HIV *infection*, but may persist even after infection, increasing the likelihood of HIV *transmission*. Specific studies of HIV-positive individuals have replicated the association between depression and sexual risk-taking (e.g., Kelly, Murphy, Bahr, Koob, et al., 1993; Kennedy et al., 1993), such as having unprotected sex with negative partners or partners of unknown serostatus, despite educational efforts to the contrary (e.g., Lehman et al., 1998). Kalichman (2000) reviewed the literature and concluded the best estimate of continued sexual risk-taking across various subgroups of HIV-positive individuals to be approximately 33%.

The association between depression, sexual risk-taking, and substance abuse has also been demonstrated among HIV-positive and HIV-negative populations (e.g., Kalichman, Kelly, & Rompa, 1997). Camacho, Brown, and Simpson (1996) found that depression was significantly related to needle risk and sexual risk-taking among over 800 daily opioid users entering methadone maintenance programs, while in a large sample of alcohol and other drug-abusing adolescent offenders (Lucenko, Malow, Sanchez-Martinez, Jennings, & Devieux, 2003), high negative affect (e.g., depression) was associated with increased susceptibility to HIV, more sexual partners, unprotected sex, and less knowledge about HIV. Although one meta-analysis to date did not support an association of depression to HIV transmission risk (Crepaz & Marks, 2001), this analysis was only sensitive to a linear relationship, and it is likely that the relationship between depression and sexual activity is curvilinear (Kalichman & Weinhardt, 2001), such that those with more severe depression may have decreased interest in sex.

The issue of whether interventions designed to reduce depressive symptoms can mitigate HIV transmission risk behavior via reductions in sexual risk-taking and substance abuse is debated and requires additional research. However, at least one study shows that addressing contributory factors to depression may result in decreased HIV transmission behaviors. Harris, Bausell, Scott, Hetherington, and Kavanagh (1998), conducted a study to evaluate the efficacy of a 16-week peer counseling and leadership intervention among African American women in methadone maintenance treatment. The group format intervention focused on building self-esteem and confidence with the goal of increasing participants' sense of control and responsibility. They reported that women randomized to the psychosocial intervention condition had significant decreases in depression and subsequently, risky sexual behaviors, relative to the control group.

6.2.4 Depression in Response to HIV Diagnosis or Treatment

Being diagnosed with HIV can be a devastating experience, and diagnosis is often associated with an increase in depressive symptoms (Folkman, 1993), though this initial increase in depressive symptoms will not result in a depressive episode for all individuals. The stress and uncertainty of living with HIV may also confer risk for depression. While most individuals will do well on treatment, routine laboratory screenings of viral load and CD4 count can be emotionally taxing, and HIV-positive individuals may feel hopeless when confronted with the idea that there are a finite number of available treatments for HIV. As HIV disease progresses, quality of life may decrease, and this too can result in depressive symptoms (see Berg, Michelson, & Safren, 2007 for a review). A more recent 2-year prospective study conducted by Atkinson et al. (2008) supports the relationship between disease progression and depression; Atkinson and colleagues found that symptomatic HIV-positive men were significantly more likely to experience an episode of major depression than asymptomatic and HIV-negative men.

Some evidence suggests that side effects of certain HIV treatments can result in a vulnerability to depression. While neurovegetative side effects of antiretroviral therapy are uncommon, use of at least one antiretroviral medication is associated with depression. Efavirenz (also known by its brand name of Sustiva) belongs to the class of medications known as the nonnucleoside reverse transcriptase inhibitors (NNRTIs) and is found in the once-daily HIV treatment known as Atripla. Efavirenz use has been associated with neuropsychiatric events, including depression, sleep disruption, and unpleasant dreams (Dong, 1998). Unlike other side effects of antiretroviral therapy which often resolve within weeks of starting treatment, efavirenz-associated depression may persist (Fumaz et al., 2002). Clinicians working with HIV-positive individuals who take efavirenz should be aware of this association and work with patients' infectious disease providers and other mental health providers to monitor the presence of depressive symptoms and to treat depression accordingly.

6.2.5 Other Considerations Related to Depression and HIV

6.2.5.1 Effects of Depression on HIV Progression

Although earlier studies failed to document an effect of depression on HIV symptoms or disease progression (Lyketsos et al., 1993; Rabkin et al., 1991), a subsequent meta-analysis found that depressive symptoms were longitudinally related to symptoms of HIV infection (Zorrilla et al., 1996). There are some studies, especially those conducted over longer intervals, that suggest depression may have direct effects on HIV outcomes, even when controlling for antiretroviral therapy use, including viral load, CD4 count, and progression to acquired immunodeficiency syndrome (AIDS) (Cook et al., 2004; Boarts, Sledjeski, Bogart, & Delahanty, 2006; Burak et al., 1993; Ickovics et al., 2001; Ironson et al., 2005; Leserman et al., 1997, 1999, 2002, 2007; Mayne, Vittinghoff, Chesney, Barrett, & Coates, 1996; Page-Shafer, Delorenze, Satariano, & Winkelstein, 1996; Patterson et al., 1996; Pence, Miller, Gaynes, & Eron, 2007). Furthermore, Ironson et al. (1994) found that men with more distress (as measured by a composite score created from self-report measures capturing symptoms of both depression and anxiety) at serostatus notification were at greater risk for HIV-related clinical symptoms 2 years later.

6.2.5.2 Depression and Immune Function in HIV

Depression and Immune Function in HIV CD4 count is one of the primary means of assessing immunity status among HIV-positive individuals, and a series of studies have attempted to characterize the relationship between depression and immunity, namely the role that depression may play in the speed of immune system decline (e.g., Burak et al., 1993; Leserman et al., 1997; Vedhara et al., 1997). Generally, existing research suggests that a relationship exists, though many studies are purely correlational in nature and cannot always control for other variables known to alter immunity. In addition, the timing of assessment varies across studies, which makes understanding the temporal relationship between depressive symptoms and CD4 count challenging. In an early study, Burak et al. (1993) found an association between depression and changes in CD4 count, but did not find an association with longevity. Another early study reported that depressive symptoms were significantly associated with declines in several lymphocyte subsets over a 2-year period (Leserman et al., 1997). General emotional distress predicted CD4 decline at 12-month follow-up in a study of HIV-positive MSM (Vedhara et al., 1997), and bereavement prior to study entry was also associated with more rapid decline in CD4+ count during 3–4-year follow-up (Kemeny & Dean, 1995). A more recent study reported that depression predicted accelerated decline of CD4 cell number and significant increases in HIV viral load over 2 years (even when controlling for the effects of antiretroviral therapy) in a multiethnic HIV-positive sample (Ironson et al., 2005).

6.2.5.3 Depression and Survival in HIV

The relationship between biological outcomes such as CD4 count and viral load and depression is particularly interesting if it translates into clinical outcomes, such as survival. Patterson et al. (1996) found that depressive symptoms predicted shorter life span over and above CD4 counts and HIV symptoms. In the San Francisco Men's Health Study, a 9-year longitudinal study, median time to first AIDS diagnosis was 1.4 years shorter for men who were depressed, compared to men who were not depressed at baseline (Page-Shafer et al., 1996). Mayne et al. (1996) found that depressive affect was related to mortality in a longitudinal study that followed 402 HIV-seropositve gay men over a period of 7.5 years: men with elevated depressive symptoms at every visit had a 1.7-times greater risk of mortality compared to those without such elevations. More recently in a cohort of 765 adult women with HIV, Ickovics et al. (2001) reported that over a 7-year period, women with chronic depressive symptoms were twice as likely to die compared with women with limited or no depressive symptoms. The importance of this finding is underscored by the fact that women tend to have higher rates of depression than men, including HIV-positive women versus HIV-positive men (Morrison et al., 2002).

In summary, the preponderance of evidence to date suggests that there is a relationship between depression and accelerated disease progression (more rapid onset of symptoms and faster progression to AIDS), more compromised immunity, and significantly decreased survival. These relationships appear to emerge most reliably in studies that favor longer follow-up periods or utilize repeated measures of depression. It should also be noted that these relationships have been observed in various subpopulations (women, gay and bisexual men, multiethnic and rural samples) and at various stages of infection, in people living with HIV.

6.2.5.4 Antiretroviral Adherence

Depression is the most robust predictor of nonadherence among persons treated for HIV disease and has been consistently identified as a factor in nonadherence to medical regimens in various other chronic disease states (DiMatteo et al., 2000). Several studies have revealed a similar association between adherence to antiretroviral therapy and symptoms or diagnosis of depression (Catz, Kelly, Bogart, Benotsch, & McAuliffe, 2000; Gordillo, del Amo, Soriano, & Gonzalez-Lahoz, 1999;

Holzemer et al., 1999; Malcolm, Ng, Rosen, & Stone, 2003; Patterson et al., 2000; Safren, Otto, & Worth, 1999; Singh et al., 1996). More recently, Boarts, Buckley-Fischer, Armelie, Bogart, and Delahanty (2009) reported that in HIV-positive persons, depressive symptoms predicted lower medication adherence and depressed persons were more likely to have detectable viral loads.

The pervasive and ubiquitous effect of depression on medication adherence is further highlighted by studies that have found negative associations between symptoms of depression and baseline adherence over and above other Axis I disorders and important psychosocial factors, including social support, adherence self-efficacy, and punishment beliefs about HIV (Safren et al., 1999). The mechanism of action may be the symptoms of depression themselves (e.g., hopelessness) or associated impairments in problem-solving and coping (Safren, Radomsky, Otto, & Salomon, 2002). Depression and posttraumatic stress disorder (PTSD) often co-occur in individuals with HIV. Studies that examine individuals with this constellation of disorders have found that depression predicts nonadherence above and beyond other severe psychopathology, such as PTSD (Sledjeski, Delahanty, & Bogart, 2005; Vranceanu et al., 2008).

Rates of depression are higher in women than men in the general population and are slightly higher among HIV-positive women versus men (Bing et al., 2001; Orlando et al., 2001; Turner, Laine, Cosler, & Hauck, 2003). Some studies have also documented poorer adherence to antiretroviral therapy among women than men (Berg, Mimiaga, & Safren, 2004; Turner et al., 2003; Van Servellen, Chang, Garcia, & Lombardi, 2002) and it is likely that depression accounts for at least some of the variance in adherence across gender. For example, Arnsten et al. (2001) examined adherence data from 85 HIV-positive individuals with current or past drug use. The mean adherence rate for the sample was 53%, and participants who were female, active cocaine users, unmarried, and depressed had lower overall rates of adherence. The authors report that their findings suggest poorer levels of adherence among HIV-positive women versus HIV-positive men and that this relationship seems to be explained by the presence of depression. Data from two large-scale studies of various HIV-related phenomena indicate that higher rates of depression are associated with lower rates of adherence in HIV-positive women (Ohmit et al., 1998), and depression was one of the most frequently cited reasons for nonadherence among a sample of women enrolled in a cognitive-behavioral intervention designed to increase adherence to antiretroviral therapy (Jones et al., 2003).

6.2.5.5 Linkage and Retention in Care

As noted above, there is growing recognition that HIV-positive individuals require frequent contact with the medical system indefinitely and that significant numbers of HIV positive individuals are not engaged in adequate care (e.g., Giordano et al., 2007; Mugavero, 2008). Linkage to care generally refers to the process of initiating contact with an infectious disease provider following diagnosis, while retention in care refers to an individual's ability to adhere to the normal schedule of visits necessary to maintain optimal well-being. Without both effective linkage to and retention in care, interventions to manage HIV (e.g., routine labs, monitoring and treatment of opportunistic infections and co-occurring conditions, delivery of antiretroviral therapy, etc.) cannot be sufficiently implemented and well-being cannot be optimized. As individuals with HIV are affected by depression at extremely high rates and depression has clearly been established as a significant barrier to adherence to antiretroviral therapy, it is prudent to examine the impact of depression on linkage and retention to HIV-related care as well.

One study by Holzemer (1999) found that not only were patients with depression less likely to be adherent to antiretroviral therapy, but they were also less likely to follow provider advice and more likely than nondepressed patients to miss regularly scheduled appointments; the alternative to missing routine visits may be higher utilization of emergency room care (Joyce et al., 2005). An additional study found that symptoms of depression and PTSD accounted for more variance in healthcare utilization than either demographic or HIV-related variables (O'Cleirigh, Skeer, Mayer, & Safren, 2009), underscoring the role of psychological factors in determining patterns of heathcare use. In this latter study, healthcare utilization was defined as number of visits to a clinic or hospital; thus, these findings may also represent more emergent-based care than retention in regular HIV care, which is undesirable.

HIV-positive persons are not homogenous with respect to their experiences with access to healthcare and associated factors, such as stigma and economic hardship. Younger MSM of color are recognized as an especially vulnerable population. In a study of characteristics associated with retention in care among young MSM from eight sites across the U.S. participating in the Special Projects of National Significance Program (SPNS), approximately half of the sample reported high levels of depressive symptomatology as measured by the Center for Epidemiologic Studies-Depression scale (CES-D) (Magnus et al., 2010). Interestingly, those who reported a higher level of depressive symptoms were less likely to fall out of care. The authors posit that this result is due to the success of the SPNS programs in engaging depressed individuals in treatment; while encouraging, this finding requires replication. Though still in its nascent stage of investigation, it appears that much like adherence to antiretroviral therapy, linkage and retention in regular HIV care is multifaceted and involves a series of system, provider, and patient-related processes. Depression likely plays a significant role in this complex interplay of factors.

6.2.6 Clinical Considerations: Assessment and Treatment of Depression in HIV-Positive Individuals

6.2.6.1 Assessment

Although depression represents one generally homogenous syndrome, there are distinct cognitive, affective, and somatic components that warrant specialized assessment. This task becomes especially challenging in the context of HIV, in which medical and psychological symptoms are often entangled. When assessing depression, it is important to make the distinction between diagnostic measures (e.g., structured clinical interview for DSM-IV disorders [SCID], mini international neuropsychiatric interview [MINI]) and symptom checklists (e.g., Beck Depression Inventory [BDI], CES-D) whereby the former measures facilitate an actual diagnosis, and the latter provide some measure of the degree to which depressive symptoms are present. In clinical settings, it is also prudent to identify the onset of depressive symptoms with respect to the timing of HIV diagnosis. This may inform the case conceptualization and may facilitate the identification of cognitions and behaviors for later intervention.

The need for careful detection of depression is evidenced by a study by Asch et al. (2003). Of 1,140 HIV-positive individuals, 37% met criteria for a diagnosis of major depressive disorder, but 45% of these patients did not have a diagnosis of depression in their medical record. This finding may suggest that depression is under recognized in this population and highlights the necessity of validating, adapting, and developing effective screening instruments in HIV-positive populations. Savard, Laberge, Gauthier, and Bergeron (1999) attempted to determine a valid cut-off score for major depression using the Hospital Anxiety and Depression Scale (HADS; Zigmond & Snaith, 1983), a clinician-administered interview designed to assess severity of depressive symptoms in an HIV-positive population. Savard and colleagues determined that a score of 7 (versus a score of 8, which is the traditional cut-off score) yielded a sensitivity of 90.9% and a specificity of 85.1%. The Depression-Dejection Scale of the Profile of Moods States (POMS; McNair, Lorr, & Droppleman, 1981) was evaluated by Patterson et al. (2006) and had a sensitivity of 55% and a specificity of 84% using SCID criteria for major depression; this scale had a sensitivity of 92% and specificity of 67% in an earlier study by Wilkins et al. (1995).

Perhaps the most ubiquitous screening instrument for depression, the BDI (Beck, Ward, Mendelson, Mock, & Erbaugh, 1961) has been used extensively in medical populations, including HIV-positive individuals. In a study investigating the potential confounds of overlapping HIV-related illness symptoms and depression-related somatic symptoms, Kalichman, Sikkema, and Somlai (1995) report exaggerated BDI scores. The authors recommend using the 12-item cognitive-affective depression subscale of the BDI with a cut-off score of 10 for clinical depression. Similar research is needed on the Beck Depression Inventory II (BDI-II) which has been available since 1996 and was developed to correspond with diagnostic criteria listed in DSM-IV (Beck, Brown, & Steer, 1996).

Although few in number, there have been efforts to develop or modify instruments to measure depression specifically in HIV-positive populations. Aidala et al. (2004) developed the Client Diagnostic Questionnaire, or the CDQ, to facilitate the identification of mental health concerns by nonmental healthcare providers. They found the CDQ to have relatively poor sensitivity for major depressive disorder (60%), but a high specificity (96%). A visual analog rating scale for mood and anxiety developed by Maruff et al. (1994) was found to correlate at .78 to the CES-D. In summary, clinicians should be aware of the potential for score inflation resulting from potential overlap between symptoms of depression and other medical side effects when assessing depressive symptoms, particularly when using self-report measures. However, standard measures of depression are likely adequate in most circumstances.

6.2.6.2 Evidenced-Based Interventions for Depression

Before clinical recommendations can be made, it is important to understand the state of the psychotherapy literature in treating depression among HIV-positive individuals. A qualitative review by Olatunji, Mimiaga, O'Cleirigh, and Safren (2006) reviewed studies that were designed to target either major depressive *disorder* or subclinical depression (depressive *symptoms*) in HIV. Of the studies for major depressive disorder, all utilized an empirically supported psychosocial treatment for depression (e.g., cognitive-behavioral therapy [CBT] or interpersonal psychotherapy), and three of the four trials utilized a randomized design that included a control group (supportive psychotherapy or no treatment). In addition, one study included use of an adjunct antidepressant in addition to a supportive therapy condition, and another added antidepressant therapy to group-based CBT treatment arm. Results suggest that psychosocial treatments that directly target depression generally improve symptoms compared to no treatment control groups. However, from this small review, it remains unclear which of the psychosocial treatments is superior among this population as participants in arms that delivered nonempirically supported therapies also improved in some cases (e.g., Kelly, Murphy, Bahr, Kalichman, et al., 1993).

Since the publication of this review, one additional trial for reducing depression has been published by Safren, Gonzalez, and Soroudi (2008), who developed a novel use of CBT to address two major concerns among individuals with HIV – depression and adherence to antiretroviral therapy. The efficacy of this treatment, which contains traditional elements of CBT (e.g., problem-solving, cognitive restructuring, behavioral activation, etc.), was recently tested (Safren et al., 2009). Forty-five participants with a depressive mood *disorder* were randomized to one of two conditions: participants in the treatment condition received 12 sessions of cognitive-behavioral therapy for depression and adherence (CBT-AD), while participants in the enhanced treatment as usual condition received one session with a study interventionist to address adherence concerns and a letter to their providers documenting depression status. Challenges to adherence were addressed in a comprehensive manner using cognitive-behavioral strategies, including problem-solving barriers to medication taking and attending medical appointments, and cognitive restructuring of maladaptive medication beliefs. Participants who were assigned to the enhanced treatment as usual group were allowed to cross over into the intervention group if they still met study inclusion criteria at the end of their participation. At the end of the study, participants in the intervention group experienced significantly lower levels of depressive symptoms and improved adherence to antiretroviral therapy, and these gains were by and large maintained up to a year posttreatment.

6.2.6.3 Treatment Considerations

When treating depression in an individual with HIV, there are a number of clinical considerations. As noted above, depression can negatively impact adherence to antiretroviral therapy. Thus, it is important for the mental health clinician to assess for any difficulties with adherence to antiretroviral medications. Depression-related difficulties with adherence may be in part related to depressed cognitions or deficits in assertiveness or problem-solving skills. For example, a patient may hold negative beliefs about their antiretrovirals, such as the medication represents a daily "reminder" of their illness. Mental health clinicians may be able to facilitate more adaptive attitudes towards antiretrovirals (e.g., they are a tool that clients can use to take control of their health). Antiretrovirals are also associated with difficult side effects for some individuals, particularly early in treatment. While these side effects often abate or resolve all together with time, it is important that the client feel empowered enough to speak with their providers about side effect management so that side effects do not negatively impact adherence or cause a client to stop taking their mediations. A mental health clinician may be able to foster effective, assertive communication with medical care providers. Finally, many individuals have difficulty with adherence due to being out of their home during dosing times, but feel unsure as to how to manage dosing outside of the home, due to privacy concerns. A mental health provider can work on problem-solving this challenge, as well as other environmental and situational barriers to adherence with HIV-positive clients.

Other psychotherapy work may focus on illness-specific cognitions or experiences, such as punishment beliefs, stigma, and discrimination. The mental health clinician should be aware and pay attention to any maladaptive thoughts around having a behaviorally transmitted chronic disease (e.g., the idea that a patient feels "dirty" or unworthy of affection from others due to their diagnosis). HIV-related stigma and discrimination are commonplace in the U.S, from family, friends, employers, and even providers. Clients of sexual, ethnic, or racial minority status may experience stigma or discrimination across one or more of these domains. Thus, mental health clinicians should be sensitive to the fact that clients' perceptions of stigma or discrimination may in fact be very real. As a result, many clients may have limited disclosure of their illness to friends, family members, or employers.

Behavioral strategies such as pleasant event scheduling or behavioral activation can be powerful tools to improve mood and increase quality of life. This is illustrated by a recent study in which behavioral activation strategies were used as part of an intervention to treat depression and suboptimal adherence in a sample of individuals engaged in residential substance abuse treatment (Daughters, Magidson, Schuster, & Safren, 2010). Mental health practitioners using such behavioral strategies should be aware that clients may have days where they do not feel well and are not able to engage in the same types of activities on days when they feel unwell. In anticipation of these periods of time, the client and therapist should work together to generate a list of activities that the client will be able to engage in, despite symptoms such as fatigue or pain. Examples may include quieter activities such as reading, watching a movie, or having a friend visit the client in their home. Behavioral activation strategies can be particularly helpful when clients are experiencing isolation, withdrawal, or any changes in their activity level due to physical symptoms or depression.

In summary, depression is highly prevalent psychological co-morbidity of HIV, with potential implications for both disease processes and self-care. However, depression is also highly treatable. To date, there is no evidence to suggest that HIV infection would reduce the effectiveness of depression treatment. Thus, mental health clinicians and HIV care providers should screen for depression in HIV-infected patients and apply evidenced-based treatments for depression in the context of HIV.

6.3 Anxiety Disorders and HIV

Relatively speaking, somewhat less research exists for anxiety in the context of HIV than depression. However, it appears that anxiety disorders are also prevalent and distressing problems for this population. *Lifetime* estimates of anxiety disorders among HIV-positive individuals in the U.S. range from 7 to 19% (e.g., Rosenberger et al., 1993; Sewell et al., 2000). Among studies using a structured clinical interview, the prevalence of any anxiety disorder among HIV-positive individuals seems to be approximately 10.8–12% (Morrison et al., 2002; Sewell et al., 2000). Individuals with HIV are disproportionately affected by certain anxiety disorders relative to the general population, including PTSD, Generalized Anxiety Disorder, and Panic Disorder, while other anxiety disorders remain understudied in HIV-positive populations. As is the case with depressive disorders, some individuals with HIV will have a preexisting DSM-IV anxiety disorder when diagnosed with HIV that impacts disease progression and management, while others will develop stress or anxiety symptoms upon diagnosis or while coping with HIV. This section begins with the epidemiology and pathophysiology of PTSD in HIV-positive individuals, followed by the epidemiology of generalized anxiety disorder, panic disorder, and other anxiety disorders, as well as what is known about the pathophysiology of these disorders in HIV-positive individuals. The consequences of anxiety in HIV-positive individuals are complex, and some of these issues will also be examined in this section. Lastly, this section will discuss clinical considerations with respect to assessment and treatment of anxiety in this population.

6.3.1 HIV and Posttraumatic Stress Disorder (PTSD)

6.3.1.1 Epidemiology

The prevalence of PTSD among HIV positive individuals seems to be higher than in the general population and among other medical patient groups (Kessler et al., 2005; Tedstone & Tarrier, 2003) with overall prevalence rates ranging from 3.2 to 60% among HIV-positive persons (e.g., Kelly et al., 1998; Kimberling, Armistead, & Forehand, 1999; Israelski et al., 2007; Martinez, Israelski, Walker, & Koopman, 2002; Morrison et al., 2002; Pence et al., 2006; Smith, 2002). Estimates of the rates of PTSD among HIV-positive individuals vary widely and seem to depend on the patient population and means of assessment. Higher rates of PTSD are detected in studies that make use of self-report measures to approximate diagnostic criteria, such as the PTSD Checklist (e.g., Smith, Egert, Winkel, & Jacobson, 2002) versus conducting structured clinical interviews. The study with the lowest rate of 3.2% utilized both a structured interview and anxiety symptom rating scales to evaluate differences in PTSD among HIV-positive women versus matched HIV-negative women (Morrison et al., 2002). The sample size was relatively small, and an active substance abuse disorder was an exclusion criterion, both of which may have impacted the lower than expected rates of PTSD. Rates may be higher among specific populations such as MSM (e.g., Kelly et al., 1998), minority women (e.g., Kimberling, Calhoun, et al., 1999), incarcerated women (Lewis, 2005), and those with persistent pain (e.g., Smith et al., 2002). In the HIV-positive population as in the general population, PTSD is often co-morbid with other psychiatric disorders, including major depressive disorder, substance abuse, and other anxiety disorders (Israelski et al., 2007; Olley, Zeier, Seedat, & Stein, 2005; Tsao, Dobalian, Moreau, & Dobalian, 2004; Tsao, Dobalian, & Naliboff, 2004).

Acute Stress Disorder is similar to PTSD, but shorter in duration; in order to meet criteria for Acute Stress Disorder, individuals must meet diagnostic criteria for a period of at least 2 days, but no longer than 4 weeks, after which time an individual may meet criteria for PTSD. Few studies have attempted to ascertain the prevalence of Acute Stress Disorder among HIV-positive individuals, but at least one study has documented rates as high as 43%, with higher rates documented in female participants, and among African-American and Caucasian participants when compared to those of mixed ethnicity or those who identified themselves as Latina/Latino (Israelski et al., 2007).

6.3.1.2 Pathophysiology

Disproportionately high numbers of HIV-positive individuals have experienced at least one traumatic event, including sexual or physical abuse (Whetten et al., 2006). Elevated rates of PTSD among individuals with HIV are possibly explained by the reported association between having experienced a traumatic event and risky sexual practices (O'Leary, Purcell, Remien, & Gomez, 2003; Purcell, Malow, Dolezal, & Carballo-Dieguez, 2004; Smith, Leve, & Chamberlain, 2006) among both HIV-negative and HIV-positive individuals. Individuals who have experienced a traumatic event and have developed PTSD may be more likely to engage in risky sexual behavior and subsequently more likely to contract HIV, though this hypothesis requires additional research. Furthermore, a history of a PTSD diagnosis has been associated with higher rates of both anal sex and sex work among HIV-positive individuals, even when controlling for factors such as drug abuse, disease related variables, and sociodemographic variables (Hutton et al., 2001), which may increase the odds of HIV transmission.

Some have posited that receiving a diagnosis of HIV constitutes a "category A," PTSD defining event. The onset of PTSD related to diagnosis of and living with HIV has not been studied widely, but initial reports suggest that significant numbers of HIV-positive individuals attribute the onset of their PTSD specifically to their HIV diagnosis; one such study documented this phenomenon in 30% of a sample of HIV-positive men (Kelly et al., 1998). Two other studies found high rates of PTSD related to HIV diagnosis (Delahanty, Bogart, & Figler, 2004; Safren, Gershuny, & Hendriksen, 2003). The latter two studies utilized self-report screening instruments and also noted adherence difficulties among those with high levels of PTSD symptoms in this context.

6.3.2 HIV and Panic Disorder

6.3.2.1 Epidemiology

Much of the research on HIV and panic disorder comes from a number of large-scale studies that document rates of 11–16% using *abbreviated* versions of structured clinical interviews (Bing et al., 2001; Orlando et al., 2002; Sherbourne et al., 2000; Tsao, Dobalian, Moreau, et al., 2004; Tsao, Dobalian, & Naliboff, 2004). These rates are considerably higher than the rate of 2.7% observed in the general population (Kessler et al., 2005). However, in a smaller sample of 148 HIV-positive individuals, only 5.4% met criteria for panic disorder based on a *full* structured clinical interview (Pence et al., 2006).

6.3.2.2 Pathophysiology

Little is known about the pathophysiology of HIV and panic disorder. No data are available to explain how the diagnosis of or living with HIV might be associated with the development of panic disorder.

6.3.3 HIV and Generalized Anxiety Disorder

6.3.3.1 Epidemiology

Reported rates of generalized anxiety disorder among HIV-positive individuals also range widely. Large-scale studies using structured clinical interviews report rates between 2.2% and 16%, (e.g., Bing et al., 2001; Morrison et al., 2002; Orlando et al., 2002). In general, these rates seem higher than that reported in the general population, where the 12-month prevalence of generalized anxiety disorder is approximately 3.1% (Kessler et al., 2005).

6.3.3.2 Pathophysiology

As with panic disorder, no formal research has been conducted with respect to the pathophysiology of generalized anxiety disorder and HIV. While it is unclear if an HIV diagnosis may lend itself to the development of generalized anxiety disorder, it would not be uncommon to see an increase in worries either immediately after an HIV diagnosis or with advanced disease progression. These scenarios may not constitute an anxiety disorder, however, if more localized to HIV.

6.3.4 *HIV and Other Anxiety Disorders*

6.3.4.1 Epidemiology

Other anxiety disorders have received less attention among HIV-positive individuals specifically, perhaps because rates are not elevated in this group. A cross-sectional study of mood and anxiety disorders in HIV positive versus HIV negative women revealed 2.2% of the sample met criteria for a specific phobia, 5.4% met criteria for social phobia, and 1.1% met criteria for obsessive compulsive disorder using a structured clinical interview (Morrison et al., 2002). Specific phobias were detected among 9% of a sample of individuals with HIV seeking care at a mental health clinic by Haller and Miles (2003). In the general population, up to 8.7% of individuals may meet criteria for a specific phobia, 6.8% for social phobia, and 1% for obsessive compulsive disorder (Kessler et al., 2005).

6.3.4.2 Pathophysiology

While no formal research has been conducted on the pathophysiology of specific phobias or obsessive compulsive disorder and HIV, some aspects of social anxiety in particular may be problematic with respect to safer sexual behavior. For example, research among gay and bisexual men has suggested that performance anxiety or embarrassment around condom use and negotiation may be related to unprotected anal intercourse, thus making one more likely to contract HIV (see O'Cleirigh, Hart, & James, 2008 for a review). In addition, fear of being sexually rejected has been associated with less frequent condom use among both HIV-positive and HIV-negative gay and bisexual men (Adam, Husbands, Murray, & Maxwell, 2005; Murray & Adam, 2001), while feelings of powerlessness have been associated with both a history of unprotected sex with high-risk partners (partners who have multiple other partners) and less frequent condom use, at least in a sample of younger age pregnant women (Kershaw et al., 2006). Fear of rejection in sexual relationships due to an HIV-positive serostatus has been documented in HIV positive MSM as well (Klitzman, 1999; Siegel & Schrimshaw, 2003).

6.3.5 *Other Considerations Related to Anxiety and HIV*

6.3.5.1 Stress and Immune Functioning

Dysregulation of the hypothalamic pituitary axis (HPA) and sympathetic adrenal medullary (SAM) system that is characteristic of several anxiety disorders may have an especially negative impact on HIV patients (O'Cleirigh et al., 2008). Specifically, dysregulation of these systems may result in elevated levels of stress hormones, including norepinephrine and cortisol which are associated with disease progression, general immune functioning, viral replication, and response to antiretroviral therapy (e.g., Cole et al., 2001; Cole, Kemeny, Fahey, Zack, & Naliboff, 2003; Cole, Korin, Fahey, & Zack, 1998; Ironson et al., 2006; Leserman et al., 2000; Schneiderman, Ironson, & Siegel, 2005). O'Cleirigh et al. (2008) thus speculate that the development and delivery of effective anxiety disorder treatments may have the potential to improve treatment and clinical outcomes in some patients.

6.3.5.2 Medication Adherence

The role of anxiety in nonadherence to antiretrovirals is less clear than the role of depression. Three studies have documented a relationship between general measures of anxiety and nonadherence to antiretroviral therapy (Ammassari et al., 2002; Schönnesson, Williams, Ross, Bratt, & Keel, 2006; Van Servellen et al., 2002), while others have examined relationships among specific anxiety disorders and adherence. One study documents a positive relationship between any anxiety disorder diagnosis (excluding PTSD) and adherence (Ingersoll, 2004), while another (Tucker, Burnam, Sherbourne, Kung, & Gifford, 2003) found that persons with a diagnosis of generalized anxiety disorder or panic disorder were 2 times more likely to report nonadherence compared to those without a psychiatric disorder. A diagnosis of social phobia has been linked to running out of medications before a refill is obtained (Ingersoll, 2004). It may be that certain types of anxiety are protective with respect to antiretroviral adherence. For example, anxiety and worry about disease progression may support adherence, while hypervigilance to bodily symptoms and worries about medication toxicity may contribute to nonadherence.

The literature on PTSD symptoms and adherence has generated conflicting data. Schönnesson et al. (2006) found the severity of intrusion and avoidance symptoms to be associated with better antiretroviral adherence. Delahanty et al. (2004) observed the opposite effect, but in a follow-up study (Boarts et al., 2006) found a modest association of PTSD symptoms with medication adherence. Vranceanu et al. (2008) recently found that PTSD did not predict adherence, either alone, or when incorporated in a model that included depressive symptoms. In theory, PTSD-related avoidance could negatively impact adherence, at least for individuals who have an association between sexually based traumas and HIV diagnosis. The relationship between PTSD and adherence to antiretroviral therapy warrants further research given the high rates of PTSD among HIV-infected individuals.

6.3.5.3 Linkage and Retention in Care

As noted above, adherence to appointments with healthcare providers is another component to successful HIV management. Van Servellen et al. (2002) found higher levels of anxiety to be associated with appointment nonadherence in HIV-positive individuals; however, a previous study found no significant relationship between appointment adherence and anxiety (McClure, Catz, & Brantley, 1999). Of note, a growing body of literature has established a link between PTSD symptoms and self-reported functional impairment, including pain (Jones et al., 2003; Simoni & Ng, 2002; Smith et al., 2002), which may actually result in greater frequency of contact with medical providers, as both a lifetime history of trauma and PTSD symptoms have been linked to increased healthcare utilization (Leserman et al., 2005; O'Cleirigh et al., 2009). Further study is required in order to fully understand the impact of anxiety on linkage to and retention in care, particularly the differential effects of various anxiety disorders that theoretically may have an impact, such as social phobia and PTSD, on appointment adherence.

6.3.6 Clinical Considerations: Assessment and Treatment of Anxiety in the Context of HIV

6.3.6.1 Assessment

Anxiety is often a broadly defined construct, and while a multitude of instruments exist by which to measure anxiety, few of these have been well validated in HIV-infected populations. When trying to choose an assessment tool, it is important to be clear on what the construct of interest is (e.g., cognitive symptoms, physiological symptoms, trait anxiety, etc.) and to differentiate anxiety disorders from general stress or HIV-related stress, as both of these factors may influence treatment decisions. As with depression, it is important to make the distinction between diagnostic measures (e.g., SCID, MINI) and symptom checklists (e.g., PTSD Checklist, beck anxiety inventory [BAI], etc.). In clinical settings, it is also prudent to identify the onset of anxiety symptoms with respect to timing of HIV diagnosis.

As in any medical illness, there is some concern that scores will be inflated due to the potential overlap between somatic symptoms of HIV infection or medication side effects, and stress or anxiety. The Beck Anxiety Inventory – Fast Screen for Medical Settings (BAI-FS) attempts to address this concern. The BAI-FS is a 7-item scale that assesses nonsomatic symptoms of anxiety and has been evaluated for use in HIV-positive individuals with chronic pain by Krefetz, Steer, Jermyn, and Condoluci (2004). In this population, the instrument was found to have an internal consistency of .8. Using a score of four, the BAI-FS has a sensitivity of 82% and a specificity of 59%.

The CDQ (Aidala et al., 2004), an instrument developed for use by non-mental health professionals, was found to have strong sensitivity (89%) for any anxiety disorder and PTSD (82%), but had poorer sensitivity for specific anxiety disorder diagnosis, such as panic disorder (55%) and generalized anxiety disorder (66%). Specificity for any anxiety disorder was 79%. A visual analog rating scale for mood and anxiety was developed by Maruff et al. (1994) and was found to correlate highly with the state anxiety subscale of the State Trait Anxiety Index (.86) but only moderately with the trait anxiety subscale (.58).

In summary, it is important to define the goal of the assessment when measuring anxiety; this will facilitate the selection of the most appropriate instrument. When possible, measures that have some validation data in an HIV-infected population are ideal. In the absence of such data, consider using an instrument that has validation data in medical populations and/or has less overlap with common somatic symptoms of the disease (i.e., difficulty sleeping, appetite changes, weight changes, fatigue). This can be challenging when trying to assess anxiety disorders with a strong physiological component, such as generalized anxiety disorder or panic disorder, and when trying to differentiate anxiety from depression. Additional research is required in order to validate common symptom checklists and self-report measures in this population in order to facilitate screening in clinical settings, as well as validity of research efforts, particularly when measuring change in response to psychosocial interventions.

6.3.6.2 Evidence-Based Treatment for Anxiety Disorders

Despite the relatively high prevalence of anxiety disorders among HIV-positive individuals, there are no published trials evaluating the efficacy of anxiety disorder treatments among HIV-positive individuals. However, numerous trials have attempted to intervene on high levels of stress, or subthreshold levels of anxiety. For example, two recent meta-analyses of stress management interventions for HIV-positive individuals conducted by Scott-Sheldon, Kalichman, Carey, and Fielder (2008) and Crepaz et al. (2008) found a small effect size for stress management interventions with respect to reductions in measures of anxiety and depressive symptoms. Of the 35 studies included in the meta-analysis, only seven studies reported data on rates of anxiety disorder diagnoses (17%). Thirty-four percent of the studies make a distinction between clinical depression versus depressive symptoms, and eight of the studies excluded participants who met criteria for a major depressive episode. The majority of the interventions were conducted in a small group format and included some element of psychoeducation (e.g., why stress management is important for HIV-positive individuals, nutrition education, importance of adherence) and "coping skills" training (e.g., formal training in relaxation strategies, assertiveness, and planning for stressful events in a deliberate way).

Moderational analyses revealed that interventions were more effective in reducing anxiety in females, those younger in age, and individuals with elevated baseline anxiety. Interventions with psychoeducational content that was solely focused on medication adherence versus education about stress were generally less effective at reducing anxiety. Given data suggesting a relationship between disruptions in the HPA and SAM systems, and disease progression and response to antiretroviral therapy, it would be of great clinical significance to demonstrate an effect of behavioral interventions on disease-specific factors; however, Scott-Sheldon et al. (2008) did not detect an effect for these interventions on immune functioning.

The meta-analysis conducted by Crepaz et al. (2008) includes 15 trials of cognitive-behavioral interventions designed to improve mental health and immune functioning in HIV-positive individuals. Of these 15 studies, ten are included in the analysis described above by Scott-Sheldon and colleagues. Results were consistent with small effect sizes for depression and anxiety in stress management interventions. Effects were only observed directly after the intervention and not at longer term follow-up assessments. All of the interventions incorporated cognitive restructuring techniques, and all but one taught coping skills. Analyses of aggregated effect sizes found that interventions were more effective in reducing depression and anxiety when ten or more intervention sessions were provided, the retention rate was greater than 80%, and fewer than 50% of participants were MSM. Five trials included CD4 count outcomes, for which the aggregated effect size was not statistically significant.

The studies in the above-captioned meta-analyses did not attempt to treat diagnostic levels of anxiety or depression. At least some of the participants in these studies met criteria for a mood and/or anxiety disorder, which may have contributed to the small effect sizes since certain symptoms of depression or anxiety (e.g., behavioral avoidance or withdrawal) could impede an individual's ability to fully engage in a stress management protocol. Furthermore, a stress management protocol cannot be assumed to treat all symptoms of depression and anxiety disorders (O'Cleirigh & Safren, 2008). Additional research evaluating interventions to treat major depressive disorder and anxiety disorders are thus needed, given the high rates of morbidity and the association with poor health behaviors such as decreased adherence to antiretroviral therapy and increased substance use (O'Cleirigh & Safren, 2008).

6.3.6.3 Treatment and Clinical Recommendations

In the absence of data supporting the best means by which to treat anxiety disorders in HIV-positive individuals, it seems that most empirically supported treatments for anxiety disorders would also be effective in this population. However, a few clinical issues are important to consider. First, a careful assessment should be conducted in order to ascertain whether a particular client meets criteria for a particular DSM anxiety disorder versus clients who are seeking treatment for better stress management skills. For the former, an empirically supported treatment, such as CBT, would likely be appropriate. CBT treatment protocols for anxiety disorders teach various skills, and many utilize exposure techniques to decrease anxiety and related avoidance. These exposure techniques would rarely be warranted for individuals without an actual anxiety disorder. However, the mental health clinician may make use of certain CBT techniques (e.g., cognitive restructuring and relaxation training) for clients with high levels of stress or subthreshold anxiety.

As reviewed in the depression section, routine laboratory monitoring may be stressful and anxiety-provoking. For clients with this experience, the mental health clinician may want to develop strategies with the client for managing the entire experience, from the blood draw to waiting for results, and actually receiving results. HIV-positive clients may also worry extensively about the way others view their appearance secondary to lipodystrophy or lipoatrophy (relatively common effects of long-term antiretroviral treatment), or about consequences of disease progression, including death. Cognitive restructuring and mindfulness-based strategies may be helpful in managing these concerns. Mental health clinicians may wish to integrate psychoeducation around HIV and anxiety when working with HIV-positive persons presenting for anxiety or stress treatment.

6.4 Schizophrenia and HIV

6.4.1 Epidemiology

The prevalence of schizophrenia among individuals with HIV appears to be substantially higher than that of the general population, with reports ranging from 4.1 to 5.7%, versus approximately 1.1% in the general population (Blank, Mandell, Aiken, & Hadley, 2002; Regier et al., 1993; Walkup, Crystal, & Sambamoorthi, 1999). Rates of HIV infection among those with a diagnosis of schizophrenia also appear to be elevated in comparison to those without a diagnosis of schizophrenia. Current studies estimate 0.5–2.8% of individuals with schizophrenia are HIV positive (Baillargeon et al., 2008; Blank et al., 2002; De Hart & Van Eyck, 2008; Himelhoch et al., 2007).

6.4.2 Pathophysiology

There is evidence that symptoms of schizophrenia may confer risk for contracting HIV (Cournos et al., 1994, 2005; Gottesman & Groome, 1997), and some research suggests that HIV in the central nervous system (CNS) may contribute to the onset of psychotic symptoms (Cournos et al., 2005; Masilah et al., 1992; Sewell, 1996). Symptoms of schizophrenia (e.g., impulse control, delusions) may contribute to sexual risk-taking or substance abuse. Although individuals with schizophrenia appear to be less sexually active than the general population (Nimgaonkar, Ward, Agarde, Weston, & Ganguli, 1997; Ritsner, Sherina, & Ginath, 1992), it appears that those who do engage in sexual activity are likely to engage in risky behaviors such as not using condoms, having multiple sex partners, using drugs or alcohol during sex, trading sex for money or goods, and having sex with a partner known to be using injection drugs (see Cournos et al., 1994 for a review). Additionally, what little research there is regarding injection drug use (IDU) in individuals with schizophrenia suggests that rates of IDU are higher in individuals with schizophrenia than the general population (Cournos et al., 1994; Gottesman & Groome, 1997; Robins & Regier, 1991).

A growing body of work indicates that individuals with severe mental illness in general, and schizophrenia in particular, are lacking important HIV knowledge and awareness, and that this may also put them at increased risk for infection (Gottesman & Groome, 1997). Aruffo, Coverdale, Chacko, and Dworkin (1990) found that patients with a diagnosis of schizophrenia knew significantly less about HIV and how it is transmitted than a control group. Kalichman, Kelly, Johnson, and Bulto (1994) also reported significant knowledge deficits in a sample of 95 psychiatric outpatients, of which 82% had schizophrenia. For example, 26% believed that one must have multiple sex partners to contract HIV, and 37% thought that showering directly following sex could prevent infection. Lack of HIV knowledge alone does not appear to account for high rates of HV infection. In a study by McKinnon, Cournos, Sugden, Guido, and Herman (1996), no correlation was found between greater knowledge and decreased HIV risk behavior.

A number of studies have investigated the link between HIV infection and the subsequent development of schizophrenia, or new-onset schizophrenia. HIV or opportunistic infections present in the CNS may have a neurological impact, and anywhere from 30 to 60% of HIV-positive individuals will experience neuropsychiatric complications (Bensalem & Berger, 2002; Pearce, 2003). Of these neuropsychiatric complications, psychosis is well documented (Sewell, 1996); however, a diagnosis of schizophrenia is not. This may be due, in part, to the focus of these studies being virus' effects on the brain rather than psychiatric diagnoses (e.g., Masilah et al., 1992). Although investigation of the temporal relationship between the onset of schizophrenia and HIV infection has been informative and clinically useful, efforts to better determine the prevalence of schizophrenia onset prior to HIV infection versus post-HIV infection are needed.

6.4.3 Treatment

Standard pharmacological treatment for schizophrenia with antipsychotic medications is recommended for individuals who are HIV positive. However, there are studies showing that certain medications may cause or exacerbate symptoms characteristic of HIV. For example, it is not uncommon for individuals with advanced HIV to exhibit motor difficulties or metabolic syndromes. Thus, newer, atypical antipsychotic medications may be preferable to the older, typical antipsychotic medications which are known to cause more Parkinsonian side effects, and antipsychotic medications associated with greater rates of metabolic syndromes should be avoided when possible (Forstein et al., 2006).

Medication adherence for both HIV and schizophrenia medication regimens is likely to be a key issue in clinical management of this population. To the extent that the patient's psychotic symptoms are well-controlled, the patient may be more capable of adhering to their HIV medication regimen. Research has demonstrated benefit from psychosocial treatments (e.g., social skills training, cognitive adaptation training) with respect to improving social functioning and self-care among those individuals with schizophrenia (Heinssen, Liberman, & Kopelwicz, 2000), though the extent to which these interventions will be effective in improving management of HIV is unknown. Additional research has evaluated the efficacy of psychosocial interventions for reducing risk of HIV infection in chronically mentally ill individuals through education and safer sex training, with some success (e.g., Kalichman, Sikkema, Kelly, & Bulto, 1995). While these investigations have produced promising results, more research is needed to address the specific needs of HIV-positive individuals with schizophrenia, both with respect to HIV care and prevention.

6.5 Other Psychological Disorders and HIV

6.5.1 Sleep Disorders and HIV

6.5.1.1 Epidemiology and Pathophysiology

There is a high occurrence of sleep disorders and subclinical sleep disruption in HIV-positive individuals, with reported rates ranging from 56 to 100% (Lee et al., 2009; Rubenstein & Selwyn, 1998; Vosvick et al., 2004). As sleep disruption is not uncommon among individuals living with a chronic illness, it may be difficult to distinguish the etiology. Although Brown, Mitler, and Atkinson (1991) found an association between CD4 count and sleep disturbance, a number of more recent studies have failed to support this association (e.g., Cohen, Ferran, Vizgirda, Kunkle, & Cloninger, 1996; Lee, Portillo, & Miramontes, 2001; Nokes & Kendrew, 2001; Perkins et al., 1995). Antiretroviral medication side effects are another potential source of sleep disruption, and studies have found a strong relation between the use of efavirenz and sleep disturbance (Fumaz et al., 2002; Nunez et al., 2001). However, it seems that co-morbid mental illness, in particular anxiety and depressive disorders, is the most significantly associated factor in sleep disorders in HIV-positive individuals (Reid & Dwyer, 2005).

6.5.1.2 Treatment

Despite the high prevalence of sleep disorders in individuals who are HIV positive, the number of treatment studies in this area is limited. Dreher (2003) investigated the effects of reduced caffeine intake in a sample of 88 HIV-positive individuals who experience sleep dysfunction and use caffeine daily. Caffeine reduction of 90% or greater resulted in a 35% improvement in sleep as measured by the Pittsburgh Sleep Quality Index (PSQI) (Buysee, Reynolds, Monk, Berman, & Kupfer, 1989). In another study, Phillips and Skelton (2001) investigated the effects of acupuncture on sleep disorders in HIV-positive individuals. Participants received 10 sessions of acupuncture over the course of 5 weeks. Sleep activity monitors (wrist actigraphs) recorded significant increases in sleep time postacupuncture intervention. Subjective sleep ratings as measured by the Current Sleep Quality Index (CSQI) (Phillips, 1996) also showed significant improvement, postacupuncture intervention. Although pharmacological treatments are the most common method of treating sleep disorders in the general population, there has yet to be a study investigating the use of medication to treat sleep disorders in an HIV-positive population (Omonuwa, Goforth, Preud'homme, & Krystal, 2009).

6.5.2 Sexual Disorders and HIV

6.5.2.1 Epidemiology and Pathophysiology

Sexual disorders encompass a wide array of symptoms, including erectile dysfunction, loss of sexual desire, and difficulties achieving orgasm. Some difficulties with sexual functioning are influenced by age and gender, which make assessment and documenting prevalence challenging. For these reasons, rates of sexual disorders among HIV-positive individuals range widely, from 21 to 90% (Asboe et al., 2007; Bouhnik et al., 2008; Collazos, 2007; Moreno-Perez et al., 2010; Trotta et al., 2008). Although studies differ in design, setting, sample characteristics, and evaluation methods, it seems clear that there are higher rates of sexual disorders in HIV-positive individuals than in the general population, where estimates for sexual disorders are between 10% and 52% for men and 25% and 63% for women (Heiman, 2002).

While it is generally believed that HIV disease progression is associated with sexual dysfunction, further research is needed. In one study by Trotta et al. (2008), no association between sexual dysfunction and CD4 count was found. Identifying the cause of sexual disorders is especially difficult in the HIV population where a number of other problems known to contribute to sexual dysfunction are fairly common, such as depression and substance use and anxiety concerning HIV transmission via sexual contact. There are also reports that antiretroviral medications, protease inhibitors in particular, may be linked to sexual dysfunction; however, the evidence is inconclusive (Collazos, 2007; Moreno-Perez et al., 2010).

6.5.2.2 Treatment

Assessment is particularly important when treating sexual disorders in HIV-positive individuals as the etiology will directly inform treatment (psychogenic versus organic). Although there are a number of psychotherapeutic interventions for a variety of sexual disorders for both men and women (see O'Donohue, Swingen, Dopke, & Regev, 1999 for review of psychotherapy for male sexual dysfunction and O'Donohue, Dopke, & Swingen, 1997 for review of psychotherapy for female sexual dysfunction), no studies have investigated such treatments in an HIV-positive population. Pharmacological treatment for erectile dysfunction is common in the general population, but it is important to be aware of potential drug–drug interactions with antiretroviral drugs (ARVs). The use of protease inhibitors has been shown to increase levels of Sildenafil (Viagra), so it is recommended that individuals taking both medications limit their Sildenafil dose to 25 mg (Piscitelli, 2000).

6.5.3 Pain Disorders and HIV

6.5.3.1 Epidemiology and Pathophysiology

Syndromes associated with chronic pain, such as neuropathy and rheumatic conditions, are commonly assessed in HIV-positive individuals (Walker, Tyndall, & Daikeler, 2008; Wulff, Wang, & Simpson, 2000). The prevalence of pain syndromes in HIV-positive individuals ranges from 35 to 80% (Dobalian, Tsao, & Duncan, 2004). Pain in the context of HIV infection can result from an extensive variety of sources both directly and indirectly related to HIV. One of the most common sources is distal symmetrical polyneuropathy (DSP), which affects over one third of all HIV-positive individuals and is often disabling (see Verma, Estanislao, & Simpson, 2005 for a review). Current prevalence estimates of rheumatic diseases (e.g., arthritis, vasculitis, diffuse infiltrative lymphocytosis syndrome) in HIV-positive individuals are 9% (Nguyen & Reveille, 2009).

6.5.3.2 Treatment

Because the etiology of pain can be variable, multidimensional assessment instruments, such as the McGill Pain Questionnaire (MPQ; Melzack & Torgenson, 1971), which includes an assessment of the affective component of pain, may be of value for this population, particularly when considering psychosocial treatments. Special attention to pain management is crucial for this population, as pain is associated with higher rates of depression in the general population (e.g., Bair et al., 2003) and in HIV-infected individuals (e.g., Rosenfield et al., 1996), as well as lower adherence to antiretroviral therapy (Berg, Cooperman, Newville, & Arnsten, 2009). Analgesic treatment is recommended for HIV-positive individuals with neuropathy (Wulff et al., 2000). Data on psychotherapy interventions for pain disorders are limited. Evans, Fishman, Spielman, and Haley (2003) compared a CBT for HIV-related neuropathic pain to a supportive psychotherapy, and while both groups experienced improvements, the CBT group showed significantly greater gains. However, the high dropout rate (over 50% of participants randomized to CBT across 6 weeks) that occurred in the CBT group raises questions of acceptability.

6.6 Cultural Considerations

The optimal treatment of mental illness within HIV-positive patients requires a consideration of patients' demographic background (e.g., race, ethnicity, culture), as this population may experience a number of factors that may increase risk for mental illness, as well as disparities in mental healthcare utilization and retention. Although the literature is sparse regarding the efficacy of evidence-based interventions with HIV-positive minorities, the available literature suggests areas for assessment, potential interventions, and treatment recommendations.

6.6.1 Factors Related to Mental Illness Within HIV-Positive Minorities

Individuals from minority backgrounds have been found to experience disparities in access to and benefit from HIV-related medical and mental health care. For example, Latinos and African Americans of both genders are disproportionately impacted by HIV (CDC, 2008a, 2008b) and, compared to non-Latino Whites, have been found to initiate medical treatment with more advanced HIV disease (e.g., AIDS diagnosis, CD4 count) and report lower adherence to HIV-related medications (see Giordano et al., 2010). Additionally, psychiatric co-morbidity and negative life experiences, such as trauma or discrimination, may place minorities at greater risk for negative outcomes. For example, HIV-positive women who have co-morbid mental and substance use disorders may be at increased risk of experiencing traumatic events that can negatively impact substance abuse treatment (see Klinkenberg & Sacks, 2004). HIV-positive African American women, in particular, have been found to be more likely to experience victimization compared to HIV-negative counterparts – an experience related to greater endorsement of psychological distress and depressive symptoms (Kimberling, Armistead, & Forehand, 1999). Discrimination may also affect HIV-positive minorities and have a negative impact on health. For example, HIV-related discrimination can negatively affect HIV-positive African American women such that those endorsing discrimination report poorer mental health (i.e., increased stress, suicidal ideation, depression, poorer self-esteem), greater HIV risk behavior (i.e., unprotected sex), and lower utilization of medical care – a relationship not found within White peers (Wingood et al., 2007). Similarly, traumatic experiences may have a stronger relationship to depression and drug use among HIV-positive Latina women as compared to those who are HIV-negative (Newcomb & Carmona, 2004), and both trauma and homophobia have been connected to psychological distress and high-risk sexual behavior in Latino gay men (Arreola, Neilands, & Diaz, 2009). Further study is needed, however, on the factors that result in resilience within HIV-positive minorities, including ways that they are able to navigate the mental healthcare system to access care and experience negative live events without developing mental illness. For example, Newcomb and Carmona (2004) found that within Latinas, though higher education was related to increased illicit drug use and acculturation, it was also associated with lower likelihood of being HIV-positive, less depression, and less trauma.

6.6.2 Treatment Utilization and Retention

Although HIV-positive minorities may be at an increased risk for factors that negatively impact mental health, this group is less likely to receive appropriate psychiatric care. Within a diverse group of HIV-positive patients, those meeting criteria for PTSD, for example, reported that 41% were not receiving either psychiatric treatment or medication (Israelski et al., 2007) and those reporting increased lifetime trauma, abuse history, and PTSD symptoms were more likely to indicate increased emergent service utilization, such as hospital emergency room visits and overnight hospitalizations, rather than consistent care (Leserman et al., 2005). Similarly, compared to HIV-positive non-Latino Whites, studies have reported that African Americans are less likely to use mental health care or psychiatric medications (Himelhoch, Josephs, Chandler, Korthuis, & Gebo, 2009), though findings on Latinos' use of medications have been mixed (Himelhoch et al., 2009; Vitiello, Burnman, Bing, Beckman, & Shapiro, 2003). In addition, Weaver et al. (2008) noted that, compared to non-Latino Whites, HIV-positive Latinos are less likely to receive concurrent mental health and substance abuse treatment, and both Latinos and African Americans are less likely to receive outpatient mental health care yet more likely to participate in substance abuse self-help groups (Weaver et al., 2008). Retention in treatment should also be addressed with this population; within a diverse group of HIV-positive adolescents, men who perceived a lack of respect or who were Latino were found less likely to be retained in treatment (Magnus et al., 2010).

6.6.3 Assessment, Intervention, and Treatment Recommendations

As mentioned above, assessment of psychiatric symptoms with HIV-positive patients requires numerous considerations: whether the assessment will be performed by a clinician through a structured interview or by the patient through a self-report symptom checklist; desire for gauging psychiatric symptoms or criteria for establishing psychiatric disorder; selecting a measure based on the distinct symptom cluster of interest; and use of a measure that, if possible, has been validated with and provides clinical cut-off scores for HIV-positive samples. Assessment with HIV-positive minorities requires that the clinician considers these factors as well as factors that may be relevant to people from diverse backgrounds such as socioeconomic status, education level, language ability and literacy, prior experience with testing, and degree of understanding of the implicit expectations inherent in completing assessments.

A limited amount of information is available on the effectiveness of evidence-based interventions within diverse HIV-positive patients, as the majority of clinical intervention research has been conducted with HIV-positive White men (Crepaz et al., 2008). For example, a recent review of clinical intervention research within HIV-positive Latinos found only one published study (Gonzalez, Hendriksen, Collins, Duran, & Safren, 2009). Examples of culturally adapted CBT are available with HIV-positive Latinos (e.g., Van Servellen et al., 2005; Durán, Stoelb, Bedoya, Antoni, & Schneiderman, 2006) and African Americans (e.g., Harris et al., 1998; Markowitz, Spielman, Sullivan, & Fishman, 2000). These examples can provide an aid to identify possible aspects of treatment that may be beneficial or counter-indicated when working with HIV-positive minorities as they are in line with recommendations for clinical practice with diverse groups in general (Hays & Iwamasa, 2006) and chronically ill minority groups in particular (Kato & Mann, 1996). Clinicians should consider whether patients' view of their symptoms, expectations of mental health care, and ability to participate in treatment are impacted by factors, such as race, ethnicity, gender, sexual orientation, socioeconomic status, language ability, and spiritual/religious beliefs. When working with HIV-positive patients in particular, clinicians can assess the patient's experience with negative life experiences (i.e., discrimination, stigma, trauma history) and possible consequences of this on the patient's view of self, as well as to assess for patient's strengths and resources. Patients may also benefit from interventions that are flexible and, as appropriate, inclusive of cultural values.

6.7 Conclusions

In summary, clinicians working with HIV-positive populations can expect to see relatively high rates of psychological co-morbidities, particularly PTSD and major depressive disorder. However, even in the absence of an anxiety or depressive disorder, persons living with HIV may experience significant distress related to stigma, economic challenges, or disease management. Clinicians caring for individuals living with HIV should carefully assess for both psychopathology and subthreshold symptoms of psychopathology using assessment tools that are validated in chronic illness populations. There are numerous treatment options (both pharmacologic and nonpharmacologic) available for many of the psychological co-morbidities reviewed in this chapter. Although psychotropic medications are indicated in some cases, clinicians may also consider skills-based psychosocial treatments. Some psychosocial treatments have documented efficacy in decreasing symptoms of anxiety and depression, and in some cases, improving adherence to life-saving antiretroviral therapy. Psychosocial treatments for anxiety and depression have particular importance in HIV because many patients prefer not to take additional medications to treat their symptoms and some psychotropic medications can be contraindicated with some antiretrovirals. While questions remain, great strides have been made over the past decade with respect to the mental health needs of those living with HIV. Treatment for HIV continues to evolve and improve, and individuals with HIV can now look forward to living longer and healthier lives. Thus, additional research into the prevalence, epidemiology, assessment, and treatment of psychological co-morbidities impacting those with HIV will be required to optimize the well-being and quality of life for these individuals.

Acknowledgments Some of the time used to create this manuscripts has supported by the Harvard University Center for AIDS Research (CFAR), an NIH funded program (P30AI060354), which is supported by the following NIH Institutes and Centers: NIAID, NCI, NIMH, NIDA, NICHD, NHLBI, NCCAM (awarded to Dr. Christina Psaros) and by NIMH grant 1R01MH084757-01A1 (awarded to Dr. Steven A. Safren).

References

Adam, B. D., Husbands, W., Murray, J., & Maxwell, J. (2005). AIDS optimism, condom fatigue, or self-esteem? Explaining unsafe sex among gay and bisexual men. *Journal of Sex Research, 42*, 238–248.

Aidala, A., Havens, J., Mellins, C. A., Dodds, S., Whetten, K., Martin, D., et al. (2004). Development and validation of the client diagnostic questionnaire (CDQ): A mental health screening tool for use in HIV/AIDS service settings. *Psychology, Health & Medicine, 9*, 362–379.

Ammassari, A., Trotta, M. P., Murri, R., Castelli, F., Narciso, P., Noto, P., et al. (2002). Corrolates and predictors of adherence to highly active antiretroviral therapy: Over view of published literature. *Journal of Acquired Immune Deficiency Syndromes, 31*(Suppl. 3), S123–S127.cbr.

Arnsten, J. H., Demas, P. A., Farzadegan, H., Grant, R. W., Gourevitch, M. N., Chang, C. J., et al. (2001). Antiretroviral therapy adherence and viral suppression in HIV-infected drug users: Comparison of self-report and electronic monitoring. *Clinical Infectious Diseases, 33*, 1417–1423.

Arreola, S. G., Neilands, T. B., & Diaz, R. (2009). Childhood sexual abuse and the sociocultural context of sexual risk among adult latino gay and bisexual men. *American Journal of Public Health, 99*, S432–S438.

Aruffo, J. F., Coverdale, J. H., Chacko, R. C., & Dworkin, R. J. (1990). Knowledge about AIDS among women psychiatric outpatients. *Hospital & Community Psychiatry, 41*, 326–328.

Asboe, D., Catalan, J., Mandalia, S., Dedes, N., Florence, E., Schrooten, W., et al. (2007). Sexual dysfunction in HIV-positive men is multi-factorial: A study of prevalence and associated factors. *AIDS Care, 19*, 955–965.

Asch, S. M., Kilbourne, A. M., Gifford, A. L., Burnam, M. A., Turner, B., Shapiro, M. F., et al. (2003). Underdiagnosis of depression in HIV: Who are we missing? *Journal of General Internal Medicine, 18*, 450–460.

Atkinson, J. H., & Grant, I. (1994). Natural history of neuropsychiatric manifestations of HIV disease. *The Psychiatric Clinics of North America, 17*, 17–33.

Atkinson, J. H., Heaton, R. K., Patterson, T. L., Wolfson, T., Deutsch, R., Brown, S. J., et al. (2008). Two-year prospective study of major depressive disorder in HIV-infected men. *Journal of Affective Disorders, 108*, 225–234.

Baillargeon, J. G., Paar, D. P., Wu, H., Giordano, T. P., Murray, O., Raimer, B. G., et al. (2008). Psychiatric disorders, HIV infection and HIV/hepatitis co-infection in the correctional setting. *AIDS Care, 20*, 124–129.

Bair, M. J., Robinson, R. L., Katon, W., & Kroenke, K. (2003). Depression and pain comorbidity: a literature review. *Archives of Internal Medicine, 163*(20), 2433–2475.

Beck, A. T., Brown, G., & Steer, R. A. (1996). *Beck depression inventory II manual*. San Antonio: The Psychological Corporation.

Beck, A. T., Ward, C. H., Mendelson, M., Mock, J., & Erbaugh, J. (1961). An inventory for measuring depression. *Archives of General Psychiatry, 4*, 561–571.

Bensalem, M. K., & Berger, J. R. (2002). HIV and the central nervous system. *Comprehensive Therapy, 28*, 23–33.

Berg, K. M., Cooperman, N. A., Newville, H., & Arnsten, J. H. (2009). Self-efficacy and depression as mediators of the relationship between pain and antiretroviral adherence. *AIDS Care, 21*, 244–248.

Berg, C. J., Michelson, S. E., & Safren, S. A. (2007). Behavioral aspects of HIV care: Adherence, depression, substance use, and HIV-transmission behaviors. *Infectious Disease Clinics of North America, 21*, 181–200.

Berg, M. B., Mimiaga, M. J., & Safren, S. A. (2004). Mental health concerns of HIV-infected gay and bisexual men seeking mental health services: An observational study. *AIDS Patient Care and STDs, 18*, 635–643.

Beyer, J. L., Taylor, L. T., Gersing, K. R., & Krishnan, R. R. (2007). Prevalence of HIV infection in a general psychiatric outpatient population. *Psychosomatics, 48*, 31–37.

Bing, E. G., Burnam, M. A., Longshore, D., Fleishman, J. A., Sherbourne, C. D., London, A. S., et al. (2001). Psychiatric disorders and drug use among human immunodeficiency virus–infected adults in the United States. *Archives of General Psychiatry, 58*, 721–728.

Blank, M. B., Mandell, D. S., Aiken, L., & Hadley, T. R. (2002). Co-occurence of HIV and serious mental illness among Medicaid recipients. *Psychiatric Services, 53*, 868–873.

Boarts, J. M., Buckley-Fischer, B. A., Armelie, A. P., Bogart, L. M., & Delahanty, D. L. (2009). The impact of HIV diagnosis-related versus non-diagnosis related trauma on PTSD, depression, medication adherence, and HIV disease markers. *Journal of Evidence-Based Social Work, 6*, 4–16.

Boarts, J. M., Sledjeski, E. M., Bogart, L. M., & Delahanty, D. L. (2006). The differential impact of PTSD and depression on HIV disease markers and adherence to HAART in people living with HIV. *AIDS and Behavior, 10*, 253–261.

Bouhnik, A., Preau, M., Schiltz, M., Obadia, Y., Spire, B., & The VESPA study group. (2008). Sexual difficulties in people living with HIV in France – results from a large representative sample of outpatients attending French hospitals. *AIDS and Behavior, 12*, 670–676.

Brienza, R. S., Stein, M. D., Chen, M., Gogineni, A., Sobota, M., Maksad, J., et al. (2000). Depression among needle exchange program and methadone maintenance clients. *Journal of Substance Abuse Treatment, 18*, 331–337.

Brown, S., Mitler, M., & Atkinson, H. (1991). Correlation of subjective sleep complaints, absolute T-4 cell number and anxiety in HIV illness. *Sleep Research, 20*, 363.

Burak, J. H., Barrett, D. C., Stall, R. D., Chesney, M. A., Ekstrand, M. L., & Coates, T. J. (1993). Depressive symptoms and CD4 lymphocyte decline among HIV-infected men. *Journal of the American Medical Association, 270*, 2563–3575.

Buysee, D., Reynolds, C., Monk, T., Berman, S., & Kupfer, D. (1989). The Pittsburgh Sleep Qualtiy Index: A new instrument for psychiatric practice. *Psychiatry Research, 28*, 193–213.

Camacho, L. M., Brown, B. S., & Simpson, D. D. (1996). Psychological dysfunction and HIV/AIDS risk behavior. *Journal of Acquired Immune Deficiency Syndromes and Human Retrovirology, 11*, 198–202.

Catz, S. L., Kelly, J. A., Bogart, L. M., Benotsch, E. G., & McAuliffe, T. L. (2000). Patterns, correlates, and barriers to medication adherence among persons prescribed new treatments for HIV disease. *Health Psychology, 19*, 124–133.

CDC. (2008a). *HIV/AIDS among women. CDC HIV/AIDS Fact Sheet*. Retrieved November 17, 2009, from http://www.cdc.gov/hiv/topics/women/resources/factsheets/pdf/women.pdf.

CDC. (2008b). *HIV/AIDS among Hispanics/Latinos. CDC HIV/AIDS Fact Sheet*. Retrieved November 17, 2009, from http://www.cdc.gov/hiv/resources/factsheets/PDF/us.pdf.

CDC. (2009a). *HIV/AIDS Surveillance Report 2007*. Atlanta.

CDC. (2009b). *HIV-associated behaviors among injection-drug users – 23 cities, United States. Morbidity and Mortality Weekly Report*. Retrieved November 17, 2009, from http://www.cdc.gov/mmwr/preview/mmwrhtml/mm5813a1.html.

CDC. (2009c). *HIV/AIDS among African-Americans. CDC HIV/AIDS Fact Sheet*. Retrieved November 17, 2009, from http://www.cdc.gov/hiv/topics/aa/resources/factsheets/pdf/aa.pdf.

Ciesla, J. A., & Roberts, J. E. (2001). Meta-analysis of the relationship between HIV infection and risk for depressive disorders. *The American Journal of Psychiatry, 158*, 725–730.

Cohen, F. L., Ferran, C. E., Vizgirda, V., Kunkle, V., & Cloninger, L. (1996). Sleep in men and women infected with human immunodeficiency virus. *Holistic Nursing Practice, 10*, 33–43.

Cole, S. W., Kemeny, M. E., Fahey, J. L., Zack, J. A., & Naliboff, B. D. (2003). Psychological risk factors HIV pathogenesis: Mediation by the autonomic nervous system. *Biological Psychiatry, 54*, 1444–1456.

Cole, S. W., Korin, Y. D., Fahey, J. L., & Zack, J. A. (1998). Norepinephrine accelerates HIV replication via protein kinase a-dependent effects on Cytokine production. *The Journal of Immunology, 161*, 610–616.

Cole, S. W., Naliboff, B. D., Kemeny, M. E., Griswold, M. P., Fahey, J. L., & Zack, J. A. (2001). Impaired response to HAART in HIV-infected individuals with high autonomic nervous system activity. *Proceedings of the National Academy of Sciences, 98*, 12695–12700.

Collazos, J. (2007). Sexual dysfunction in the highly active antiretroviral therapy era. *AIDS Reviews, 9*, 237–245.

Cook, J. A., Grey, D., Burke, J., Cohen, M. H., Gurtman, A. C., Richardson, J. L., et al. (2004). Depressive symptoms and AIDS-related mortality among a multisite cohort of HIV-positive women. *American Journal of Public Health, 94*, 1133–1140.

Cournos, F., Guido, J. R., Coomaraswamy, S., Meyer-Bahlburg, H., Sugden, R., & Horwatch, E. (1994). Sexual activity and risk of HIV infection among patients with schizophrenia. *The American Journal of Psychiatry, 151*, 228–232.

Cournos, F., McKinnon, K., & Sullivan, G. (2005). Schizophrenia and comorbid human immunodeficiency virus or hepatitis C virus. *Journal of Clinical Psychiatry, 66*(Suppl. 6): 27–33.

Crepaz, N., & Marks, G. (2001). Are negative affective states associated with HIV sexual risk behaviors? A meta-analytic review. *Health Psychology, 20*, 291–299.

Crepaz, N., Passin, W. F., Herbst, J. H., Rama, S. M., Malow, R. M., Purcell, D. W., et al. (2008). Meta-analysis of cognitive behavioral interventions on HIV-positive persons' mental health and immune functioning. *Health Psychology, 27*, 4–14.

Cruess, D. G., Evans, D. L., Repetto, M. J., Gettes, D., Duoglas, S. D., & Petitto, J. M. (2003). Prevalence, diagnosis, and pharmacological treatment of mood disorders in HIV disease. *Biological Psychiatry, 54*, 307–316.

Daughters, S. B., Magidson, J. M., Schuster, R. M., & Safren, S. (2010). ACT HEALTHY: A combined cognitive-behavioral depression and medication adherence treatment for HIV-infected substance users. *Cognitive and Behavioral Practice, 17*, 309–321.

Davidson, K. M., & Ritson, E. B. (1993). The relationship between alcohol dependence and depression. *Alcohol and Alcoholism, 28*, 147–155.

De Hart, M., & Van Eyck, D. (2008). Prevalence of HIV and hepatitis C infection among patients with schizophrenia. *Schizophrenia Research, 108*, 307–308.

Delahanty, D. L., Bogart, L. M., & Figler, J. L. (2004). Posttraumatic stress disorder symptoms, salivary cortisol, medication adherence, and CD4 levels in HIV-positive individuals. *AIDS Care, 16*, 247–260.

Dew, M. A., Becker, J. T., Sanchez, J., Caldararo, R., Lopez, O. L., Wess, J., et al. (1997). Prevalence and predictors of depressive, anxiety, and substance use disorders in HIV-infected and uninfected men: A longitudinal evaluation. *Psychological Medicine, 27*, 395–409.

DiMatteo, M. R., Lepper, H. S., & Croghan, T. W. (2000). Depression is a risk factor for noncompliance with medical treatment: Meta-analysis of the effects of anxiety and depression on patient adherence. *Archives of Internal Medicine, 160*, 2101–2107.

Dixit, A. R., & Crum, R. M. (2000). Prospective study of depression and the risk of heavy alcohol use in women. *The American Journal of Psychiatry, 157*, 751–758.

Dobalian, A., Tsao, J. C. I., & Duncan, R. (2004). Pain and the use of outpatient services among persons with HIV results from a nationally representative survey. *Medical Care, 42*, 129–138.
Dong, B. J. (1998). Efavirenz (DuPong Pharmaceuticals Co.). *IDrugs, 1*, 700–711.
Dreher, H. M. (2003). The effect of caffeine reduction on sleep quality and well-being in persons with HIV. *Journal of Psychosomatic Research, 54*, 191–198.
Durán, R., Stoelb, B., Bedoya, C. A., Antoni, M., & Schneiderman, N. (2006). *Adapting a manulaized group intervention for Spanish speaking adults living with HIV: El proyecto ARMESE.* Paper presented at the annual American Group Psychotherapy Association meeting, San Francisco.
Evans, S., Fishman, B., Spielman, L., & Haley, A. (2003). Randomized trial of cognitive behavioral therapy versus supportive psychotherapy for HIV-related peripheral neuropathic pain. *Psychosomatics, 44*, 44–50.
Folkman, S. (1993). Psychosocial effects of HIV infection. In L. Goldberger & S. Breznitz (Eds.), *Handbook of stress: Theoretical and clinical aspects* (pp. 658–681). New York: The Free Press.
Forstein, M., Cournos, F., Douaihy, A., Goodkin, K., Wainberg, M. L., & Wapenyi, K. H. (2006). *Guideline watch: Practice guideline for the treatment of patients with HIV/AIDS.* Arlington: American Psychiatric Association.
Fumaz, C. R., Tuldra, A., Ferrer, M. J., Paredes, R., Bonjoch, A., Toni, J., et al. (2002). Quality of life, emotional status, and adherence of HIV-1-infected patients treated with efavierenz versus protease inhibitor-containing regiments. *Journal of Acquired Immune Deficiency Syndromes, 29*, 244–253.
Giordano, T. P., Bartsch, G., Zhang, Y., Tedaldi, E., Absalon, J., Mannheimer, S., et al. (2010). Disparities and outcomes for African American and Latino subjects in the flexible initial retrovirus suppressive therapies (FIRST) trial. *AIDS Patient Care and STDs, 24*, 1–9.
Giordano, T. P., Gifford, A. L., White, A. C., Jr., Suarez-Almazor, M. E., Rabeneck, L., Hartman, C., et al. (2007). Retention in care: A challenge to survival with HIV infection. *Clinical Infectious Diseases, 44*, 1493–1499.
Gonzalez, J. S., Hendriksen, E. S., Collins, E. M., Duran, R. E., & Safren, S. A. (2009). Latinos and HIV/AIDS: Examining factors related to disparity and identifying opportunities for psychosocial intervention research. *AIDS and Behavior, 13*, 582–602.
Gordillo, V., del Amo, J., Soriano, V., & Gonzalez-Lahoz, J. (1999). Sociodemographic and psychological variables influencing adherence to antiretroviral therapy. *AIDS, 13*, 1763–1769.
Gottesman, I. I., & Groome, C. S. (1997). HIV/AIDS risks as a consequence of schizophrenia. *Schizophrenia Bulletin, 23*, 675–684.
Haller, D. L., & Miles, D. R. (2003). Suicidal ideation among psychiatric patients with HIV: Psychiatric morbidity and quality of life. *AIDS and Behavior, 7*, 101–108.
Harris, R. M., Bausell, R. B., Scott, D. E., Hetherington, S. E., & Kavanagh, K. H. (1998). An intervention for changing high-risk HIV behaviors of African American drug-dependent women. *Research in Nursing & Health, 21*, 239–250.
Hays, P. A., & Iwamasa, G. Y. (Eds.). (2006). *Culturally responsive cognitive-behavioral therapy: Assessment, practice, and supervision.* Washington: American Psychological Association.
Heiman, J. R. (2002). Sexual dysfunction: Overview of prevalence, etiological factors, and treatments. *Journal of Sex Research, 39*, 73–78.
Heinssen, R. K., Liberman, R. P., & Kopelwicz, A. (2000). Psychosocial skills training for schizophrenia: Lessons from the laboratory. *Schizophrenia Bulletin, 26*, 21–46.
Himelhoch, S., Josephs, J. S., Chandler, G., Korthuis, P. T., & Gebo, K. A. (2009). Use of outpatient mental health services and psychotropic medications among HIV-infected patients in a multisite, multistate study. *General Hospital Psychiatry, 31*, 538–545.
Himelhoch, S., McCarthy, J. F., Ganoczy, D., Medoff, D., Dixon, L. B., & Blow, F. C. (2007). Understanding associations between serious mental illness and HIV among patients in the VA health system. *Psychiatry Services, 58*, 1165–1172.
Holden, A. E. C., Shain, R. N., Miller, W. B., Piper, J. M., Perdue, S. T., Thurman, A. R., et al. (2008). The influence of depression on sexual risk reduction and STD infection in a controlled, randomized intervention trial. *Sexually Transmitted Diseases, 35*, 898–904.

Holzemer, W. L., Corless, I. B., Nokes, K. M., Turner, J. G., Brown, M. A., Powell-Cope, G. M., et al. (1999). Predictors of self-reported adherence in persons living with HIV disease. *AIDS Patient Care and STDs, 13*, 185–197.

Hutton, H. E., Treisman, G. J., Hunt, W. R., Fishman, M., Kendig, N., Swetz, A., et al. (2001). HIV risk behaviors and their relationship to posttraumatic stress disorder among women prisoners. *Psychiatric Services, 52*, 508–513.

Ickovics, J. R., Hamburger, M. E., Vlahov, D., Schoenbaum, E. E., Schuman, P., Boland, R. J., et al. (2001). Mortality, CD4 cell count decline, and depressive symptoms among HIV-seropositive women: Longitudinal analysis from the HIV Epidemiology Research Study. *Journal of the American Medical Association, 285*, 1460–1465.

Ingersoll, K. (2004). The impact of psychiatric symptoms, drug use, and medication regimen on non-adherence to HIV treatment. *AIDS Care, 16*, 199–211.

Ironson, G., Friedman, A., Klimas, N., Antoni, M., O'Hearn, P., Fletcher, M. A., et al. (1994). Distress, denial, and low adherence to behavioral interventions predict faster disease progression in gay men infected with human immunodeficiency virus. *International Journal of Behavioral Medicine, 1*, 90–105.

Ironson, G., O'Cleirigh, C., Fletcher, M. A., Laurenceau, J. P., Balbin, E., Klimas, N., et al. (2005). Psychosocial factors predict CD4 and viral load change in men and women with human immunodeficiency virus in the era of highly active antiretroviral treatment. *Psychosomatic Medicine, 67*, 1013–1021.

Ironson, G., O'Cleirigh, C., Kumar, M., Balbin, E., Schneiderman, N., & Fletcher, M. (2006). *Depression, Coping, and Neurohormonal Predictors of HIV Disease Progression over 4 years in a Diverse Sample*. Presented at XVI International AIDS Conference, Toronto.

Israelski, D. M., Prentiss, D. E., Lubega, S., Balmas, G., Garcia, P., & Muhammad, M. (2007). Psychiatric comorbidity in vulnerable populations receiving primary care for HIV/AIDS. *AIDS Care, 19*, 220–225.

Jones, E., Vermaas, R. H., McCartney, H., Beech, C., Palmer, I., Hyams, K., et al. (2003). Flashbacks and post-traumatic stress disorder: The genesis of a 20th-century diagnosis. *The British Journal of Psychiatry, 182*, 158–163.

Joyce, G. F., Chan, K. S., Orlando, M., & Burnam, M. A. (2005). Mental health status and use of general medical services for persons with human immunodeficiency virus. *Medical Care, 43*, 834–839.

Kalichman, S. C. (2000). HIV transmission risk behaviors of men and women living with HIV-AIDS: Prevalence, predictors, and emerging clinical interventions. *Clinical Psychology: Science and Practice, 7*, 32–47.

Kalichman, S. C., Kelly, J. A., Johnson, J. R., & Bulto, M. (1994). Factors associated with risk for HIV infection among chronic mentally ill adults. *The American Journal of Psychiatry, 151*, 221–227.

Kalichman, S. C., Kelly, J. A., & Rompa, D. (1997). Continued high-risk sex among HIV seropositive gay and bisexual men seeking HIV prevention services. *Health Psychology, 16*, 369–375.

Kalichman, S. C., Sikkema, K. J., Kelly, J. A., & Bulto, M. (1995). Use of a brief behavioral skills intervention to prevent HIV infection among chronic mentally ill adults. *Psychiatric Services, 46*, 275–280.

Kalichman, S. C., Sikkema, K. J., & Somlai, A. (1995). Assessing persons with human immunodeficiency virus (HIV) using the beck depression inventory: Disease processes and other potential confounds. *Journal of Personality Assessment, 64*, 86–100.

Kalichman, S. C., & Weinhardt, L. (2001). Negative affect and sexual risk behavior: Comment on Crepaz and Marks. *Health Psychology, 20*, 300–301.

Kato, P. M., & Mann, T. (Eds.). (1996). *Handbook of diversity issues in health psychology*. New York: Plenum Press.

Kelly, J. A., Murphy, D. A., Bahr, G. R., Kalichman, S. C., Morgan, M. G., Stevenson, L. Y., et al. (1993). Outcome of cognitive-behavioral and support group brief therapies for depressed, HIV-infected persons. *The American Journal of Psychiatry, 150*, 1679–1686.

Kelly, J. A., Murphy, D. A., Bahr, G. R., Koob, J. J., Morgan, M. G., Kalichman, S. C., et al. (1993). Factors associated with severity of depression and high-risk sexual behavior among persons diagnosed with human immunodeficiency virus infection. *Health Psychology, 12*, 215–219.

Kelly, B., Raphael, B., Judd, F., Perdices, M., Kernutt, G., Burnett, P., et al. (1998). Posttraumatic stress disorder in response to HIV infection. *General Hospital Psychiatry, 20*, 345–352.

Kemeny, M. E., & Dean, L. (1995). Effects of AIDS-related bereavement on HIV progression among New York City gay men. *AIDS Education and Prevention, 7*, 36–47.

Kennedy, C. A., Skurnick, J., Wan, J. Y., Quattrone, G., Sheffet, A., Quionenes, M., et al. (1993). Psychological distress, drug and alcohol use as correlates of condom use in HIV serodiscordant heterosexual couples. *AIDS, 7*, 1493–1499.

Kershaw, T., Small, M., Joseph, G., Theodore, M., Bateau, R., & Frederic, R. (2006). The influence of power on HIV risk among pregnant women in rural Haiti. *AIDS and Behavior, 10*, 309–318.

Kessler, R. C., Chiu, W. T., Demler, O., & Walters, E. E. (2005). Prevalence, severity, and comorbidity of 12-month DSM-IV disorders in the national comorbidity survey replication. *Archives of General Psychiatry, 62*, 617–627.

Kilbourne, A. M., Justice, A. C., Rabeneck, L., Rodriguez-Barradas, M., & Weissman, S. (2001). General medical and psychiatric comorbidity among HIV-infected veterans in the post-HAART era. *Journal of Clinical Epidemiology, 54*(Suppl. 1), S22–S28.

Kimberling, R., Armistead, L., & Forehand, R. (1999). Victimization experiences and HIV infection in women: Associations with serostatus, psychological symptoms, and health services. *Journal of Traumatic Stress, 12*, 41–58.

Kimberling, R., Calhoun, K. S., Forehand, R., Armistead, L., Morse, E., Morse, P., et al. (1999). Traumatic stress in HIV-infected women. *AIDS Education and Prevention, 11*, 321–330.

Klinkenberg, W. D., & Sacks, S. (2004). Mental disorders and drug abuse in persons living with HIV/AIDS. *AIDS Care, 16*, S22–S42.

Klitzman, R. L. (1999). Self-disclosure of HIV status to sexual partners: A qualitative study of issues faced by gay men. *Journal of Gay and Lesbian Medical Association, 3*, 39–49.

Knowlton, A. R., Latkin, C. A., Chung, S., Hoover, D. R., Ensminger, M., & Celentano, D. D. (2000). HIV and depressive symptoms among low-income illicit drug users. *AIDS and Behavior, 4*, 353–360.

Krefetz, D. G., Steer, R. A., Jermyn, R. T., & Condoluci, D. V. (2004). Screening HIV-infected patients with chronic pain for anxiety and mood disorders with the Beck Anxiety and Depression Inventory–fast screens for medical settings. *Journal of Clinical Psychology in Medical Settings, 11*, 283–289.

Lee, K. A., Gay, C., Portillo, C. J., Coggins, T., Davis, H., Pullinger, C. R., et al. (2009). Symptom experience in HIV-infected adults: A function of demographic and clinical characteristics. *Journal of Pain and Symptom Management, 38*, 882–893.

Lee, K. A., Portillo, C. J., & Miramontes, H. (2001). The influence of sleep and activity patterns on fatigue in women with HIV/AIDS. *The Journal of the Association of Nurses in AIDS Care, 12*(Suppl), 19–27.

Lehman, J. S., Hecht, F. M., Fleming, P. L., Coleman, S., Chesney, M., Bindman, A., et al. (1998). HIV testing behavior among at-risk populations: Why do persons seek, defer, or avoid getting tested in the United States? *International Conference on AIDS, 12*, 867.

Leserman, J., Jackson, E. D., Petitto, J. M., Golden, R. N., Silva, S. G., Perkins, D. O., et al. (1999). Progression to AIDS: The effects of stress, depressive symptoms, and social support. *Psychosomatic Medicine, 61*, 397–406.

Leserman, J., Petitto, J. M., Golden, R. N., Gaynes, B. N., Gu, H., Perkins, D. O., et al. (2000). The impact of stressful life events, depression, social support, coping, and cortisol on progression to AIDS. *The American Journal of Psychiatry, 157*, 1221–1228.

Leserman, J., Petitto, J. M., Gu, H., Gaynes, B. N., Barroso, J., Golden, R. N., et al. (2002). Progression to AIDS, a clinical AIDS condition and mortality: Psychosocial and physiological predictors. *Psychosomatic Medicine, 32*, 1059–1073.

Leserman, J., Petitto, J. M., Perkins, D. O., Folds, J. D., Golden, R. N., & Evans, D. L. (1997). Severe stress, depressive symptoms, and changes in lymphocyte subsets in human immunodeficiency virus-Infected men. *Archives of General Psychiatry, 54*, 279–285.

Leserman, J., Whetten, K., Lowe, K., Stangl, D., Swartz, M., & Theilman, N. (2005). How trauma, recent stressful events, and PTSD affect functional health and health utilization in HIV-infected patients in the South. *Psychosomatic Medicine, 67*, 500–507.

Leserman, J., Pence, B. W., Whetten, K., Mugavero, M. J., Thielman, N. M., Swartz, M. S., et al. (2007). Relation of lifetime trauma and depressive symptoms to mortalilty in HIV. *The American Journal of Psychiatry, 164*, 1707–1713.

Lewis, C. F. (2005). Post-traumatic stress disorder in HIV-positive incarcerated women. *The Journal of the American Academy of Psychiatry and the Law, 33*, 455–464.

Low-Beer, S., Yip, B., O'Shaughnessy, M. V., Hogg, R. S., & Montaner, J. S. (2000). Adherence to triple therapy and viral load response. *Journal of Acquired Immune Deficiency Syndromes, 23*, 360–361.

Lucenko, B., Malow, R., Sanchez-Martinez, M., Jennings, T., & Devieux, J. (2003). Negative affect and HIV risk in alcohol and other drug (AOD) abusing adolescent offenders. *Journal of Child & Adolescent Substance Abuse, 13*, 1–17.

Lyketsos, C. G., Hoover, D. R., Guccione, M., Senterfitt, W., Dew, M. A., Wesch, J., et al. (1993). Depressive symptoms as predictors of medical outcomes in HIV infection. Multicenter AIDS Cohort Study. *The Journal of the American Medical Association, 270*, 2563–2567.

Lyketsos, C. G., Hutton, H., Fishman, M., Schwartz, J., & Treisman, G. J. (1996). Psychiatric morbidity on entry to an HIV primary care clinic. *AIDS, 10*, 1033–1039.

Magnus, M., Jones, K., Phillips, G., Binson, D., Hightow-Wiedman, L. B., Richards-Clarke, C., et al. (2010). Characteristics associated with retention among African American and Latino adolescent HIV-positive men: Results from the outreach, care, and prevention to engage HIV-seropositive young MSM of color special projects of national significance initiative. *Journal of Acquired Immune Deficiency Syndromes, 53*, 529–536.

Maj, M., Satz, P., Janssen, R., Zaudig, M., Starace, F., D'Elia, L., et al. (1994). WHO neuropsychiatric AIDS study, cross sectional phase 1. Study design and psychiatric findings. *Archives of General Psychiatry, 51*, 39–49.

Malcolm, S. E., Ng, J. J., Rosen, R. K., & Stone, V. E. (2003). An examination of HIV/AIDS patients who have excellent adherence to HAART. *AIDS Care, 15*, 251–261.

Markowitz, J. C., Spielman, L. A., Sullivan, M., & Fishman, B. (2000). An exploratory study of ethnicity and psychotherapy outcome among HIV-positive patients with depressive symptoms. *The Journal of Psychotherapy Practice and Research, 9*, 226–231.

Martinez, A., Israelski, D., Walker, C., & Koopman, C. (2002). Posttraumatic stress disorder in women attending human immunodeficiency virus outpatient clinics. *AIDS Patient Care and STDs, 16*, 283–291.

Maruff, P., Wood, S., Currie, J., McArthur-Jackson, C., Malone, V., & Benson, E. (1994). Computer-administered visual analogue mood scales: Rapid and valid assessment of mood in HIV positive individuals. *Psychological Reports, 74*, 39–42.

Masilah, E., Achim, C. L., Ge, N., DeTeresa, R., Terry, R. D., & Wiley, C. A. (1992). Spectrum of human immunodeficiency virus – associated neocortical damage. *Annals of Nuerology, 32*, 321–329.

Mayne, T. J., Vittinghoff, E., Chesney, M. A., Barrett, D. C., & Coates, T. J. (1996). Depressive affect and survival among gay and bisexual men infected with HIV. *Archives of Internal Medicine, 156*, 2233–2238.

McClure, J. B., Catz, S. L., & Brantley, P. J. (1999). Early appointment adherence among persons living with HIV. *AIDS and Behavior, 3*, 157–165.

McKinnon, K., Cournos, F., Sugden, R., Guido, J. R., & Herman, R. (1996). The relative contributions of psychiatric symptoms and AIDS knowledge to HIV risk behaviors among people with severe mental illness. *The Journal of Clinical Psychiatry, 57*, 506–513.

McNair, P. M., Lorr, M., & Droppleman, L. F. (1981). *POMS manual* (2nd ed.). San Diego: Educational and Industrial Testing Service.

Melzack, R., & Torgenson, W. S. (1971). On the language of pain. *Anesthesiology, 34*, 50–59.

Moreno-Perez, O., Escoin, C., Serna-Candel, C., Pico, A., Alfayate, R., Merino, E., et al. (2010). Risk factors for sexual and erectile dysfunction in HIV-infected men: The role or protease inhibitors. *AIDS, 24*, 255–264.

Morrison, M. F., Petitto, J. M., Have, T. T., Gettes, D. R., Chiappini, M. S., Weber, A. L., et al. (2002). Depressive and anxiety disorders in women with HIV infection. *The American Journal of Psychiatry, 159*, 789–796.

Mugavero, M. J. (2008). Improving engagement in HIV care: What can we do? *Topics in HIV Medicine, 16*(5), 156–161.

Murray, J., & Adam, B. D. (2001). Aging, sexuality, and HIV issues among older gay men. *The Canadian Journal of Human Sexuality, 10*, 75–90.

Newcomb, M. D., & Carmona, J. V. (2004). Adult trauma and HIV status among Latinas: Effects upon psychological adjustment and substance use. *AIDS and Behavior, 8*, 417–428.

Nguyen, B. Y., & Reveille, J. D. (2009). Rheumatic manifestations assocated with HIV in the highly active antiretroviral therapy era. *Current Opinion in Rheumatology, 21*, 404–410.

Nimgaonkar, V. L., Ward, S. E., Agarde, H., Weston, N., & Ganguli, R. (1997). Fertility in schizophrenia: Results from a contemporary US cohort. *Acta Psychiatrica Scandinavica, 95*, 364–369.

Nokes, K. M., & Kendrew, J. (2001). Correlates of sleep quality in persons with HIV disease. *The Journal of the Association of Nurses in AIDS Care, 12*, 17–22.

Nunez, M., de Requena, D. G., Gallego, L., Jimenez-Nacher, I., Gonzalez-Lahoz, J., & Soriano, V. (2001). Higher efavirenz plasma levels correlate with development of insomnia. *Journal of Acquired Immune Deficiency Syndromes and Human Retrovirology, 28*, 399.

O'Cleirigh, C., Hart, T. A., & James, C. A. (2008). HIV and Anxiety. In M. J. Zvolensky & J. A. J. Smits (Eds.), *Health behaviors and physical illness in anxiety and its disorders: Contemporary theory and research*. New York: Springer.

O'Cleirigh, C., & Safren, S. A. (2008). Optimizing the effects of stress management interventions in HIV. *Health Psychology, 27*, 297–301.

O'Cleirigh, C., Skeer, M., Mayer, K. H., & Safren, S. A. (2009). Functional impairment and health care utilization among HIV-infected men who have sex with men: The relationship with depression and post-traumatic stress. *Journal of Behavioral Medicine, 36*, 466–477.

O'Donohue, W., Dopke, C. A., & Swingen, D. N. (1997). Psychotherapy for female sexual dysfunction: A review. *Clinical Psychology Review, 17*, 537–566.

O'Donohue, W., Swingen, D. N., Dopke, C. A., & Regev, L. G. (1999). Psychotherapy for male sexual dysfuction: A review. *Clinical Psychology Review, 19*, 591–630.

O'Leary, A., Purcell, D., Remien, R. H., & Gomez, C. (2003). Childhood sexual abuse and sexual transmission risk behavior among HIV-positive men who have sex with men. *AIDS Care, 15*, 17–26.

Ohmit, S., Schuman, P., Schoenbaum, E., Rompalo, A., Cohen, M., Richardson, J., et al. (1998). Adherence to antiretroviral therapy (ART) among women in the HIV Epidemiology Research Study (HERS) and Women's Inter-Agency HIV Study (WIHS). *International Conference on AIDS, 12*, 590.

Olatunji, B. O., Mimiaga, M. J., O'Cleirigh, C., & Safren, S. A. (2006). A review of treatment studies of depression in HIV. *Topics in HIV Medicine, 14*(3), 112–124.

Olley, B. O., Zeier, M. D., Seedat, S., & Stein, D. J. (2005). Post-traumatic stress disorder among recently diagnosed patients with HIV/AIDS in South Africa. *AIDS Care, 17*, 550–557.

Omonuwa, T. S., Goforth, H. W., Preud'homme, X., & Krystal, A. D. (2009). The pharmacologic management of insomnia in patients with HIV. *Journal of Clinical Sleep Medicine, 5*, 251–262.

Orlando, M., Burnam, A. M., Beckman, R., Morton, S. C., London, A. S., Bing, E. G., et al. (2002). Re-estimating the prevalence of psychiatric disorders in a nationally representative sample of persons receiving care for HIV: Results from the HIV costs and services utilization study. *International Journal of Methods in Psychiatric Research, 11*, 75–82.

Orlando, M., Burnam, M. A., Sherbourne, C. D., Morton, S. A., London, A. S., Hays, R. D., et al. (2001). Brief screening of psychiatric disorders among a national sample of HIV-positive adults: Concordance between the composite international diagnostic interview (CIDI) and CIDI short form (CIDI-SF). *International Journal of Methods in Psychiatric Research, 10*, 97–107.

Page-Shafer, K., Delorenze, G. N., Satariano, W., & Winkelstein, W., Jr. (1996). Comorbidity and survival in HIV infected men in the San Francisco Men's Health Survey. *Annals of Epidemiology, 6*, 420–430.

Panel on Antiretroviral Guidelines for Adults and Adolescents. (2011). *Guidelines for the use of antiretroviral agents in HIV-1-infected adults and adolescents. Department of Health and Human Services*. December 1, 2009; 1–174. Updated version available at http://www.aidsinfo.nih.gov/ContentFiles/AdultandAdolescentGL.pdf. Accessed July 22, 2011.

Patterson, T. L., Shaw, W. S., Semple, S. J., Cherner, M., McCutchan, A., Atkinson, J. H., et al. (1996). Relationship of psychosocial factors to HIV disease progression. *Annals of Behavioral Medicine, 18*, 30–39.

Patterson, D. L., Swindells, S., Mohr, J., Vergis, E. N., Squire, C., Wagener, M. M., et al. (2000). Adherence to protease inhibitor therapy and outcomes in patients with HIV infection. *Annals of Internal Medicine, 133*, 21–30.

Patterson, K., Young, C., Woods, S. P., Vigil, O., Grant, I., Atkinson, J. H., et al. (2006). Screening for major depression in person with HIV infection: The concurrent predictive validity of the profile of mood states depression-dejection scale. *International Journal of Methods in Psychiatric Research, 15*, 75–82.

Pearce, B. D. (2003). *Can a virus cause schizophrenia? Facts and hypotheses*. Boston: Kluwer.

Pence, B. W., Miller, W. C., Gaynes, B. N., & Eron, J. J. (2007). Psychiatric illness and virologic response in patients initiating highly active antiretroviral therapy. *Journal of Acquired Immune Deficiency Syndromes, 44*, 159–166.

Pence, B. W., Miller, W. C., Whetten, K., Eron, J. J., & Gaynes, B. N. (2006). Prevalence of DSM-IV– defined mood, anxiety, and substance use disorders in an HIV clinic in the southeastern United States. *Journal of Acquired Immune Deficiency Syndromes, 42*, 298–306.

Perkins, D. O., Leserman, J., Stern, R. A., Baum, S. F., Liao, D., Golden, R. N., et al. (1995). Somatic symptoms and HIV infection: Relationship to depressive symptoms and indicators of HIV disease. *The American Journal of Psychiatry, 152*, 1776–1781.

Phillips, K. D. (1996). *Development of an instrument to measure current sleep quality*. Unpublished manuscript, University of South Carolina.

Phillips, K. D., & Skelton, W. D. (2001). Effects of individualized acupuncture on sleep quality in HIV disease. *The Journal of the Association of Nurses in AIDS Care, 12*, 27–39.

Piscitelli, S. C. (2000). *Antiretroviral pharmacology: Issues and management. The Body: The Complete HIV/AIDS Resouce*. Retrieved May 11, 2010, from http://www.thebody.com/content/art2574/html.

Purcell, D. W., Malow, R. M., Dolezal, C., & Carballo-Dieguez, A. (2004). Sexual abuse of boys: Short- and long-term associations and implications for HIV prevention. In L. J. Koenig, L. S. Doll, A. O'Leary, & W. Pequegnat (Eds.), *From child sexual abuse to adult sexual risk: Trauma, revictimization, and intervention* (pp. 93–114). Washington: American Psychological Association.

Rabkin, J. G. (1996). Prevalence of psychiatric disorders in HIV illness. *International Review of Psychiatry, 8*, 157–166.

Rabkin, J. G., Williams, J. B. W., Remien, R. H., Goetz, R., Kertzner, R., & Gorman, J. M. (1991). Depression, distress, lymphocyte subsets, and human immunodeficiency virus symptoms on two occasions in HIV positive homosexual men. *Archives of General Psychiatry, 48*, 111–119.

Regier, D. A., Narrow, W. E., Rae, D. S., Manderscheid, R. W., Locke, B. Z., & Goodwin, F. K. (1993). The de facto mental and addictive disorders service system. Epidemiologic Catchment Area prospective 1-year prevalence rates of disorders and services. *Archives of General Psychiatry, 50*(2), 85–94.

Reid, S., & Dwyer, J. (2005). Insomnia in HIV infection: A systematic review of prevalence, correlates, and management. *Psychosomatic Medicine, 67*, 260–269.

Reisner, S. L., Mimiaga, M. J., Skeer, M., Bright, D., Cranston, K., Isenberg, D., et al. (2009). Clinically significant depressive symptoms as a risk factor for HIV infection among black MSM in Massachusetts. *AIDS and Behavior, 13*, 798–810.

Ritsner, M., Sherina, O., & Ginath, Y. (1992). Genetic epidemiological study of schizophrenia: Reproduction behavior. *Acta Psychiatrica Scandinavica, 85*, 423–429.

Robins, L. N., & Regier, D. A. (1991). *Psychiatric disorders in America – The Epidemiologic Catchment Area Study*. New York: Free Press.

Rosenberger, P. H., Bornstein, R. A., Nasrallah, H. A., Para, M. F., Whitaker, C. C., Fass, R. J., et al. (1993). Psychopathology in human immunodeficiency virus infection: Lifetime and current assessment. *Comprehensive Psychiatry, 34*, 150–158.

Rosenfeld, B., Breitbart, W., McDonald, M. V., Passik, S. D., Thaler, H., & Portenoy, R. K., (1996). Pain in ambulatory AIDS patients II: Impact of pain on psychological functioning and quality of life. *Pain, 68*(2–3), 323–328.

Rubenstein, M. L., & Selwyn, P. A. (1998). High prevalence of insomnia in an out-patient population with HIV infection. *Journal of Acquired Immune Deficiency Syndromes and Human Retrovirology, 19*, 260–265.

Safren, S. A., Gershuny, B. S., & Hendriksen, E. S. (2003). Symptoms of post traumatic stress and death anxiety in persons with human immunodeficiency virus and medication adherence difficulties. *AIDS Patient Care and STDs, 17*, 657–664.

Safren, S. A., Gonzalez, J. S., & Soroudi, N. (2008). *Coping with chronic illness: A cognitive-behavioral approach for adherence and depression*. New York: Oxford University Press.

Safren, S. A., O'Cleirigh, C., Tan, J. Y., Raminani, S. R., Reilly, L. C., Otto, M. W., et al. (2009). A randomized controlled trial of cognitive behavioral therapy for adherence and depression (CBT-AD) in HIV-infected individuals. *Health Psychology, 28*, 1–10.

Safren, S. A., Otto, M. W., & Worth, J. (1999). Life-Steps: Applying cognitive-behavioral therapy to patient adherence to HIV medication treatment. *Cognitive and Behavioral Practice, 6*, 332–341.

Safren, S. A., Radomsky, A. S., Otto, M. W., & Salomon, E. (2002). Predictors of psychological well-being in a diverse sample of HIV-positive patients on highly active antiretroviral therapy. *Psychosomatics, 43*, 478–485.

Savard, R., Laberge, B., Gauthier, J. G., & Bergeron, M. G. (1999). Screening clinical depression in HIV-seropositive patients using the hospital anxiety and depression scale. *AIDS and Behavior, 3*, 167–175.

Schneiderman, N., Ironson, G., & Siegel, S. (2005). Stress and health: Psychological, behavioral, and biological determinants. *Annual Review of Clinical Psychology, 1*, 607–628.

Schönnesson, L. N., Williams, M. L., Ross, M. W., Bratt, G., & Keel, B. (2006). Facotrs associated with suboptimal antiretroviral therapy adherence to dose, schedule, and dietary instructions. *AIDS and Behavior, 11*, 175–183.

Scott-Sheldon, L. A. J., Kalichman, S. C., Carey, M. P., & Fielder, R. L. (2008). Stress management interventions for HIV+ adults: A meta-analysis of randomized controlled trials, 1989 to 2006. *Health Psychology, 27*, 129–139.

Sewell, D. D. (1996). Schizophrenia and HIV. *Schizophrenia Bulletin, 22*, 465–473.

Sewell, M. C., Goggin, K. J., Rabkin, J. G., Ferrando, S. J., McElhiney, M. C., & Evans, S. (2000). Anxiety syndromes and symptoms among men with AIDS: A longitudinal controlled study. *Psychosomatics, 41*, 294–300.

Sherbourne, C. D., Hays, R. D., Fleishman, J. A., Vitiello, B., Magruder, K. M., Bing, E. G., et al. (2000). Impact of psychiatric conditions on health-related quality of life in persons with HIV infection. *The American Journal of Psychiatry, 157*, 248–254.

Siegel, K., & Schrimshaw, E. W. (2003). Reasons for adopting celibacy among older men and women living with HIV/AIDS. *Journal of Sex Research, 40*, 189–200.

Simoni, J. M., Frick, P. A., Pantalone, D. W., & Turner, B. J. (2003). Antiretroivral adherence interventions: A review of current literature and ongoing studies. *Topics in HIV Medicine, 11*(6), 185–198.

Simoni, J. M., & Ng, M. T. (2002). Abuse, health locus of control, and perceived health among HIV-positive women. *Health Psychology, 21*, 89–93.

Singh, N., Squier, C., Sivek, C., Wagener, M., Nguyen, M. H., & Yu, V. L. (1996). Determinants of compliance with antiretroviral therapy in patients with human immunodeficiency virus: Prospective assessment with implications for enhancing compliance. *AIDS Care, 10*, 1033–1039.

Sledjeski, E. M., Delahanty, D. L., & Bogart, L. M. (2005). Incidence and impact of posttraumatic stress disorder and comorbid depression on adherence to HAART and CD4+ counts in people living with HIV. *AIDS Patient Care and STDs, 19*, 728–736.

Smith, M. Y., Egert, J., Winkel, G., & Jacobson, J. (2002). The impact of PTSD on pain experience in persons with HIV/AIDS. *Pain, 98*, 9–17.

Smith, D. K., Leve, L. D., & Chamberlain, P. (2006). Adolescent girls' offending and health-risking sexual behavior: The predictive role of trauma. *Child Maltreatment, 11*, 346–353.

Substance Abuse and Mental Health Services Association. (2002). *Results from the 2001 National Household Survey on Drug Abuse: Volume I. Summary of National Findings*. Retrieved November, 17, 2009, from http://www.oas.samhsa.gov/nhsda/2k1nhsda/PDF/01SOFfrontmatter_W.pdf.

Tedstone, J. E., & Tarrier, N. (2003). Posttraumatic stress disorder following medical illness and treatment. *Clinical Psychology Review, 23*, 409–448.

Trotta, M. P., Ammassari, A., Murri, R., Marconi, P., Zaccarelli, M., Cozzi-Lepri, A., et al. (2008). Self-reported sexual dysfunction is frequent among HIV-infected persons and is associated with suboptimal adherence to antiretrovirals. *AIDS Patient Care and STDs, 22*, 291–299.

Tsao, J. C. I., Dobalian, A., Moreau, C., & Dobalian, K. (2004). Stability of anxiety and depression in a national sample of adults with human immunodeficiency virus. *The Journal of Nervous and Mental Disease, 192*, 111–118.

Tsao, J. C. I., Dobalian, A., & Naliboff, B. D. (2004). Panic disorder and pain in a national sample of persons living with HIV. *Pain, 109*, 172–180.

Tucker, J. S., Burnam, A. M., Sherbourne, C. D., Kung, F., & Gifford, A. L. (2003). Substance use and mental health correlates of nonadherence to antiretroviral medications in a sample of patients with human immunodeficiency virus infection. *The American Journal of Medicine, 114*, 573–580.

Turner, B. J., Laine, C., Cosler, L., & Hauck, W. W. (2003). Relationship of gender, depression, and health care delivery with antiretroviral adherence in HIV-infected drug users. *Journal of General Internal Medicine, 18*, 248–257.

Turrina, C., Fiorazzo, A., Turano, A., Cacciani, P., Regini, C., Castelli, F., et al. (2001). Depressive disorders and personality variables in HIV positive and negative intravenous drug-users. *Journal of Affective Disorders, 65*, 45–53.

Van Servellen, G., Chang, B., Garcia, L., & Lombardi, E. (2002). Individual and system level factors associated with treatment nonadherence in human immunodeficiency-infected men and women. *AIDS Patient Care and STDs, 16*, 269–281.

Van Servellen, G., Nyamathi, A., Carpio, F., Pearce, D., Garcia-Teague, L., Herrera, G., et al. (2005). Effects of a treatment adherence enhancement program on health literacy, patient-provider relationships and adherence to HAART among low-income HIV-positive Spanish-speaking Latinos. *AIDS Patient Care and STDs, 19*, 745–759.

Vedhara, K., Nott, K. H., Bradbeer, C. S., Davidson, E. A., Ong, E. L., Snow, M. H., et al. (1997). Greater emotional distress is associated with accelerated CD4+ cell decline in HIV infection. *Journal of Psychosomatic Research, 42*, 379–390.

Verma, S., Estanislao, L., & Simpson, D. (2005). HIV-associated neuropathic pain epidemiology, Pathophysiology and management. *CNS Drugs, 19*, 325–334.

Vitiello, B., Burnman, M. A., Bing, E. G., Beckman, R., & Shapiro, M. F. (2003). Use of psychotropic medications among HIV-infected patients in the United States. *The American Journal of Psychiatry, 160*, 547–554.

Vosvick, M., Gore-Felton, C., Ashton, E., Koopman, C., Fluery, T., Israelski, D., et al. (2004). Sleep disturbance among HIV-positive adults the role of pain, stress, and social support. *Journal of Psychosomatic Research, 57*, 459–463.

Vranceanu, A. M., Safren, S. A., Lu, M., Coady, W. M., Skolnik, P. R., Rogers, W. H., et al. (2008). The relationship of post-traumatic stress disorder and depression to antiretroviral medication adherence in persons with HIV. *AIDS Patient Care and STDs, 22*, 313–321.

Walker, U. A., Tyndall, A., & Daikeler, T. (2008). Rheumatic conditions in human immunodeficiency virus infection. *Rheumatology, 47*, 952–959.

Walkup, J., Crystal, S., & Sambamoorthi, U. (1999). Schizophrenia and major affective disorder among Medicaid recipients with HIV/AIDS in New Jersey. *American Journal of Public Health, 89*, 1101–1103.

Weaver, M. R., Conover, C. J., Proescholdbell, R. J., Arno, P. S., Ang, A., Ettner, S. L., et al. (2008). Utilization of mental health and substance abuse care for people living with HIV/AIDS, chronic mental illness, and substance abuse disorders. *Journal of Acquired Immune Deficiency Syndromes, 47*, 449–458.

Whetten, K., Leserman, J., Lowe, K., Stangl, D., Thielman, N., Swartz, M., et al. (2006). Prevalence of childhood sexual abuse and physical trauma in an HIV-positive sample from the deep south. *American Journal of Public Health, 96*, 1028–1030.

Wilkins, J. W., Hamby, S. L., Robertson, K. R., Seillier-Moiseiwitsch, F., Knorr, K. L., Barry, N. S., et al. (1995). The Profile of Mood States as a screening test for major depression in HIV+ patients. *Assessment, 2*, 181–188.

Williams, C. T., & Latkin, C. A. (2005). The role of depressive symptoms in predicting sex with multiple high-risk partners. *Journal of Acquired Immune Deficiency Syndromes, 38*, 69–73.

Wingood, G. M., DiClemente, R. J., Mikhail, I., McCree, D. H., Davies, S. L., Hardin, J. W., et al. (2007). HIV discrimination and the health of women living with HIV. *Women & Health, 46*, 99–112.

Wulff, E. A., Wang, A. K., & Simpson, D. M. (2000). HIV-associated peripheral neuropathy: Epidemiology, pathophysiology, and treatment. *Drugs, 59*, 1251–1260.

Zigmond, A. S., & Snaith, R. P. (1983). The hospital anxiety and depression scale. *Acta Psychiatrica Scandinavica, 67*, 361–370.

Zorrilla, E. P., McKay, J. R., Luborsky, L., & Schmidt, K. (1996). Relation of stressors and depressive symptoms to clinical progression of viral illness. *The American Journal of Psychiatry, 153*, 626–635.

Chapter 7
Psychological Co-morbidities in Patients with Pain

B. Van Dorsten and James N. Weisberg

7.1 Introduction: The Biopsychosocial Nature of Pain

Chronic pain is one of the most common, disabling, and expensive medical conditions in the world. A host of epidemiological studies report that approximately 15% of US adults report experiencing chronic pain each year (Andersson, 1999) and a lifetime prevalence of back pain in nearly 80% of adults (Lanes et al., 1995). Gatchel and Turk (1996) estimated that 80% of all physician visits are for the complaint of pain, and physical symptoms such as pain are the leading reason that patients seek medical care (Komaroff, 1990; Kroenke, 2001). In 2007, nearly 12% of US adults reported having back pain and medical spending for back pain assessment and treatment alone exceeded $30 billion in that year (Soni, 2010). Over one third of primary care visits in the United States are for the primary complaint of pain (Upshur, Luckmann, & Savageau, 2006), consistent with wide-ranging epidemiological estimates from 5 to 55% of the adult US population.

The most commonly used definition of pain is that proposed by Merskey and Bogduk (1994) and endorsed by the International Association for the Study of Pain: "an unpleasant sensory and emotional experience associated with actual or potential tissue damage, or described in terms of such damage." This definition recognizes pain as a multifactorial construct whose expression may be influenced by a host of anatomical, physiological, and psychosocial factors (Loeser & Melzack, 1999). Historically, the biologic or medical model of pain embraced a

B. Van Dorsten (✉)
Department of Physical Medicine and Rehabilitation, F-493,
University of Colorado School of Medicine, 1635 Aurora Court, Aurora, CO 80045, USA
e-mail: brent.vandorsten@ucdenver.edu

S. Pagoto (ed.), *Psychological Co-morbidities of Physical Illness: A Behavioral Medicine Perspective*, DOI 10.1007/978-1-4419-0029-6_7,

dualistic understanding of the mind and body as functionally distinct entities. For centuries, pain models followed traditional disease models, represented by a Cartesian dualistic view that mind and body were distinct and did not interact. This view adopted the premise that the symptom of pain represented a correlating tissue injury that could be identified and eradicated, but the philosophical and empirical limitations of the dualistic model yielded to recognition and acceptance that psychological and social factors could influence the course of pain (Gatchel, Peng, Fuchs, Peters, & Turk, 2007). The strict illness model has generally been replaced by the biopsychosocial model of pain (Engel, 1977) which equally considers biological, social, and psychological factors as potential contributors to the etiology, maintenance, and presentation of pain (Gatchel & Okifuji, 2006; Turk & Flor, 1999).

Conceptualizing pain as a biopsychosocial phenomenon obviates the need for a biopsychosocial treatment approach, which encourages patients to focus on self-management and functional improvement over complete pain alleviation (Bruns & Disorbio, 2009; Gatchel et al., 2007; Turk & Okifuji, 2002; Van Dorsten, 2006). The biopsychosocial model of pain management has the strongest empirical support for long-term patient benefits (Ojifuji, Turk, & Kalauokalani, 1999). Physicians appear in increasing agreement with the parameters of multidisciplinary treatment of pain as evidenced by survey results reported by Berman, Bausell, & Lee (2000). The authors surveyed 362 physicians specializing in pain management regarding which of 22 non-pharmacological adjuvant treatment strategies they considered to be "legitimate" treatments for patients with pain. Results indicated strong recognition and support for a host of psychosocial approaches and interventions including counseling (81%), biofeedback (83%), behavioral medicine (78%), relaxation instruction (61%), and hypnosis (64%). Results indicate widespread pain physician acceptance of psychosocial, cognitive, and behavioral strategies as adjuvant therapies in the management of pain.

Perhaps even more than for other medical conditions, psychosocial factors have been determined to strongly contribute to pain onset, severity, chronicity, and disability. Severe pain has been associated in the literature with a host of negative emotional conditions including depression, anxiety, and anger (McCracken, Faber, & Janeck, 1998; Pincus, Burton, Vogel, & Field, 2002; Van Dorsten, 2006; Wade, Price, Hamer, Schwartz, & Hart, 1990). den Boer et al. (2006) reported the results of a systematic review which identified depression, anxiety, somatization, pain, job dissatisfaction, and passive coping among the factors which predicted poor surgical outcome. Patients with psychological disorders have been shown to consistently use medical services more than those without (Barsky, Orav, & Bates, 2005; O'Donohue & Cucciare, 2005; Sansone, Sansone, & Wiederman, 1996), and approximately 20% of the population accounted for 88% of healthcare expenditures in 1998 (Ash, Zhao, Ellis, & Kramer, 2001). Naessens, Baird, Van Hourten, Vanness, and Campbell (2005) reported that only 2–3% of primary care patients accounted for more than 20% of all medical visits in 1997, and even minor psychological stressors increased medical visits by up to 50%.

7.2 Pain Epidemiology

Summarizing the aggregate of epidemiological studies published to date, as many as half of the general population of adults experience chronic pain at any given time (Gatchel et al., 2007). Torrence, Smith, Bennett, and Lee (2006) reported results of a survey of 6,000 UK family practice adult patients and indicated a 48% prevalence rate of any chronic pain, with 8% being reported having pain of neuropathic origin. Several additional large-scale population surveys have reported varying prevalence rates dependent upon pain type and assessment strategy. Between 5 and 55% of general population adults have been shown to acknowledge chronic widespread musculoskeletal pain depending upon survey methods and definitions of pain (Andersson, 1994; Hunt, Silman, & Benjamin, 1999). In a large literature review, Gran et al., (2003) estimated chronic widespread musculoskeletal pain in 10% of general population and the prevalence of fibromyalgia symptoms in 3–5% of the general population with a strong predominance in females. Elliott, Smith, Penny, Smith, and Chambers (1999) reported that 45.6% of 3,605 adult community residents surveyed reported chronic pain (e.g., present for at least 3 months), with low back and arthritis pain being the most common conditions cited. Walker (2000) conducted a systematic review of the pain epidemiology literature and reported a 12-month general population prevalence of low back pain between 22 and 65%. Most recently, Johannes, Le, Zhou, Johnston, and Dworkin (2010) conducted an internet-based survey of 27,035 US adults and reported a 30.7% point prevalence of chronic pain (34.3% for females, 26.7% for males). Half of respondents acknowledging pain reported daily pain and 32% estimated their pain as severe (e.g., ≥7 on a 0–10 point rating scale). These numbers compared similarly to a large population survey of Canadian adults which reported 29% of adults reporting chronic pain in the past year (Moulin, Clark, Speechley, & Morley-Foster, 2002).

7.3 Physician Challenges in Managing Patients with Pain

As will be delineated in several sections throughout this chapter, substantial obstacles are faced by physicians attempting to accurately assess and comprehensively treat the heterogeneous population of patients with pain. Several of these obstacles appear imbedded in the perspectives and biases of the physician population itself. Significant numbers of physicians in multiple specialties have admitted to opiophobia (e.g., prejudice against prescribing opioid medications for patients with pain), displayed lack of knowledge about pain treatment, and had negative views about patients with pain (Weinstein et al., 2000). Women are more likely than men to be inappropriately diagnosed and undertreated, more likely to receive sedatives than opioids, more discounted in their report of pain, and more likely to have pain complaints attributed to emotional factors (Cepeda & Carr, 2003; Hoffman & Tarzian, 2001). It has also been reported that physicians consistently underestimate pain intensity compared with patient ratings, and that physician experience was actually associated with greater underestimates (Marquie et al., 2003).

Physician education in pain might improve physician performance and confidence in managing pain. An abundance of literature confirms that pain is underassessed and undertreated in virtually all patient populations (Hirsch et al., 2009; Paquet, Kergoal, & Dube, 2005; Simmonds & Scudds, 2001), and this circumstance has prompted multiple calls for improvements in pain education for physicians (IOM, 2004; JCAHO, 2000; Peter & Watt-Watson, 2008). Given that pain is the principal reason for the majority of visits to a physician, it stands to reason that physicians should receive extensive educational training in the assessment and management of pain. However, prior published surveys of practicing physicians and those in training conclude that a majority believe their training in pain is inadequate (Cleeland, Cleeland, Dar, & Rinehardt, 1986; Sengstaken & King, 1994; Von Roenn, Cleeland, Gonin, Hatfield, & Pandya, 1993). Astonishingly, prior survey studies have shown that the average primary care physician receives less than 2 hours of residency instruction in pain management per year (Sengstaken & King, 1994; Van Dorsten et al., 2005). According to new newly released recommendations from the Institute of Medicine (2011; page 4–11), "The case for including comprehensive education about pain in medical education is powerful ... Pain treatment is an essential component of clinical practice. A variety of clinical practice guidelines are available to direct improvements in clinical practice (Bigos, Bowyer, & Braen, 1994), but survey evidence suggests that these guidelines have had minimal impact in improving care (Di Iorio, Henley, & Doughty, 2000; Jackson & Browning, 2005). Since up to 85% of patients presenting with back pain have no abnormal findings on diagnostic testing (Deyo, 1986), the opportunity for a multidisciplinary approach appears rich.

One of the principle initiatives in the past decade to improve pain assessment and treatment was the publication of new standards for pain assessment and treatment in JCAHO-accredited hospitals (Joint Commission on Accreditation of Healthcare Organizations, 2000). This initiative was intended to promote pain as the "5th vital sign" and make standardized pain assessment and treatment a component of the management of all chronic disease states. This initiative also appeared progressive in that it called for the inclusion of psychological assessments to be conducted in addition to patient histories and physical examination of complaints. Unfortunately, initial evidence suggests that this initiative has been unsuccessful in changing the effectiveness of pain assessment (Lucas, Vlahos, & Ledgerwood, 2007; Mularski et al., 2006). Mularski et al. (2006) conducted comprehensive chart reviews of 300 patient visits before and after the implementation of the "Pain as the 5th Vital Sign" initiative at a veteran's hospital. Despite the initiative's intent, the investigators found no significant improvements on any of seven quality of care indicators variably including provider assessment, pain examinations, medication changes in response to pain, and initiation of additional pain treatment. Despite this lack of initial inertia, it remains hopeful that consistent documentation of pain severity and treatment efforts, along with the standard incorporation of psychological assessment data, might vastly improve the management of pain for future populations.

7.4 Depression and Pain

Over the past several decades, depression has consistently been identified in the literature as perhaps the most frequent co-morbid condition in patients with chronic pain. Significant variability appears in estimated prevalence due to discrepant patient populations and means of assessing depression across studies (Bair, Robinson, Katon, & Kroenke, 2003; Romano & Turner, 1985). In an attempt to clarify prevalence of mood diagnoses in the US general population, Kessler, Berglund, et al. (2005) reported a reevaluation of results from the National Co-morbidity Survey Replication (Kessler et al., 2003) to determine both the lifetime and 12-month prevalence rates of US adults meeting a DSM-IV disorder. These estimates better allow us to adequately appreciate the magnitude of the prevalence of depressive disorders in patients with pain. Kessler, Berglund, et al. (2005) reported the lifetime prevalence rate of a US adult reporting symptoms meeting the DSM-IV criteria for an Axis I diagnosis to be 46.4%, and the lifetime prevalence of a depressive disorder at 20.8% with the bulk of this prevalence being accounted for by major depressive disorder (16.6%). Kessler, Wat Tat Chiu, Demler, and Walters (2005) authored an additional report of the 12-month prevalence of depression in this cohort of US adults at 9.5%. Comparing these community adult prevalence numbers with published literature for medical patients yields surprising findings. Decades of published prevalence rates of depression in patients with pain have suggested rates as high as 30–56%; widely variable again by patient population and assessment strategy (Bair et al., 2003; Reid et al., 2002; Romano & Turner, 1985). As such, general conclusion from this data supports that depression rates in patients experiencing pain may reach 2–3-fold the prevalence in community adults. Further, Bair et al. (2003) reported mean prevalence rates for concurrent depression in patients with pain dependent upon the treatment environment or specialty care clinics in which they were assessed. These authors reported depression prevalence rates of 52% for patients treated in pain clinics or inpatient pain programs; 56% for Orthopedic or Rheumatology clinics (i.e., excluding patients with fibromyalgia); 85% for facial pain patients treated in dental clinics, and 27% for patients in primary care clinics. The authors report that medically unexplained pain complaints were associated with higher levels of depression than pain of specific etiology.

7.4.1 Diagnosing Depression in Medical Patients

Despite evidence suggesting that depression is the third most common reason for patients to seek a primary care visit (Shah, 1992), primary care physician training has historically not been extensive as it relates to mood disorders and available literature suggests that primary care physicians accurately diagnose only 35–50% of major depressive disorder cases (Badger et al., 1994; Coyne, Schwenk, & Fechner-Bates, 1995; Gerber et al., 1989; Perez-Stable, Miranda, Munoz, & Ying, 1990; Von Korff, Shapiro, & Burke, 1987). Patients with depression typically present to primary medical providers with symptoms which include emotional and physical components including medically unexplained pain (Katon, Sullivan, & Walker, 2001). Bair et al. (2003) reported that 65% or more of patients with depression present with at least one pain complaint and as many as 75% of primary care patients with depression present to physicians with exclusively physical complaints (Kroenke, Jackson, & Chamberlin, 1997; Simon, Von Korff, Piccinelli, Fullerton, & Ormel, 1999). As a potential cue to physician providers, available data suggest that as the severity of pain and as the number of pain complaints increase, the probability of contributing depressive symptoms increases exponentially (Dworkin & Gitlin, 1991; Kroenke, Spitzer, & Williams, 1994). Primary care patients with two or more different pain complaints have been shown to be six times more likely to be depressed, while patients with three or more different pain complaints are eight times more likely to meet diagnostic criteria for depression (Katon & Sullivan, 1990). The proportion of depression-related physician visits increased from 50% in 1987 to 64% in 2001, with patients likely to approach primary care physicians for diagnosis and treatment more so than mental health specialists (Gaynes et al., 2007; Middleton, Gunnell, Whitley, Darling, & Fankel, 2001; Stafford, MacDonald, & Finkelstein, 2001). Even more difficult for the primary care physician or mental health specialist in differentiating complaints from a diagnostic standpoint is the high symptom concordance between major depressive disorders and many medical conditions. For example, there is high symptom concordance between medically diagnosable depression and many somatic illness variables including appetite or weight changes, poor sleep, lethargy, reduced libido, and decreased optimism or activity levels (American Psychiatric Association, 1994; Boyd & Weisman, 1986; Van Dorsten, 2006).

7.4.2 *Impact of Depression on Medical Treatment Outcome*

In accordance with the historical medical model of illness, there is an implicit assumption that eradicating a medical complaint would eliminate any associated psychological symptoms (Gatchel et al., 2007; Turk & Okifuji, 2002; Turk, Swanson, & Tunks, 2008). Often in the reality of medical care, the ultimate issue in mood disorders can be reduced to the relative impact of a mood condition on medical treatment outcome. The presence of depression is well substantiated in the pain treatment literature as posing a significant obstacle to achieving improvements in pain severity and functional outcomes. Across decades, depression has been empirically shown to adversely influence medical treatment outcome in multiple ways including impaired rehabilitation (Frank, Elliott, Corcoran, & Wonderlich, 1987), early treatment termination (Katon, Lin, & Kroenke, 2007; Painter, Seres, & Newman, 1980), decreased adherence with medications (Bane et al., 2006; Cramer & Rosenheck, 1998; DiMatteo, Lepper, & Croghan, 2000; Gehi, Haas, Pipkin, & Whooley, 2005), increased utilization of healthcare services (Barsky et al., 2005; Forrest & Wolkind, 1974), higher relapse following treatment

(Kerns & Haythornthwaite, 1988; Painter et al., 1980), and decreased return to work and higher unemployment rates (Dolce, Crocker, & Doleys, 1986; Sullivan, Reesor, Mikail, & Fisher, 1992). Depression has also been shown to associate with other unhealthy lifestyle behaviors including smoking, sexual dysfunction, less exercise, and alcohol use (Niles, Mori, Lambert, & Wolf, 2005).

Specific to the pain treatment literature, presence of depression has been associated with a variety of negative outcomes including increased number of pain complaints (Betrus, Elmore, & Hamilton, 1995), higher reported pain severity (Lamb, Guralnik, & Buchner, 2000; Wells, Golding, & Burnam, 1989), higher post-operative pain (Taenzer, Melzack, & Jeans, 1986), longer duration of pain (Burton, Tillotson, Main, & Hollus, 1995), and greater levels of functional limitation and disability (Dionne et al., 1997; Lamb et al., 2000). A curious finding in the depression and pain literature centers around the evidence that depressed chronic pain patients are more likely to be prescribed and use opioid medications than pain patients without depressive symptoms (Breckenridge & Clark, 2003; Reid et al., 2002; Sullivan, Edlund et al., 2005; Turk & Okifuji, 1997). These patients are also more likely to be prescribed opioid medications than antidepressant medications (Doan & Wadden, 1989). Sullivan, Edlund et al. (2005) reported that the presence of a common depressive or anxiety disorder increased the odds of receiving opioid medications by 3–6-fold, and increased report of emotional distress or worsening mental health status were associated with increased likelihood of opioid prescription for even acute worker compensation patients with acute low back pain (Stover et al., 2006). These authors reported that 53% of workers compensation patients with acute low back who reported emotional distress obtained opioids at their first physician visit. It may be considered that the clinical presentation of patients with both mood and pain disorders demonstrates greater levels of suffering leading to intervention, or that any of the myriad of factors discussed above regarding the presentation of these patients to physician providers influence treatment choice. Taken in aggregate, the available literature suggests that depression may pose the most significant threat to medical treatment outcome for patients with pain.

7.4.3 Reciprocal Improvements in Pain with Depression Treatment

Several studies have reported that pain severity is associated with poor depression treatment outcomes (Bair et al., 2004; Cherkin, Deyo, Street, & Barlow, 1996; Sullivan et al., 1992; Von Korff, Ormel, Katon, & Lin, 1992; Von Korff & Simon, 1996). Bair et al. (2003) summarized results of 22 studies investigating the effect of antidepressant medication therapy – 18 tricyclic antidepressants (TCA) in 18 studies, selective serotonin reuptake inhibitors (SSRI) in four studies – on pain and co-morbid depression. The authors reported that TCAs were associated with improvements in both pain and depression in the vast majority of studies (15 of 18), while efficacy of SSRIs in this circumstance remained unsettled. Kroenke et al. (2008) reported the results of a prospective randomized clinical trial of depression treatment in 405 patients with pain, Major Depressive Disorder, or Dysthymia. In this study, patients were randomized to intervention consisting of primary care physician visits plus telephone counseling providing strategies for depression management vs. usual care consisting of primary care physician visit only. Intervention patients received telephone calls from case managers 1 week after primary care visit, then monthly until this regimen could be faded if remission of depression symptoms was achieved. Depression case managers were supervised by psychiatrists and counseled patients with respect to overcoming barriers to adherence and adopting depression self-management strategies such as exercise or increasing social activities. Results indicated that pain severity was sufficient to produce at least moderate interference with daily activities for 42% of patients, and that pain modestly improved in both groups over 6 months (e.g., no group differences). Multivariate modeling controlling for age, gender, and medical co-morbidities indicated a significant improvement in depression severity in the collaborative care intervention group, but that depression severity increased with higher pain interference and decreased with passage of time for both groups.

Lin et al. (2003) reported modest improvement in pain severity and pain-related interference with daily activities with a similar counseling intervention in 1,001 adults with arthritis. In this study, patients were randomly assigned to either a 12-month intervention consisting of antidepressant therapy and/or (patient preference) 6–8 in-person or telephone counseling visits with a nurse case manager or to a usual care condition consisting of antidepressant therapy and referral to mental health care if deemed necessary. Case managers again provided counseling regarding regimen adherence, education, and strategies to increase adaptive behaviors. Main outcome measures were collected at baseline, and 3-, 6-, and 12-month intervals and variously included depression severity as measured by the Hopkins Symptom Checklist (Derogatis, Lipman, & Covi, 1973), pain severity, general health status, and interference with daily activities secondary to arthritis. Results indicated that the percentage of patients using antidepressant medications increased over the course of 12 months for both groups (e.g., 5% increase to 52% in usual care; 23% increase to 66% in intervention patients), while percent receiving counseling increased 9% to 16% in usual care versus a 39% increase to 47% in intervention patients. Forty-one percent of intervention patients achieved a 50% reduction in depression severity vs. 18% of usual care patients. At 12-month follow-up, intervention patients reported significant lower pain intensity and interference with activity due to pain than usual care patients. Authors concluded that benefits of improved depression care in patients with arthritis extended beyond mood improvements to include decreased pain and improved functional status. As is reported later in this chapter, cognitive-behavioral therapies designed to address pain and mood have been shown to be successful in improving both pain severity and emotional distress, while minimal data regarding the impact of anxiety treatment on pain severity or chronicity restricts conclusions regarding reciprocal affects.

7.5 Anxiety and Pain

While the bulk of literature published to date on mood and pain has focused exclusively on depression, comparatively less study has been done in the area of anxiety and pain. As in the previous section, the magnitude of the prevalence of anxiety disorders in patients with pain may be best appreciated by comparing it to that of the general US adult population.

7.5.1 Anxiety Prevalence

Within the National Co-morbidity Survey Study previously discussed, Kessler, Berglund, et al. (2005) reported a lifetime general population prevalence of 28.8% for any DSM-IV anxiety disorder with specific phobia (12.5%) and social phobia (12.1%) being most prevalent. Kessler, Wat Tat Chiu, et al. (2005) subsequently reported the 12-month prevalence of diagnostic anxiety disorders in this cohort of US adults at 18.1% – nearly twice the 12-month prevalence of depressive disorder. Comparing this community adult anxiety prevalence with published literature for medical patients again yields surprising results. Available literature estimates the prevalence of anxiety diagnoses in up to 49% in primary care patients (Gaynes et al., 2007), and as high as 20–62% in patients with pain (Atkinson, Slater, Patterson, Grant, & Garfin, 1991; Reid et al., 2002).

Gaynes et al. (2007) reported the results of a large survey study of 1,063 adult primary care patients and 1,478 patients receiving care in specialty medical clinics for a variety of medical conditions including pain. The authors reported overall prevalence rates of anxiety diagnoses at 49% for primary care patients and 52% for patients receiving care in specialty medical clinics. Social phobia (25.3%) and post-traumatic stress disorder (16.5%) were identified as the two most prevalent anxiety disorder diagnoses in primary care, and social phobia (32.1) and generalized anxiety disorder (21.2) were the most prevalent in specialty care medical clinics. Gureje et al. (2008) reported a lesser prevalence of specific anxiety diagnosis ranging from 8% for Panic Disorder to 11.7% for Social Phobia in a US community cohort of 5,692 adults who report pain in two or more body areas. Fleet et al. (1996) reported that 25% of patients seeking emergency room evaluation for chest pain fulfilled the DSM criteria for panic disorder. These aggregate 50% rates of co-morbid anxiety in medical patients are similar to prior published rates (Gaynes et al., 1995; Stein, Kirk, Prabhu, Grott, & Terepa, 1995).

While depression has again received the bulk of empirical attention in patients with pain, recent data suggest that anxiety may be equally as prevalent and problematic globally for these patients. Specifically, Gureje et al. (2008) reported the results of a worldwide, 17-nation survey study of 85,088 community dwelling adults investigating differences in the prevalence of mood, anxiety, and substance use disorders exist for individuals reporting pain at one vs. multiple sites. Both single and multiple pain complaints were associated with increased prevalence of depression and anxiety disorders. Compared to those without pain, patients with a single pain complaint achieved odds ratios of 1.8 for mood disorders and 1.9 for anxiety disorders; while patients with multisite pain complaints achieved odds rations of 3.7 for depression and 3.6 for anxiety disorders. These results suggested equally strong proportions of both anxiety and depression for patients with multisite pain across genders and cultures. Chronic pain appears no less related to anxiety than depression with multiple pain sites nearly doubling the likelihood of an anxiety disorder.

7.5.2 *Impact of Anxiety on Medical Treatment Outcome*

Available research supports a negative association between the presence of anxiety and pain treatment outcome. Available data have shown anxiety to be associated with increased reports of pain, pain severity, pain behaviors, postoperative pain levels, increased nonspecific physical complaints, and decreased functional outcome (de Groot et al., 1997; Granot & Ferber, 2005; Hagg, Fritzell, Ekselius, & Nordwall, 2003; Kalkman et al., 2003; Mannion et al., 2007; McCracken et al., 1998). Further, patients with anxiety and pain have been shown to report an increased number of diffuse and medically unexplained somatic symptoms (Henningsen, Zimmerman, & Sattel, 2003; Katon et al., 2001, 2007); and to demonstrate increased health care utilization (Simon, 1992; Simpson, Kazmierczak, Power, & Sharp, 1994). As anxiety and arousal increases in patients with pain and medical issues, Ley 1982 (c.f. Belar & Deardorff, 1995) suggested that patients attending clinic visits reported decreased recall of information provided, potentially affecting adherence with recommendations. This collective influence of depression and anxiety on medical and pain treatment outcomes is summarized in Fig. 7.1.

7.6 Somatoform Disorders and Pain

In the DSM-IV, somatoform disorders are defined as consisting of persistent physical complaints, which suggests a medical condition, but that are not fully explained by any specific medical findings or diagnosis. The symptoms become diagnostic when they reach an intensity that causes clinically significant emotional distress or impairment in occupational, social, or other types of daily functioning (DSM-IV, p. 445). Seven individual somatoform disorders exist to differentiate the array of clinical phenomena, symptom complaints, and medical and psychiatric factors implicated in the etiology and expression of the condition. For the purpose of this chapter on pain, two somatoform disorders, somatization disorder and pain disorder, are of particular interest. The essential diagnostic feature of *somatization disorder* is a chronic pattern of multiple clinically significant medical complaints which require medical attention. The complaints are not fully explained by medical findings, and

INCREASED:

Number of pain complaints

Pain severity

Post-operative pain report

Duration of pain

Functional limitation and disability

Health care utilization

Subjective pain intensity and duration

Medication use (3-6 fold increase in opioid prescriptions)

Number of diffuse health and pain complaints

Premature treatment drop-out, relapse after treatment

Sedentary activity, alcohol/drug use

DECREASED:

Return to work

Adherence with medication

Rehabilitative outcome

Comprehension of information provided at visits

Fig. 7.1 Collective influence of depression and anxiety disorders on medical and pain treatment outcome

associated impairments are often in excess of what might be expected by available evidence. An important component of the diagnosis of somatization disorder is that the physical complaints involve multiple body systems (e.g., neurological, gastrointestinal) and that these complaints include pain in at least four different body regions. As such, patients with somatization disorder would be expected to readily offer frequent and multiple complaints of pain to physician providers.

The second somatoform disorder of prominent interest is *pain disorder* in which the complaint of pain is the dominant symptom which prompted the patient to seek professional attention. As with somatization disorder, the pain complaints must cause significant distress and impairment at any of several levels of functioning. Three diagnostic subtypes of pain disorder exist and are differentiated by provider interpretation of the significance of psychological factors in the etiology or maintenance of the pain complaint. One subtype associates pain directly to an identifiable medical condition and psychological factors are determined to have minimal or no role in the onset or persistence of symptoms. A second subtype takes the diametric view and is diagnosed upon the perception that medical findings have little influence on the presentation of symptoms, while psychological factors are interpreted to have significant influence on symptom production. The third subtype of pain disorder assumes prominent roles by both medical and psychological factors in combination and is that which most likely represents the majority of pain data discussed in this chapter and the professional literature as a whole. This constellation of somatoform disorder symptoms is commonly referred to in the professional literature as *medically unexplained symptoms* (MUS) in reference to physical symptom complaints for which there are no associated or confirmatory biological, pathological, or physical findings (Nezu, Nezu, & Lombardo, 2001). These symptoms are typically chronic in nature and patients may demand repeat diagnostic testing and conservative treatment without diagnostic confirmation or symptom improvement. Somatization and the somatoform disorders are among the most common "mental health disorders" confronted in medicine estimated at a prevalence of 10–25% of primary care visits (Gureje, Simon, & Ustun, 1997; Ormel et al., 1994; Spitzer et al., 1994) and with health care system costs exceeding $100 billion annually (Barsky et al., 2005). The literature suggests a strong association between patterns of somatization and mood disorder. As many as 80% of patients diagnosed with somatization disorder, fibromyalgia, chronic fatigue syndrome, or irritable bowel syndrome meet criteria for a DSM-IV disorder in their lifetime (Bass & Murphy, 1991; Clark et al., 1995; Epstein et al., 1999), with up to 50% having a current co-morbid DSM-IV diagnosis (Allen, Gara, & Escobar, 2001; Simon & Von Korff, 1991)

Excessive healthcare use is an expensive hallmark of somatoform disorder patients, and somatizing patients have been reported to amass over two times the number of inpatient and outpatient medical visits compared to nonsomatizing patients (Kroenke, 2007). Patients with MUS accumulate over two times the annual cost of nonsomatizing patients (Barsky et al., 2005) and have been shown to incur lifetime healthcare expenses that are 6–14 times the US average (Smith, Monson, & Ray, 1986). Significant functional limitations are common in these patients who report on average being bedridden 2–7 days per month by their diffuse symptoms (Katon et al., 1991; Woolfolk & Allen, 2007). Up to 25% of visits to physicians are for physical complaints that lack a clear organic etiology (Gureje, 1997).

7.6.1 Treatment of Somatization Disorders

Patients presenting to physicians with medically unexplained symptoms pose significant challenges for treatment and physicians are often frustrated with multiple and frequent complaints and dissatisfaction with care (Hahn, 2001; Lin, Katon, & Von Korff, 1991). Longitudinal studies suggest that only 31% of patients with somatization disorder receiving standard medical care but no specific treatment for somatization symptoms evidenced diminished complaints after 15 years (Coryell & Norton, 1981). Investigations utilizing cognitive-behavioral therapy (CBT) for somatization symptoms have proliferated in light of the high prevalence of somatization symptoms in medical patients and dearth of evidence of the efficacy of conventional medical care to improve symptoms. In the treatment outcome literature, CBT is a widely used term to describe an intervention strategy designed to address physical symptoms, maladaptive cognitions, health behaviors, healthcare utilization, social influences on symptoms, and emotional factors. Multiple combinations of CBT strategies have been tested and generally include some combination of relaxation training, coping/cognitive restructuring, problem solving, and assertiveness training to increase the occurrence of self-management behaviors and reinforce their long-term durability. Overall, the following summary provides encouraging support for the efficacy of broad-based CBT packages in improving outcomes for patients with medically unexplained symptoms.

Kroenke (2007) reported meta-analysis results of 34 randomized clinical trials involving 3,922 adult somatoform patients. Results reported that CBT-based treatments with a median number of eight sessions were effective in 11 of 13 studies and the best empirically established treatment for somatoform symptoms to date. Nezu et al. (2001) published an extensive critical review of the CBT literature for medically unexplained symptoms and reported CBT to be an effective treatment. The authors reported CBT to produce moderate effect sizes for reduction of physical symptoms and mood disturbances. Allen and Woolfolk (2010) published a recent review of the efficacy of CBT treatment for somatization and concluded that patients treated with CBT demonstrated significant reductions in somatic complaints and mood disturbances and improved functioning.

Finally, Escobar et al. (2007) tested a ten-session CBT-based intervention focusing on reduction of distress via relaxation training, activity regulation, and cognitive restructuring plus a consultation letter to physicians with recommendations for physician management of patients with medically unexplained symptoms. This treatment was compared with standard medical care plus the consultation letter for 172 adult primary care patients meeting diagnosis of somatization disorder. Results of this brief intervention suggested significant physician ratings of "much improved" or "very improved" for treatment group patients. Intervention patients showed decreased physical complaints and improvement in self-reported depression. This study replicated and expanded upon similar results using a similar intervention by Allen, Woolfolk, Escobar, Gara, and Hamer (2006).

7.7 Axis II Personality Disorders Co-morbidities in Pain

The relationship between chronic pain and personality traits, characteristics, and disorders has long been researched and debated. While a relatively solid body of research exists regarding the prevalence and possible causal relationships between chronic pain and clinical disorders such as depression and anxiety, the interaction between chronic pain and Axis II Personality Disorders is much less clear. A brief introduction to the basic terms and concepts in the literature on pain and personality follows along with a brief historical overview. Recent hypotheses and research investigating the relationship between chronic pain and personality disorders and review of nonpathological personality characteristics such as perceived optimism and resiliency are provided. A comprehensive discussion of these issues has been previously published (Gatchel & Weisberg, 2000).

The term "personality trait" generally refers to relatively enduring patterns of perception, interpersonal relations, and thoughts about oneself and about one's world. When these traits become inflexible and maladaptive and cause significant functional impairment or subjective distress, they are considered to be DSM-IV personality disorders (American Psychiatric Association, 1994). The DSM-IV uses a categorical, or dichotomous, system for determining the presence of a personality disorder, and many have argued this is an artificial distinction assuming that personality and personality disorders lie on a spectrum and do not lend themselves well to dichotomous categorization (Reich & Thompson, 1987; Widiger, Trull, Hurt, Clarkin, & Frances, 1987). The DSM-IV lists ten distinct personality disorders. In addition, personality disorder not otherwise specified (PDNOS) is used when an individual displays features of more than one personality disorder, but not to the necessary extent to fulfill full criteria for any specific personality disorder category.

Historically, the topic of personality traits and disorders in chronic pain has been given considerable professional attention dating to Freud and the psychoanalytic tradition (Breuer and Freud, 1893; cited by Gentry, Shows, & Thomas, 1974). Breuer and Freud proposed that unresolved emotional issues such as guilt were believed to be the root of chronic pain and that emotional pain was being expressed through physical mechanisms. Since Freud, several theorists have postulated that certain personality characteristics or traits may predispose one to chronic pain (Engel, 1959; Sternbach, 1974). Between the 1950s and the 1970s, psychoanalytic research was devoted to identifying personality patterns or styles that might confirm or disconfirm the existence of physiologically based pain; that is, to distinguish between "real" or organic pain and "psychogenic" or functional pain syndromes (Engel, 1959; Hanvik, 1951; McCreary, Turner, & Dawson, 1977; Sternbach, 1974). The Minnesota Multidimensional Personality Inventory (MMPI; Hathaway & McKinley, 1943) was the most widely used measure of personality in these studies, despite the fact that it was not intended for use with pain patients. The ability of the MMPI to distinguish between organic and nonorganic pain patients has yielded conflicting and controversial results. Results were also generally mixed as to whether certain MMPI profiles could predict treatment outcome (Gentry et al., 1974; McCreary, Turner, & Sawson, 1979; Wiltse & Rocchio, 1975).

While the MMPI focuses primarily on psychopathology, the NEO Personality Inventory (NEO-PI; Costa & McCrae, 1992) assesses a continuum of personality function based on five domains of personality. These domains include: (1) Neuroticism (emotional stability), (2) Extroversion, (3) Openness (to new experiences), (4) Conscientiousness, and (5) Agreeableness. The NEO-PI represents one of the most widely used instruments in chronic pain research to assess both nonpathological and pathological personality traits. In many studies, Neuroticism has emerged as a significant predictor of both illness behavior (Lauver & Johnson, 1997) and increased psychological distress (Affleck, Tennen, Urrows, & Higgens, 1992; BenDebba, Torgerson, & Long, 1997). In a study of injured workers in

Australia, Wall, Ogloff, and Morrissey (2006) used the Structured Clinical Interview for DSM Disorders (SCID-II; First, Gibbon, Spitzer, Williams, & Benjamin, 1997) and Neo-FFI (Costa & McCrae, 1992) with workers having all types of injuries (not limited to pain) and found that injured workers with higher levels of personality dysfunction on the SCID-II had poorer outcomes and greater costs than those with lower levels. These researchers also reported that individuals who were high on the Neuroticism scale and low on the Extraversion scale of the NEO-FFI also had poorer health outcomes. The author's note that the pattern seen on the NEO-FFI is similar to those seen to be anxious and socially avoidant which is consistent with studies discussed below.

In addition to the MMPI and NEO-PI, other measures of personality dysfunction and of the normal realm personality traits and functioning exist. Some researched and validated measures used to assess personality pathology in chronic pain patients include the Millon Clinical Multiaxial Inventory-III (Millon, Davis, Millon, & Grossman, 2009), The Temperment and Character Inventory (C. Cloninger, 1994), and the Battery for Health Improvement-II (BHI-II; Bruns & Disorbio, 2003). As these inventories attest, the topic of personality can be viewed narrowly and discretely as in the DSM-IV diagnostic criteria, or much more broadly including various additional constructs such as "neuroticism," "introversion", "harm avoidance," "trait anxiety," "anger," "inhibition," and "sensitivity" (Applegate, Keefe, & Siegler, 2005; Calabrese, Lyness, Sorensen, & Duberstein, 2006; Dworkin, Hetzel, & Banks, 1999; Krueger, Tackett, & Markon, 2004; Vossen, Van Os, Hermens, & Lousberg, 2006). Available research suggests that certain characteristics may increase an individual's proclivity towards developing chronic pain. Gatchel (1996) reported it unlikely that any single personality variable may be independently predictive, but more likely that patients with pain compose a heterogeneous group of personality traits and disorders. Similarly, no single personality style, trait, or disorder is likely to predispose an individual to the development of chronic pain. An emerging area of interest centers on personality traits which might positively impact the experience of chronic pain and function. Some novel traits gaining investigative attention include "optimism," "self-efficacy" (Peters & Vancleef, 2008), and "resiliency" (Peters, 2009).

7.7.1 *Personality Disorders*

Research suggests a significantly higher prevalence of personality disorders in chronic pain patients (31–59%) as compared to individuals presenting to psychiatric clinics for treatment, various medical populations, and the general population (Weisberg, 2000; Weisberg & Keefe, 1997). Recent literature on personality traits and disorders in chronic pain suggests that a diathesis-stress framework may account for the high co-morbidity of personality disorders observed in chronic pain patients (Weisberg & Keefe, 1997). That is, there are likely to be underlying genetic and perhaps early-life predispositions to personality disorders that may or may not become expressed under the stress of chronic pain arises with the associated biological, psychological, and social consequences of long-standing pain. Others suggest that many aspects of personality represent "states" or changeable characteristics, rather than "traits," or stable characteristics (Fishbain et al., 2006) and that these "states" are influenced by an individual's level of emotional distress at the time of personality assessment. Given that roughly 50% of chronic pain sufferers have co-morbid depression and/or anxiety disorders, it may be important to account for acute emotional states at the time of assessment. Emerging research findings on several individual personality constructs (e.g., optimism, self-efficacy, resiliency, conscientiousness) are important as they have been preliminarily suggested to correlate, and potentially predict, treatment outcome. In a recent article investigating temperament, character, and personality disorders in chronic pain patients, Conrad et al. (2007) took a novel approach to the diagnosis of personality in the chronic pain population by using the Temperament and Character Inventory (TCI; Cloninger, Svrakic, & Przybeck, 1993), based on his psychobiological model of personality which distinguishes between temperament and character dimensions. In this model, temperament is considered to represent stable stimulus-response patterns that can be considered to be the basis for personality "traits." Character dimensions are conceptualized as "states" and represent differences in goals, values, attitudes, and self-concept. Conrad et al. (2007) successfully brought together the co-morbidity between clinical psychiatric disorders and personality and the notion that certain personality traits are stable while others may be more likely to change over time affected by co-morbid depression and anxiety. A unique finding by Cloninger and colleagues was that even when controlling for mood and anxiety, the Harm Avoidance scale of the TCI was significantly higher in chronic pain patients than in control subjects. According to authors, Harm Avoidance is related to early emotion, fear, and autonomic arousal, all of which are often clinically observed in chronic pain sufferers and are similar to the concept of fear-avoidance. There remains much work to be done to improve our understanding of the complex interactions between pain, clinical "states," and personality and in understanding the potential causal relationship between pain and personality.

7.8 Fear-Avoidance of Pain or "Kinesiophobia"

"Kinesiophobia" was first defined by Kori, Miller, and Todd (1990, p. 36) as an "irrational and debilitating fear of physical movement and activity resulting from a feeling of vulnerability to painful injury or (re)injury." This term has been widely used in the literature to describe fear-related avoidance of physical activity or movement in response to concern that activity will increase pain to unmanageable levels or promote actual tissue damage (Van Dorsten & Lindley, 2010; Vlaeyen, Kole-Snijders, Boeren, & van Eck, 1995). Avoidance of movement has been shown to associate with catastrophic thoughts about pain and depression and may readily lead to the adoption of passive activity and hypervigilance of pain sensation (Van Dorsten & Lindley, 2010).

There are three scales commonly used in the professional literature to assess fear of pain and fear-avoidance of movement including the Tampa Scale for Kinesiophobia (TSK; Vlaeyen et al., 1995), the Fear Avoidance Belief Questionnaire (FABQ; Waddell, Newton, Henderson, Somerville, & Main, 1993), and the Fear of Pain Questionnaire (FPQ; McNeil & Rainwater, 1998). The Tampa Scale for Kinesiophobia was originally developed by Miller, Kori, and Todd in 1991, but was unpublished until Vlaeyen and colleagues published with permission in 1995. The TSK is a 17-item self-report inventory that assesses fear of injury related to movement. The Fear Avoidance Beliefs Questionnaire is a 16-item self-report measure containing two subscales designed to assess beliefs about how physical activity and work influence low back pain and whether they should be avoided. The TSK and FABQ have been shown to have acceptable reliability and validity for patients with both chronic and acute pain (Crombez, Vlaeyen, Heuts, & Lysens, 1999; Roelofs, Goubert, Peters, Vlaeyen, & Crombez, 2004; Swinkels-Meewisse, Swinkels, Verbeek, Vlaeyen, & Oostendorp, 2003). The Fear of Pain Questionnaire (McNeil & Rainwater, 1998) is a 30-item self-report questionnaire and is unique in that it assesses avoidance/escape behaviors associated with fear of specific pain circumstances. Three factors derived from the scale – Fear of Severe Pain (e.g., breaking one's leg), Fear of Minor Pain (e.g., getting a paper cut) and Fear of Medical Pain (having one's blood drawn) – assess fear-avoidance responses and anxiety in pain patients in specific situations.

Literature over 15 years has shown fear-avoidance of pain to be a powerful predictor of functional disability in both adults and children (Grotle, Vollstad, Veierod, & Brox, 2004; Miro, Huguet, & Nieto, 2007; Samwel, Kraaimaat, Crul, & Evers, 2007; Vlaeyen & Linton, 2000). Incredibly, pain-related fear as assessed by the TSK and FABQ has been shown to be a greater predictor of subjective disability than pain severity itself (Crombez et al., 1999) and a strong predictor of poor behavioral efforts including functional capacity measurement, walking speed, and avoidance of simple movement (Al-Obaidi et al., 2000; Crombez et al., 1999; Vlaeyen et al., 1995). Fear-avoidance of activity has been empirically associated with increased pain and functional disability following spine surgery (den Boer et al., 2006; Mannion et al., 2007).

7.8.1 Treatment of Fear-Avoidance

In a review of 16 studies utilizing CBT strategies to reduce fear-avoidance, Lohnberg (2007) reported that in vivo exposure strategies, in which the patient is sequentially exposed to those specific physical activities which are avoided in anticipation that they might produce intolerable pain, were found to be more effective than traditional CBT for pain coping, education, physical therapy, or nonspecific graded activity increase. Several additional studies have reported in vivo exposure to decrease fear-avoidance beliefs and increase functional capacity in pain patients with high fear-avoidance scores (Boersma et al., 2004; Linton, Overmeer, Janson, Vlaeyen, & de Jong, 2002; Vlaeyen et al., 2001a, 2001b; Linton et al., 2002).

7.9 Catastrophizing

Catastrophizing has been defined by Sullivan et al. (2001; p. 52) as "an exaggerated negative mental set brought to bear during actual or anticipated painful experience." The term is widely used to describe the tendency of some patients with pain to experience exaggeratedly negative or catastrophic thoughts about pain (e.g., "I feel I can't stand it anymore"; "it's terrible and I think it's never going to get any better") which in turn may magnify the threat or seriousness of pain sensations. Empirical literature has documented a strong relationship between high catastrophizing scores and pain intensity and subjective disability in several differing pain populations (Butler et al., 1989; Jacobson & Butler, 1996; Thorn et al., 2007).

7.9.1 Assessment of Catastrophizing

Two scales are predominately used in the literature to assess catastrophizing in response to pain including the Coping Strategies Questionnaire (CSQ; Rosenstiel & Keefe, 1983) and the Pain Catastrophizing Scale (PCS; Sullivan et al., 1995). The Coping Strategies Questionnaire is the most widely used measure of pain *coping* in the professional literature, and the relationship between CSQ scores and multiple measures of pain and functioning are well documented for several pain populations (Boothby, Thorn, Stroud, & Jensen, 1999; Jensen & Karoly, 1991). Six items extracted from the CSQ constitute the Catastrophizing scale and this subscale has received suitable empirical support as a stand-alone scale (Keefe, Brown, Wallston, & Caldwell, 1989). The CSQ Catastrophizing scale assesses frequency of catastrophic thoughts when one is in pain, helplessness and extent of perceived control over pain. This scale has been extracted for use in many studies of pain coping (Keefe et al., 2001; Turner, Dworkin, Mancl, Huggins, & Truelove, 2001) and has been empirically shown to moderately predict pain intensity and disability and to be the single most powerful predictor of pain severity in 564 veterans with chronic pain (Tan, Jensen, Robinson-Whelen, Thornby, & Monga, 2001).

The Pain Catastrophizing Scale is the most widely published measure of pain *catastrophizing* in the professional literature. The PCS is composed of 13 items which assess the degree to which individuals experience catastrophic thoughts when they feel pain. Factor analytic investigations of the PCS suggest that catastrophizing may be conceived as a unitary construct composed of three dimensions – magnification, rumination, and helplessness (Osman et al., 2000; Sullivan et al., 2000). This scale has been widely used since its inception and an abundance of research has shown catastrophic thoughts about pain to significantly correlate with increased pain severity, perceived disability, increased analgesic use, hopelessness, referral to specialists, healthcare system use, hospitalization, emotional distress, postsurgical pain, and activity interference (Bishop & Warr, 2003; Butler et al., 1989; Gil, Abrams, & Phillips, 1993; Gil, Thompson, & Keith, 1992, 1993; Granot & Ferber, 2005; Jacobson & Butler, 1996; Severeijns et al., 2004; Sullivan et al., 2001; Turner et al., 2001).

7.9.2 *Treatment of Catastrophizing*

CBT interventions have extensive empirical support as being highly successful in assisting patients with pain to manage pain and increase function. However, as with all treatments, not all patients equally benefit and little is known about why treatments are less efficacious for some or what treatment might be best for any given individual patient (Turk & Okifuji, 2002). In fact, meta-analytic investigations of the efficacy of CBT for pain have repeatedly identified the limitation that CBT is composed of multiple variations of treatment strategies (Eccleston, Morley, Williams, Yorke, & Mastroyannopoulou, 2002; Ostelo et al., 2005; Thorn et al., 2002). Thorn et al., (2002) postulated that traditional forms of CBT may be less effective for individuals scoring high on catastrophizing in that these patients may increasingly ruminate about pain and its consequences or be highly hypervigilant to pain sensation with limited ability to distract from pain. The authors suggested that typical adaptations of CBT are not designed to specifically target catastrophic thinking as an outcome measure and proposed a step-wise CBT treatment algorithm designed to reduce pain catastrophizing. The efficacy of this proposed treatment was tested by Thorn et al. (2007) in a randomized controlled trial of 34 individuals with headache who were randomized to 10 weekly sessions of CBT or wait list control. Results indicated that the active CBT treatment produced significant reductions in anxiety and pain catastrophizing. Although significant differences were not found for headache intensity, the authors reported that half of participants demonstrated meaningful differences in other headache indices (e.g., headache frequency, medication use).

In another investigation of factors affecting catastrophizing, Smeets et al. (2006) reported that pain catastrophizing scores were improved in patients with chronic low back pain who were randomized to active physical therapy, CBT, or CBT plus physical therapy, but not in wait list control patients. The authors reported that pre- to post-treatment change in pain catastrophizing scores mediated reduction in disability and pain complaints, and in contrast to Thorn et al. (2007), concluded that treatment elements not specifically targeted to pain catastrophizing may reduce this phenomenon in patients with pain. While the treatment literature regarding pain catastrophizing is in its infancy, there appears to be growing scientific support for the use of cognitive and behavioral treatments aimed at reducing pain catastrophizing to improve medical treatment outcome (Buer & Linton, 2002; Jensen, Turner, & Romano, 2001; Spinhoven et al., 2004; Sullivan, Adams, Rhodenizer, & Stanish, 2006).

7.10 Psychological Treatment of Pain and Co-morbidities

Consistent with the theoretical underpinnings of the Gate Control Theory (Melzack & Wall, 1965), cognitive and affective factors are postulated to modulate pain sensation via descending analgesic pathways. While the specific mechanism of action of most psychological processes remains unknown, Williams (1999) identified three potential pathways in which psychosocial factors may dampen afferent signals. Via the endorphin-mediated analgesic system, the production of endogenous opioids may be facilitated by changes in serotonin and norepinephrine levels, as suggested by the efficacy of antidepressant medications and psychological therapies in decreasing pain. Second, Williams identified a nonendogenous opioid-mediated descending pathway in which excitatory amino acids are released and bind to NMDA receptors to dampen afferent signals. Third, additional investigation is needed to improve our understanding of the ability of estrogen-mediated factors to inhibit firing of pain neurons.

7.10.1 Patient-Centered Outcomes for Pain Treatment

Pain treatment programs commonly assess patient outcomes in a variety of similar fashions focusing on pain reduction, reduction in medication intake, decreased healthcare use and increased functional activities. It has been assumed that patients prioritize these same endpoints when evaluating the success of treatment, but until recently little research regarding patient-derived goals for pain care has existed. In an initial investigation of patient goals for pain treatment, Casarett, Karlawish, Sankar, Hirschman, and Asch (2001) interviewed 40 patients attending an outpatient pain service regarding their most highly desired improvements associated with treatment. Eighty percent of patients desired pain decrease, while 70% identified decreased frequency of medication doses and 68% decreased opioid intake. Additional goals identified included improved sleep (32%), decreased interference with daily activities by pain (30%), and improved mood (8%). These authors concluded that evaluation of pain treatment should involve specific patient goals and that patient goals may extend well beyond pain reduction.

This investigation of specific patient goals for pain treatment was expanded upon by Robinson et al. (2005) who surveyed 100 patients with pain regarding their goals for treatment improvement in four domains including pain (intensity), fatigue/tiredness, emotional distress, and interference with daily activities. Participants were requested to complete the Patient-Centered Outcomes Questionnaire, a five-item inventory which requested patients to rate each domain from 0 to 10 to identify pretreatment usual levels (baseline), desired levels, levels at which the patient would consider treatment successful, expected levels after treatment, and the subjective importance that these levels be achieved. Results reported that patients rated it as very important (e.g., 7.2–9.2 across domains) that greater than 50% improvement was achieved in all domains to consider treatment a success. Patients did not expect treatment to fulfill their goals. The authors concluded that pain patients desire substantially broader-based treatment improvements and of a considerably greater magnitude than previously thought to consider pain treatment successful.

O'Brien et al. (2010) also used the Patient-Centered Outcomes Questionnaire to determine pretreatment goals for 248 patients diagnosed with fibromyalgia and 54 low back pain patients prior to receiving care at tertiary care clinics. Results reported that fibromyalgia patients desired greater than 50% reductions in subjective pain and over 60% reduction in emotional distress, fatigue, and interference with daily activities to consider treatment a success; while back pain patients desired between 58–68% reductions in these same content areas. Results again suggested that patients did not expect treatment to achieve these goals. In aggregate, the collective results of these preliminary studies suggest that broad-based psychosocial and medical goals need to be defined and evaluated as a standard part of treatment for patients with pain so as to better account for specific patient goals and outcomes when devising treatment.

7.10.2 Efficacy of Cognitive-Behavioral Therapy for Pain

As per the multiple treatment reviews provided throughout this chapter, the strong emphasis in cognitive-behavioral pain management programs is to comprehensively address the aggregate of maladaptive beliefs (e.g., invalid attributions of the cause of pain, activity will worsen pain), expectations which guide illness behavior (e.g., chronicity, treatment failure), maladaptive short-term coping strategies (e.g., excessive reclining, drug/alcohol use), mood influences (e.g., depression, anxiety, catastrophizing), social influences (e.g., family/social reinforcement of sick role behaviors, litigation/unemployment), and behavioral practices (e.g., medication and healthcare system use) which may perpetrate pain and disability. To achieve these objectives, CBT approaches employ a wide range of cognitive and behavioral intervention strategies including psychoeducation, relaxation training, sleep hygiene, selective self-monitoring, managing mood, development of adaptive coping strategies (e.g., distraction, assertiveness training, replacing self-defeating negative thoughts), graded activity increases (or graded exposure in the context of fear-avoidance of activity), and goal setting to increase participation in quality of life activities (Gatchel & Okifuju, 2006; Sullivan, Feuerstein, Gatchel, Linton, & Pransky, 2005; Van Dorsten, 2006). Cognitive-behavioral therapies formulate the cornerstone of multidisciplinary "functional restoration" programs which have substantial empirical support of efficacy in treating the multiple phenomena associated with chronic pain (Dworkin et al., 2002; Gatchel & Okifuji, 2006; Turk, Loeser, & Monarch, 2002; Turk & Okifuji, 1998). Throughout this chapter, significant evidence supporting the efficacy for CBT, behavioral therapy, or their combination for improving pain and disability is provided. Comprehensive published literature reviews and meta-analyses of the literature have concluded these therapies to be efficacious in both adults (Allen & Woolfolk, 2010; Brox et al., 2003; Morley, Eccleston, & Williams, 1999; Turner & Jensen, 1993) and children and adolescents (Eccleston et al., 2002; Palermo, Eccleston, Lewandowski, Williams, & Morley, 2010). Ostelo et al. (2005) conducted a Cochrane review of behavioral treatments for low back pain and importantly pointed out that results support the efficacy of CBT and relaxation strategies for short-term improvements in pain, but that long-term improvement awaits further verification.

7.10.3 *Efficacy of Psychodynamic Therapy for Pain*

Few studies utilizing psychodynamic therapy for patients with pain have been published and with highly variable results. Bassett and Pilowsky (1985) reported the results of a small study ($n = 26$) comparing six 30-min sessions of supportive psychotherapy vs. twelve 60-min sessions of psychodynamic therapy in patients with pain. The authors reported 22% of supportive therapy patients reported feeling subjectively improved vs. 54% of psychodynamic therapy patients. A variety of methodological concerns were noted including a high drop-out rate, small number of participants, generally incomparable treatment lengths, and the inherent difficulties in investigating several basic principles of psychodynamic therapy. The authors recognized that few controlled studies exist to evaluate the efficacy of psychodynamic therapy, the challenge of many indefinable outcomes in assessing this therapy, and the time-consuming nature of this therapy approach which renders it inaccessible to large numbers of patients.

Pilowsky and Barrow (1990) tested 12 weekly psychodynamic psychotherapy sessions in patients with chronic intractable pain without identifiable organic basis. This study utilized a four-group randomized design comparing Amitriptyline or placebo paired with psychodynamic therapy or unstructured "supportive" contacts with a physician. Psychodynamic therapy emphasized reconceptualizing pain as unexpressed emotional dynamic and attempting to resolve it through therapy, while the "supportive contact" was designed as an unstructured assessment by the physician of pain symptom and medication' effects. Results were unique in that psychotherapy patients demonstrated modest functional improvement, despite reporting a significant pain *increase* over the course of therapy.

Monsen and Monsen (2000) reported a prospective investigation of subjective pain in 40 patients with diffuse musculoskeletal pain of unknown etiology who were randomized to receiving either 33 sessions of psychodynamic body therapy (e.g., psychodynamic psychotherapy coupled with physical activity therapies) or to a treatment-as-usual medical care control. Results indicated significant decreases in pain severity and emotional distress (e.g., depression, anxiety, somatization) for treatment patients compared with controls. Interestingly, the authors reported 50% of the treatment sample to be pain-free following psychodynamic treatment, and that treatment-related improvements were sustained 1 year posttreatment. These significant and unusual findings would appear to emphasize the need for replication and further investigation.

7.11 Summary and Future Directions

This chapter reviews a vast literature which emphasizes a very strong influence of psychological disorders and other psychosocial factors on pain expression, assessment, and treatment outcomes. Many psychological influences on medical treatment outcome have been identified in the literature and have been shown to predict treatment failure more accurately than medical factors (Bruns & Disorbio, 2009; Van Dorsten & Lindley, 2010). Considerable evidence exists to suggest that multidisciplinary treatment efforts are more effective than single provider approaches in producing positive functional treatment outcomes (Flor, Fydrich, & Turk, 1992; Guzman et al., 2002; Lang, Leibig, Kastner, Neundorfer, & Heuschmann, 2003; Van Dorsten, 2006; van Tulder, Koes, & Malmivaara, 2005). The aggregate of available literature appears to strongly suggest that physicians intending to optimize treatment outcomes may necessarily wish to partner with pain psychologists to efficiently identify patients experiencing psychosocial challenges and formulate broad-based treatment outcome targets. Treatment outcome goals should encompass both professional provider goals and patient-centered goals to improve patient satisfaction with care. Towards this end, it appears increasingly critical to have psychologists closely integrated into the treatment system so as to be seen as an integral component of comprehensive treatment (Van Dorsten, 2006). Traditional outpatient consultation approaches appear unlikely to suffice as up to 50–80% of patients referred for mental health intervention fail to pursue care (Escobar, Waitzkin, & Silver, 1998). Cognitive and behavioral treatments can offer valuable improvements for patients with pain, but despite recent initiatives to improve pain assessment and treatment, an insufficient number of patients are receiving comprehensive multidisciplinary evaluation and treatment. Given the sheer magnitude of the numbers of patients with pain and the high prevalence of contributing psychosocial factors, the need to increase the numbers of specially training psychologists to provide this service is obviated.

A significant number of psychosocial variables including mood, personality, beliefs, expectations, and employment and litigation factors have been abundantly shown in the literature as threatening positive medical treatment outcome (Bruns & Disorbio, 2009; Van Dorsten & Lindley, 2010). In order to better understand and increase the specificity and utility of this literature, significantly more research is needed to identify specific factors which might predict the progression from acute to chronic pain and to clarify which variables constitute the strongest risk factors for specific patient populations (e.g., primary care, surgery) or for specific outcomes (e.g., return to work, medication intake, decreased use of the healthcare system). Turk and Okifuji (2002) rightfully emphasized the need to further clarify CBT treatment results via future research to specify which treatment components might be most important to achieve specific outcomes for specific types of patients. These authors acknowledged that psychosocial treatment is most commonly offered in a manualized format with little tailoring to specific patients or diagnostic subgroups and emphasized the need for continued research in treatment *matching* to improve both clinical and cost effectiveness of psychological treatments. The significant presence of psychosocial and behavioral co-morbidities in medical patients obviates the need to continue creative empirical exploration of various treatment formats which might allow us to provide psychosocial assessment and treatment to greater numbers of patients. Clinicians and researchers are encouraged to unite their efforts to identify effective treatment formats to allow care access to larger numbers of patients by utilizing alternate technologies.

Considering the massive numbers of patients with medically unexplained pain complaints, the utility of the current diagnostic classification system for patients with pain and medically unexplained symptoms has been called to question. Wise and Birket-Smith (2002) reported that the DSM-III and IV classification systems have done little to improve our understanding of the somatoform disorders and have had little influence in guiding new research or treatment insights for this set of heterogeneous patients and their heterogeneous complaints. Primary concerns identified by these authors include the heterogeneity of symptoms, the unreliability of diagnostic subcategories in the DSM-III and DSM-IV somatoform disorder section, and the lack of treatment guidance inherent in the diagnoses (Mayou et al., 2005; Smith et al., 1986). Birket-Smith and Mortenson (2002) reported an attempt to differentiate psychiatric symptoms among 127 patients who met the diagnosis of any somatoform disorder following structured diagnostic interview. These authors found no data to differentiate mood or personality characteristics for patients with pain complaints vs. without. Some have opined that historically the classification system for medically unexplained symptoms has simplistically relied heavily on symptom counting (Fava et al., 1995), while others have proposed the elimination of the somatoform category from the DSM-V in favor of a new system which might relate more readily to the functional disorder classifications used by physicians (Mayou, Kirmayer, Simon, Kroenke, & Sharpe, 2005). No doubt, the somatoform disorders will continue to pose a significant and controversial taxonomic challenge in DSM-V and medicine as a whole (Wise & Birket-Smith, 2002).

Both clinical observation and published surveys of practicing psychiatrists suggest that use of the somatoform diagnoses in clinical practice appears quite rare (Mayou et al., 2005; Stern, Murphy, & Bass, 1993). While the factors discussed above may influence this low utilization rate, realistic concerns regarding the potential clinical impact of these diagnoses may also affect use. For example, many neurological disorders (e.g., multiple sclerosis) can have long periods of expression in which various symptoms may wax and wane from minor to debilitating before diagnostic confirmation of the disease is made. Many healthcare providers may be realistically apprehensive regarding use of a psychiatric diagnosis (e.g., somatization disorder) to describe the medically unexplained (as yet) symptoms and the patient's current clinical presentation in light of the potentially deleterious effect on future medical assessment and treatment. Concern exists that labeling a patient's symptom presentation with a psychiatric diagnosis might unduly be accepted as a "confirmation" that symptoms are produced via psychiatric mechanisms and minimize the vigor of future medical investigation of symptoms. The significant presence of affective and behavioral factors in patients presenting to medical practitioners is apparent, and failure to implement psychological assessment and treatment into mainstream medical care has yielded frustrating and failing result. Little progress appears to have been made via a single provider approach or treatment via consultation and as such the data in this chapter strongly support the groundswell of activity in including mental health providers in the establishment of the new medical home for medical patients.

References

Affleck, G., Tennen, H., Urrows, S., & Higgens, P. (1992). Neuroticism and the pain-mood relation in rheumatoid arthritis: Insights from a prospective daily study. *Journal of Consulting and Clinical Psychology, 60*, 119–126.

Allen, L. A., Gara, M. A., & Escobar, J. I. (2001). Somatization: A debilitating syndrome in primary care. *Psychosomatics, 42*, 63–67.

Allen, L. A., & Woolfolk, R. L. (2010). Cognitive behavioral therapy for somatoform disorders. *Psychiatric Clinics of North America, 33*, 579–593.

Allen, L. A., Woolfolk, R. L., Escobar, J. I., Gara, M. A., & Hamer, R. M. (2006). Cognitive-behavioral therapy for somatization disorder: A randomized clinical trial. *Archives of Internal Medicine, 166*, 1512–1518.

Al-Obaidi, S. M., Nelson, R. M., Al-Awadhi, S., & Al-Shuwaie, N. (2000). The role of anticipation and fear of pain in the persistence of avoidance behavior in patients with chronic low back pain. *Spine, 25*, 1126–1131.

American Psychiatric Association. (1994). *Diagnostic and Statistical Manual of Mental Disorders* (4th ed.). Washington: American Psychological Association.

Andersson, H. I. (1994). The epidemiology of chronic pain in a Swedish rural area. *Quality of Life Research, 3*, S19–S26.

Andersson, G. B. (1999). Epidemiological features of chronic low back pain. *The Lancet, 354*, 581–585.

Applegate, K., Keefe, F., & Siegler, I. (2005). Does personality at college entry predict number of reported pain conditions at mid-life? A longitudinal study. *The Journal of Pain, 6*(2), 92–97.

Ash, A., Zhao, Y., Ellis, R. P., & Kramer, M. S. (2001). Finding future high cost cases: Comparing prior cost versus diagnosis-based methods. *Health Services Research, 36*, 194–206.

Atkinson, J. H., Slater, M. A., Patterson, T. L., Grant, I., & Garfin, S. R. (1991). Prevalence, onset, and risk of psychiatric disorders in men with chronic low back pain: A controlled study. *Pain, 45*, 111–121.

Badger, L. W., deGruy, F. V., Hartman, J., Plant, M. A., Leeper, J., Ficken, R., et al. (1994). Psychosocial interest, medical interviews, and the recognition of depression. *Archives of Family Medicine, 3*, 862–864.

Bair, M. J., Robinson, R. L., Eckert, G. J., Stang, P. E., Croghan, T. W., & Kroenke, K. (2004). Impact of pain on depression treatment response in primary care. *Psychosomatic Medicine, 66*, 17–22.

Bair, M. J., Robinson, R. L., Katon, W. J., & Kroenke, K. (2003). Depression and pain comorbidity: A literature review. *Archives of Internal Medicine, 163*, 2433–2445.

Bane, C., Hughes, C. M., & McElnay, J. C. (2006). The impact of depressive symptoms and psychosocial factors on medication adherence in cardiovascular disease. *Patient Education and Counseling, 60*, 187–193.

Barsky, A. J., Orav, E. J., & Bates, D. W. (2005). Somatization increases medical utilization and costs independent of psychiatric and medical comorbidity. *Archives of General Psychiatry, 62*, 903–910.

Bass, C., & Murphy, M. (1991). Somatization disorder in a British teaching hospital. *British Journal of Clinical Practice, 45*, 237–244.

Bassett, D. L., & Pilowsky, I. (1985). A study of brief psychotherapy for chronic pain. *Journal of Psychosomatic Research, 29*, 259–264.

Belar, C. D., & Deardorff, W. W. (1995). *Clinical health psychology in medical settings*. Washington: American Psychological Association.

BenDebba, M., Torgerson, W., & Long, D. (1997). Personality traits, pain duration and severity, functional impairment, and psychological distress in patients with persistent low back pain. *Pain, 72*, 115–125.

Berman, B. M., Bausell, R. B., & Lee, W. L. (2000). Use and referral patterns for 22 complimentary and alternative medical therapies by members of the American College of Rheumatology: Results of a national survey. *Archives of Internal Medicine, 162*, 766–770.

Betrus, P. A., Elmore, S. K., & Hamilton, P. A. (1995). Women and somatization: Unrecognized depression. *Health Care for Women International, 16*, 287–297.

Bigos, S. J., Bowyer, O. R., & Braen, G. R. (1994). *Acute low back problems in adults: Clinical practice guideline.* No. 14. Rockville, MD: US Department of Health and Human Services, Public Health Service, Agency for Health Care Policy and Research; Publication 95-0642.

Birket-Smith, M., & Mortenson, E. L. (2002). Pain in somatoform disorders: Is somatoform pain disorder a valid diagnosis? *Acta Psychiatrica Scandinavica, 106*, 103–108.

Bishop, S. R., & Warr, D. (2003). Coping, catastrophizing and chronic pain in breast cancer. *Journal of Behavioral Medicine, 26*, 265–281.

Boersma, K., Linton, S., Overmeer, T., Jansson, M., Vlaeyen, J., & de Jong, J. (2004). Lowering fear-avoidance and enhancing function through exposure in vivo: A multiple baseline study across six patients with back pain. *Pain, 108*, 8–16.

Boothby, J. L., Thorn, B. E., Stroud, M. W., & Jensen, M. P. (1999). Coping with pain. In R. J. Gatchel & D. C. Turk (Eds.), *Psychosocial factors in pain: Critical perspectives* (pp. 345–359). New York: Guilford.

Boyd, J. H., & Weisman, M. M. (1986). Epidemiology. In E. S. Payke (Ed.), *Handbook of affective disorders*. New York: Guilford.

Breckenridge, J., & Clark, J. D. (2003). Patient characteristics associated with opioid versus nonsteroidal anti-inflammatory drug management of chronic low back pain. *The Journal of Pain, 4*, 344–350.

Brox, J. L., Sorenson, R., Friis, P. T., Nygaard, O., Indahl, A., & Keller, A. (2003). Randomized clinical trials of lumbar instrumented fusion and cognitive intervention and exercises in patients with chronic low back pain and disc degeneration. *Spine, 28*, 1913–1921.

Bruns, D., & Disorbio, J. M. (2003). *The battery for health improvement-II*. Minneapolis: NCS Pearson.

Bruns, D., & Disorbio, J. M. (2009). Assessment of biopsychosocial risk factors for medical treatment: A collaborative approach. *Journal of Clinical Psychology in Medical Settings, 16*, 127–147.

Butler, R. W., Damarin, F. L., Beaulieu, C., Schwebel, A. I., & Thorn, B. E. (1989). Assessing cognitive coping strategies for acute postsurgical pain. *Psychol Assess, 1*, 41–45.

Buer, N., & Linton, S. J. (2002). Fear-avoidance beliefs and catastrophizing: Occurrence and risk factor in back pain and ADL in the general population. *Pain, 99*, 485–491.

Burton, A. K., Tillotson, K. M., Main, C. J., & Hollus, S. (1995). Psychosocial predictors of outcome in acute and subchronic low back trouble. *Spine, 20*, 722–728.

Calabrese, S., Lyness, J., Sorensen, S., & Duberstein, P. (2006). Personality and the association of pain and depression. *The American Journal of Geriatric Psychiatry, 14*(6), 546–549.

Casarett, D., Karlawish, J., Sankar, P., Hirschman, K., & Asch, D. A. (2001). Designing pain research for the patient's perspective: What trial end points are important to patients with chronic pain? *Pain Medicine, 2*, 309–316.

Cepeda, M. S., & Carr, D. B. (2003). Women experience more pain and require more morphine than men to achieve similar degree of analgesia. *Anesthesia and Analgesia, 97*, 1464–1468.

Cherkin, D. C., Deyo, R. A., Street, J. H., & Barlow, W. (1996). Predicting poor outcomes from back pain seen in primary care using patients' own criteria. *Spine, 21*, 2900–2907.

Clark, M. R., Katon, W., Russo, J., Kith, P., Sintay, M., & Buchwalk, D. (1995). Risk factors for symptom persistence in a 2½ year follow-up study. *The American Journal of Medicine, 98*, 187–195.

Cleeland, C. S., Cleeland, L. M., Dar, R., & Rinehardt, L. C. (1986). Factors influencing physician management of cancer pain. *Cancer, 58*, 796–800.

Cloninger, C. (1994). *The temperment and character inventory (TCI): A guide to its development and use*. St. Louis: Center for Psychobiology of Personality, Washington University.

Cloninger, C., Svrakic, D. M., & Przybeck, T. R. (1993). A psychobiological model of temperment and character. *Archives of General Psychiatry, 50*, 975–990.

Conrad, R., Schilling, G., Bausch, C., Nadstawek, J., Wartenberg, H., & Wegener, I. (2007). Temperament and character personality profiles and personality disorders in chronic pain patients. *Pain, 133*, 192–199.

Coryell, W., & Norton, S. G. (1981). Briquet's syndrome (somatization disorder) and primary depression: Comparison of background and outcome. *Comprehensive Psychiatry, 22*, 249–256.

Costa, P., & McCrae, R. (1992). *NEO PI-R professional manual: Revised NEO personality inventory (NEO PI-R) and NEO five-factor inventory (NEO-FFI)*. Odessa: Psychological Assessment Resources.

Coyne, J. C., Schwenk, T. L., & Fechner-Bates, S. (1995). Nondetection of depression by primary care physicians reconsidered. *General Hospital Psychiatry, 17*, 3–12.

Cramer, J. A., & Rosenheck, R. (1998). Compliance with medication regimens for mental and physical disorders. *Psychiatric Services, 49*, 196–201.

Crombez, G., Vlaeyen, J. W., Heuts, P. H., & Lysens, R. (1999). Pain-related fear is more disabling than pain itself: Evidence on the role of pain-related fear in chronic back pain disability. *Pain, 80*, 329–339.

de Groot, K. I., Boeke, S., van den Berge, H. J., Duivenvoorden, H. J., Bonke, B., & Passchier, J. (1997). The influence of psychological variables on postoperative anxiety and physical complaints in patients undergoing lumbar surgery. *Pain, 69*, 19–25.

den Boer, J. J., Oostendorp, R. A., Beems, T., Munneke, M., Oerlemans, M., & Evers, A. W. (2006). A systematic review of bio-psychosocial risk factors for an unfavourable outcome after lumbar disc surgery. *Euro Spine J, 15*, 527–536.

Derogatis, L. R., Lipman, R. S., & Covi, L. (1973). SCL-90: An outpatient psychiatric rating scale – preliminary report. *Psychopharmacology Bulletin, 9*, 13–28.

Deyo, R. A. (1986). The early diagnostic evaluation of patients with low back pain. *Journal of General Internal Medicine, 1*, 328–335.

Di Iorio, D., Henley, E., & Doughty, A. (2000). A survey of primary care physician practice patterns and adherence to acute low back problem guidelines. *Archives of Family Medicine, 9*, 1015–1021.

DiMatteo, M. R., Lepper, H. S., & Croghan, T. W. (2000). Depression is a risk factor for noncompliance with medical treatment: Meta-analysis of the effects of anxiety and depression on patient adherence. *Archives of Internal Medicine, 160*, 2101–2107.

Dionne, C. E., Koepsell, T. D., Von Korff, M., Deyo, R. A., Barlow, W. E., & Checkoway, H. (1997). Predicting long-term functional limitations among back pain patients in primary care settings. *Journal of Clinical Epidemiology, 50*, 31–43.

Doan, B. D., & Wadden, N. P. (1989). Relationship between depressive symptoms and descriptions of chronic pain. *Pain, 36*, 75–84.

Dolce, J. J., Crocker, M. F., & Doleys, D. M. (1986). Prediction of outcome among chronic pain patients. *Behaviour Research and Therapy, 24*, 313–319.

Dworkin, R. H., & Gitlin, M. J. (1991). Clinical aspects of depression in chronic pain patients. *The Clinical Journal of Pain, 7*, 79–94.

Dworkin, R., Hetzel, R., & Banks, S. (1999). Toward a model of the pathogenesis of chronic pain. *Seminars in Clinical Neuropsychiatry, 4*(3), 176–185.

Dworkin, S. F., Turner, J. A., Mancl, L., Wilson, L., Massoth, D., Huggins, K. H., et al. (2002). A randomized clinical trial of a tailored comprehensive care treatment program for temporomandibular disorders. *Journal of Orofacial Pain, 16*, 259–276.

Eccleston, C., Morley, S., Williams, A., Yorke, L., & Mastroyannopoulou, K. (2002). Systematic review of randomised controlled trials of psychological therapy for chronic pain in children and adolescents, with a subset of meta-analysis of pain relief. *Pain, 99*, 157–165.

Elliott, A. M., Smith, B. H., Penny, K. I., Smith, W. C., & Chambers, W. A. (1999). The epidemiology of chronic pain in the community. *The Lancet, 354*, 1248–1252.

Engel, G. L. (1959). "Psychogenic" pain and the pain-prone patient. *American Journal of Medicine, 26*, 899–918.

Engel, G. L. (1977). The need for a new medical model: A challenge for biomedicine. *Science, 196*, 129–136.

Epstein, S. A., Kay, G., Clauw, D., Heaton, R., Klein, D., & Krupp, L. (1999). Psychiatric disorders in patients with fibromyalgia: A multicenter investigation. *Psychosomatics, 40*, 57–63.

Escobar, J. I., Gara, M. A., Diaz-Martinez, A. M., Interian, A., Warman, M., & Allen, L. A. (2007). Effectiveness of a time-limited cognitive behavior therapy-type intervention among primary care patients with medically unexplained symptoms. *Annals of Family Medicine, 5*, 328–335.

Escobar, J. I., Waitzkin, H., & Silver, R. C. (1998). Abridged somatization: A study in primary care. *Psychosomatic Medicine, 60*, 466–472.

Fava, G. A., Freyberger, H. J., Bech, P., Ghristodoulou, T., Sensky, T., Theorell, T., et al. (1995). Diagnostic criteria for use in psychosomatic research. *Psychotherapy and Psychosomatics, 63*, 1–8.

First, M., Gibbon, M., Spitzer, R., Williams, J., & Benjamin, L. (1997). *Structured clinical interview for DSM-IV axis II personality disorders (SCID-II)*. Washington: American Psychiatric Publishers.

Fishbain, D., Cole, B., Cutler, R., Lewis, J., Rosomoff, H., & Rosomoff, R. (2006). Chronic pain and the measurement of personality: Do states influence traits? *Pain Medicine, 7*, 509–529.

Fleet, R. P., Dupuis, G., Marchand, A., Burelle, D., Arsenault, A., & Bernard, D. (1996). Panic disorder in emergency department chest pain patients: Prevalence, comorbidity, suicidal ideation, and physician recognition. *The American Journal of Medicine, 101*, 371–380.

Flor, H., Fydrich, T., & Turk, D. C. (1992). Efficacy of multidisciplinary pain treatment centers: A meta-analytic review. *Pain, 49*, 221–230.

Forrest, A. J., & Wolkind, S. N. (1974). Masked depression in men with low back pain. *Rheumatology and Rehabilitation, 13*, 148–153.

Frank, R. G., Elliott, T., Corcoran, J., & Wonderlich, S. (1987). Depression following spinal cord injury: Is it necessary? *Clinical Psychology Review, 7*, 611–630.

Gatchel, R. J. (1996). Psychological disorders and chronic Pain: Cause and effect relationships. In D. C. Turk & R. Gatchel (Eds.), *Psychosocial approaches to pain management: A practitioner's handbook* (pp. 33–52). New York: Guilford.

Gatchel, R. J., Peng, Y. B., Fuchs, P. N., Peters, M. L., & Turk, D. C. (2007). The biopsychosocial approach to chronic pain: Scientific advances and future directions. *Psychological Bullentin, 133*, 581–624.

Gatchel, R. J., & Turk, D. (1996). *Psychological approaches to pain management: A practitioner's handbook*. New York: Guilford.

Gatchel, R. J., & Weisberg, J. (2000). *Personality characteristics of patients with pain*. Washington: American Psychological Association.

Gatchel, R. J., & Okifuji, A. (2006). Evidence-based scientific data documenting the treatment and cost-effectiveness of comprehensive pain programs for chronic pain management. *J Pain, 7*, 779–793.

Gaynes, B. N., Magruder, K. M., & Burns, B. J. (1995). Does a coexisting anxiety disorder predict persistence of depressive illness in primary care patients with major depression? *General Hospital Psychiatry, 21*, 158–167.

Gaynes, B. N., Rush, A. J., Trivedi, M. H., Wisniewski, S. R., Balasubramani, G. K., & Spencer, D. C. (2007). Major depression symptoms in primary care and psychiatric settings: A cross-sectional analysis. *Annals of Family Medicine, 5*, 126–134.

Gehi, A., Haas, D., Pipkin, S., & Whooley, M. A. (2005). Depression and medication adherence in outpatients with coronary heart disease. *Archives of Internal Medicine, 165*, 2508–2515.

Gentry, W. D., Shows, W. D., & Thomas, M. (1974). Chronic low back pain: A psychological profile. *Psychosomatics, XV*, 174–177.

Gerber, P. D., Barrett, J., Barrett, J., Manheimer, E., Whitting, R., & Smith, R. (1989). Recognition of depression by internists in primary care: A comparison of internist and "gold standard" psychiatric assessments. *Journal of General Internal Medicine, 4*, 7–13.

Gil, K. M., Abrams, M. R., & Phillips, G. (1993). Sickle cell disease pain: Predicting health care use and activity level at 0-month follow-up. *Journal of Consulting and Clinical Psychology, 60*, 267–273.

Gil, K. M., Thompson, R. J., & Keith, B. R. (1992). Sickle cell disease pain in children and adolescents: Change in pain frequency and coping strategies over time. *Journal of Pediatric Psychology, 18*, 621–637.

Gran, J. T. (2003). The epidemiology of chronic generalized musculoskeletal pain. *Best Practice & Research. Clinical Rheumatology, 17*, 547–561.

Granot, M., & Ferber, S. G. (2005). The roles of pain catastrophizing and anxiety in the prediction of postoperative pain intensity: a prospective study. *The Clinical Journal of Pain, 21*, 439–445.

Grotle, M., Vollstad, N. K., Veierod, M. B., & Brox, J. I. (2004). Fear-avoidance beliefs and distress in relation to disability in acute and chronic low back pain. *Pain, 112*, 343–352.

Gureje, O., Simon, G. E., & Ustun, T. (1997). Somatization in cross-cultural perspective: A World Health Organization study in primary care. *The American Journal of Psychiatry, 154*, 989–995.

Gureje, O., Von Korff, M., Kola, L., Demyttenaere, K., He, Y., & Posada-Villa, J. (2008). The relation between multiple pains and mental disorders: Results for the World Mental Health Surveys. *Pain, 135*, 82–91.

Guzman, J., Esmail, R., Karjalainen, K., Malmivaara, A., Irvin, E., & Bombardier, C. (2002). Interdisciplinary bio-psycho-social rehabilitation for chronic low back pain. *Cochrane Database of Systemic Reviews, 1*, CD000963.

Hagg, O., Fritzell, P., Ekselius, L., & Nordwall, A. (2003). Predictors of outcome in fusion surgery for chronic low back pain. A report from the Swedish Lumbar Spine Study. *European Spine Journal, 12*, 22–33.

Hahn, S. R. (2001). Physical symptoms and physician-experienced difficulty in the physician-patient relationship. *Annals of Internal Medicine, 134*, 897–904.

Hanvik, L. J. (1951). MMPI profiles in patients with low back pain. *Journal of Consulting Psychology, 15*, 350–353.

Hathaway, S. R., & McKinley, J. (1943). *Minnesota multiphasic personality inventory*. Minneapolis: University of Minnesota Press.

Henningsen, P., Zimmerman, T., & Sattel, H. (2003). Medically unexplained physical symptoms, anxiety, and depression: A meta-analytic review. *Psychosomatic Medicine, 65*, 528–533.

Hirsch, A. T., George, S. Z., & Robinson, M. E. (2009). Pain assessment and treatment disparities: A virtual human technology investigation. *Pain, 143*, 106–113.

Hoffman, D. E., & Tarzian, A. J. (2001). The girl who cried pain: A bias against women in the treatment of pain. *The Journal of Law, Medicine & Ethics, 29*, 12–27.

Hunt, I. M., Silman, A. J., & Benjamin, S. (1999). The prevalence and associated features of chronic widespread pain in the community using the "Manchester" definition of chronic widespread pain. *Rheumatology, 38*, 275–279.

Institute of Medicine. (2004). *Improving medical education: Enhancing the behavioral and social science content of medical school curricula*. Washington: The National Academies Press.

IOM (Institute of Medicine). (2011). *Relieving pain in America: A blueprint for transforming prevention, care, education, and research*. Washington DC: The National Academies Press.

Jackson, J., & Browning, R. (2005). Impact of national low back pain guidelines on clinical practice. *Southern Medical Journal, 98*, 139–142.

Jacobson, P. B., & Butler, R. W. (1996). Relation of cogntive coping and catastrophizing to acute pain and analgesic use following breast cancer surgery. *J Behav Med, 19*, 17–29.

Jensen, M. P., & Karoly, P. (1991). Control beliefs, coping efforts, and adjustment to chronic pian. *Journal of Consulting and Clinical Psychology, 59*, 431–438.

Jensen, M. P., Turner, J. A., & Romano, J. M. (2001). Change in beliefs, catastrophizing, and coping are associated with improvement in multidisciplinary pain treatment. *Journal of Consulting and Clinical Psychology, 69*, 655–662.

Johannes, C. B., Le, T. K., Zhou, X., Johnston, J. A., & Dworkin, R. H. (2010). The prevalence of chronic pain in United States adults: Results of an internet based study. *The Journal of Pain, 11*, 1230–1239.
Joint Commission on Accreditation of Healthcare Organizations. (2000). *Implementing the new pain management standards*. Oakbrook Terrace: JCAHO.
Kalkman, C. J., Visser, K., Moen, J., Bonsel, G. J., Grobbee, D. E., & Moons, K. G. (2003). Preoperative prediction of severe postoperative pain. *Pain, 105*, 415–423.
Katon, W. J., Lin, E., & Kroenke, K. (2007). The association of depressive and anxiety with medical symptom burden in patients with chronic medical illness. *General Hospital Psychiatry, 29*, 147–155.
Katon, W. J., Lin, E., Von Korff, M., Russo, J., Lipscomb, P., & Bush, T. (1991). Somatization: A spectrum of severity. *The American Journal of Psychiatry, 148*, 34–40.
Katon, W. J., & Sullivan, M. D. (1990). Depression and chronic medical illness. *The Journal of Clinical Psychiatry, 51*, 3–11.
Katon, W. J., Sullivan, M. D., & Walker, E. (2001). Medical symptoms without identified pathology: Relationship to psychiatric disorders, childhood and adult trauma and personality traits. *Annals of Internal Medicine, 134*, 917–925.
Keefe, F. J., Brown, G. K., Wallston, K. A., & Caldwell, D. S. (1989). Coping with rheumatoid arthritis pain: Catastrophizing as a maladaptive strategy. *Pain, 37*, 51–56.
Keefe, F. J., Lebebvre, J. C., Egert, J. R., Affleck, G., Sullivan, M. J., & Caldwell, D. S. (2001). The relationship of gender to pain, pain behavior, and disability in osteoarthritis patients: The role of catastrophizing. *Pain, 87*, 325–334.
Kerns, R. D., & Haythornthwaite, J. A. (1988). Depression among chronic pain patients: Cognitive-behavioral analysis and effect on rehabilitation outcome. *Journal of Consulting and Clinical Psychology, 56*, 870–876.
Kessler, R. C., Berglund, P., Demler, O., Jin, R., Koretz, D., Merikangas, K. R., et al. (2003). The epidemiology of major depressive disorder: Results from the National Comorbidity Survey Replication (NCS-R). *JAMA, 289*, 3095–3105.
Kessler, R. C., Berglund, P., Demler, O., Jin, R., & Walters, E. E. (2005). Lifetime prevalence and age-of-onset distributions of DSM-IV disorders in the National Co-morbidity Survey Replication. *Archives of General Psychiatry, 62*, 593–602.
Kessler, R. C., Wat Tat Chiu, A. M., Demler, O., & Walters, E. E. (2005). Prevalence, severity, and co-morbidity of 12-month DSM-IV disorders in the National Co-morbidity Survey Replication. *Archives of General Psychiatry, 62*, 617–627.
Komaroff, A. L. (1990). "Minor" illness symptoms: The magnitude of their burden and of our ignorance. *Archives of Internal Medicine, 150*, 1586–1587.
Kori, S. H., Miller, R. P., & Todd, D. D. (1990). Kinesiophobia: A new view of chronic pain behavior. *Pain Manage, 3*, 35–43.
Kroenke, K. (2001). Studying symptoms: Sampling and measuring issues. *Annals of Internal Medicine, 134*, 844–853.
Kroenke, K. (2007). Efficacy of treatment for somatoform disorders: A review of randomized controlled trials. *Psychosomatic Medicine, 69*, 881–888.
Kroenke, K., Jackson, J. L., & Chamberlin, J. (1997). Depressive and anxiety disorders in patients presenting with physical complaints: Clinical predictors and outcomes. *American Journal of Medicine, 103*, 339–347.
Kroenke, K., Shen, J., Oxman, T. E., Williams, J. W., & Dietrich, A. J. (2008). Impact of pain on the outcomes of depression treatment: Results from the RESPECT trial. *Pain, 134*, 209–215.
Kroenke, K., Spitzer, R. L., & Williams, J. B. (1994). Physical symptoms in primary care: Predictors of psychiatric disorders and functional impairment. *Archives of Family Medicine, 3*, 774–779.
Krueger, R., Tackett, J., & Markon, K. (2004). Structural models of comorbidity among common mental disorders: Connections to chronic pain. *Advances in Psychosomatic Medicine, 25*, 63–77.

Lamb, S. E., Guralnik, J. M., & Buchner, D. M. (2000). Factors that modify the association between knee pain and mobility limitation in older women: The Women's Health and Aging Study. *Annals of the Rheumatic Diseases, 59*, 331–337.

Lanes, T. C., Gauron, E. F., Spratt, K. F., Wernimont, T. J., Found, E. M., & Weinstein, J. N. (1995). Long-term follow-up of patients with chronic back pain treated in a multidisciplinary rehabilitation program. *Spine, 20*, 801–806.

Lang, E., Leibig, K., Kastner, S., Neundorfer, B., & Heuschmann, P. (2003). Interdisciplinary rehabilitation versus usual care for chronic low back pain in the community: Effects of quality of life. *The Spine Journal, 3*, 270–276.

Lauver, S., & Johnson, J. (1997). The role of neuroticism and social support in older adults with chronic pain behavior. *Personality and Individual Differences, 23*, 165–167.

Lin, E. H., Katon, W., & Von Korff, M. (1991). Frustrated patients: Physician and patient perspectives among distressed high users of medical services. *Journal of General Internal Medicine, 6*, 241–246.

Lin, E. H., Katon, W., Von Korff, M., Tang, L., Willimas, J. W., & Kroenke, K. (2003). Effect of improving depressoin care on pain and functioal outcomes among older adults with arthritis. *JAMA, 290*, 2428–2434.

Linton, S. J., Overmeer, T., Janson, M., Vlaeyen, J. W., & de Jong, J. R. (2002). Graded in vivo exposure treatment for fear-avoidant pain patients with functional disability: A case study. *Cognitive Behaviour Therapy, 31*, 49–58.

Loeser, J. D., & Melzack, R. (1999). Pain: An overview. *The Lancet, 3535*, 1607–1609.

Lohnberg, J. A. (2007). A review of outcomes studies on cognitive-behavioral therapy for reducing fear-avoidance beliefs among individuals with chronic pain. *Journal of Clinical Psychology in Medical Settings, 14*, 113–122.

Lucas, C. E., Vlahos, A. L., & Ledgerwood, A. M. (2007). Kindness kills: The negative impact of pain as the fifth vital sign. *Journal of the American College of Surgery, 205*, 101–107.

Mannion, A. F., Elfering, A., Staerkle, R., Junge, A., Grob, D., Dvorak, J., et al. (2007). Predictors of multidimensional outcome after spinal surgery. *European Spine Journal, 16*, 777–786.

Marquie, L., Raufaste, E., Lauque, D., Marine, C., Ecoiffier, M., & Sorum, P. (2003). Pain ratings by patients and physicians: Evidence of a systematic pain miscalibration. *Pain, 102*, 289–296.

Mayou, R., Kirmayer, L. J., Simon, G., Kroenke, K., & Sharpe, M. (2005). Somatoform disorders: Time for a new approach in DSM-V. *American Journal of Psychiatry, 162*, 847–855.

McCracken, L. M., Faber, S. D., & Janeck, A. S. (1998). Pain-related anxiety predicts non-specific physical complaints in persons with chronic pain. *Behaviour Research and Therapy, 36*, 621–630.

McCreary, C., Turner, J., & Dawson, E. (1977). Differences between functional versus organic low back pain patients. *Pain, 4*, 73–78.

McCreary, C., Turner, J., & Sawson, E. (1979). The MMPI as a predictor of response to conservative treatment for low back pain. *Journal of Clinical Psychology, 3*, 278–284.

McNeil, D. W., & Rainwater, A. J. (1998). Development of the Fear of Pain Questionnaire-III. *Journal of Behavioral Medicine, 21*, 389–410.

Melzack, R., & Wall, P. D. (1965). Pain mechanisms: A new theory. *Science, 150*, 971–979.

Middleton, N., Gunnell, D., Whitley, E., Darling, D., & Fankel, S. (2001). Secular trends in antidepressant prescribing in the IK, 1975-1998. *Journal of Public Health Medicine, 23*, 262–267.

Millon, T., Davis, R., Millon, C., & Grossman, S. (2009). *The Millon Clinical Mulitaxial Inventory-III* (3rd ed.). Minneapolis: National Computer Systems.

Miro, J., Huguet, A., & Nieto, R. (2007). Predictive factors of chronic pediatric pain and disability: A delphi poll. *The Journal of Pain, 8*, 774–792.

Monsen, K., & Monsen, J. T. (2000). Chronic pain and psychodynamic body therapy: A controlled outcome study. *Psychotherapy, 37*, 257–269.

Morley, S., Eccleston, C., & Williams, A. (1999). Systematic review and meta-analysis of randomized controlled trials of cognitive behavioral therapy and behavior therapy for chronic pain in adults, excluding headache. *Pain, 80*, 1–13.

Moulin, D. E., Clark, A. J., Speechley, M., & Morley-Foster, P. K. (2002). Chronic pain in Canada: Prevalence, treatment, impact and the role of opioid analgesia. *Pain Research and Management, 7*, 179–184.

Mularski, R. A., White-Chu, F., Overbay, D., Miller, L., Asch, S. M., & Ganzini, L. (2006). Measuring pain as the 5th vital sign does not improve quality of pain management. *Journal of General Internal Medicine, 21*, 607–612.

Murskey, H., & Bogduk, N. (1994). *Classification of chronic pain* (p. 210). Seattle: International Association for the Study of Pain Press.

Naessens, J. M., Baird, M. A., Van Hourten, H. K., Vanness, D. J., & Campbell, C. R. (2005). Predicting persistently high primary care use. *Annals of Family Medicine, 3*, 324–330.

Nezu, A. M., Nezu, C. M., & Lombardo, E. R. (2001). Cognitive-behavior therapy for medically unexplained symptoms: A critical review of the treatment literature. *Behavior Therapy, 32*, 537–583.

Niles, B. L., Mori, D. L., Lambert, J. F., & Wolf, E. J. (2005). Depression in primary care: Comorbid disorders and related problems. *Journal of Clinical Psychology in Medical Settings, 12*, 71–77.

O'Brien, E. M., Staud, R. M., Hassinger, A. D., McCulloch, R. C., Craggs, J. G., Atchison, J. W., et al. (2010). Patient-centered perspective on treatment outcomes in chronic pain. *Pain Medicine, 11*, 6–15.

O'Donohue, W., & Cucciare, M. A. (2005). The role of psychological factors in medical presentations. *Journal of Clinical Psychology in Medical Settings, 12*, 13–24.

Ojifuji, A., Turk, D. C., & Kalauokalani, D. (1999). Clinical outcomes and economic evaluation of the multidisciplinary pain centers. In A. Block, E. Kremer, & E. Fernandez (Eds.), *Handbook of pain syndromes* (pp. 77–99). Mahwah: Lawrence Erlbaum.

Osman, A., Barrios, F. X., Gutierrez, P. M., Kopper, B., Merrifield, T., & Grittmann, L. (2000). The Pain Catastrophizing Scale: Further psychometric evaluation with adult samples. *Journal of Behavioral Medicine, 23*, 351–365.

Ostelo, R.W., van Tulder, M.W., Vlayen, J.W., Linton, S.J., Morley, S.J., & Assendelft, W.J. (2005). Behavioural treatment for chronic low back pain. *Cochrane Database of Systemic Review,* 1, CD002014. DOI: 10.1002/14651858.CD002014.pub2.

Painter, J. R., Seres, J. L., & Newman, R. I. (1980). Assessing the benefits of the pain center: Why some patients regress. *Pain, 8*, 101–113.

Palermo, T. M., Eccleston, C., Lewandowski, A. S., Williams, A., & Morley, S. (2010). Randomized controlled trials of psychological therapies for management of chronic pain in children and adolescents: An updated meta-analytic review. *Pain, 148*, 387–397.

Paquet, C., Kergoal, M. J., & Dube, L. (2005). The role of everyday emotion regulation on pain in hospitalized elderly: Insights from a prospective within-day assessment. *Pain, 115*, 355–363.

Perez-Stable, E. J., Miranda, J., Munoz, R. F., & Ying, Y. (1990). Depression in medical outpatients: Underrecognition and misdiagnosis. *Archives of Internal Medicine, 150*, 1083–1088.

Peter, E., & Watt-Watson, J. (2008). Improving pain management eduction. In S. Rachiq, D. Schlopflocher, P. Taenzer, & E. Jonsson (Eds.), *Chronic pain: A health policy perspective*. New York: Wiley-Blackwell.

Peters, M. (2009). Optimism as a resiliency for chronic pain. *European Journal of Pain, 13*, S7.

Peters, M. L., & Vancleef, L. M. G. (2008). The role of personality traits in pain perception and disability. *Review in Analgesia, 10*, 11–22.

Pilowsky, I., & Barrow, C. (1990). A controlled study of psychotherapy and Amitriptyline used individually and in combination in the treatment of chronic intractable "psychogenic" pain. *Pain, 40*, 3–19.

Pincus, T., Burton, K., Vogel, S., & Field, A. P. (2002). A systematic review of psychological factors as predictors of chronicity/disability in prospective cohorts of low back pain. *Spine, 27*, E109–E120.

Reich, J., & Thompson, D. (1987). DSM-III personality disorder clusters in three populations. *British Journal of Psychiatry, 150*, 471–475.

Reid, M. C., Engles-Horton, L. L., Weber, M. B., Kerns, R. D., Rogers, E. L., & O'Connor, P. G. (2002). Use of opioid medications for chronic noncancer pain syndromes in primary care. *Journal of General Internal Medicine, 17*, 173–179.

Robinson, M. E., Brown, J. L., George, S. Z., Edwards, P. S., Atchison, J. W., Hirsh, A. T., Waxenberg, L. B., Wittmer, V., & Fillingham, R. B. (2005). Multidimensional success criteria and expectations for treatment of chronic pain: The patient perspective. *Pain Med, 6*, 336–345.

Roelofs, J., Goubert, L., Peters, M. L., Vlaeyen, J. W., & Crombez, G. (2004). The Tampa Scale for Kinesiophobia: Further examination of psychometric properties in patients with chronic low back pain and fibromyalgia. *European Journal of Pain, 8*, 495–502.

Romano, J. M., & Turner, J. A. (1985). Chronic pain and depression: Does the evidence support a relationship? *Psychological Bulletin, 97*, 18–34.

Rosenstiel, A. K., & Keefe, F. J. (1983). The use of coping strategies in chronic low back pain: Relationship to patient characteristics and current adjustment. *Pain, 17*, 33–44.

Samwel, H. J., Kraaimaat, F. W., Crul, B. J., & Evers, A. W. (2007). The role of fear avoidance and helplessness in explaining functional disability in chronic pain: A prospective study. *International Journal of Behavioral Medicine, 14*, 237–241.

Sansone, R. A., Sansone, L. A., & Wiederman, M. W. (1996). Borderline personality disorder and health care utilization in a primary care setting. *Southern Medical Journal, 89*, 1367–1372.

Sengstaken, E. A., & King, S. A. (1994). Primary care physicians and pain: Education during residency. *The Clinical Journal of Pain, 10*, 303–308.

Severeijns, R., Vlaeyen, J. W., & van den Hout, M. (2004). Do we need a communal coping model of pain catastrophizing? An alternative explanation. *Pain, 111*, 226–229.

Shah, A. (1992). The burden of psychiatric disorders in primary care. *International Review of Psychiatry, 4*, 243–250.

Simmonds, M. J., & Scudds, R. J. (2001). Pain, disability, and physical therapy in older adults: Issues of patients and pain, practitioners and practice. *Topics in Geriatric Rehabilitation, 16*, 12–23.

Simon, G. E. (1992). Psychiatric disorder and functional somatic symptoms as predictors of health care use. *Psychiatric Medicine, 10*, 49–59.

Simon, G. E., & Von Korff, M. (1991). Somatization and psychiatric disorder in the NIMH epidemiological catchment area study. *The American Journal of Psychiatry, 148*, 1494–1500.

Simon, G. E., Von Korff, M., Piccinelli, M., Fullerton, C., & Ormel, J. (1999). An international study of the relationship between somatic symptoms and depression. *The New England Journal of Medicine, 341*, 1329–1335.

Simpson, R. J., Kazmierczak, T., Power, K. G., & Sharp, D. M. (1994). Controlled comparison of the characteristics of patients with panic disorder. *British Journal of General Practice, 44*, 352–356.

Smith, G. R., Monson, R. A., & Ray, D. C. (1986). Patients with multiple unexplained symptoms: Their characteristics, functional health, and health care utilization. *Archives of Internal Medicine, 146*, 69–72.

Smeets, R. J., Vlaeyen, J. W. S., Kester, A. D., & Knottnerus, J. A. (2006). Reduction of pain catastrophizing mediates the outcome of both physical and cognitive-behavioral treatment in chronic low back pain. *J Pain, 7*, 261–271.

Soni, A. (2010). *Back problems: Use and expenditures for the U.S. adult population, 2007.* Statistical brief #289, July 2010. Rockville: Agency for Healthcare Research and Quality, from http://www.meps.ahrq.gov/mepsweb/data_files/publications/st289/stat289.shtml

Spinhoven, P., ter Kuile, M., Kole-Snijders, A. M., Mansfield, M. H., den Ouden, D. J., & Vlaeyen, J. W. (2004). Catastrophizing and internal pain control as mediators of outcome in the multidisciplinary treatment of low back pain. *European Journal of Pain, 8*, 211–219.

Stafford, R. S., MacDonald, E. A., & Finkelstein, S. N. (2001). National patterns of medication treatment for depression, 1987-2001. *Primary Care Companion to the Journal of Clinical Psychiatry, 3*, 232–235.

Stein, M. B., Kirk, P., Prabhu, V., Grott, M., & Terepa, M. (1995). Mixed anxiety-depression in a primary care clinic. *Journal of Affective Disorders, 34*, 79–84.

Stern, J., Murphy, M., & Bass, C. (1993). Attitudes of British psychiatrists to the diagnosis of somatization disorder: A questionnaire survey. *The British Journal of Psychiatry, 162*, 463–466.

Sternbach, R. A. (1974). *Pain patients: Traits and treatment*. New York: Academic.

Stover, B. D., Turner, J. A., Franklin, G., Gluck, J. V., Fulton-Kehoe, D., Sheppard, L., et al. (2006). Factors associated with early opioid prescription among workers with low back injuries. *The Journal of Pain, 7*, 718–725.

Sullivan, M. J., Tripp, D. A., & Santor, D. (2000). Gender differences in pain and pain behavior: The role of catastrophizing. *Cog Res Ther, 21*, 555–568.

Sullivan, M. J., Adams, H., Rhodenizer, T., & Stanish, W. D. (2006). A psychosocial risk factor-targeted intervention for the prevention of chronic pain and disability following whiplash injury. *Physical Therapy, 86*, 8–18.

Sullivan, M. D., Edlund, M. J., Steffick, D., & Unutzer, J. (2005). Regular use of prescribed opioids: Association with common psychiatric disorders. *Pain, 119*, 95–103.

Sullivan, M. J., Feuerstein, M., Gatchel, R. J., Linton, S. J., & Pransky, G. (2005). Integrating psychosocial and behavioral interventions to achieve optimal rehabilitation outcomes. *Journal of Occupational Rehabilitation, 15*, 475–489.

Sullivan, M. J., Reesor, K., Mikail, S., & Fisher, R. (1992). The treatment of depression in chronic low back pain: Review and recommendations. *Pain, 50*, 5–13.

Sullivan, M. J., Thorn, B. E., Haythornthwaite, J. A., Keefe, F., Martin, M., Bradley, L. A., et al. (2001). Theoretical perspectives on the relation between catastrophizing and pain. *The Clinical Journal of Pain, 17*, 52–64.

Swinkels-Meewisse, E. J., Swinkels, R. A., Verbeek, A. L., Vlaeyen, J. W., & Oostendorp, R. A. (2003). Psychometric properties of the Tampa Scale of Kinesiophobia and the fear-avoidance beliefs questionnaire in acute low back pain. *Manual Therapy, 8*, 29–36.

Taenzer, P., Melzack, R., & Jeans, M. E. (1986). Influence of psychological factors on postoperative pain, mood and analgesic requirements. *Pain, 24*, 331–342.

Tan, G., Jensen, M. P., Robinson-Whelen, S., Thornby, J. I., & Monga, T. N. (2001). Coping with chronic pain: A comparison of two measures. *Pain, 90*, 127–133.

Torrence, N., Smith, B. H., Bennett, M. I., & Lee, A. J. (2006). The epidemiology of chronic pain of predominately neuropathic origin. Results from a general population study. *Journal of Pain, 7*, 281–289.

Thorn, B. E., Boothy, J. L., & Sullivan, M. J. (2002). Targeted treatment of catastrophizing for the management of pain. *Cog Beh Prac, 9*, 127–138.

Thorn, B. E., Pence, L. B., Ward, L. C., Kilgo, G., Clements, K. L., Cross, T. H., Davis, A. M., & Tsui, P. W. (2007). A randomized clinical trial of targeted cognitive behavioral treatment to reduce catastrophizing in chronic headache sufferers. *J Pain, 8*, 938–949.

Turk, D. C., & Flor, H. (1999). Chronic pain: A biobehavioral perspective. In R. J. Gatchel & D. C. Turk (Eds.), *Psychosocial factors in pain: Critical perspectives* (pp. 18–34). New York: Guilford.

Turk, D. C., Loeser, J. D., & Monarch, E. S. (2002). Chronic pian: Purposes and costs of interdisciplinary pain rehabilitation programs. *Trends in Evidence Based Neuropsychiatry, 4*, 64–69.

Turk, D. C., & Okifuji, A. (1997). What factors affect physicians' decisions to prescribe opioids for chronic non-cancer pain patients? *The Clinical Journal of Pain, 13*, 330–336.

Turk, D. C., & Okifuji, A. (1998). Treatment of chronic pain patients: Clinical outcomes, cost-effectiveness and cost-benefits of multidisciplinary pain centers. *Critical Reviews in Physical and Rehabilitation Medicine, 10*, 181–208.

Turk, D. C., & Okifuji, A. (2002). Psychological factors in chronic pain: Evolution and revolution. *Journal of Consulting and Clinical Psychology, 70*, 678–690.

Turk, D. C., Swanson, K. S., & Tunks, E. R. (2008). Psychological approaches in the treatment of chronic pain patients – When pills, scalpels and needles are not enough. *Canadian Journal of Psychiatry, 53*, 213–223.

Turner, J. A., Dworkin, S. F., Mancl, L., Huggins, K. H., & Truelove, E. L. (2001). The role of beliefs, catastrophizing, and coping in the functioning of patients with temporomandibular disorders. *Pain, 92*, 41–51.

Turner, J. A., & Jensen, M. P. (1993). Efficacy of cognitive therapy for chronic low back pain. *Pain, 52*, 169–177.

Upshur, C. C., Luckmann, R. S., & Savageau, J. A. (2006). Primary care provider concerns about management of chronic pain in community clinic populations. *Journal of General Internal Medicine, 21*, 652–655.

Van Dorsten, B. (2006). Psychological considerations in preparing patients for implantation procedures. *Pain Medicine, 7*, S47–S57.

Van Dorsten, B., Dingmann, C., Brewer, A., Bridgewater, J., Davies, H.R., & Benchekroun, S. (2005). A re-assessment of pain education in primary care residency in the United States. *11th World Congress on Pain, International Association for the Study of Pain*, Sydney, Australia.

Van Dorsten, B., & Lindley, E. M. (2010). *Improving outcomes via behavioral assessment of spine surgery candidates* (pp. 15–20). Jan/Feb: SpineLine.

van Tulder, M. W., Koes, B., & Malmivaara, A. (2005). Outcome of non-invasive treatment modalities on back pain: An evidence-based review. *European Spine Journal, 10*, 1017–1045.

Vlaeyen, J. W. S., de Jong, J., Geilen, M., Heuts, P. H., & Van Breukelen, G. (2001a). Graded exposure in vivo in the treatment of pain related fear: A replicated single-case experimental design in four patients with chronic low back pain. *Behaviour Research and Therapy, 39*, 151–166.

Vlaeyen, J. W. S., de Jong, J., Geilen, M., Heuts, P. H., & Van Breukelen, G. (2001b). The treatment of fear of movement/(re)injury in chronic low back pain: Further evidence on the effectiveness of exposure in vivo. *The Clinical Journal of Pain, 18*, 251–261.

Vlaeyen, J. W., Kole-Snijders, A. M., Boeren, R. G., & van Eck, H. (1995). Fear of movement/(re) injury in chronic low back pain and its relation to behavioral performance. *Pain, 62*, 363–373.

Vlaeyen, J. W., & Linton, S. J. (2000). Fear avoidance and its consequences in chronic musculoskeletal pain: A state of the art. *Pain, 85*, 317–332.

Von Korff, M., Ormel, J., Katon, W., & Lin, E. H. (1992). Disability and depression among hugh utilizers of health care: A longitudinal analysis. *Archives of General Psychiatry, 49*, 91–100.

Von Korff, M., Shapiro, S., & Burke, J. D. (1987). Anxiety and depression in a primary care clinic: Comparison of Diagnostic Interview Schedule, General Health Questionnaire and practitioner assessments. *Archives of General Psychiatry, 44*, 152–156.

Von Korff, M., & Simon, G. (1996). The relationship between pain and depression. *The British Journal of Psychiatry. Supplement, 30*, 101–108.

Von Roenn, J. H., Cleeland, C. S., Gonin, R., Hatfield, A. K., & Pandya, K. J. (1993). Physician attitudes and practice in cancer pain management: A survey from the Eastern Cooperative Oncology Group. *Annals of Internal Medicine, 119*, 121–126.

Vossen, H., Van Os, J., Hermens, H., & Lousberg, R. (2006). Evidence that trait-anxiety and trait-depression differentially moderate cortical processing of pain. *Clinical Journal of Pain, 22*, 725–729.

Waddell, G., Newton, M., Henderson, I., Somerville, D., & Main, C. J. (1993). A Fear Avoidance Beliefs Questionnaire (FABQ) and the role of fear avoidance beliefs in chronic pain and disability. *Pain, 52*, 157–168.

Wade, J. B., Price, D. D., Hamer, R. M., Schwartz, S. M., & Hart, R. P. (1990). An emotional component analysis of chronic pain. *Pain, 40*, 303–310.

Walker, B. F. (2000). The prevalence of low back pain: A systematic review of the literature from 1966-1998. *Journal of Spinal Disorders, 13*, 205–217.

Wall, C., Ogloff, J., & Morrissey, S. (2006). The psychology of injured workers: Health and cost of vocational rehabilitation. *Journal of Occupational Rehabilitation, 16*, 513–528.

Weinstein, S. M., Laux, L. F., Thornby, J. L., Lorimor, R. J., Hill, C. S., Thorpe, D. M., et al. (2000). Physician's attitudes toward pain and the use of opioid analgesics: Results of a survey from the Texas Cancer Pain Initiative. *Southern Medical Journal, 93*, 479–487.

Weisberg, J. (2000). Personality and personality disorders in chronic pain. *Current Review of Pain, 4*(1), 60–70.

Weisberg, J., & Keefe, F. (1997). Personality disorders in the chronic pain population: basic concepts, empirical findings, and clinical implications. *The Journal of Pain, 6*, 1.

Wells, K. B., Golding, J. M., & Burnam, M. A. (1989). Affective, substance use, and anxiety disorders in persons with arthritis, diabetes, heart disease, high bold pressure, or chronic lung conditions. *General Hospital Psychiatry, 11*, 320–327.

Widiger, T. A., Trull, T. J., Hurt, S. W., Clarkin, J., & Frances, A. (1987). A multidimensional scaling of the DSM-III personality disorders. *Archives of General Psychiatry, 44*, 557–563.

Williams, D. A. (1999). Acute pain (with emphasis on painful medical procedures). In R. J. Gatchel & D. C. Turk (Eds.), *Psychosocial factors in pain: Critical perspectives* (pp. 151–163). New York: Guilford.

Wiltse, L. L., & Rocchio, P. D. (1975). Preoperative psychological tests as predictors of success of chemonucleolysis in the treatment of the low back syndrome. *Journal of Bone and Joint Surgery, 57*, 478–483.

Wise, T. N., & Birket-Smith, M. (2002). The somatoform disorders for DSM-V: The need for changes in process and content. *Psychosomatics, 43*, 437–440.

Woolfolk, R. L., & Allen, L. A. (2007). *Treating somatization: A cognitive-behavioral approach*. New York: Guilford.

Chapter 8
Psychiatric Disorders, Stress, and Their Treatment Among People with Multiple Sclerosis

David C. Mohr

8.1 Introduction: Multiple Sclerosis

Multiple sclerosis (MS) is a chronic, often inflammatory disorder involving the CNS, that affects approximately 400,000 people in the United States and 2.5 million worldwide (Compston et al., 2006). It is believed to begin as an autoimmune disease, in which the immune system attacks the myelin sheath around the axons of the CNS, which results in plaques or lesions. As the disease progresses, it is believed to shift from an inflammatory disease to one with neurodegenerative features. Because MS is a disease of the CNS, symptoms are highly heterogonous. Common symptoms include, but are not limited to, debilitating fatigue, loss of function or feeling in limbs, loss of bowel or bladder control, sexual dysfunction, blindness due to optic neuritis, loss of balance, pain, cognitive dysfunction, and emotional changes (Noseworthy, Lucchinetti, Rodriguez, & Weinshenker, 2000).

The clinical course has two general clinical features: exacerbation and progression. Exacerbation is characterized by a sudden onset or increase of symptoms within 24 h, which if left untreated can last for weeks or months. Exacerbation is preceded by an autoimmune process in which the immune system mistakes a protein in the myelin sheath around the axons of the neurons of the CNS as foreign. Inflammation increases the permeability of the blood-brain barrier (BBB), allowing activated autoaggressive immune cells to gain access to the CNS, which then attack the myelin sheath. While autoaggressive immune activity often occurs without the individual noticing, if it causes sufficient damage, clinical symptoms of exacerbation can occur. As the inflammation subsides, the myelin can be repaired to some extent. Depending on the degree of repair, symptoms remit either fully or partially,

D.C. Mohr (✉)
Department of Preventive Medicine, Northwestern University, Feinberg School of Medicine, 680 N. Lakeshore Drive, Suite 1220, Chicago, IL 60611, USA
e-mail: d-mohr@northwestern.edu

S. Pagoto (ed.), *Psychological Co-morbidities of Physical Illness: A Behavioral Medicine Perspective*, DOI 10.1007/978-1-4419-0029-6_8,

leaving residual symptoms that are unlikely to improve. Progression refers to the steady worsening of symptoms that can occur in the absence of exacerbation, which is now believed to be a neurodegenerative process.

MS can take several possible courses (Lublin & Reingold, 1996). Approximately 85% of MS begins with a relapsing-remitting course characterized by periodic disease exacerbations with no progression. Approximately 10–15% begin with a primary progressive course in which there is a steady progression of symptoms with no exacerbations. It is very common for relapsing-remitting patients, as the disease worsens, to begin showing signs of progression between exacerbations and for the frequency of exacerbations to decline or even cease. This is referred to as a shift to secondary progressive MS and is believed to reflect a shift from an autoimmune process to a neurodegenerative process. A small percentage of patients with primary progressive MS begin showing exacerbations after a period of time, a course that is referred to as progressive-relapsing. These distinctions have significance in the medical treatment for MS. For example, medications that are effective for one course are often not effective for another course. However, for the purposes of this chapter, we will not make these distinctions except when necessary.

8.1.1 Epidemiology of MS

MS clearly has a genetic component, with 25–30% concordance rates among monozygotic twins (Milo & Kahana, 2009). MS is usually diagnosed between the ages of 20 and 40. Prevalence among women is about twice that found in men. MS is most common among Caucasians and is comparatively rare among other races. However, prevalence among African-Americans, while lower than European-Americans, is higher than among Africans. Asians who have immigrated to North America have rates that are higher than Asians who live in Asia. People who are born in more northern latitudes in the northern hemisphere (and more southern latitudes in the southern hemisphere) have greater risk of developing MS. Migration studies show that people who move in their youth (usually prior to age 10) acquire the risk of the new environment, while people who migrate at an older age (typically after age 15) are more likely to retain the risk of the environment that they move from. This has led to a variety of environmental theories of etiology. For example, a growing body of work suggests the lower exposure to sunlight in the northern latitudes and the resulting deficits in vitamin D could increase risk among genetically vulnerable individuals (Ascherio & Munger, 2007b). A variety of infectious agents have also been implicated. For example, people infected with the Epstein Barr virus at an early age are 10 times more likely to develop MS than those who are never infected, and 2–3 times more likely than those infected later in life (Ascherio & Munger, 2007a). Stress has also been implicated as a risk factor. For example, an epidemiological study using a large population-based register found that parents who lost a child under the age of 18 showed a more than 50% increased risk of subsequently developing MS compared to parents who did not lose a child (Li et al., 2004).

Furthermore, parents whose child died suddenly were more than twice as likely to develop MS, compared to those who did not lose their children. As sudden death (e.g., through accident, suicide, or homicide) is far more traumatic than death after a prolonged illness, this can be seen as a dose effect for the effects of stress.

While the etiology of MS remains very unclear, a growing body of evidence suggests a variety of causes that include genetic vulnerability, environmental exposures, and potentially even psychological factors.

8.1.2 Epidemiology of Psychological Disorders in MS

Depression is common among people with MS. Among a wide range of studies evaluating prevalence of depression, two stand out as having good methodology. A population-based epidemiological study found that the 12-month prevalence of major depressive disorder was 15.7% among people with MS, compared to 7.4% in the general population (Patten, Beck, Williams, Barbui, & Metz, 2003). Among people with MS of age 18–45, depression was particularly high, affecting 25.7% in a 12-month period. Lifetime risk of major depressive disorder was 50.3% (Sadovnick et al., 1996). Few studies have evaluated the frequency of other mood disorders such as dysthymia (Chwastiak & Ehde, 2007).

The literature on the prevalence of anxiety disorders in MS is smaller and there are no high quality studies. Estimates of prevalence rates range from 19 to 90% (Jose Sa, 2008), although most point prevalence rates for a clinically significant level of symptoms are in the 25–41% range (Feinstein, O'Connor, Gray, & Feinstein, 1999; Janssens et al., 2003; Zorzon et al., 2001).

In a study of 140 consecutive clinic MS patients, 35.7% were found to have a lifetime history of an anxiety disorder (Korostil & Feinstein, 2007). The period following diagnosis may be a time when patients are particularly vulnerable to anxiety. In the months following diagnosis, 36% showed clinically significant levels of anxiety (Janssens et al., 2003) which persisted for at least 2 years (Janssens et al., 2006).

Several studies have reported that bipolar disorder occurs at approximately twice the rate in MS than in the general population (Edwards & Constantinescu, 2004; Marrie et al., 2009; Schiffer, Wineman, & Weitkamp, 1986). Bipolar signs may precede other neurological symptoms of MS (Chwastiak & Ehde, 2007; Kwentus, Hart, Calabrese, & Hekmati, 1986). While the reasons for this remain unclear, there has been speculation that this may be due to the specific location of brain lesions as well as shared genetic etiology (Schiffer et al., 1986).

Dysregulation of affect is common as MS progresses. Euphoria, referring to an overly optimistic state, is estimated to occur in as many as 25% of MS patients, although these patients tend to have more advanced cognitive and physical impairment and to have greater numbers of brain lesions and loss of gray matter (Rabins et al., 1986; Sanfilipo, Benedict, Weinstock-Guttman, & Bakshi, 2006). Pseudobulbar affect, also referred to as pathological laughter and crying, refers to a syndrome in which expressions of affect occur in the absence of subject experiences of the emotions – laughter without mirth and tears without sadness (Korostil & Feinstein, 2007). This occurs in approximately 10% of patients and typically involves considerable loss of tissue over broad areas of the brain (Feinstein, Feinstein, Gray, & O'Connor, 1997).

8.1.2.1 Neuropsychological Functioning

While it is beyond the scope of this chapter to thoroughly review neuropsychological functioning, it is important that providers and researchers have some familiarity with cognitive impairment in MS. Estimates of the prevalence of cognitive impairment ranges from 43 to 70% (Chiaravalloti & DeLuca, 2008). It is not strongly correlated with physical impairment and can occur early in the disease or later. The speed at which information is processed and memory tend to be the areas that are most commonly affected. Memory problems tend to result from difficulty recalling information, rather than recognizing information. That is, it tends to be a problem of forgetfulness and rarely is a frank amnestic dementia. Many patients have greater difficult with more complex sustained or divided attentional tasks. These attentional problems can also interfere with learning new information and the formation of memories. Simple attention, comprehension, and general intelligence usually remain intact. It should be noted that the presentation of cognitive problems, like much of MS, can be quite heterogeneous.

Self-reported cognitive functioning tends to be very inaccurate, while reports of spouses tend to be more reliable (Benedict et al., 2003). Depression and fatigue can greatly inflate self-reported estimates of the severity of cognitive impairment (Julian, Merluzzi, & Mohr, 2007; Kinsinger & Mohr, 2010), while patients with significant cognitive impairment are more likely to show euphoria and underestimate their level of impairment.

8.1.3 Biobehavioral Mechanisms of Co-morbidity

This section will focus on the biopsychosocial mechanisms of the co-morbidity between MS and psychiatric disorders. The discussion will focus primarily on depression, as this is the area where most of the research has been conducted. We will review the literature on the role of genetics, MS pathogenic factors, MS pathology, MS symptoms, MS treatments, psychosocial factors, and stress.

8.1.3.1 Genetic Factors

There has been very little work examining the genetic underpinnings of depression among people with MS. The genetic factors that are associated with depression among medically health individuals are likely also associated with depression among people with MS. However, the data are mixed on whether or not there is a genetic link between MS and depression. One study found that close relatives of depressed MS patients were more likely to be depressed than relatives of a depressed control group, suggesting that some shared genetic etiology between MS and depression (Salmaggi et al., 1998). However, a second study found that the frequency of depression among first-degree relatives of depressed MS patients was lower than among control patients, suggesting that the increased rates of depression among MS patients do not have a genetic basis (Sadovnick et al., 1996). The one study examining depression and apolipoprotein (Apo) E alleles found that ApoE ε2 alleles was associated with greater positive affect and potentially decreased depression, suggesting a protective effect (Julian et al., 2009). While consistent with literature outside of MS, this was a small study and as such should be reproduced.

8.1.3.2 MS Pathogenesis

Inflammation is a major pathogenic component of MS, particularly during the relapsing phases of the disease (e.g., relapsing-remitting MS and early secondary progressive MS). A growing body of literature outside of MS has implicated such inflammation as an etiologic factor in depression (Capuron & Dantzer, 2003). Increased proinflammatory cytokine production, including interleukin (IL)-1, IL-6, tumor necrosis factor (TNF)-α, and interferon (IFN)-γ, have been shown to be associated with depression. Proinflammatory cytokines have been show to produce "sickness behaviors" in animals and humans that are similar to symptoms of depression, including decreased appetite, weight loss, sleep disturbance, psychomotor retardation, reduced interest in the physical and social environment, and loss of libido. In humans, proinflammatory cytokines also produce reduced mood, anxiety, and memory impairment.

There is circumstantial support for the cytokine-driven depression among people with MS. More than 90% of MS patients in exacerbation (the clinical manifestation of an inflammatory process) experience significant levels of distress, compared with 39% of MS patients who are not in exacerbation and 12% of spinal cord-injured patients (Dalos, Rabins, Brooks, & O'Donnell, 1983). While the symptoms of an exacerbation may be distressing, the consistency of distress in the presence of exacerbation suggests that these symptoms are not simply a psychosocial reaction, but likely have some biological etiology related to the exacerbation. Depression is more common among patients who are younger and are at earlier stages in the disease when it is more likely to be inflammatory (Patten et al., 2003), which is also consistent with the cytokine hypothesis. Indeed, proinflammatory cytokines such as TNF-α and IFN-γ are associated with both exacerbation and depression (Kahl, Kruse, Faller, Weiss, & Rieckmann, 2002). Furthermore, high levels of TNF-α 6 months after exacerbation continued to be significantly associated with continuing depression. Certainly, the data to date are not conclusive and much work remains. However, emerging evidence supports the hypothesis that the increased rates of depression among people with MS compared to medically healthy populations are likely due in part to underlying inflammatory processes (Gold & Irwin, 2009). Thus, depression should be seen not just as a reaction to MS, but as a symptom of MS that should be managed as part of the MS care team (Mohr, 2007).

8.1.3.3 MS Pathology

The pathological sequelae of MS pathogenic factors, particularly in terms of loss and damage to brain tissue, have long been a focus of research. Early studies of global brain atrophy did not show a relationship to psychiatric disturbance (Ron & Logsdail, 1989). However, more recent studies that located lesions in specific brain regions have found that depression is associated with very focal lesions in the arcuate fasciculus (Pujol, Bello, Deus, Marti-Vilalta, & Capdevila, 1997) as well as areas in the frontal, temporal, and parietal areas (Bakshi et al., 2000; Zorzon et al., 2002). Indeed, using conventional imaging, lesion volume in the frontal, prefrontal, and anterior temporal regions has been reported to account for as much as 40% of depression (Feinstein et al., 2004, 2010). Using a newer neuroimaging technique, diffusion tensor imaging, changes in the left anterior temporal region were seen where no changes were evident by conventional imaging (Feinstein et al., 2010). Thus, there is emerging evidence that damage to specific brain regions can increase risk of depression symptoms. Advances in neuroimaging technology such as diffusion tensor imaging, magnetic transfer imaging, and spectroscopy will likely provider greater insights into neuroanatomical involvement in depression.

While it is increasingly clear that lesions in these specific brain regions can increase risk of depressive symptoms, it remains unclear whether the lesions increase risk of depressive symptoms that are similar in etiology and response to treatment to symptoms of depression among medically health people, or if these symptoms represent a substantially different etiology and pathogenesis, and would not respond to antidepressant treatment (Alexopoulos, 2006; Julian & Mohr, 2006). Studies examining the moderating effects of lesions in specific brain regions on response to treatments will be important to determine their prognostic value as well as to characterize the nature of depressive symptoms resulting from these lesions.

8.1.3.4 Physical and Cognitive Symptom Severity

A common assumption is that greater symptom severity will result in greater distress and depression. In general, research has found that the association between severity of physical impairment and depression ranges from small to nonexistent (Stenager, Knudsen, & Jensen, 1994; Zorzon et al., 2002). A relatively large portion of this literature has focused on the relationship between fatigue and depression, where some investigators have found a relationship (Ford, Trigwell, & Johnson, 1998; Schwartz, Coulthard-Morris, & Zeng, 1996). However, clinical trials of pharmacologic treatments for fatigue have shown no effect on depression (Krupp et al., 1995), while treatments for depression consistently show improvements in fatigue (Mohr, Hart, & Goldberg, 2003; Mohr, Hart, & Vella, 2007). This suggests that to the degree that fatigue and depression are associated, it is more likely that depression affects fatigue than the reverse.

Similarly, a number of reviews of the literature have concluded that there is no evidence of a relationship between neuropsychological impairment and depression (Brassington & Marsh, 1998; Mohr & Cox, 2001). However, some recent research examining more refined areas of information processing suggest that specific areas of cognitive functioning may be related to depression and anxiety. It is hypothesized, based on work in geriatric populations, that fronto-subcortical brain pathology can produce both impairments in executive function and symptoms that mimic depression (Alexopoulos, 2006). Executive functioning is a cluster of high-order capacities, which include selective attention, behavioral planning and response inhibition, and the manipulation of information in problem-solving tasks. Preliminary work in this area has found an association between impairment in executive functioning and depression in MS (Julian & Arnett, 2009; Julian & Mohr, 2006).

A similar but separate line of work has suggested that while performance on routine cognitive tasks may not be affected by depression, more effortful tasks that place a demand on attentional resources, such as executive functioning or speeded tasks, are more impaired among MS patients who are depressed (Arnett, Barwick, & Beeney, 2008; Arnett et al., 1999). Thus, while there is a growing, literature supporting the relationship between depression and specific neuropsychological impairment, principally executive function, there is little information regarding the nature of this relationship. It is unclear to what degree the relationship between depression and executive functioning is the result of a common neuropathological etiology and to what degree depression increases neuropsychological deficits in effortful tasks.

8.1.3.5 MS Treatments

In rare cases, depression may be an iatrogenic effect of medications. Oral or IV glucocorticoids are used to treat exacerbations, which can produce changes in mood and cognition (Medical Economics, 1998). There has also been some speculation that new-onset or increased depression may be an iatrogenic effect associated with some of the disease-modifying treatments (DMTs) commonly used to treat MS. Specifically, early uncontrolled studies suggested that the interferon-betas may be associated with increased risk of depression (Mohr et al., 1996, 1998; Neilley, Goodin, Goodkin, & Hauser, 1996). More recent studies have consistently shown that interferon-betas do not cause increases in depressive symptoms (Borràs et al., 1999; Feinstein, O'Connor, & Feinstein, 2002). However, given the initial concerns, many of these clinical trials excluded patients with severe, active depression. Thus, while the preponderance of evidence suggests that DMTs do not cause depression, one cannot rule out the possibility that DMTs may activate depression among vulnerable patients.

8.1.3.6 Psychosocial Factors

A variety of psychosocial factors have been identified that are associated with depression, anxiety, and emotional adjustment (Dennison, Moss-Morris, & Chalder, 2009). While these factors are similar to those found to be associated with increased risk of depression and anxiety among people without medical illness, many of these factors can be augmented by the difficulties and burden posed by MS. Psychosocial factors are particularly important because they are potentially modifiable through psychological and behavioral intervention.

Stress and Coping

A large literature has examined adjustment from a stress and coping model, which defines coping as "constantly changing cognitive and behavioral efforts to manage specific external and/or internal demands that are appraised as taxing or exceeding the resources of the person" (Lazarus & Folkman, 1984, p. 141). A stressor, typically an external event, must be appraised as having two qualities to be stressful. First, the event must threaten something valued. Certainly, threats to health or financial stability can be stressful. However, a growing body of evidence indicates that socially evaluative threats – threats from the judgment of others, can cause significant stress responses (Dickerson & Kemeny, 2004). Second, an event must be perceived as uncontrollable.

A fairly large literature indicated that stressful life events, as well as perceived stress, are associated with increase risk of depression (Aikens, Fischer, Namey, & Rudick, 1997; Gilchrist & Creed, 1994; McCabe, 2005; Pakenham, 1999; Patten, Metz, & Reimer, 2000). The appraisal of threat and accountability, a potential mediator of the effects of stress on well-being, has also been linked to depression and emotional well-being (Pakenham, 1999; Pakenham, Stewart, & Rogers, 1997; Wineman, Durand, & Steiner, 1994).

Many studies have examined the relationship between coping and a variety of mental health outcomes, including depression, anxiety, and adjustment. In general, avoidant coping is associated with greater levels of depression. More active, problem-focused coping tends to be less related to depression or not related at all (Aikens et al., 1997; McCabe, McKern, & McDonald, 2004; Mohr, Goodkin, Gatto, & Van der Wende, 1997). This literature, however, has not demonstrated causality. Many of these studies suggest that poor coping skills lead to greater depression. However, it is just as possible that depression causes greater avoidant coping and decreases an individual's capacity to engage in more active, problem-focused coping.

Social Support

A large literature on social support suggests that it can moderate the effects of stressful events by providing active, tangible help as well as emotional support.

Most studies do not find a significant independent relationship between social support and emotional well-being or depression. Studies examining the relationship between social support and depression have been mixed (McCabe et al., 2004; Pakenham, 1999). More focused studies suggest perceived unsupportiveness is associated with greater depression, while perceived positive support is unrelated to depression (Wineman, 1990). However, as with coping, these studies do not suggest causality. While negative social support may increase distress and depression, a substantial literature outside of MS also has found that depressed individuals can elicit negative interactions from people in their social networks (Coyne & Downey, 1991).

8.1.4 The Effect of Stress and Depression on MS

While stress and coping have been examined as contributors to depression, a growing literature has also examined the relationship between stress, coping and distress, and exacerbation in MS. Charcot, who first characterized MS in the nineteenth century, wrote that grief, vexation, and adverse changes in social circumstance were related to the onset of MS (Charcot, 1877). Many people with MS believe that stress and distress make their MS worse, particularly by increasing the risk of exacerbation. These beliefs are supported by a meta-analysis that found a consistent association across studies between stressful life events and an increased risk of MS exacerbations (Mohr, Hart, Julian, Cox, & Pelletier, 2004). In addition, stressful life events, primarily in the form of family and work conflicts, are associated with a significant increase in the risk of the occurrence of a new gadolinium-enhancing (Gd+) MRI brain lesions 8 weeks later (Mohr, Goodkin, et al., 2000). Gd+MRI brain lesions are believed to be a neuroimaging marker of MS autoimmune activity in the brain.

It should be emphasized that while there is substantial evidence of an *association* between stress and MS exacerbation, there is not yet any evidence that stress *causes* exacerbation. Even longitudinal studies in which the occurrence of stress precedes the onset of disease activity does not demonstrate disease activity.

The relationship between a stressor and a disease outcome is commonly conceptualized as a simple relationship in which the onset of a stressor initiates the onset of a disease process or outcome. The temporal model of stress and disease outcomes posits that this relationship can be far more complex (Mohr & Pelletier, 2006). Both the course of the exacerbation and the course of the stressor occur over varying lengths of time, with different pathogenic processes at different stages. Figure 8.1 displays a model of the relationship between a stressor and the disease event. Both the disease event (in this case exacerbation) and stress (particularly chronic stress) occur over time, having an onset, a period during which the pathognomic features are present more or less continuously, and a resolution. This model facilitates consideration of the relationship between the pathogenic features of stress and exacerbation at each stage of development.

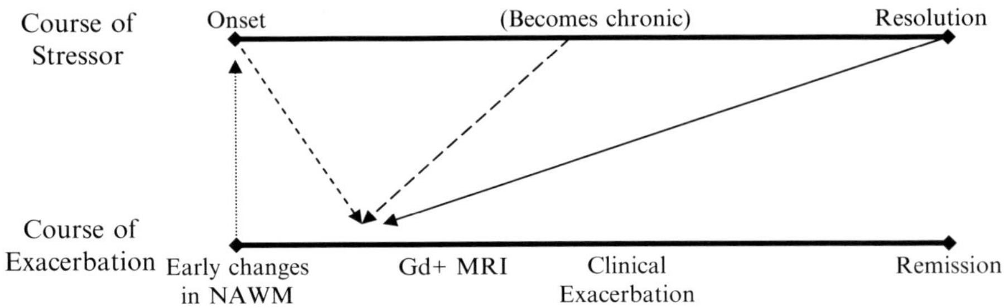

Fig. 8.1 Temporal model of stress and exacerbation

Stressors occur over a period of time and can be highly variable. Generally, the onset is accompanied by sympathetic activation, increases in epinephrine and norepinephrine, and activation of the hypothalamic-pituitary-adrenal (HPA) axis. As the stressor becomes chronic, the HPA axis can become dysregulated, resulting in higher levels of circulating cortisol (Sapolsky, Romero, & Munck, 2000). Resolution or adaptation to the stressor under normal circumstances results in reregulation of the HPA axis and return of circulating levels of cortisol to baseline.

MS exacerbation, as displayed in Fig. 8.1, is preceded by changes in normal-appearing white matter in the CNS that later becomes the target of autoaggressive immune activity (Goodkin et al., 1998). Once there is BBB breakdown and active inflammation at that site, attempts at regulation of the inflammation occur, including the production of Th2 cytokines such as IL-10. If regulation is not successful within that period of time, clinical signs of exacerbation occur. Even in the absence of treatment with glucocorticoids, these symptoms will resolve partially or fully over a period of weeks or months.

As one can see from Fig. 8.1, the potential interactions between a stressor and the course of exacerbation are manifold. For example, as shown with the dotted line, the onset of the stressor could potentially be associated with the early changes in normal-appearing brain tissue, the beginnings of inflammation, the failure of regulatory efforts and subsequent exacerbation, or the remission of exacerbation. Thus, a patient's or subject's experience of stress could be an early sign of underlying disease activity. The short dashed line represents a common belief that the onset of stress contributes to the initiation of MS disease activity. The long dashed line indicates a hypothesis that it is the transition from acute to chronic stress that increases risk of MS disease activity. Finally, the solid line represents the hypothesis that it is the cessation of stress which increases risk of MS disease activity. This hypothesis suggests that patients' beliefs that stress causes disease activity are the result of an attributional bias that leads people to attribute negative outcomes to negative events.

There are data from both human and animal models supporting an effect from each of the critical time points in the evolution of a stressor, the onset, change from acute to chronic, and the resolution (Mohr & Pelletier, 2006). Furthermore, these temporal relationships are not mutually exclusive.

8.1.4.1 Psychosocial Models

While the findings of an association between stressful life events and exacerbation have been consistent, the effects sizes tend to be modest, with considerable variability. This suggests that there are likely a number of moderators. Certainly, there may be genetic and disease-related factors that influence an individual's susceptibility to stress. There may also be psychosocial factors that affect the relationship between stress and MS inflammation. We will review four of these here.

Depression

One study examined immune function among patients with MS involved in a trial comparing treatments for depression (Mohr & Cox, 2001). Patients showed significant reductions in T cell production of IFN-γ, which is a critical cytokine believed to be a lynchpin in the immune cascade that leads to exacerbation. While there was no control condition, the reductions in IFN-γ were related to improvements in depression, suggesting that depression or distress may be related to IFN-γ production.

Attributional Style

In the study described above (Mohr & Cox, 2001), change in IFN-γ production and change in three components of depression, vegetative symptoms, affective symptoms, and negative attributions or beliefs not significantly related to either vegetative or affective symptoms. However, reductions in IFN-γ production were significantly related to improvements in the negative attributions that are common in depression. The sample size was too small to infer that affective or vegetative symptoms are unimportant. However, the findings suggest that negative attributions or expectations about threat and ability to manage threat may have distinct effects on immune functioning in MS.

Coping

Coping has been examined as a potential moderator between the occurrence of stressful life events and the subsequent development of new Gd+MRI brain lesions (Mohr, Goodkin, Nelson, Cox, & Weiner, 2002). Greater use of distraction as a method of managing problems was associated with a weaker association between stress and subsequent Gd+MRI, while less use of distraction tended to increase this association. Distraction is considered a generally adaptive coping strategy in which a person consciously shifts attention away from a problem that is not resolvable to something else, such as something pleasurable or something that is resolvable. There were similar trends for problem-solving strategies, which tended to reduce the relationship between stress and subsequent Gd+MRI, and rumination or worry, which tended to increase the relationship between stress and subsequent Gd+MRI.

This is somewhat consistent with a previous study showing less adaptive, avoidant coping was associated with increased exacerbation rates (Warren, Warren, & Cockerill, 1991). Thus, the data to date suggest that the use of more adaptive coping strategies may affect the relationship between stress and MS inflammation.

Social Support

Social support is increasingly being viewed as an important resource for patients to manage stressors (Uchino, Cacioppo, & Kiecolt-Glaser, 1996). Supportive relationships can provide practical support (e.g., help with chores) and emotional support (e.g., someone to talk with about problems). Social support has been found to be a significant moderator of the relationship between IFN-γ and depression (Mohr & Genain, 2004). Depression is strongly related to IFN-γ production among patients with low social support, while for patients with good social support there is no significant relationship between depression and IFN-γ production. This suggests that good social support may buffer any effects of depression or distress on IFN-γ production

Biological Models

While psychosocial models can take us from external events to biological stress response systems, biological models are required that can explain the interaction between these stress response systems and MS pathogenic factors. The last few years have witnessed the development of credible, testable biological models for how stressful life events might result in inflammation (Gold et al., 2005; Mohr & Pelletier, 2006; Morale et al., 2001). One such model that is beginning to show support is the glucocorticoid resistance hypothesis.

Cortisol is the end effector in a primary stress response system, the HPA axis (Chrousos, 1995). One paradox for stress research in MS is that stress generally is believed to increase circulating cortisol, and cortisol is a principal endogenous method of controlling inflammation. However, most studies suggest that less stress produces quite the opposite effect. The glucocorticoid resistance hypothesis is one potential explanation. Over time, increased circulating cortisol secondary to chronic stress can reduce the number and function of glucocorticoid receptors on immune cells, thereby making them less responsive to regulatory control by cortisol (Miller, Cohen, & Ritchey, 2002). The immune cells of patients with MS have been shown to be less sensitive to the regulatory effects of glucocorticoids than the cells of healthy individuals (DeRijk, Eskandari, & Sternberg, 2004), particularly during the more inflammatory stages of the illness (van Winsen et al., 2005). Furthermore, this glucocorticoid resistance is independent of history of treatment with glucocorticoids.

Under conditions of downregulated glucocorticoid receptors, if there is a small increase in autoreactive inflammation, immune cells would be less responsive to the regulatory effects of cortisol. The autoreactive immune cascade would be able to continue uncontrolled until a full-blown exacerbation had occurred. Thus, chronic stress, while not causing exacerbation, may leave patients less able to regulate autoreactive MS immune processes once they are initiated.

8.1.5 Psychiatric Diagnosis

As noted above, while patients with MS can show a variety of psychiatric symptoms, virtually all of the attention on diagnosis has occurred in depression. To diagnose MDD, a patient must have had either depressed mood or decreased interest or pleasure in activities (anhedonia) for at least 2 weeks, plus at least four additional symptoms including among the following: change in appetite, change in sleep, psychomotor retardation or agitation, fatigue, sense of worthlessness, problems in concentration, and thoughts of suicide. Other depressive diagnoses such as dysthymia or subthreshold depressions may include subsets of these symptoms. It is important to note that the cardinal symptoms are depressed mood *or* anhedonia. Many depressed MS patients may not feel sad, but may have lost motivation or interest in engaging in activities.

There have been some suggestions that some symptoms of depression are confounded with symptoms of MS (Mohr, Goodkin, Likosky, et al., 1997). For example, fatigue, cognitive impairment, insomnia, and change in weight could all potentially be symptoms of either MDD or MS. However, more recent evidence suggests that these symptoms may not be due to only one source, but may be multiply determined. Indeed, a recent study has shown that all symptoms of depression improve with treatment for depression, including those that might be confounded with MS (Moran & Mohr, 2005). Thus, in diagnosing depression, symptoms used in the diagnosis of MDD should not be excluded just because they may also be related to MS. Any symptom of depression may be considered to contribute to a diagnosis of MDD if it occurs in the presence of either depressed mood or anhedonia.

Depression is underdiagnosed in MS, with as many as 67% of depression going undetected (Marrie et al., 2009; Minden, Orav, & Reich, 1987; Mohr, Hart, Fonareva, & Tasch, 2006). A taskforce on depression in MS recommended routine screening for depression. A number of screening questionnaires have been shown to effectively identify MS patients who likely have MDD, including both longer questionnaires such as the Beck Depression Inventory (Sullivan, Weinshenker, Mikail, & Bishop, 1995) as well as two item questions modeled on the PHQ-2 (Kroenke, Spitzer, & Williams, 2003; Mohr, Hart, Julian, & Tasch, 2007). However, it should be noted that outside MS, a growing number of studies indicated that without organizational enhancements and accessible systems of care, such screening tools will have little or no impact (Gilbody, Sheldon, & House, 2008).

8.1.6 Treatment for Depression

The literature on treatment of psychiatric disorders has focused principally on depressive symptoms. As such, discussion of treatment will focus on depression. Evidence suggests that depression in MS, left untreated, will not improve (Mohr & Goodkin, 1999). While the etiology of depression in MS may include disease-specific factors such as brain lesions or inflammation, the treatment literature suggests that, as a group, patients with MS respond to treatment for depression as well as patients without MS.

8.1.6.1 Antidepressant Medications

Open label studies have suggested treatment with serotonin-specific reuptake inhibitors, tricyclics, and other classes of antidepressant medications are effective at reducing depression (Flax, Gray, & Herbert, 1991; Scott, Allen, Price, McConnell, & Lang, 1996). The first small placebo-controlled trial of the tricyclic, desimpramine, with 28 depressed MS patients showed mixed outcomes (Schiffer & Wineman, 1990). While 5 weeks of treatment showed significant improvements on an interviewer-rated measure, there was no significant improvement, compared to placebo, on self-reported severity. At the end of the trial, most patients were receiving either the minimal clinical dosage of 150 mg per day or less. A more recent trial compared 12 weeks of a flexible dose of paroxetine (10–40 mg) to placebo in 42 MS patients with MDD. Both groups improved and there were no significant differences between the treatment arms (Ehde et al., 2008). However, effect sizes were similar to those seen in larger trials. It is possible that the failure to find significant effects was due both to the short treatment duration and the small sample sizes.

Another trial compared three 16-week treatments for major depressive disorder among MS patients: sertraline, cognitive behavioral therapy (CBT) tailored to the needs of people with MS (Mohr, 2010a, 2010b), and group supportive expressive therapy (Spiegel & Classen, 2000). Sertraline produced significant reductions in depressive symptoms on both objective and subjective measures of depression which were significantly larger than the group supportive expressive therapy, and equivalent to CBT (Mohr, Boudewyn, Goodkin, Bostrom, & Epstein, 2001). Physicians met every 4 weeks with patients to evaluate progress and side effects, and to adjust dosage accordingly. The median daily dosage by the end of treatment was 150 mg, or three times the minimal clinical dosage. To the best of our knowledge, there is no indication in the literature that there is any difference in efficacy between sertraline, paroxetine, or desimpramine. Thus, the difference between the trials is likely that patients in the sertraline trial received more potent dosing over a longer period of time, compared to the other two trials.

8.1.6.2 Physician Care for Depression

The vast majority treatment for depression is administered by nonmental health physicians (Regier et al., 1993) and there is no reason to think this is not true in MS (Mohr, Hart, Fonareva, et al., 2006). A study of 260 patients with MS cared for by neurologists in a large health maintenance organization found that 26% of patients met MDD criteria as judged by an evaluation independent from the physician (Mohr, Hart, Fonareva, et al.). Of those patients meeting MDD criteria, 67% received no antidepressant, 30% received antidepressant treatment that was at or below minimal clinical dosage, and only 3% received doses that exceeded minimal clinical dosages. As noted above, adequate symptom remission is only likely to occur at higher dosages of antidepressant medication. These results suggest that inadequate treatment and failure to adhere to treatment guidelines for pharmacotherapy, which require frequent follow-up and dose adjustment, are a substantial problem in the management of depression in MS (AHCPR, 1999).

8.1.6.3 Psychotherapy for Depression

Two early trials comparing group administered CBT to a waitlist or treatment as usual control conditions showed strong improvements in depressive symptoms (Foley, Bedell, LaRocca, Scheinberg, & Reznikoff, 1987; Larcombe & Wilson, 1984). Early trials comparing insight-oriented group treatments to no treatment controls also demonstrated reductions in depression (Crawford & McIvor, 1985, 1987); however, in a meta-analysis, these effect sizes were found to be significantly smaller than outcomes for group CBT (Mohr & Goodkin, 1999).

The first comparative outcome trial randomized patients who received 16 weeks of a manualized individual CBT (Mohr, 2010a, 2010b), a manualized supportive expressive group therapy (Spiegel & Classen, 2000), or a pharmacotherapy with sertraline with a standardized follow-up protocol. The CBT and pharmacotherapy produced significant improvement in depression, compared to the group supportive expressive treatment, which produced no significant improvement (Mohr, Boudewyn, Goodkin, et al., 2001).

While most patients with depression want psychological treatments (Dwight-Johnson, Sherbourne, Liao, & Wells, 2000), most have barriers that prevent access, such as cost, transportation, and time constraints (Mohr, Hart, Howard, et al., 2006; Mohr et al., 2010). This is particularly true of patients with MS and depression (Marrie et al., 2009). In an effort to overcome structural barriers to care, we investigated the use of the telephone to extend care. An initial pilot of an 8-week telephone-administered CBT (T-CBT) intervention produced significant improvement, compared to treatment as usual (Mohr, Likosky, et al., 2000). A follow-up study compared a 16-week manualized individual T-CBT intervention with a 16-week manualized individual telephone-administered supportive emotion-focused therapy (T-SEFT) (Mohr, Hart, Julian, et al., 2005). While patients showed significant improvements in both treatments, on most measures of depression, T-CBT produced significantly greater improvements than T-SEFT.

The evidence indicates the psychological interventions can be effective for the treatment of depression among patient with MS. There also is some suggestion that cognitive behavioral interventions may be somewhat more effective than other emotion-focused treatments. This is notable, as such treatment differences have not been found among depressed but medically healthy people (Watson, Gordon, Stermac, Kalogerakos, & Steckley, 2003). It may be that concerns related to the disease, as well as management of the symptoms and social sequelae, are more amenable to a cognitive behavioral focus. However, it is also true that many people improved in emotion-focused treatments, and the differences between the treatments disappeared rapidly after the cessation of treatment (Mohr, Hart, Julian, et al., 2005). Thus, at this point the data would suggest patient treatment preferences should play a significant role in the selection of treatment modality, but that in the absence of strong preferences, CBT should be the default treatment of choice.

Our group recently published the therapist manual (Mohr, 2010a) and patient workbook (Mohr, 2010b) for a CBT-based "Stress and Mood Management Program for Individuals with MS." This is the treatment model that has been validated in several of the clinical trials described above (Mohr, Boudewyn, Goodkin, et al., 2001; Mohr, Hart, Julian, et al., 2005; Mohr, Likosky, et al., 2000). The treatment uses standard behavioral activation and cognitive restructuring as part of the core intervention. The core treatment also includes several features that we have found useful and important to people with MS. The treatment teaches problem solving and goal setting. As part of behavioral activation, the treatment also focuses on increasing awareness of positive events that occur routinely in the patient's life. This has been shown to be important in improving positive affect (Mohr, Hart, Julian, et al., 2005), which, while independent of negative affect, may increase resilience to stressful events (Folkman, 1997; Folkman & Moskowitz, 2000). Because of the significant impact MS can have on social supports and networks, social support is a core module of the treatment. Finally, a variety of optional modules are available to allow the patient and therapist to tailor the treatment to the patient's needs. These include modules that focus on MS symptom management, including fatigue, pain, cognitive impairment, and injection anxiety (discussed in more detail below). There are also modules that address psychosocial co-morbidities common among people with MS, including anxiety reduction, communication and assertiveness training, and relaxation skills.

8.1.6.4 Prediction of Response and Relapse in Treatment for Depression

In general, research has found no evidence that any global measures of physical or cognitive impairment disease predict initial responses to pharmaco- and psychotherapies. However, patients with greater lesion load and greater levels of cognitive impairment are significantly less likely to maintain the treatment gains at 6-month follow-up (Mohr, Epstein, et al., 2003). This suggests that MS patients with cognitive impairment and high lesion load who are treated for depression should be followed closely to ensure maintenance of treatment gains.

While psychotherapy and antidepressant medications produce similar results in populations of depressed patients, there may be some instances when one is preferable to the other. There is an emerging literature suggesting that antidepressant medications may be less effective than psychotherapy among patients with one specific class of neuropsychological deficits, executive dysfunction (e.g., deficits in planning, organizing, sequencing, and problem solving), which is associated with frontal and fronto-subcortical brain lesions. This effect was first seen in the treatment of depression in the elderly (Alexopoulos, Kiosses, Choi, Murphy, & Lim, 2002;

Alexopoulos et al., 2000; Kalayam & Alexopoulos, 1999). Similarly in MS, executive dysfunction is significantly associated with response to pharmacotherapy, with greater executive dysfunction predicting less response to pharmacotherapy. However, executive dysfunction is unrelated to response to psychotherapy (Julian & Mohr, 2006). This suggests that for depressed patients with executive dysfunction, psychotherapy may be the treatment of choice.

If indeed psychological treatments are superior to pharmacotherapy for patients with executive dysfunction, it will be important to understand why this is the case. One hypothesis is that depression resulting from fronto-subcortical brain lesions has a very different etiology for standard depression. It is marked by greater levels of anhedonia and difficulties initiating behavior (Alexopoulos, 2006). Thus, psychological and behavioral treatments that focus on behavior activation and engagement with the environment may better address pathology underlying this form of depression than would pharmacotherapy.

8.1.6.5 Secondary Outcomes

Treatments for depression can have a variety of ancillary benefits for patients with MS. Improvements in depression result in significant improvements in quality of life and well-being (Cosio, Siddique, Jin, & Mohr, 2011; Hart, Fonareva, Merluzzi, & Mohr, 2005). Successful treatment for depression has been shown to result in significant improvements in disability (Mohr, Hart, & Vella, 2007). Treating depression can also improve some MS symptoms, most notably fatigue (Mohr, Hart, et al., 2003). Successful treatment for depression may also improve patient adherence to DMTs (Mohr, Likosky, et al., 2000).

8.1.6.6 Anxiety

As noted above, anxiety is likely as prevalent as depression, but has received far less attention. No treatments for general anxiety have been examined among people with MS. However, one specific form of anxiety has received some attention.

Self-Injection Anxiety (SIA)

Most of the DMTs for MS require injections on a regular basis, ranging from daily to once per week. It is recommended that patients learn to self-inject. A partner or caregiver can give the injections; however, reliance on such assistance is believed to result in decreased adherence as adherence depends on the initiative and reliability of two people instead of one (Mohr, Boudewyn, Likosky, Levine, & Goodkin, 2001).

While injection phobia is a recognized diagnosis, self-injection anxiety (SIA) is not part of the DSM-IV diagnostic criteria (Mohr & Cox, 2003). We have defined SIA as subjective anxiety that is sufficient to prevent self-injection. Most people with SIA do not meet DSM-IV criteria for injection phobia, as they are able to receive injections. Nevertheless, SIA has consistently been shown to be a principal cause of nonadherence to injectable medications (Mohr, Boudewyn, Likosky, et al., 2001; Turner, Williams, Sloan, & Haselkorn, 2009).

To address SIA, we developed a manualized 6-session treatment that tailors standard cognitive behavioral procedures used in the treatment of phobias (Mohr, 2010a, 2010b). An initial pilot of SIA counseling (SIAC) administered by psychologists found that 7 out of 8 patients were able to learn to self-inject within the six sessions, and the eighth patient was able to self-inject with an additional session (Mohr, Cox, Epstein, & Boudewyn, 2002). It should be noted that several of these patients showed significant signs of anxiety, including frank injection phobia and vasovagal reactions to the sight of needles. A second trial comparing SIAC administered by nurses to a relaxation intervention supported the efficacy of SIAC (Mohr, Cox, & Merluzzi, 2005), although the remission rates were lower than those obtained by psychologists.

8.1.7 Summary

In summary, psychiatric disorders and symptoms are more common among people with MS, compared to healthy populations, most notably including depression, anxiety, and possibly bipolar disorders. The increased prevalence of depression may be due to inflammation and lesion volume in specific frontal, temporal, and/or parietal brain regions. As in depression generally, genetic and psychosocial factors also contribute to depression, but it is unclear if they account for the greater prevalence of psychiatric disorders and distress among people with MS. While depression and possibly other psychiatric disorders may result from etiologies that differ from etiologies of these disorders in healthy populations, evidence suggests that people with MS can respond to pharmacotherapeutic and psychotherapeutic interventions.

References

AHCPR. (1999). *Treatment of depression: Newer pharmacotherapies (No. AHCPR Publication No. 99-E014)*. Washington: Agency for Health Care Policy and Research.

Aikens, J. E., Fischer, J. S., Namey, M., & Rudick, R. A. (1997). A replicated prospective investigation of life stress, coping, and depressive symptoms in multiple sclerosis. *Journal of Behavioral Medicine, 20*(5), 433–445.

Alexopoulos, G. S. (2006). The vascular depression hypothesis: 10 years later. *Biological Psychiatry, 60*(12), 1304–1305.

Alexopoulos, G. S., Kiosses, D. N., Choi, S. J., Murphy, C. F., & Lim, K. O. (2002). Frontal white matter microstructure and treatment response of late-life depression: A preliminary study. *The American Journal of Psychiatry, 159*(11), 1929–1932.

Alexopoulos, G. S., Meyers, B. S., Young, R. C., Kalayam, B., Kakuma, T., Gabrielle, M., et al. (2000). Executive dysfunction and long-term outcomes of geriatric depression. *Archives of General Psychiatry, 57*(3), 285–290.

Arnett, P. A., Barwick, F. H., & Beeney, J. E. (2008). Depression in multiple sclerosis: Review and theoretical proposal. *Journal of the International Neuropsychological Society, 14*(5), 691–724.

Arnett, P. A., Higginson, C. I., Voss, W. D., Wright, B., Bender, W. I., Wurst, J. M., et al. (1999). Depressed mood in multiple sclerosis: Relationship to capacity-demanding memory and attentional functioning. *Neuropsychology, 13*, 434–446.

Ascherio, A., & Munger, K. L. (2007a). Environmental risk factors for multiple sclerosis. Part I: The role of infection. *Annals of Neurology, 61*(4), 288–299.

Ascherio, A., & Munger, K. L. (2007b). Environmental risk factors for multiple sclerosis. Part II: Noninfectious factors. *Annals of Neurology, 61*(6), 504–513.

Bakshi, R., Czarnecki, D., Shaikh, Z. A., Priore, R. L., Janardhan, V., Kaliszky, Z., et al. (2000). Brain MRI lesions and atrophy are related to depression in multiple sclerosis. *Neuroreport, 11*(6), 1153–1158.

Benedict, R. H., Munschauer, F., Linn, R., Miller, C., Murphy, E., Foley, F., et al. (2003). Screening for multiple sclerosis cognitive impairment using a self-administered 15-item questionnaire. *Multiple Sclerosis, 9*(1), 95–101.

Borràs, C., Río, J., Porcel, J., Barrios, M., Tintoré, M., & Montalbon, X. (1999). Emotional state of patients with relapsing-remitting MS treated with interferon beta-1b. *Neurology, 52*, 1636–1639.

Brassington, J. C., & Marsh, N. V. (1998). Neuropsychological aspects of multiple sclerosis. *Neuropsychology Review, 8*(2), 43–77.

Capuron, L., & Dantzer, R. (2003). Cytokines and depression: The need for a new paradigm. *Brain, Behavior, and Immunity, 17*(Suppl 1), S119–S124.

Charcot, J. M. (1877). *Lectures on diseases of the nervous system* (G. Sigerson, Trans.). London: New Sydenham Society.

Chiaravalloti, N. D., & DeLuca, J. (2008). Cognitive impairment in multiple sclerosis. *Lancet Neurology, 7*(12), 1139–1151.

Chrousos, G. P. (1995). The hypothalamic-pituitary-adrenal axis and immune-mediated inflammation. *The New England Journal of Medicine, 332*(20), 1351–1362.

Chwastiak, L. A., & Ehde, D. M. (2007). Psychiatric issues in multiple sclerosis. *The Psychiatric Clinics of North America, 30*(4), 803–817.

Compston, A., Confavreux, C., Lassmann, H., McDonald, I., Miller, D., Noseworthy, J., et al. (2006). *McAlpine's multiple sclerosis*. Philadelphia: Churchill Livingston/Elsevier.

Cosio, D., Siddique, J., Jin, L., & Mohr, D. C. (2011). The effect of telephone-administered cognitive-behavioral therapy on quality of life among patients with multiple sclerosis. *Annals of Behavioural Medicine, 41*(2), 227–234.

Coyne, J. C., & Downey, G. (1991). Social factors and psychopathology: Stress, social support, and coping processes. *Annual Review of Psychology, 42*, 401–425.

Crawford, J. D., & McIvor, G. P. (1985). Group psychotherapy: Benefits in multiple sclerosis. *Archives of Physical Medicine and Rehabilitation, 66*(12), 810–813.

Crawford, J. D., & McIvor, G. P. (1987). Stress management for multiple sclerosis patients. *Psychological Reports, 61*(2), 423–429.

Dalos, N. P., Rabins, P. V., Brooks, B. R., & O'Donnell, P. (1983). Disease activity and emotional state in multiple sclerosis. *Annals of Neurology, 13*(5), 573–577.

Dennison, L., Moss-Morris, R., & Chalder, T. (2009). A review of psychological correlates of adjustment in patients with multiple sclerosis. *Clinical Psychology Review, 29*(2), 141–153.

DeRijk, R. H., Eskandari, F., & Sternberg, E. M. (2004). Corticosteroid resistance in a subpopulation of multiple sclerosis patients as measured by ex vivo dexamethasone inhibition of LPS induced IL-6 production. *Journal of Neuroimmunology, 151*(1–2), 180–188.

Dickerson, S. S., & Kemeny, M. E. (2004). Acute stressors and cortisol responses: A theoretical integration and synthesis of laboratory research. *Psychological Bulletin, 130*(3), 355–391.

Dwight-Johnson, M., Sherbourne, C. D., Liao, D., & Wells, K. B. (2000). Treatment preferences among depressed primary care patients. *Journal of General Internal Medicine, 15*(8), 527–534.

Edwards, L. J., & Constantinescu, C. S. (2004). A prospective study of conditions associated with multiple sclerosis in a cohort of 658 consecutive outpatients attending a multiple sclerosis clinic. *Multiple Sclerosis, 10*(5), 575–581.
Ehde, D. M., Kraft, G. H., Chwastiak, L., Sullivan, M. D., Gibbons, L. E., Bombardier, C. H., et al. (2008). Efficacy of paroxetine in treating major depressive disorder in persons with multiple sclerosis. *General Hospital Psychiatry, 30*(1), 40–48.
Feinstein, A., Feinstein, K., Gray, T., & O'Connor, P. (1997). Prevalence of neurobehavioral correlates of pathological laughing and crying in multiple sclerosis. *Archives of Neurology, 54*, 1116–1121.
Feinstein, A., O'Connor, P., Akbar, N., Moradzadeh, L., Scott, C. J., & Lobaugh, N. J. (2010). Diffusion tensor imaging abnormalities in depressed multiple sclerosis patients. *Multiple Sclerosis, 16*(2), 189–196.
Feinstein, A., O'Connor, P., & Feinstein, K. (2002). Multiple sclerosis, interferon beta-1b and depression. A prospective investigation. *Journal of Neurology, 249*(7), 815–820.
Feinstein, A., O'Connor, P., Gray, T., & Feinstein, K. (1999). The effects of anxiety on psychiatric morbidity in patients with multiple sclerosis. *Multiple Sclerosis, 5*, 323–326.
Feinstein, A., Roy, P., Lobaugh, N., Feinstein, K., O'Connor, P., & Black, S. (2004). Structural brain abnormalities in multiple sclerosis patients with major depression. *Neurology, 62*(4), 586–590.
Flax, J. W., Gray, J., & Herbert, J. (1991). Effect of fluoxetine on patients with multiple sclerosis. *The American Journal of Psychiatry, 148*(11), 1603.
Foley, F. W., Bedell, J. R., LaRocca, N. G., Scheinberg, L. C., & Reznikoff, M. (1987). Efficacy of stress-inoculation training in coping with multiple sclerosis. *Journal of Consulting and Clinical Psychology, 55*(6), 919–922.
Folkman, S. (1997). Positive psychological states and coping with severe stress. *Social Science & Medicine, 45*, 1207–1221.
Folkman, S., & Moskowitz, J. T. (2000). Positive affect and the other side of coping. *American Psychologist, 55*, 647–654.
Ford, H., Trigwell, P., & Johnson, M. (1998). The nature of fatigue in multiple sclerosis. *Journal of Psychosomic Research, 45*(1 Spec No.), 33–38.
Gilbody, S., Sheldon, T., & House, A. (2008). Screening and case-finding instruments for depression: A meta-analysis. *Canadian Medical Association Journal, 178*(8), 997–1003.
Gilchrist, A. C., & Creed, F. H. (1994). Depression, cognitive impairment and social stress in multiple sclerosis. *Journal of Psychosomatic Medicine, 38*, 193–201.
Gold, S. M., & Irwin, M. R. (2009). Depression and immunity: Inflammation and depressive symptoms in multiple sclerosis. *Immunology and Allergy Clinics of North America, 29*(2), 309–320.
Gold, S. M., Mohr, D. C., Huitinga, I., Flachenecker, P., Sternberg, E. M., & Heesen, C. (2005). The role of stress-response systems for the pathogenesis and progression of MS. *Trends in Immunology, 26*(12), 644–652.
Goodkin, D. E., Rooney, W. D., Sloan, R., Bacchetti, P., Gee, L., Vermathen, M., et al. (1998). A serial study of new MS lesions and the white matter from which they arise. *Neurology, 51*, 1689–1697.
Hart, S., Fonareva, I., Merluzzi, N., & Mohr, D. C. (2005). Treatment for depression and its relationship to improvement in quality of life and psychological well-being in multiple sclerosis patients. *Quality of Life Research, 14*(3), 695–703.
Janssens, A. C., Buljevac, D., van Doorn, P. A., van der Meche, F. G., Polman, C. H., Passchier, J., et al. (2006). Prediction of anxiety and distress following diagnosis of multiple sclerosis: A two-year longitudinal study. *Multiple Sclerosis, 12*(6), 794–801.
Janssens, A. C., van Doorn, P. A., de Boer, J. B., van der Meche, F. G., Passchier, J., & Hintzen, R. Q. (2003). Impact of recently diagnosed multiple sclerosis on quality of life, anxiety, depression and distress of patients and partners. *Acta Neurologica Scandinavica, 108*(6), 389–395.
Jose Sa, M. (2008). Psychological aspects of multiple sclerosis. *Clinical Neurology and Neurosurgery, 110*(9), 868–877.

Julian, L., Merluzzi, N. M., & Mohr, D. C. (2007). The relationship among depression, subjective cognitive impairment, and neuropsychological performance in multiple sclerosis. *Multiple Sclerosis, 13*(1), 81–86.

Julian, L. J., & Arnett, P. A. (2009). Relationships among anxiety, depression, and executive functioning in multiple sclerosis. *Clinical Neuropsychology, 23*(5), 794–804.

Julian, L. J., & Mohr, D. C. (2006). Cognitive predictors of response to treatment for depression in multiple sclerosis. *The Journal of Neuropsychiatry and Clinical Neurosciences, 18*, 356–363.

Julian, L. J., Vella, L., Frankel, D., Minden, S. L., Oksenberg, J. R., & Mohr, D. C. (2009). ApoE alleles, depression and positive affect in multiple sclerosis. *Multiple Sclerosis, 15*(3), 311–315.

Kahl, K. G., Kruse, N., Faller, H., Weiss, H., & Rieckmann, P. (2002). Expression of tumor necrosis factor-alpha and interferon-gamma mRNA in blood cells correlates with depression scores during an acute attack in patients with multiple sclerosis. *Psychoneuroendocrinology, 27*(6), 671–681.

Kalayam, B., & Alexopoulos, G. S. (1999). Prefrontal dysfunction and treatment response in geriatric depression. *Archives of General Psychiatry, 56*(8), 713–718.

Kinsinger, S., & Mohr, D. C. (2010). Relationship between depression, fatigue, subjective cognitive impairment, and objective neuropsychological functioning in patients with multiple sclerosis. *Neuropsychology, 24*(5), 573–580.

Korostil, M., & Feinstein, A. (2007). Anxiety disorders and their clinical correlates in multiple sclerosis patients. *Multiple Sclerosis, 13*(1), 67–72.

Kroenke, K., Spitzer, R. L., & Williams, J. B. (2003). The Patient Health Questionnaire-2: Validity of a two-item depression screener. *Medical Care, 41*(11), 1284–1292.

Krupp, L. B., Coyle, P. K., Doscher, C., Miller, A., Cross, A. H., Jandorf, L., et al. (1995). Fatigue therapy in multiple sclerosis: Results of a double-blind, randomized, parallel trial of amantadine, pemoline, and placebo. *Neurology, 45*(11), 1956–1961.

Kwentus, J. A., Hart, R. P., Calabrese, V., & Hekmati, A. (1986). Mania as a symptom of multiple sclerosis. *Psychosomatics, 27*(10), 729–731.

Larcombe, N. A., & Wilson, P. H. (1984). An evaluation of cognitive-behaviour therapy for depression in patients with multiple sclerosis. *The British Journal of Psychiatry, 145*, 366–371.

Lazarus, R. S., & Folkman, S. (1984). *Stress, appraisal, and coping*. New York: Springer.

Li, J., Johansen, C., Bronnum-Hansen, H., Stenager, E., Koch-Henriksen, N., & Olsen, J. (2004). The risk of multiple sclerosis in bereaved parents: A nationwide cohort study in Denmark. *Neurology, 62*(5), 726–729.

Lublin, F. D., & Reingold, S. C. (1996). Defining the clinical course of multiple sclerosis: Results of an international survey. National Multiple Sclerosis Society (USA) advisory committee on clinical trials of new agents in multiple sclerosis. *Neurology, 46*(4), 907–911.

Marrie, R. A., Horwitz, R., Cutter, G., Tyry, T., Campagnolo, D., & Vollmer, T. (2009). The burden of mental comorbidity in multiple sclerosis: Frequent, underdiagnosed, and undertreated. *Multiple Sclerosis, 15*(3), 385–392.

McCabe, M. P. (2005). Mood and self-esteem of persons with multiple sclerosis following an exacerbation. *Journal of Psychosomatic Research, 59*(3), 161–166.

McCabe, M. P., McKern, S., & McDonald, E. (2004). Coping and psychological adjustment among people with multiple sclerosis. *Journal of Psychosomatic Research, 56*(3), 355–361.

Medical Economics. (1998). *Physicians' desk reference* (52nd ed.). Montvale: Medical Economics Data Production Company.

Miller, G. E., Cohen, S., & Ritchey, A. K. (2002). Chronic psychological stress and the regulation of pro-inflammatory cytokines: A glucocorticoid-resistance model. *Health Psychology, 21*(6), 531–541.

Milo, R., & Kahana, E. (2010). Multiple sclerosis: Geoepidemiology, genetics and the environment. *Autoimmunity Reviews, 9*(5), 387–394.

Minden, S. L., Orav, J., & Reich, P. (1987). Depression in multiple sclerosis. *General Hospital Psychiatry, 9*(6), 426–434.

Mohr, D. C. (2007). Stress and multiple sclerosis. *Journal of Neurology, 254*(Suppl 2), II65–II68.

Mohr, D. C. (2010a). *The stress and mood management program for individuals with multiple sclerosis: Therapist guide*. New York: Oxford Press.
Mohr, D. C. (2010b). *The stress and mood management program for individuals with multiple sclerosis: Workbook*. New York: Oxford Press.
Mohr, D. C., Boudewyn, A. C., Goodkin, D. E., Bostrom, A., & Epstein, L. (2001). Comparative outcomes for individual cognitive-behavior therapy, supportive-expressive group psychotherapy, and sertraline for the treatment of depression in multiple sclerosis. *Journal of Consulting and Clinical Psychology, 69*(6), 942–949.
Mohr, D. C., Boudewyn, A. C., Likosky, W., Levine, E., & Goodkin, D. E. (2001). Injectable medication for the treatment of multiple sclerosis: The influence of self-efficacy expectations and injection anxiety on adherence and ability to self-inject. *Annals of Behavioral Medicine, 23*(2), 125–132.
Mohr, D. C., & Cox, D. (2001). Multiple sclerosis: Empirical literature for the clinical health psychologist. *Journal of Clinical Psychology, 57*(4), 479–499.
Mohr, D. C., & Cox, D. (2003). Managing difficulties with adherence to injectable medications due to blood, injection, and injury phobia and self-injection anxiety. *American Journal of Drug Delivery, 1*, 215–221.
Mohr, D. C., Cox, D., Epstein, L., & Boudewyn, A. (2002). Teaching patients to self-inject: Pilot study of a treatment for injection anxiety and phobia in multiple sclerosis patients prescribed injectable medications. *Journal of Behavior Therapy and Experimental Psychiatry, 33*(1), 39–47.
Mohr, D. C., Cox, D., & Merluzzi, N. (2005). Self-injection anxiety training: A treatment for patients unable to self-inject injectable medications. *Multiple Sclerosis, 11*(2), 182–185.
Mohr, D. C., Epstein, L., Luks, T. L., Goodkin, D., Cox, D., Goldberg, A., et al. (2003). Brain lesion volume and neuropsychological function predict efficacy of treatment for depression in multiple sclerosis. *Journal of Consulting and Clinical Psychology, 71*(6), 1017–1024.
Mohr, D. C., & Genain, C. (2004). Social support as a buffer in the relationship between treatment for depression and T-cell production of interferon gamma in patients with multiple sclerosis. *Journal of Psychosomatic Research, 57*(2), 155–158.
Mohr, D. C., & Goodkin, D. E. (1999). Treatment of depression in multiple sclerosis: Review and meta-analysis. *Clinical Psychology: Science and Practice, 6*, 1–9.
Mohr, D. C., Goodkin, D. E., Bacchetti, P., Boudewyn, A. C., Huang, L., Marrietta, P., et al. (2000). Psychological stress and the subsequent appearance of new brain MRI lesions in MS. *Neurology, 55*(1), 55–61.
Mohr, D. C., Goodkin, D. E., Gatto, N., & Van der Wende, J. (1997). Depression, coping and level of neurological impairment in multiple sclerosis. *Multiple Sclerosis, 3*(4), 254–258.
Mohr, D. C., Goodkin, D. E., Likosky, W., Beutler, L., Gatto, N., & Langan, M. K. (1997). Identification of Beck depression inventory items related to multiple sclerosis. *Journal of Behavioral Medicine, 20*(4), 407–414.
Mohr, D. C., Goodkin, D. E., Likosky, W., Gatto, N., Neilley, L. K., Griffin, C., et al. (1996). Therapeutic expectations of patients with multiple sclerosis upon initiating interferon beta-1b: Relationship to adherence to treatment. *Multiple Sclerosis, 2*(5), 222–226.
Mohr, D. C., Goodkin, D. E., Nelson, S., Cox, D., & Weiner, M. (2002). Moderating effects of coping on the relationship between stress and the development of new brain lesions in multiple sclerosis. *Psychosomatic Medicine, 64*(5), 803–809.
Mohr, D. C., Hart, S. L., Fonareva, I., & Tasch, E. S. (2006). Treatment of depression for patients with multiple sclerosis in neurology clinics. *Multiple Sclerosis, 12*(2), 204–208.
Mohr, D. C., Hart, S. L., & Goldberg, A. (2003). Effects of treatment for depression on fatigue in multiple sclerosis. *Psychosomatic Medicine, 65*(4), 542–547.
Mohr, D. C., Hart, S. L., Howard, I., Julian, L., Vella, L., Catledge, C., et al. (2006). Barriers to psychotherapy among depressed and nondepressed primary care patients. *Annals of Behavioral Medicine, 32*(3), 254–258.
Mohr, D. C., Hart, S. L., Julian, L., Catledge, C., Honos-Webb, L., Vella, L., et al. (2005). Telephone-administered psychotherapy for depression. *Archives of General Psychiatry, 62*(9), 1007–1014.

Mohr, D. C., Hart, S. L., Julian, L., Cox, D., & Pelletier, D. (2004). Association between stressful life events and exacerbation in multiple sclerosis: A meta-analysis. *British Medical Journal, 328*(7442), 731.

Mohr, D. C., Hart, S. L., Julian, L., & Tasch, E. S. (2007). Screening for depression among patients with multiple sclerosis: Two questions may be enough. *Multiple Sclerosis, 13*(2), 215–219.

Mohr, D. C., Hart, S. L., & Vella, L. (2007). Reduction in disability in a randomized controlled trial of telephone-administered cognitive-behavioral therapy. *Health Psychology, 26*(5), 554–563.

Mohr, D. C., Ho, J., Duffecy, J., Baron, K. G., Lehman, K. A., Jin, L., et al. (2010). Perceived barriers to psychological treatments and their relationship to depression. *Journal of Clinical Psychology, 66*(4), 394–409.

Mohr, D. C., Likosky, W., Bertagnolli, A., Goodkin, D. E., Van Der Wende, J., Dwyer, P., et al. (2000). Telephone-administered cognitive-behavioral therapy for the treatment of depressive symptoms in multiple sclerosis. *Journal of Consulting and Clinical Psychology, 68*(2), 356–361.

Mohr, D. C., Likosky, W., Boudewyn, A. C., Marietta, P., Dwyer, P., Van der Wende, J., et al. (1998). Side effect profile and adherence to in the treatment of multiple sclerosis with interferon beta-1a. *Multiple Sclerosis, 4*(6), 487–489.

Mohr, D. C., & Pelletier, D. (2006). A temporal framework for understanding the effects of stressful life events on inflammation in patients with multiple sclerosis. *Brain, Behavior, and Immunity, 20*(1), 27–36.

Morale, C., Brouwer, J., Testa, N., Tirolo, C., Barden, N., Dijkstra, C. D., et al. (2001). Stress, glucocorticoids and the susceptibility to develop autoimmune disorders of the central nervous system. *Neurological Sciences, 22*(2), 159–162.

Moran, P. J., & Mohr, D. C. (2005). The validity of Beck Depression Inventory and Hamilton Rating Scale for Depression items in the assessment of depression among patients with multiple sclerosis. *Journal of Behavioral Medicine, 28*(1), 35–41.

Neilley, L. K., Goodin, D. S., Goodkin, D. E., & Hauser, S. L. (1996). Side effect profile of interferon beta-1b in MS: Results of an open label trial. *Neurology, 46*, 552–554.

Noseworthy, J. H., Lucchinetti, C., Rodriguez, M., & Weinshenker, B. G. (2000). Multiple sclerosis. *The New England Journal of Medicine, 343*(13), 938–952.

Pakenham, K. I. (1999). Adjustment to multiple sclerosis: Application of a stress and coping model. *Health Psychology, 18*(4), 383–392.

Pakenham, K. I., Stewart, C. A., & Rogers, A. (1997). The role of coping in adjustment to multiple sclerosis-related adaptive demands. *Psychology, Health & Medicine, 2*, 197–211.

Patten, S. B., Beck, C. A., Williams, J. V., Barbui, C., & Metz, L. M. (2003). Major depression in multiple sclerosis: A population-based perspective. *Neurology, 61*(11), 1524–1527.

Patten, S. B., Metz, L. M., & Reimer, M. A. (2000). Biopsychosocial correlates of lifetime major depression in a multiple sclerosis population. *Multiple Sclerosis, 6*(2), 115–120.

Pujol, J., Bello, J., Deus, J., Marti-Vilalta, J. L., & Capdevila, A. (1997). Lesions in the left arcuate fasciculus region and depressive symptoms in multiple sclerosis. *Neurology, 49*, 1105–1110.

Rabins, P. V., Brooks, B. R., O'Donnell, P., Pearlson, G. D., Moberg, P., Jubelt, B., et al. (1986). Structural brain correlates of emotional disorder in multiple sclerosis. *Brain, 109*, 585–597.

Regier, D. A., Narrow, W. E., Rae, D. S., Manderscheid, R. W., Locke, B. Z., & Goodwin, F. K. (1993). The de facto US mental and addictive disorders service system. Epidemiologic catchment area prospective 1-year prevalence rates of disorders and services. *Archives of General Psychiatry, 50*(2), 85–94.

Ron, M. A., & Logsdail, S. J. (1989). Psychiatric morbidity in multiple sclerosis: A clinical and MRI study. *Psychological Medicine, 19*(4), 887–895.

Sadovnick, A. D., Remick, R. A., Allen, J., Swartz, E., Yee, I. M., Eisen, K., et al. (1996). Depression and multiple sclerosis. *Neurology, 46*(3), 628–632.

Salmaggi, A., Palumbo, R., Fontanillas, L., Eoli, M., La Mantia, L., Solari, A., et al. (1998). Affective disorders and multiple sclerosis: A controlled study on 65 Italian patients. *Italian Journal of Neurological Sciences, 19*(3), 171–175.

Sanfilipo, M. P., Benedict, R. H., Weinstock-Guttman, B., & Bakshi, R. (2006). Gray and white matter brain atrophy and neuropsychological impairment in multiple sclerosis. *Neurology, 66*(5), 685–692.

Sapolsky, R. M., Romero, L. M., & Munck, A. U. (2000). How do glucocorticoids influence stress responses? Integrating permissive, suppressive, stimulatory, and preparative actions. *Endocrine Reviews, 21*(1), 55–89.
Schiffer, R. B., & Wineman, N. M. (1990). Antidepressant pharmacotherapy of depression associated with multiple sclerosis. *The American Journal of Psychiatry, 147*, 1493–1497.
Schiffer, R. B., Wineman, N. M., & Weitkamp, L. R. (1986). Association between bipolar affective disorder and multiple sclerosis. *The American Journal of Psychiatry, 143*(1), 94–95.
Schwartz, C. E., Coulthard-Morris, L., & Zeng, Q. (1996). Psychosocial correlates of fatigue in multiple sclerosis. *Archives of Physical Medicine and Rehabilitation, 77*(2), 165–170.
Scott, T. F., Allen, D., Price, T. R., McConnell, H., & Lang, D. (1996). Characterization of major depression symptoms in multiple sclerosis patients. *The Journal of Neuropsychiatry and Clinical Neurosciences, 8*(3), 318–323.
Spiegel, D., & Classen, C. (2000). *Group therapy for cancer patients: A research-based handbook of psychosocial care*. New York: Basic Books.
Stenager, E., Knudsen, L., & Jensen, K. (1994). Multiple sclerosis: Correlation of anxiety, physical impairment and cognitive dysfunction. *Italian Journal of Neurological Sciences, 15*(2), 97–101.
Sullivan, M. J., Weinshenker, B., Mikail, S., & Bishop, S. R. (1995). Screening for major depression in the early stages of multiple sclerosis. *The Canadian Journal of Neurological Sciences, 22*(3), 228–231.
Turner, A. P., Williams, R. M., Sloan, A. P., & Haselkorn, J. K. (2009). Injection anxiety remains a long-term barrier to medication adherence in multiple sclerosis. *Rehabilitation Psychology, 54*(1), 116–121.
Uchino, B. N., Cacioppo, J. T., & Kiecolt-Glaser, J. K. (1996). The relationship between social support and physiological processes: A review with emphasis on underlying mechanisms and implications for health. *Psychological Bulletin, 119*, 488–531.
van Winsen, L. M., Muris, D. F., Polman, C. H., Dijkstra, C. D., van den Berg, T. K., & Uitdehaag, B. M. (2005). Sensitivity to glucocorticoids is decreased in relapsing remitting multiple sclerosis. *The Journal of Clinical Endocrinology and Metabolism, 90*(2), 734–740.
Warren, S., Warren, K. G., & Cockerill, R. (1991). Emotional stress and coping in multiple sclerosis (MS) exacerbations. *Journal of Psychosomatic Research, 35*(1), 37–47.
Watson, J. C., Gordon, L. B., Stermac, L., Kalogerakos, F., & Steckley, P. (2003). Comparing the effectiveness of process-experiential with cognitive-behavioral psychotherapy in the treatment of depression. *Journal of Consulting and Clinical Psychology, 71*(4), 773–781.
Wineman, N. M. (1990). Adaptation to multiple sclerosis: The role of social support, functional disability, and perceived uncertainty. *Nursing Research, 39*(5), 294–299.
Wineman, N. M., Durand, E. J., & Steiner, R. P. (1994). A comparative analysis of coping behaviors in persons with multiple sclerosis or a spinal cord injury. *Research in Nursing and Health, 17*, 185–194.
Zorzon, M., de Masi, R., Nauelli, D., Ukmar, J., Mucelli, R. P., Cazzato, G., et al. (2001). Depression and anxiety in multiple sclerosis. A clinical and MRI study in 95 subjects. *Journal of Neurology, 248*, 416–421.
Zorzon, M., Zivadinov, R., Nasuelli, D., Ukmar, M., Bratina, A., Tommasi, M. A., et al. (2002). Depressive symptoms and MRI changes in multiple sclerosis. *European Journal of Neurology, 9*(5), 491–496.

Chapter 9
Psychological Co-morbidities of Dementia

Carla Bejjani and Mark E. Kunik

9.1 Introduction

Dementia is a clinical syndrome characterized by a gradually progressing cognitive impairment. This impairment is commonly manifested by memory deficits; but the presence of one or more additional cognitive disturbances, including aphasia, agnosia, apraxia or executive dysfunction, is required to make the diagnosis, according to the *Diagnostic and Statistical Manual of Mental Disorders, 4th Edition, Text Revision* (*DSM-IV-TR*) criteria. Those disturbances should be a change from the previous baseline and should cause significant distress to the patient and caregivers. Medical problems that can cause memory impairment, substance abuse and a psychiatric axis I diagnosis need to be ruled out before making the diagnosis of dementia (Rabins et al., 2007).

Alzheimer's disease (AD) is the most frequent type and is present in 50% of cases. Vascular dementia (including mixed AD and vascular dementia) accounts for 25% of cases, and Lewy body dementia 15% of cases. Other dementias include frontotemporal dementia, progressive aphasia, alcohol-related dementia, Parkinson's dementia, and secondary cases of dementia syndrome such as intracranial lesions (Burns & Iliffe, 2009). Although there are differences in pathophysiology, clinical symptoms and course of dementia, there are only small differences in the prevalence of behavioral symptoms across the dementias. Kunik et al. looked at those differences in a study comparing 150 dementia patients with AD, vascular dementia and alcohol-related dementia. They found that neither the characteristics nor severity of agitation differed among the different subtypes, but that the patients admitted for behavioral disturbances with a diagnosis of vascular dementia were less cognitively impaired (Kunik et al., 2000).

C. Bejjani (✉)
Psychiatry and Behavioral Sciences, Baylor College of Medicine, Houston, TX, USA
e-mail: carlabejjani@hotmail.com

S. Pagoto (ed.), *Psychological Co-morbidities of Physical Illness: A Behavioral Medicine Perspective*, DOI 10.1007/978-1-4419-0029-6_9,

Dementia is a global problem, and approximately 12 million people in the world are currently diagnosed. This number is expected to reach 25 million by the year 2040 (Ferri et al., 2005). Prevalence estimates of dementia in the United States range from 5% in those aged 71–79 years to 25–50% in those 90 or older (Shub & Kunik, 2009). From a financial perspective, dementia is a heavy burden, with estimates of annual cost at $57,000 per patient in the United States (Ferri et al., 2005). In 2005 an estimated $315.4 billion was spent worldwide for the care of dementia patients, with 33% of the cost provided by family members (Wimo, Winblad, & Jonsson, 2007).

The global burden of dementia is very high, as dementia contributes to 11.2% of the total years lived with disability (Alzheimer's Society, 2007). Dementia is also the number one reason for institutionalization in the elderly population (Aguero-Torres, von Strauss, Viitanen, Winblad, & Fratiglioni, 2001). Approximately 20% of patients are institutionalized the first year after their diagnosis, but this percentage increases to 50% after 5 years and to almost 90% after 8 years (Aguero-Torres et al.).

Behavioral and psychiatric co-morbidities are very frequent in dementia, affecting as many as 90% of patients (Plassman et al., 2007); and, along with other factors, including the severity of cognitive and functional deficits, they are strongly associated with earlier institutionalization (Luppa, Luck, Brähler, König, & Riedel-Heller, 2008); they are also important contributors to caregiver stress and depression. From a financial standpoint, the management of neuropsychiatric disturbances in dementia accounts for 33% of the global cost of dementia and is associated with low income and unemployment in caregivers (Sink, Holden, & Yaffe, 2005).

Researchers of the Cache County Study (Lyketsos et al., 2000) looked at the prevalence of neuropsychiatric disturbances in community-dwelling patients with dementia. They found that almost 61% of the patients had at least one disturbance and that 32% of those were considered serious. Apathy was the most frequently encountered psychiatric co-morbidity, occurring in 27% of patients; whereas depression and agitation/aggression occurred in 24%. Other symptoms reported were delusions (18.5%), hallucinations (13.7%), anxiety (17%), irritability (20.4%), aberrant motor behavior (14.3%), disinhibition (9.1%) and elation (1%). In this chapter we review the most frequent disturbances in dementia, not distinguishing by specific type of dementia unless it is crucial for management.

9.2 Apathy

Apathy lacks a standardized definition and is not a diagnosis in the *DSM-IV*, which is a barrier to basic clinical and epidemiologic research, as well as clinical management (Lerner, Strauss, & Sami, 2007). Stuss et al. suggested that it is defined as a lack of responsiveness to stimuli that is demonstrated by a lack of self-initiated behavioral, cognitive or affective actions (Stuss, van Reekum, & Murphy, 2000). Others have suggested that apathy encompasses diminished initiation and diminished persistence of thoughts and actions. Patients with apathy have low interest and social engagement and are, in general, indifferent to their surroundings. Their emotions are blunted, and they are not bothered by their disease, as they lack insight. It is usually the family members or caregivers who seek treatment (Landes, Sperry, Milton, Strauss, & Geldmacher, 2001).

9.2.1 *Epidemiology*

Apathy is the most common behavioral symptom in AD (Lerner et al., 2007). Researchers from the Cache County epidemiologic study reported that 27% of community-dwelling dementia patients were found to have apathy (Lyketsos et al., 2000). The prevalence of apathy was higher (65.1%) when the subjects were outpatients with AD (van Reekum, Stuss, & Ostrander, 2005). Other authors reported numbers as high as 92% (Mega, Cummings, Fiorello, & Gornbein, 1996). The prevalence of apathy in long-term settings has not been well studied (van Reekum et al., 2005), but it is expected to be higher than in outpatient settings because its severity increases with the progression of the disease (Mega et al., 1996). This suggests that the overall prevalence of apathy in AD will increase when data from inpatient settings are added.

9.2.2 *Pathophysiology*

9.2.2.1 Neuropathological Disturbances

Several studies suggest that apathy is very common in lesions of the frontal regions (Lerner et al., 2007). Judgment, planning, insight and abstraction are executive functions mediated by the dorsolateral prefrontal circuit (Chow et al., 2009). The lateral orbital prefrontal circuit mediates self-regulation, and lesions result in disinhibition; whereas lesions of the anterior cingulate circuit are associated with disturbances of activation, motivation and goal-directed activities (Chow et al.). For example, in the course of AD, when the medial frontal and orbitofrontal region are affected, the patient will exhibit extreme apathy, especially when the lesions are bilateral (Lerner et al., 2007).

9.2.2.2 Neurochemical Disturbances

Evidence suggests that deregulations in both the dopaminergic and cholinergic systems are involved in the development of apathy. Dopamine might act independently or via its interaction with the cholinergic system (Boyle & Malloy, 2004). Apathy is more frequent in patients with extrapyramidal symptoms than in patients without these symptoms (Gilley, Wilson, Bennett, & Fox, 1991), and it has been found to improve when treated with agents that modulate dopaminergic neurotransmission (Lerner et al., 2007).

Of the neuropsychiatric symptoms of dementia, apathy has been shown to respond best to treatment with cholinesterase inhibitors (Boyle & Malloy, 2004), favoring the hypothesis that the cholinergic system is implicated in the pathology of apathy. This theory is further encouraged by the correlation between frontal activation and apathy demonstrated by neuroimaging studies (Craig et al., 1996; Sultzer et al., 1995), as well as by findings that the frontal lobes are more severely affected by the cholinergic depletion than the rest of the brain in AD (Cummings, 2000).

9.2.3 Clinical Care

9.2.3.1 Assessment

Several standardized instruments have been developed recently to permit a more specific assessment of apathy. Prior to that, clinicians used routine psychiatric interviews and global behavioral scales to identify apathy (Landes et al., 2001). The Composite Apathy and Irritability Scale is an informant questionnaire (Landes et al.) that contains 14 questions on apathy and 14 on irritability. It has been used by researchers in both AD and Huntington's disease (Chatterjee, Anderson, Moskowitz, Hauser, & Marder, 2005). The Dementia Apathy Interview and Rating has an additional advantage, as it compares the frequency of specific events in the previous month vs. that prior to memory loss. It relies on the caregiver's report during the interview, which is structured around 16 questions. Its internal consistency is strong (α=0.89), as well as its temporal reliability (0.85 over 2 months) (Strauss & Sperry, 2002).

The Neuropsychiatric Inventory (NPI) is one of the instruments used most often to assess several behavioral aspects of dementia, including apathy. It evaluates ten items, hallucinations, delusions, dysphoria, euphoria, anxiety, apathy, agitation, irritability, disinhibition and aberrant motor behavior (pacing and rummaging). With it, the caregiver or family member is asked to rate on a scale from 0 to 4 and 0 to 3, respectively, the frequency and severity of certain symptoms; and a total score is summed up. It has four screening questions for apathy, loss of motivation, interest, indifference or difficulty in engaging. When the screening is positive for any of these questions, the subscale of apathy is then administered. It is an eight-question questionnaire that helps confirm apathy and evaluate its frequency and severity, as well as how distressing it is to the caregiver. The NPI has excellent interrater reliability (98–100%), and high concordance with other behavioral instruments has demonstrated its validity (Cummings, 1997; Cummings et al., 1994). It is also helpful in distinguishing apathy from depression, as it also has a subscale for depression (Boyle & Malloy, 2004). However, one potential limitation is the lack of consensus as to what the cutoff score for apathy should be (van Reekum et al., 2005).

Depression is the main differential diagnosis to consider, as many patients with apathy exhibit symptoms that are also common to depression, such as excessive sleep, anhedonia, psychomotor retardation and fatigue. Although the patient can be diagnosed with depression according to *DSM-IV* criteria, it is important to distinguish the two entities, as they may respond differently to treatment (Lerner et al., 2007). However, to help with this distinction, it is useful to keep in mind that depression is primarily a mood disturbance usually characterized by dysphoria; whereas apathy is primarily a motivational loss and an emotional indifference (Boyle & Malloy, 2004). The presence of one of the neurologic disorders typically associated with apathy should help the clinician with this distinction (Lerner et al., 2007). The following clinical questions may help to differentiate apathy from depression: "Are you content with your life? (Yes = apathy)," and "Is there anything that you would like to change in your life? (No = apathy)."

Another distinction needs to be made with anhedonia, which is most commonly defined as the subjective "inability to experience pleasure." Anhedonia is a symptom and not a syndrome and can be part of the presentation in many syndromes, including apathy, dementia, major depression and schizophrenia. The lack of a universal definition of anhedonia has made the development of rating scales for anhedonia very challenging. The Snaith Hamilton Pleasure Scale is the most widely used and has proven to be of a certain value in patients with Parkinson's disease, but no research has studied its validity in patients with dementia. A clear definition of *anhedonia* is a necessary first step to facilitate the development of anhedonia rating scales.

9.3 Evidence-Based Treatment (Brief and Intensive Approaches)

9.3.1 Pharmacological Therapy

Very little research has looked at the pharmacological treatment of apathy in patients with dementia, and no specific guidelines or recommendations have been issued yet. Although no data exist on the safety of medications used, at times they appear to be the only available option. Selective serotonin reuptake inhibitors (SSRIs) are among the medications frequently used to treat apathy; however, no clear evidence supports that they help reduce apathy in patients with dementia (Boyle & Malloy, 2004). A recent study looked at the effects of treatment with citalopram on some behavioral disturbances encountered in patients with dementia. These researchers reported a 60% improvement in apathy scores (using the NPI apathy subscale) in the group taking citalopram. These results appear promising, and a randomized controlled trial (RCT) might help shed more light on this area (Siddique, Hynan, & Weiner, 2009).

Providers should, however, be aware that, because of their interference with the dopaminergic system, SSRIs can produce apathy and agitation. Therefore, if a depressed patient does not respond to treatment or develops apathy after being started on an SSRI, the clinician should reconsider the diagnosis and switch medications (Lerner et al., 2007).

Cholinesterase inhibitors were primarily developed to slow the cognitive decline in dementia, but it appears that they also help with the behavioral co-morbidities of dementia (Cummings, 2000, 2003), with apathy benefiting the most (Boyle & Malloy, 2004). After reviewing several studies, Boyle & Malloy concluded that donepezil reduced apathy in moderate-to-severe dementia (Boyle & Malloy).

Galantamine has also been used, and in a recent study rivastigmine improved apathy as well as other behavioral symptoms in patients with probable AD after 26 weeks of treatment (Onyike et al., 2007). The data seem promising, but more studies are needed to confirm efficacy and generate specific recommendations.

Dopaminergic agents, such as bupropion and amantadine, have been shown to reduce apathy in AD (Lerner et al., 2007). Patients with apathy have improved when treated with psychostimulants such as dextroamphetamine and methylphenidate. This class of medication has potential side-effects, such as agitation and irritability, in patients with dementia (Boyle & Malloy, 2004), as well as an increased risk for arrhythmias and myocardial infarction. Therefore, low doses of the medications should be administered in patients with cardiac risk factors (Lerner et al., 2007).

9.3.1.1 Behavioral Interventions

Unlike most other neuropsychiatric co-morbidities of dementia, apathy has not been shown to improve in studies comparing a combination of behavioral interventions and pharmacological treatment with a pharmacological treatment alone (Boyle & Malloy, 2004). Chapman et al. found that apathy did not improve when cognitive communication stimulation techniques were used with donepezil compared with donepezil alone, although the global functional ability improved (Chapman, Weiner, Rackley, Hynan, & Zientz, 2004).

Few RCTs of behavioral interventions targeting apathy in patients with dementia have been conducted, and most have been negative. In a 4-week RCT, Politis et al. compared a reminiscence-based kit intervention supposed to provide mental stimulation to a time and attention one-on-one control in a population of patients with dementia residing in long-term care facilities. The activity lasted 30 min, during which the therapist asked questions of different levels about five topics: geography, fun foods, farm animals, vegetables, and musical instruments. In the control intervention the therapist and patient chose how to spend 30 min together. The time spent did not encompass a structured activity and could involve discussion or random activities. Apathy, as measured by the NPI apathy subscale, improved with both interventions; but no significant difference was noted between groups. This might suggest that any kind of planned activity can improve apathy; however, this possibility needs to be confirmed by a comparison with a nontreated arm, and further studies should be done to determine the required frequency and length of such an intervention. Another finding from this RCT is that the reduction in apathy was correlated with improvement in the global NPI scale, which raises the question whether this improvement is a direct consequence of the intervention or the effect of the reduction of apathy (Politis et al., 2004).

Multisensory behavioral therapy (MSBT) uses automatic reinforcement (Skinner, 1953; Vaughan & Michael, 1982) and the physiological model of the relaxation response (Benson & Klipper, 1975). The sensory preference assessment procedure consists of two phases. The first phase consists of introducing several individual stimuli, one at a time, while observing "approach responses" consisting of positive initiation by patients or "avoidance" "evidenced by any negative behavior." If the patient exhibits a positive approach, the stimulus is presented for 5 s (or 30 s for musical stimuli); otherwise, the presentation is immediately stopped. The next step consists of multiple pairing trials within the same class of stimulus, which is usually started with the visual stimuli and not recommended for the auditory stimuli. Once the preferred combination of shapes, intensity, colors, positions and symmetry of the visual stimuli is determined, a second class of stimuli, usually music, is assessed with the preferred visual combination. Using the same procedure, tactile then olfactory stimuli are assessed in combination with the already selected stimuli to reach the optimal individualized multisensory combination preferred by the patient (Staal, Pinkney, & Roane, 2003).

A study compared the efficacy of standard inpatient psychiatric treatment alone, which encompasses occupational therapy, a structured hospital setting, and use of standard pharmacological therapy, with standard treatment in combination with MSBT. In this study the intervention was individualized to the patient with a new sensory-assessment method that matched the patient's preferences in terms of sensory stimuli (visual, tactile, auditory or olfactory) over the first two to three sessions. Once the preference was established, the patients underwent six 25–30 min sessions of MSBT. Agitation improved in both groups; however, MSBT was found to reduce apathy, whereas standard inpatient care did not. Although the mechanism of action is unknown, Staal et al. suggested that, when combined with standard care, MSBT can improve apathy by evoking interest/focusing on the environment (Staal et al., 2007). Some behavioral approaches appear promising. However, studies comparing pharmacological treatment with nonpharmacological treatment with apathy as the outcome have not been conducted yet. If similar or greater efficacy is demonstrated, advancements might be expected, as very little data exist regarding the safety and efficacy of pharmacological interventions in the treatment of apathy (Lerner et al., 2007).

9.4 Depressive Disorders

9.4.1 Epidemiology

Depressive syndromes affect 40–55% of patients with AD, 20–25% with major depressive disorder and an additional 20–30% with other depressive symptoms, including minor depression (Lyketsos & Olin, 2002; Zubenko et al., 2003).

There is no consensus about the natural history of depression in dementia. Some data suggest that depression increases as dementia progresses from mild to moderate but decreases in severe stages (Forsell, Jorm, Fratiglioni, Grut, & Winblad, 1993), whereas other studies report that it increases in severe stages (Zubenko et al., 2003), and others fail to demonstrate a consistent association between the stage of dementia and depression (Payne et al., 1998).

The course of depression in AD is also still unknown, with some studies suggesting that it is of shorter duration and can resolve without treatment (Brodaty & Luscombe, 1996); whereas Devanand et al. found, in a large study, that 30–40% of cases persisted beyond 6 months (Devanand et al., 1997).

Depression in dementia has very negative consequences, such as early placement in a nursing home, greater disability in performing activities of daily living (Lyketsos et al., 1997), physical aggression towards the caregiver (Lyketsos, Steele, et al., 1999), depression and increased burden for caregivers (González-Salvador et al., 2000) and increased mortality in patients (Bassuk, Berkman, & Wypij, 1998).

9.4.2 Pathophysiology

The prevalence of depression in the population of patients with dementia is more elevated than in the nondemented population of the same age, and most patients with depression and dementia do not report mood problems prior to the onset of the cognitive decline (Zubenko et al., 2003), suggesting that depression is not simply a result of chance alone in these patients. It is also likely that depression is not a simple psychological reaction to the knowledge of having dementia, as most studies do not show a correlation between insight about dementia and depression (Lyketsos & Lee, 2004).

Postmortem studies have shown that depression in dementia is associated with selective loss of neuradrenergic cells of the locus cereleus of the brain. It is also associated with loss of the dorsal raphe serotoninergic nuclei (Förstl et al., 1992).

It is unclear whether there is a genetic susceptibility to developing depression, as some studies have demonstrated that a family history of mood disorder in a first-degree relative is associated with greater risk for depression (Fahim et al., 1998); whereas others have not found an association (Heun, Papassotiropoulos, Jessen, Maier, & Breitner, 2001). ApoE4 was studied as a potential susceptibility gene for depression in AD, and one study found its frequency to be related to the development of late-onset depression (Krishnan et al., 1996) and hippocampal volume reduction in late-onset depression (Kim, Payne, Levy, MacFall, & Steffens, 2002); but a review of several other studies was not in favor of associating the ApoE4 genotype with depressive symptoms (Lyketsos & Lee, 2004).

Defects in the serotoninergic system have been implicated in the development of major depressive disorder, but studies so far have not been able to find an association between the 5HTTLPR serotonin transporter gene polymorphism and depression in AD (Zill et al., 2000). Some 5HT 2 receptor variants have been found to be associated with depression in AD (Holmes, Arranz, Collier, Powell, & Lovestone, 2003), but results still need to be replicated before they can be generalized.

9.4.3 Assessment

Assessing depression in patients with dementia can be challenging. Depressive symptoms can be the initial presentation of dementia and can fluctuate over time (Lyketsos & Olin, 2002; Rabins et al., 2007). Compared with older patients with intact cognition, patients with dementia are more likely to report a diminished ability to concentrate or indecisiveness during a major depressive episode (Zubenko et al., 2003). On the other hand, patients with dementia are less likely to report insomnia/hypersomnia, feelings of worthlessness and guilt, thoughts of death/suicide (Zubenko et al.) or frank sadness but instead report anxiety, irritability, worry or fear (Lyketsos & Lee, 2003). Of note, psychotic symptoms such as hallucinations and delirium are more frequent in depressed persons with dementia than in the comparable population; and this can be a source of misdiagnosis (Lyketsos et al., 2001). To account for these differences, revised diagnostic criteria have been proposed for depression in patients who have AD. Specifically, participants in the National Institute of Mental Health Depression of AD Workshop suggested adding irritability, social withdrawal and isolation (Olin, Katz, Meyers, Schneider, & Lebowitz, 2002; Olin, Schneider, et al., 2002). Further confounders of assessment include symptoms of apathy and anxiety. These symptoms frequently coexist with depression but are also independent behavioral dimensions (Starkstein, Ingram, Garau, & Mizrahi, 1983).

Several measures are available for screening and diagnosing depression. In the early stages of the disease, the Geriatric Depression Scale, which relies on patient self report, can be used (Yesavage et al., 1983). In more advanced stages, patients may be unable to reliably respond to self-rating questionnaires; and depression may go undetected or underestimated. Some clinician-administered instruments, such as a modified version of the Hamilton Rating Scale for Depression (HAM-D) (Zubenko et al., 2003) or the Cornell Scale for Depression in Dementia (CSDD), are more practical, as they elicit information from both the patient and caregiver. Both scales have been validated in patients with a broad range of cognitive impairment (Alexopoulos, Abrams, Young, & Shamoian, 1988; Mulsant, Sweet, & Rifal, 1994). The CSDD, which is interviewer administered, might be more sensitive to the detection of treatment effect than the HAM-D (Mayer et al., 2006). Patients with depression should always be evaluated for suicide risk.

In a review of the literature looking at suicide and nonfatal self-injurious behavior in dementia, Haw et al. concluded that suicide appears to be increased soon after the diagnosis in patients suffering from mild dementia as well as in patients suffering from Huntington's disease or when the diagnosis of dementia is made during a hospitalization. Depression appears to be a risk factor for suicide in dementia patients, as well as young age; hopelessness; good insight into the illness; failure to respond to anti-dementia drugs; and, as stated above, mild cognitive impairment. One should keep in mind, however, that many studies used in this review had serious methodological limitations; more research is needed for a better understanding of the association of suicide with dementia in general and the association with certain subtypes of dementia such as vascular or Lewy Body, in which suicide rates are high (Haw, Harwood, & Hawton, 2009).

9.4.4 Evidence-Based Treatment (Brief and Intensive Approaches)

As a first step a complete evaluation should be done to clarify the diagnosis and rule out exacerbating factors such as primary medical problems (Lyketsos & Lee, 2003). For example, an occult anemia can cause a patient to be constantly tired and possibly cause him/her to decrease physical activities and stay home or sleep. This can be easily mistaken for depression, simple lab work can identify the problem, and treatment might improve the symptoms as well as the patient's mood. Hypothyroidism is another medical problem that frequently presents as depression in the elderly. Constipation and urinary tract infections are benign in the younger population and will rarely lead to mood or behavioral problems. Older adults, however, have fragile health that can be easily affected. This is especially a problem in patients with dementia, who may have difficulty communicating with their caregivers. In cases when pathology often manifests with behavioral problems and eliciting the symptoms to make the correct diagnosis is difficult, a simple urinary exam or physical exam might be valuable; life stressors and possible problems with the caregiver also need to be assessed and addressed when possible, as patients can react to those with symptoms of depression. For example, a patient with dementia who has issues with his/her caregiver can elect to limit conversations and interactions, be difficult to engage, and/or refuse to eat food prepared by this caregiver. All these symptoms are very common in depression, and changing the caregiver or trying to work out the issues might be more beneficial than a trial of antidepressant medication.

Several approaches can be used to treat depression in patients with dementia. These include electroconvulsive therapy (ECT), pharmacotherapy, and psychosocial modalities. Psychosocial interventions are the first-line treatment.

9.4.4.1 Psychosocial Modalities

Nonpharmacological interventions include supportive-therapy techniques, such as reminding the patient of previous accomplishments, focusing on positive aspects of life, instilling hope and promoting enjoyable activities. Simple activities are recommended, such as self-expression and crafts, music, mild exercise, reminiscing with photos, participating in religious activities, and visiting people and places.

Caregivers can support the patient by giving him/her one-on-one attention, acknowledging his/her feelings, finding ways that he/she can contribute to family life, and showing him/her love and appreciation (Nguyen, Love, & Kunik, 2008).

Of the 11 randomized controlled studies of psychosocial treatments of depression in older adults with dementia, seven showed significant improvement in the treatment group compared with the control group. In eight of these groups, improvements were maintained beyond the active-treatment period (Teri et al., 2005). Most of these RCTs used depression scales, validated in patients with dementia.

The psychosocial treatments studied were diverse. They included interventions based on behavioral approaches that focus on training caregivers to problem-solve and communicate effectively. Therapists taught caregivers in the community behavioral techniques, either by increasing pleasant activities or by problem solving in 9 weekly 1-h sessions over 9 weeks (Teri et al., 1997).

An important strategy was to teach caregivers how to approach specific problem behaviors and avoid disruption, which would negatively impact the affect. Exercise programs were implemented, and caregivers were taught by masters-level social workers and physical therapists how to address the behavioral disturbances that usually arise with increased physical activities. This intervention was conducted in the patients' homes, in twelve 1-h sessions over 3 months.

Other interventions were geared towards nursing staff taking care of patients with depression and dementia. In a protocol developed by Lawton et al. over 12 months, research staff conducted twice-monthly administrative planning sessions, human-relations training with nurses, and 7 h of training with direct-care staff on the stimulation-retreat approach. They also improved interdisciplinary care planning and developed activity programming. This was in addition to family support through phone calls, discussion groups, and social gatherings (Lawton et al., 1998).

Distraction techniques and developing realistic, individualized goals for behavioral improvement with close supervision to help the achievement of these goals also proved effective in reducing depression after implementing the interventions for 12 weeks. Strategies included training nurse assistants to assist in activities of daily living for 45–60 min per day, help meeting psychosocial needs using 25 modules for 25 min every day or both these interventions (Beck et al., 2002).

Structured programs were also used to promote social engagement by decreasing social isolation and increasing patients' sense of control over their environment. Some examples proven effective include having two patients participate in the same activity (for example, riding a special bicycle attached to a wheelchair), which is likely to stimulate social interaction during the activity and later during a group designed to have patients share their personal experience. Initially research staff used the wheelchair bicycle with the patients for an hour, 5 times a week for 2 weeks; then for the last 10 weeks, volunteers, family members or staff members participated with the patients twice a week (Buettner & Fitzsimmons, 2002). Another example of successful intervention is evidenced by a decrease in emerging withdrawal and irritability when a recording of family members' voices was played by nursing staff at least twice every day (Camberg et al., 1999).

Other interventions were employed to modify sensory or environmental stimulation. An approach that proved successful was identifying specific sensory needs of each patient and then developing specific strategies and environmental modifications to meet the particular needs of each patient, whether it was increasing or decreasing sensory stimulation. This was conducted by facility staff in 30-min sessions over 4 weeks (Baker et al., 2003).

Group reminiscence therapy also improved cognitive and affective function in a recent RCT undertaken by Wang (2007). Although these interventions have proven effective in reducing depression in patients with dementia, they rely on the presence and important commitment and availability of caregivers, which makes their implementation very challenging. Currently, no studies in the literature suggest possible options for situations for which caregivers are not available.

9.4.4.2 Antidepressants

If depression is severe or the patient is having suicidal, homicidal ideations and/or is not eating or drinking, pharmacological therapy should start early (Lyketsos & Lee, 2003). Although placebo-controlled studies of antidepressants have produced contradictory results, as many of them failed to prove efficacy, the American Psychiatric Association (APA) practice guidelines support a trial of an antidepressant to treat clinically significant depressive symptoms in patients with dementia (Lyketsos & Olin, 2002).

SSRIs are generally the first-line agents because they have a better safety and tolerability profile than tricyclics and monoamine oxidase inhibitors, which have cardiovascular and anticholinergic adverse effects. Among the SSRIs, citalopram (starting dose of 10 mg daily) and sertraline (starting dose of 25 mg daily) appear to have the strongest efficacy data, based on limited clinical trials (Lyketsos & Lee, 2003; Shub & Kunik, 2009). They may also be preferred because they are least likely to induce or inhibit the cytochrome P-450 liver enzyme that affects the hepatic metabolism of most drugs, thus preventing interaction with other drugs (Lyketsos & Olin, 2002; Rabins et al., 2007).

Alternative agents, including serotonin norepinephrine reuptake inhibitors (venlafaxine, duloxetine), mirtazapine and bupropion, may be second-line treatment options. However, data from controlled studies in adults with dementia are lacking. Patients with dementia are particularly prone to medication adverse effects. Whichever agent is chosen, the paradigm of "start low and go slow" should be followed (Shub & Kunik, 2009).

The efficacy of treatment should be monitored by frequent measures on standardized symptom-rating scales. A good response might take up to 9–12 weeks of full-dose treatment. If by 6 weeks there is not partial improvement, then switching medication class should be a consideration. If there is partial improvement after 6 weeks, adding a second agent might be beneficial (Lyketsos et al., 2003). If nonpharmacological treatments and two subsequent trials of medications fail, hospitalization or referral to a specialist in geriatric psychiatry may be indicated. In this case, ECT might be an alternative (Lyketsos & Lee, 2003).

9.4.4.3 ECT

ECT, also known as electroshock, is a well-established psychiatric treatment in which seizures are electrically induced in normal neurons by applying pulses of current through the scalp of anesthetized patients for therapeutic effect (Kaplan & Sadock, 2007). If pharmacological interventions are ineffective or contraindicated, ECT can be an alternative. A chart review of patients with depression and dementia at Johns Hopkins Hospital showed a statistically significant improvement in depression in those who were treated with ECT (Rao & Lyketsos, 2000). Risks (including high rates of delirium in dementia patients) and benefits (including improved cognition when depression is successfully treated) must be carefully weighed on an individual basis (Lyketsos & Olin, 2002).

9.5 Behavioral/Aggressive Disorders

In persons with dementia, agitation may manifest in a variety of behaviors, including verbal aggression (e.g., yelling), physical aggression, combativeness or resistance to care, psychomotor hyperactivity, and disinhibition. Although we will refer to these behaviors as agitation, it is important when addressing behavioral disturbances to specify the target behavior (Braun & Kunik, 2004). Disruptive behaviors are a frequent cause of caregiver stress and burnout; nursing-home placement or hospitalization; injuries to patients, other residents, and caregivers; property damage; and decreased quality of life for all involved (Kunik et al., 2003; Tariot, 1999). Disruptive behaviors may trigger inappropriate medication administration by healthcare providers. Such behaviors can also lead to potential civil lawsuits or regulatory problems for long-term care facilities, home-care providers, and day centers (Kapp, 2000).

9.5.1 Epidemiology

Population-based studies of community-dwelling older adults find that as many as 24% of patients with dementia experience agitation/aggression during the course of their illness (Lyketsos et al., 2000). The prevalence of agitation increases with dementia severity and in institutionalized patients, but no differences have been found in the prevalence or phenomenology of agitation across types of dementia (Cohen-Mansfield, Marx, & Rosenthal, 1989; Kapp, 2000; Kunik et al., 2000).

9.5.2 Pathophysiology

Behavioral symptoms often have multiple causes and can be affected by different factors related to the patient, caregiver or environment. Some factors are modifiable, while others are not.

9.5.2.1 Patient Factors

One of the main differential diagnoses in agitated patients with dementia is delirium. Delirium is a life-threatening condition that occurs frequently in demented patients and usually leads to their admission to an acute hospital setting. Delirium usually presents with agitation and combativeness, as well as confusion and fluctuating levels of arousal. Perception and cognition are also affected, as delirious patients might experience auditory and visual hallucinations and a precipitous decline in cognitive functioning. Many of these symptoms are also present in dementia, but the sudden occurrence of the symptomatology should prompt the clinician to make the diagnosis of delirium. Distinguishing agitation in the context of delirium from agitation as a consequence of dementia is important because delirium is the manifestation of an acute, usually treatable medical condition rather than the inevitable progression of dementia. Although the occurrence of delirium in dementia has been shown to be related to worsened cognition in the long run, it is necessary to treat delirium and its underlying cause, as this is likely to reverse the acute agitation (Macdonald, 1999).

Pain is very frequent among patients with dementia, as they tend to be advanced in age and are likely to have medical conditions that can cause pain, such as arthritis, musculoskeletal pain, scars and so forth. In a recent study, Kunik et al. found that it is the worst pain over the past week rather than current pain that is best correlated with predicting aggression (Kunik et al., 2010). Demented patients may have difficulty articulating their pain to caregivers; instead, they often try to communicate their discomfort via aggressive behaviors (Nguyen et al., 2008). For this reason, it is of utmost importance to assess pain, even if it is at times hard to completely reverse it, because even a mild reduction in pain will likely manifest with decreased agitation and aggressive behavior.

Often patients with dementia have medical and psychiatric co-morbidities that need to be treated with medications. Some of these medications have side-effects that can precipitate or aggravate agitation and aggression. For example, if a demented patient is suffering from insomnia and is treated with antihistamines, which are very common over-the-counter medications, the anticholinergic effects of the sleep aid will probably lead to disinhibition, inappropriate behavior and agitation. This also is a highly modifiable cause of aggression or agitation (Braun & Kunik, 2004).

Psychosis and depression are two psychiatric conditions associated with agitation in patients with dementia. They are discussed elsewhere in the chapter, but it is important to screen for them when a demented patient presents with agitation or aggression, as they are modifiable factors, and their treatment will have a positive impact on those behaviors.

Some factors related to the patient are difficult to change and are proven to be associated with worsened agitation in the context of dementia. The patient's personality prior to the onset of dementia is, for instance, very hard to modify at an advanced age. Agitation is associated with the severity of dementia, and it might help a frustrated caregiver to understand that this is a contributor that can be barely modified. Low socioeconomic status, poor education and male gender are characteristics of patients that are unmodifiable and are associated with agitation (Braun & Kunik, 2004).

9.5.2.2 Caregiver Factors

Agitation can also stem from factors affecting the caregiver. Research suggests that increased burden at baseline and poor relationship of caregiver with patient later on are associated with behavioral problems (Kunik et al., 2010). Caregivers of patients with dementia have higher rates of depression, anxiety, sleep and appetite problems, prescription-drug usage, medical illnesses and mortality than noncaregivers (Kunik et al., 2008; Nguyen et al., 2008). Those psychological and emotional needs and the quality of their current relationship with patients are modifiable factors that should be addressed as developed below. The caregiver's skills and coping mechanisms can also be improved, whereas the quality of his/her past relationship with the patient, gender, race and socioeconomic status are important unmodifiable factors.

9.5.2.3 Environmental Factors

Some environmental factors can predispose for agitation. It is important to assess the physical aspect of a facility (i.e., lighting, noise), social interaction and stimulation of the patient, use of restraints and traffic flow, as well as the change of environment, because addressing these factors can result in decreased agitation. The staffing ratio and the setting are also very important environmental factors, but they are very difficult to modify (Braun & Kunik, 2004).

9.5.2.4 Sundowning

Sundowning occurs in almost 45% of patients diagnosed with AD. It is a period of the day, usually late afternoon, evenings and nights, when patients exhibit agitation, confusion, mood swings, hallucinations and other disruptive behaviors. Although we don't have a clear understanding of this phenomenon, it is thought to be associated with the circadian cycle. Some possible explanations include decreased exposure to light, difficulty adapting to the decreased activity level in the evening and sleep disturbances related to dementia. Sundowning is frequently associated with wandering, which increases the risk of nighttime elopement (Wick & Zanni, 2005).

9.5.3 Clinical Care

9.5.3.1 Assessment

Patients who exhibit agitation warrant a detailed evaluation, including a description of the behavior, its timing, frequency and chronology (Lesser & Hughes, 2006). Instruments to quantify agitation/aggression and monitor target behaviors in patients with dementia include the NPI Questionnaire (Cummings et al., 1994), the Behavioral Pathology in Alzheimer's Disease Rating Scale (BEHAVE-AD) and the Cohen-Mansfield Agitation Inventory. The latter is a clinician- or caregiver-rated questionnaire that categorizes disruptive behaviors (either verbal or physical) on a spectrum from nonaggressive to aggressive (Cohen-Mansfield, 2000). Ideally, these instruments should be completed with interviews with different caregivers (Kalapatapu & Neugroschl, 2009).

Triggers should be looked for, and a causality or association elicited. Any changes in the environment, including staff changes or overstimulation (Kalapatapu & Neugroschl, 2009), should be monitored and addressed as needed. Changes in medication (e.g., anticholinergic side-effects) and the patient's medical condition should be carefully reassessed, and a complete medical evaluation can be warranted. Further evaluation includes a thorough physical exam and baseline lab work, including a complete blood count, basic metabolic panel, urine analysis, chest X-ray, and EkG that can help rule out an occult medical condition. For example, abdominal palpation can easily help rule out urinary retention; and a digital rectal exam, although not very comfortable, can reveal a fecal impaction with resolution of agitation once the impaction is resolved. A complete blood count can very easily detect anemia or an infection, and a chest X-ray or urine analysis will help localize the infectious source. At times a patient may be delirious; and if the initial work is nonrevealing, the provider should pursue the underlying cause with other lab work, such as liver-function tests; B12, folate and ammonia levels; and, eventually, a computed tomography head scan. The possibility of substance use (illicit drugs or alcohol) should not be overlooked and can be scanned for with a urine drug screen. All efforts should be geared towards finding a potentially modifiable cause, but one should keep in mind that, in the absence of such a cause, agitation can be a manifestation of the progression of dementia (Lesser & Hughes, 2006).

Pain is another factor that can cause agitation frequently in persons with dementia. It can be very challenging to assess because of patients' cognitive impairment and difficulty in verbalizing their complaints. Several assessment tools have been designed to meet their special needs. The Iowa Pain Thermometer is a validated self-report tool that allows the patient to indicate the degree of pain by marking on a thermometer graphic with verbal descriptors of pain intensity. In addition, because older adults often deny experiencing pain, clinicians may consider asking the patient whether he or she experiences "aching" or "hurting" instead of "pain." In some cases, primary care providers (PCPs) must rely more on observation-based assessments for cognitively impaired patients who cannot verbalize pain (Nguyen et al., 2008). Common pain behaviors include facial expressions (e.g., frowning, grimacing, having a distorted expression, rapid blinking), verbalizations/vocalizations (e.g., sighing, moaning, calling out, verbal abuse), body movements (e.g., tension, guarding, fidgeting, increased pacing/rocking, gait or mobility changes), changes in interpersonal interactions (e.g., being aggressive, resisting care, being disruptive, being withdrawn), and changes in activity patterns (e.g., appetite change, sleep change, sudden cessation of common routines) and mental status (e.g., crying, increased confusion, irritability, distress) (AGS Panel on Persistent Pain in Older Persons, 2002). The Non-Communicative Patient's Pain Assessment Instrument is an example of a valid observational scale that evaluates some of these behaviors and is appropriate for use with dementia patients (Snow et al., 2004). It is a brief measure that can be easily administered. Regardless of the type of screen, positive screens should be followed by careful, comprehensive physical and psychosocial evaluation to detect causes for reported pain or observed behaviors (Nguyen et al., 2008). As mentioned above, depression and psychosis cause agitation in dementia patients. We will not expand on their assessment, as it is discussed in other parts of the chapter.

9.5.3.2 Caregiver Burden and Relationship

As noted previously, caregiver burden and the relationship of the caregiver with the patient are predictive factors for aggression/ agitation. Every visit with a patient with dementia should include screening the caregiver by asking questions to determine how he/she is coping, whether he/she needs more support, and how healthy his/her relationship is with the patient. Questions can be simple, such as, "Tell me what it was like when your loved one developed memory problems"; "How are you able to care for him/her?" or "Describe your relationship." One-on-one interviews allow caregivers to be truthful about problems. Clinicians should also be vigilant in screening for signs of caregiver burden. Common signs include feelings of exhaustion, guilt, anger and anxiety; social withdrawal and isolation; impaired sleep and concentration; increased health problems; and a decline in caregiving (Rabins et al., 2007). Two brief assessment tools are available to evaluate burden and relationship. Five questions from the Margaret Blenkner Research Center (MBRC) Caregiver Strain Instrument assess for strain in the caregiver-patient relationship (Bass, McClendon, Deimling, & Mukherjee, 1994; Bass, Noelker, & Rechlin, 1996). The Mini-Burden Interview has seven questions to assess the caregiver's perception and experience of burden (e.g., "Have you had difficulty sleeping? Eating?") with three more questions on potential causes of burden (e.g., "Does your loved one have behavioral problems? Paranoia?") (Agronin, 2004).

9.5.3.3 Evidence-Based Treatment (Brief and Intensive Approaches)

Because of effectiveness and safety concerns of medication use, especially with antipsychotics, there is a need to emphasize nonpharmacological interventions in treating behavioral disturbances (Shub & Kunik, 2009).

Nonpharmacological Treatment

Behavioral Approaches for the Patient

Two behavioral approaches are possible: a systematic *ABC* approach to implementing a behavioral plan helps individualize treatment and monitor improvement. This entails identifying specific *A*ntecedents of target problem *B*ehavior and their *C*onsequences and devising specific strategies to address these (Rabins et al., 2007). For example, repetitive screaming (depending on the antecedent identified) can be treated by fulfilling unmet needs (e.g., pain, toileting), providing increased socialization, or reducing overstimulation in the environment (not going out in a crowd, for example) (Agronin, 2004; Shub & Kunik, 2009).

The Three *R*s approach (repeat, reassure and redirect) is also a method to minimize medication use. For example, if a patient is getting upset because he/she thinks it is time to go to a doctor's appointment, the caregiver could reassure him/her by saying that the appointment isn't until much later and then redirecting him/her to another activity, such as watching TV, listening to music or doing crafts (Kalapatapu & Neugroschl, 2009).

Having to decide between multiple choices can frustrate a cognitively impaired patient and lead to agitation or aggression; limiting choices can be successful in decreasing agitation. Patients can also feel overwhelmed by multistep activities, such as dressing or brushing teeth, leading them to be agitated or aggressive. Simplifying the task (for example, using Velcro on clothing to facilitate dressing/undressing) or breaking an activity down into several simple tasks can minimize behavioral disturbances (e.g., instead of saying, "Go brush your teeth," say "Take the toothbrush, take the toothpaste, put the toothpaste on the toothbrush and then brush your upper teeth, then your bottom teeth, then rinse your mouth") (Kalapatapu & Neugroschl, 2009). As a general rule, limit arguing with an agitated patient unless he/she is an immediate danger to self or others (Lesser & Hughes, 2006). Caregivers should also try to minimize patients' interactions with strangers and facilitate orientation by making digital clocks and calendars easily available (Lesser & Hughes, 2006).

In addition to individual behavioral plans, some persons with dementia also benefit from activity- or sensory-oriented psychosocial treatments. In a recent review of five randomized clinical trials and 14 observational studies of activity interventions, significant decreases in problem behaviors or aggression/agitation were seen with sensory-stimulating activities (helping patients reexperience familiar smells, movements, textures, sights, sounds and tastes by concentrating on one sense at a time) and sensory-calming activities (such as listening to relaxing music), physical activities-based interventions (including exercise and walking programs), and recreational activities. A review of three randomized clinical trials and 21 observational studies of sensory-therapy interventions (many of which involved music interventions) also largely favored intervention groups on measures of agitation. Studies have failed to show benefit with aromatherapy and bright-light therapy (Bharani & Snowden, 2005).

Approaches to Care for the Caregiver

Another important aspect in caring for patients with dementia is to care for the caregiver because caregiver burden and the quality of the relationship between the caregiver and the patient are predictor factors for aggression. The clinician can listen, offer practical advice and be emotionally supportive to the caregiver and refer him/her to the appropriate resources. When distress is significant and persistent, referral to mental health professionals and/or pharmacologic treatment is indicated (Nguyen et al., 2008).

Nonpharmacologic interventions with the caregiver can be summed up in the mnemonic: Educate, Empower, Environmental, Engage, Energize, and End points (Agronin, 2004). Educate caregivers about the disease and resources. Empower the caregiver with skills to improve dementia care. This may involve developing a flexible daily routine, using simple language to enhance communication, and labeling items to facilitate memory. Assist caregivers in identifying potential environmental hazards in the home to protect the patient. Engage caregivers and patients with stimulating and pleasurable activities. Encourage the caregiver to take respite time and tend to his/her needs, thereby energizing his/her ability to be a better caregiver (Nguyen et al., 2008). A daycare program for the loved one with dementia provides, in addition to a structured activity, a much-needed respite for caregivers (Lesser & Hughes, 2006). Lastly, gradually prepare the caregiver for end points, such as hospice or long-term care. Keep in mind that monitoring the caregiver's personal level of frustration and burnout will help him/her control inappropriate behavior and enhance reinforcement when a patient exhibits a positive behavior (Lesser & Hughes).

In addition to these strategies, healthcare professionals can refer caregivers to programs to reduce burden and strengthen the caregiver-patient relationship. These include strategies for coping with frustration or depression, exercise interventions, stress-management techniques, and support groups (American Psychiatric Association, 2007). Organizations such as the Alzheimer's Association (http://www.alz.org) and the Alzheimer's Disease Education and Referral Center (http://www.nia.nih.gov/Alzheimers) provide valuable information about local resources and offer caregiver-support services, hot-lines, and educational information (Nguyen et al., 2008). Of the many interventions geared towards caregivers, three types have been shown to be effective: psychoeducational skill building, psychotherapy (mainly cognitive behavioral), and multicomponent (using a combination of at least two approaches such as education, family meetings, and skill building; Coon & Evans, 2009).

CBT for Treating Pain in Patients with Dementia

In a pilot study, cognitive behavioral therapy (CBT) has been found to be effective in treating pain in persons with mild and moderate dementia (Keefe, 1996; Kraus et al., 2008). Components include relaxation techniques, distraction methods, pleasant activity scheduling and pacing, and cognitive restructuring to help patients recognize the relationship between pain symptoms, cognitions and behaviors, and to challenge negative pain thoughts (Hadjistavropoulos & Hadjistavropoulos, 2008; Keefe, 1996).

Cognitive restructuring techniques can also be used in the primary care setting. By asking a few questions during a regular office visit, the physician can identify erroneous thoughts stemming from false pain-related beliefs and attempt to generate more realistic thinking (Hadjistavropoulos & Hadjistavropoulos, 2008) by educating patients about their pain and teaching them how to come up with coping self-statements, e.g., "I will never be happy because I have pain" will be replaced with "I have pain, but there are things I can do to improve my quality of life" (Nguyen et al., 2008). Simple distraction techniques, such as focusing on a hobby or movie, counting, or performing imagery exercises, can also be useful. The latter can help counter negative images of pain and give mental relief. For example, ask the patient to describe what the pain feels like. A reply might be, "It feels like my back is on fire" (Hadjistavropoulos & Hadjistavropoulos, 2008). Encourage the patient to imagine taking a bucket of water to douse the pain or being in a comfortable environment, such as the beach. In addition, relaxation techniques, such as diaphragmatic abdominal breathing, can be taught in a few minutes by a PCP (Hadjistavropoulos & Hadjistavropoulos). Instruct the patient to take slow, deep breaths to the diaphragm, not the chest. Chest breathing can worsen pain and is associated with anxiety and tension. Place the patient's hand on his/her abdomen; and say that, while he/she is breathing, he/she should notice the hand moving. With practice, the patient should be able to achieve a state of relaxation and have better control over pain. Lastly, exercise and paced-activity scheduling are essential in managing chronic pain. Clinicians, including physical therapists, can create a modified exercise plan to meet the patient's capabilities, needs, and interests (Nguyen et al., 2008).

9.5.3.4 Pharmacotherapy

The consequences of untreated agitation/aggression can be very serious; agitation may lead to disability, threats to personal health and the safety of others, increased caregiver burden, and institutionalization (Agronin, 2004). Thus, despite the well-established risk of pharmacotherapy in this population, when behavioral measures alone are insufficient, APA guidelines support the use of antipsychotic medications (Rabins et al., 2007). The atypical antipsychotics risperidone and olanzapine have the best evidence for efficacy (Sink et al., 2005). Antidepressants (SSRIs and trazodone) are relatively safe, and a therapeutic trial might be warranted, especially for nonpsychotic patients with mild agitation (Shub & Kunik, 2009), those who cannot tolerate antipsychotics or are nonresponders and those who have mild symptoms (Rabins et al., 2007). Sink et al. found in an evidence-based review in 2005 that citalopram has better efficacy in treating agitation and other behavioral aspects of dementia other than depression (Sink et al., 2005). Pollock et al. found in a clinical trial comparing rispedal with citalopram for treating behavioral and psychotic symptoms in patients with dementia that citalopram was as effective for psychotic symptoms as risperdal (Pollock et al., 2007). Given the better side-effect profile of citalopram, it might be a reasonable first-choice alternative, especially in patients with depression and/or anxiety (Kalapatapu & Neugroschl, 2009). SSRIs can also be used in sexually disinhibited patients, as decreasing libido is a frequent side-effect (Kalapatapu & Neugroschl, 2009).

Results from a small, randomized clinical trial with trazodone were promising for decreasing problematic behaviors in patients with frontotemporal dementia (Sultzer, Gray, Gunay, Berisford, & Mahler, 1997). Sultzer et al. found that trazodone reduced perseveration and oppositionality in sundowning; whereas Haldol was more efficient in reducing elopement, restlessness and pacing.

Evidence exists of modest, but statistically significant, efficacy of cholinesterase inhibitors (donepezil and memantin; Sink et al., 2005) on agitation. There is limited evidence of efficacy for anticonvulsants, lithium, and alpha blockers. All these agents can cause adverse effects and thus are not recommended, except for patients who have not responded to, or tolerated, other treatments (Rabins et al., 2007). Patients exhibiting chronic disinhibition agitation might be less responsive to antipsychotics, and a trial of 50–100 mg of valproate might be beneficial (Herrmann, 1998). However, the US Food and Drug Administration issued a warning about emerging or worsening suicidal ideations and mood or behavioral changes with anticonvulsant treatment and recommends monitoring target symptoms and behaviors (Kalapatapu & Neugroschl, 2009).

Benzodiazepines, because of their severe side-effect profile, are not recommended for elderly patients. They can, however, be useful as a short-term treatment in agitated patients with severe anxiety. If given for more than a month, they should be tapered down, and long-term benzodiazepines such as diazepam or Librium should be avoided (Rabins et al., 2007).

The use of physical restraints should be restricted to behavioral emergencies if the patient is combative and puts self or others at imminent risk (Rabins et al., 2007). Their use beyond these circumstances may increase risk of falls and contribute to cognitive decline. In fact, restraint reduction has been shown to decrease serious injuries in nursing-home residents (Burton, German, Rovner, & Brant, 1992).

9.6 Psychotic Disorders

The *DSM IV-TR* includes under the term *psychosis* the presence of certain symptoms, such as delusions, hallucinations, disorganized speech or behavior (American Psychiatric Association, 2000). In the context of dementia, delusions tend to be simple, nonbizarre and paranoid in nature (Schneider & Dagerman, 2004). When compared with other neuropsychiatric co-morbidities of dementia, psychosis is less prevalent; but it is a commonly associated behavioral problem (Aalten et al., 2008).

9.6.1 Epidemiology

Delusions of theft are the most frequent (Ropacki & Jeste, 2005). Other types of delusions include patients thinking that they are not in their home, that their spouses are having an affair, and that familiar figures are imposters (Lesser & Hughes, 2006; Reisberg et al., 1987). Delusions fluctuate and are usually not systemized. Hallucinations are more frequently visual than auditory (Finkel, Burns, & Cohen, 2000).

In a review of 55 studies looking at psychosis in dementia, Ropacki et al. found that 41.1% of patients with AD experience psychotic symptoms at some point over the course of their disease (Ropacki & Jeste, 2005). Delusions were the most frequent psychotic symptom encountered (36%). Patients experienced hallucinations 18% of the time, and both hallucinations and delusions 7.8–20.8% of the time. Psychosis occurred less frequently in outpatient settings (prevalence 12.2–65.2%) than in inpatient settings such as hospitals, nursing homes and neurobehavioral units (prevalence of 31.2–74.1) (Ropacki & Jeste, 2005). Psychosis developed in 20–25% of the patients during the first year of diagnosis and in 32.5–36.1% over a 2-year period and stabilized at around 50% after the third year (Paulsen et al., 2000; Ropacki & Jeste, 2005). Once developed, psychotic symptoms persist for several months, decrease in intensity after a year and rarely persist for more than 2 years. They are associated with a greater decline in cognitive function and a high rate of extrapyramidal symptoms (Ropacki & Jeste, 2005; Stern et al., 1994).

Psychosis occurs more frequently in African Americans and those with greater severity of cognitive deficit. However, no clear association was elicited with other risk factors such as age, age at onset of AD, duration of AD, education, gender or family history of dementia or psychiatric illness (Ropacki & Jeste, 2005).

9.6.2 Pathophysiology

Based on clinical differences, psychosis in the context of dementia seems to be distinct from schizophrenia. Several studies have attempted to elucidate a neuropathological theory of psychosis in dementia, but inconsistencies predominate (Bondareff, 1996). Increased neurodegenerative changes in the cortex (but not in the aminergic nuclei), increased subcortical norepinephrine, and reduced cortical and subcortical serotonin/5-HIAA have been found in patients with dementia who had associated psychosis (Zubenko et al., 1991). Those patients also have four to five times higher levels of abnormal paired helical filament-tau protein in the entorhinal and temporal cortices (Mukaetova-Ladinska, Harrington, Xuereb, Roth, & Wischik, 1995).

Several findings implicate the frontal lobe. For example, on neuropsychological testing, the frontal lobe and executive functions were more impaired in patients with psychosis than in those without (Schneider & Dagerman, 2004). Advances in neuroimaging further suggest involvement of frontal-lobe dysfunction in development of psychotic symptoms in AD. On a florodeoxyglucose study, a decreased metabolism in the right superior dorsal lateral cortex and the anterior cingulated appeared to be associated with the presence of delusions (Schneider & Dagerman), whereas the severity of the delusions was related to hypometabolism in the right inferior frontal pole and orbital frontal areas (Sultzer et al., 2003). Psychotic symptoms, especially delusions, are more frequently seen in patients in more severe stages of dementia, which led Lesser et al. to see their development as an intrinsic part of the dementia (Aalten et al., 2008; Lesser & Hughes, 2006).

9.6.3 Clinical Care

9.6.3.1 Assessment

No specific criteria have been established for the diagnosis of psychosis in the context of dementia as a separate entity. Some authors have proposed criteria (Jeste, Sanford, & Finkel, 2000), but they have not been officially recommended. As a general rule, patients who present with psychotic symptoms should first undergo a thorough medical and neurological evaluation to rule out a possible underlying medical illness (Madhusoodanan, Shah, Brenner, & Gupta, 2007). Specific attention should be geared towards delirium, as many psychotic symptoms occur in that context. The psychiatric status of the patient should also be assessed and a previous psychiatric diagnosis such as schizophrenia ruled out. Once all other causes of psychosis are ruled out, the patient is considered to have psychosis of AD. The BEHAVE-AD (Reisberg et al., 1987) and the NPI are standardized rating scales that can be used to target and evaluate the severity of psychotic symptoms (Madhusoodanan et al., 2007). The BEHAVE-AD is a 25-item scale administered to the caregiver that measures behavioral disturbances. Symptoms are grouped in seven categories and rated from 0 to 3, depending on severity. The seven categories are as follows: paranoid and delusional ideation, hallucinations, activity disturbances such as wandering, aggressiveness, diurnal rhythm disturbances, affective disturbances and anxieties and phobias (Harwood, Ownby, & Barker, 1998). The BEHAVE-AD has good validity (Sclan et al., 1996) and inter-rater reliability (Mack & Patterson, 1994). The NPI (Cummings et al., 1994) can also be used in the assessment of psychosis, as it targets hallucinations and delusions among other neuropsychiatric disturbances. Another instrument is the Dementia Psychosis Scale, an 18-item scale rated with the caregiver to quantify the severity and types of delusions (Rayner, O'Brien, & Schoenbachier, 2006).

9.6.3.2 Evidence-Based Treatment (Brief and Intensive Approaches)

Nonpharmacological Treatment

Behavioral and environmental interventions, including redirection and reassurance, are recommended as first-line treatment for psychotic symptoms that do not cause significant danger or distress. Such interventions can also be important adjuncts to psychopharmacological therapy (Rabins et al., 2007; Rayner et al., 2006).

A large RCT stressing nonpharmacological management in older adults with AD demonstrated the effectiveness of collaborative care in reducing behavioral symptoms, reflected by significant improvements in NPI scores (Callahan al., 2006). This collaborative-care intervention included caregiver instructions and handouts about AD and ways to seek legal advice for financial and end-of-life issues, as well as a protocol to address hallucinations and delusions; the protocol entailed using reassuring touch; keeping familiar objects around; establishing a daily routine; having adequate light to reduce shadows; giving noncommittal answers; attempting to distract the patient; and avoiding direct confrontation, arguments, reasoning or rationalization and changes in surroundings (Callahan et al.). Arguing with a patient who is experiencing psychotic symptoms will lead to further agitation and aggression; the caregiver might want to consider showing understanding and validating the patient's perception. Patients with dementia are likely to have sensory deficits; and environmental objects such as mirrors, stuffed animals and dolls can easily provoke illusions and worsen delusions and hallucinations. Distracting patients with simple activities such as walking or eating and reassuring them that they are safe and that doors and windows are locked to prevent intrusions can help address paranoia (Lesser & Hughes, 2006). One should keep in mind that the improvement in behavioral symptoms reported after using collaborative care was based on improvements of the total NPI scores, which include several neuropsychiatric disturbances in addition to psychotic disturbances (Callahan et al., 2006). Studies focusing on improvement of specific psychosis scores are still needed to permit conclusions about the use of nonpharmacological techniques in treating the psychosis of dementia (Madhusoodanan et al., 2007).

Pharmacological Treatment

The APA recommends treating psychotic symptoms with nonpharmacological measures when they are not associated with agitation and/or aggression and when they do not cause significant distress to the patient. However, it supports the addition of low doses of antipsychotic medications when severe distress occurs and/or there is concern about the safety of patients or caregivers (Rabins et al., 2007). A great deal of caution is indicated when starting these medications. Increased mortality rates of 1.6–1.7 greater odds, particularly from cerebrovascular events, has now been well documented in a large meta-analysis of randomized clinical trials (Schneider, Dagerman, & Insel, 2005). The FDA conducted an assessment reviewing several studies; and results suggested that causes of death are variable, with most cases being cardiovascular or infectious in nature. No differences in mortality between different drugs were noted (Stone, 2005). Research suggests that the rate of cerebrovascular events varies from 1.3 to 4% and is related to the presence of vascular dementia and older age (Greenspan, Eerdekens, & Mahmoud, 2004). Although the mechanism of action is still unknown, several hypotheses have been postulated, including the possibility of incriminating metabolic effects, serotoninergic effect on vessels, increased platelet aggregation and increased thrombosis and orthostasis via action on $alpha_1$-adrenergic receptors (Madhusoodanan et al., 2007).

These results led the FDA in April 2005 to mandate a black-box warning about increased risk of death and cerebrovascular events in elderly patients with dementia who are taking conventional or atypical antipsychotics. The American Association of Geriatric Psychiatry issued a letter to healthcare professionals in which it stated that the black-box warning should not preclude professionals from prescribing antipsychotics when needed, as they have been proven to be efficacious in treating the behavioral aspects of dementia. However, they strongly emphasized the importance of discussing potential side-effects, including increased mortality and cerebrovascular events, with patients and caregivers and including an informed consent in the chart (American Association for Geriatric Psychiatry, 2005).

The multicenter, double-blind, placebo-controlled Clinical Antipsychotics Trials of Intervention Effectiveness in Patients with AD, which assessed the efficacy of atypical antipsychotics in outpatients with AD, further suggests that the risk of adverse effects may outweigh the benefits. The discontinuation rate for any reason was not different among treatments and placebo, but the discontinuation rate because of lack of efficacy was lower with olanzapine and risperidone than with placebo (Sultzer et al., 2008). When it is decided to initiate treatment, the choice of medication should be individualized (Shub & Kunik, 2009). Special attention should be directed to patients with dementia with Lewy bodies, as patients with this type of dementia are very sensitive to extrapyramidal side-effects (Shub & Kunik), and cholinesterase inhibitors have been shown to improve hallucinations (Weintraub & Hurtig, 2007). Typical antipsychotics were found to be more effective than placebo in treating psychosis in dementia in a meta-analysis of controlled trials (Lanctot et al., 1998; Schneider, Pollack, & Lyness, 1990), but they have many serious side-effects that make them less desirable in an elderly population. Some of these include extrapyramidal symptoms, Tardive dyskinesia, and anticholinergic and cardiovascular side-effects (Madhusoodanan et al., 2007).

Among the atypical antipsychotics no agent has been approved by the FDA for the treatment of psychosis in dementia (Alexopoulos et al., 2005), but a Cochrane Collaboration review of placebo-controlled trials concluded that risperidone and olanzapine may improve aggression more than placebo and that risperidone may improve psychosis relative to placebo (Ballard, 2006). Atypical antipsychotics tend to have fewer side-effects than typical antipsychotics and have the least drug-drug interaction among the psychotropics, which is an important consideration in a population in which polypharmacy is very common (Madhusoodanan et al., 2007).

Clozapine and ziprazidone have not been studied in AD (Madhusoodanan et al., 2007). An alternative to antipsychotic medications includes SSRIs. Data suggest that in AD serotoninergic deficits may contribute to depression and also to psychosis and aggression (Pollock et al., 2002). One short-term, randomized, double-blind, placebo-controlled study demonstrated that citalopram was more effective in diminishing psychosis and agitation than either placebo or pherphenazine (Pollock et al.). Mood stabilizers have not been proven to be beneficial in treating psychotic symptoms in patients with dementia, and there are very limited data on the use of cholinesterase inhibitors for psychotic problems in dementia patients (Shub & Kunik, 2009).

9.7 Anxiety Disorders

Anxiety is more common in individuals with dementia than in individuals without dementia (Bungener, Jouvent, & Derouesne, 1996; Hwang, Masterman, Ortiz, Fairbanks, & Cummings, 2004; Lyketsos et al., 2000; Porter et al., 2003; Wands et al., 1990), and it is associated with worse quality of life (QoL), problem behaviors, limitations in activities of daily living, nighttime awakenings and poorer neuropsychological performance, even after controlling for depression (Hoe, Hancock, Livingston, & Orrell, 2006; McCurry, Logsdon, Vitiello, & Teri, 2004; Starkstein, Jorge, Petracca, & Robinson, 2007; Teri et al., 1999). Anxiety in dementia has also been associated with future nursing-home placement, suggesting that it represents a particularly burdensome problem for caregivers (Gibbons, Teri, & Logsdon, 2002). Much of the literature on anxiety in dementia has focused on clinically significant anxiety, and little has focused on anxiety disorders.

9.7.1 Epidemiology

Anxiety is very common in the dementia population, with prevalence estimates ranging from 5 to 21% for anxiety disorders and from 8 to 71% for anxiety symptoms (Seignourel, Kunik, Snow, Wilson, & Stanley, 2008). A prospective study looking at the prevalence of anxiety upon referral to nursing homes found anxiety to be present in 41.6% of cases (Bakker, Duivenvoorden, van der Lee, & Trijsburg, 2005). The prevalence of anxiety ranged from 7 to 69% in a nursing-home population (Zuidema, Koopmans, & Verhey, 2007), which is comparable to the prevalence reported in the outpatient population. After reviewing the literature, Kunik et al. suggested that anxiety is relatively stable across the range of dementia severity, until the profound/terminal stage, when it decreases (Seignourel et al., 2008) and that individuals with retained insight experience greater anxiety.

9.7.2 Pathophysiology

Little is known about the pathophysiology of anxiety in dementia. Several hypotheses have been proposed, but no definite conclusion has been reached. The association found in several studies between awareness of cognitive deficits and anxiety in dementia raises interesting possibilities. First, being aware of one's cognitive decline may generate anxiety (Aalten, van Valen, Clare, Kenny, & Verhey, 2005). Second, both awareness of deficits and anxiety may be related to preserved expressive language abilities. On the other hand, it is still unclear whether anxiety in dementia can be considered a separate clinical entity or whether it is part of a broader syndrome. The literature has mostly looked at the relationship of anxiety in dementia with depression and agitation. Some authors have suggested that there is strong overlap between anxiety and agitation (Yesavage & Taylor, 1991) and that perhaps agitation may be a symptom of generalized anxiety (Mintzer & Brawman-Mintzer, 1996). To determine whether anxiety is distinct from other neuropsychiatric symptoms in dementia, Seignourel et al. reviewed factor analyses pertaining to this question. They concluded, after reviewing six studies, that existing evidence provides more support for the distinctiveness of anxiety and agitation than for their equivalence (Seignourel et al., 2008).

Another possibility suggested by the literature is that anxiety is confounded with depression in individuals with dementia. In dementia, between 68% and 75% of individuals with dementia and generalized anxiety disorder (GAD) also meet criteria for a major depressive disorder (Ferretti, McCurry, Logsdon, Gibbons, & Teri, 2001; Starkstein et al., 2007), and GAD is associated with greater depressive symptoms in AD (Chemerinski, Petracca, Manes, Leiguarda, & Starkstein, 1998). After reviewing the literature, Seignourel et al. concluded that the bulk of the evidence suggests that depression and anxiety are highly comorbid in individuals with dementia but could not comment further on whether they form distinct constructs, as existing studies provide conflicting evidence, and no study to date has focused specifically on this question (Seignourel et al., 2008).

From a neurobiological perspective, very few studies have been conducted to evaluate the structural changes associated with anxiety in dementia. Some research has shown that the dorsolateral region of the prefrontal cortex, which mediates several cognitive processes, especially executive functions, appears to be hyperactive in patients with GAD (Mathew et al., 2004). A reduction in the volume of the amygdala, which is part of the fear and stress neurocircuitry, might also be a major component of chronic distress in dementia patients (Wilson, Arnold, Schneider, & Bennett, 2007). Neurochemical imbalance is also implicated in development of GAD in patients with dementia. For example, on the basis of animal studies, researchers have found that serotonergic dysfunction in the hippocampal and frontal region is associated with GAD (Graeff, Guimaraes, De Andrade, & Deakin, 1996). Furthermore, the reduction of cholinergic pathways to the hippocampus in AD probably reduces the brain's capacity to handle anxiety and also contributes to excessive distress in dementia patients (Beaudreau & O'Hara, 2008). This might have a therapeutic implication, as it has been shown that isolated activation of the cholinergic pathways to the hippocampus has reduced anxiety (Millan, 2003). Genetic susceptibility such as presence of the short allele of 5HTTLPR and APOE e4 might contribute to the development of anxiety and other comorbid neuropsychiatric symptoms in the context of dementia over time, but this hypothesis still needs further exploration and confirmation (Beaudreau & O'Hara, 2008).

9.7.3 Clinical Care

9.7.3.1 Assessment

Due to the symptom overlap between anxiety and dementia, it can be difficult to define anxiety in dementia. Common symptoms include restlessness, being easily fatigued and having difficulty concentrating, all of which can occur in dementia without the presence of an anxiety disorder. Unfortunately, the hallmark of GAD, excessive anxiety or worry that is difficult to control, cannot always be assessed reliably in individuals with dementia, particularly those with expressive or receptive language difficulties. Defining anxiety based solely on behavioral observations or caregiver report may be insufficient. On the basis of these difficulties, Seignourel et al. suggested a few criteria that would help when evaluating anxiety in the context of dementia. They first recommended that it be assessed independently because it is still unclear whether anxiety is part of a broader syndrome (agitation or depression) in the dementia population. Second, they recommended that instruments should focus on symptoms of anxiety that are less likely to be affected by the presence of dementia. Concentration difficulties, in particular, are not likely to discriminate well between anxious and nonanxious individuals with dementia (Starkstein et al., 2007). Third, instruments should, whenever possible, be scored based on information from multiple sources, including at least the patient him- or herself and a caregiver. Finally, instruments should have strong psychometric properties, i.e., reliability, validity and sensitivity to change (Seignourel et al., 2008).

Modified criteria for GAD have been suggested (Starkstein et al., 2007), although they probably require expert consensus for greater validity and wide adoption. The revised criteria for GAD in individuals with dementia consist of (a) excessive anxiety/worry that is difficult to control (criteria A and B of the *DSM-IV*); and (b) three of the following five symptoms: restlessness, irritability, muscle tension, fears and respiratory symptoms, which were found to independently predict GAD diagnosis.

Four instruments have been widely used to assess anxiety in patients with dementia. The NPI (Cummings et al., 1994) comprises ten domains, with a later version adding two additional domains (Cummings, 1997) including an anxiety scale. Symptoms are assessed for the last 30 days, and the NPI is scored based on an interview with a caregiver. In an attempt to differentiate symptoms specific to anxiety from those that can commonly occur in pure dementia, the NPI assesses specific somatic symptoms (e.g., butterflies in stomach) in addition to anxiety and fears. Good interrater reliabilities have been reported for the anxiety domain for frequency (93.6% agreement) and severity (100% agreement), and test-retest reliabilities range from 0.64 to 0.71 (Cummings et al., 1994; Fuh, Liu, Meg, Wang, & Cummings, 2001). Large correlations have been reported between the anxiety domains of the NPI and the BEHAVE-AD, but they provide little information about construct validity because the rate of overall neuropsychiatric symptoms was not controlled. A shorter, self-administered version of the NPI (NPI-Q) has been developed (Kaufer et al., 2000) and the anxiety domains are highly correlated (0.82–0.84) with those of the original NPI. Researchers also developed the Caregiver-Administered NPI (Kang et al., 2004), which contains all the original items of the NPI. Administered by the caregiver, it also is highly correlated with the original NPI on prevalence ($\kappa=0.62$), frequency ($r=0.69$), severity ($r=0.64$) and caregiver burden ($r=0.61$) of anxiety.

The BEHAVE-AD (Reisberg, Auer, & Monteiro, 1996; Reisberg et al., 1987) is a caregiver interview comprising seven domains. The anxiety domain includes four items: anxiety regarding upcoming events, other anxieties, fear of being left alone, and other phobias. Thus, rather than inquiring about specific symptoms (e.g., sweating), the BEHAVE-AD asks the caregiver to make broad judgments about the presence of anxieties and fears, which shifts the responsibility of defining anxiety and distinguishing between symptoms of anxiety and symptoms of dementia to the caregiver. The anxiety score is obtained by adding the individual scores from each item. Estimates of interrater reliability have ranged from good (0.60) to excellent (0.89) across studies (Patterson et al., 1990; Sclan et al., 1996). Construct validity has not been fully examined, and information about differential relationships with other neuropsychiatric symptoms is not available.

The Worry scale (LaBarge, 1993) and the Rating for Anxiety in Dementia (RAID) (Shankar, Walker, & Frost, 1999) have been designed specifically to assess anxiety or worry in dementia. The Worry Scale (LaBarge, 1993), a self-report measure for use in individuals with mild dementia, has good internal consistency ($\alpha=0.85$) and correlates strongly with measures of trait and state anxiety (0.55 for both). However, it also correlates strongly with measures of depression (0.66) and moderately with measures of state and trait anger (0.32 and 0.31, respectively). Moreover, an examination of scale items reveals that they cover a wide range of coping and emotional responses to dementia, including anger ("I feel resentful and angry"), embarrassment ("I feel embarrassed"), and confidence in one's abilities ("I can handle changes in my life as they come"). By inquiring mostly about subjective emotional states, it is likely to minimize overlap with dementia symptoms. Because it relies solely on self-report, it can be used only with individuals with mild dementia, which limits its usefulness. Such an approach also ignores difficulties related to lack of insight, which is common in dementia, even in the mild stage (Derouesné et al., 1999; Zanetti, Vallotti, & Frisoni, 1999). The Worry Scale also correlates as strongly with measures of depression as it does with measures of anxiety (Gibbons, Teri, Logsdon, & McCurry, 2006), which raises questions about its discriminant validity. The Worry Scale also correlates strongly with measures of state and trait anger, and individual items cover a wide range of coping and emotional responses to dementia.

The RAID (Shankar et al., 1999) includes 20 items, each scored on a 4-point scale. Several items inquire about worry (worry about physical health, finances, etc.), while others include sleep disturbance, irritability, and a number of somatic symptoms (palpitations, dry mouth, shortness of breath), which could overlap with other medical or psychiatric conditions. The last two items, which are not included in the total score, inquire about phobias and panic attacks. Information is gathered about the patient's symptoms over the past 2 weeks from all available sources, including the patient, the caregiver, clinical observations and medical records, which is an advantage when compared with other instruments in use, which use only one source of information each. A total score is obtained by adding scores for the first 18 items. Scale items show fair-to-excellent interrater and test-retest reliability, and the scale has satisfactory internal consistency (α=0.83). Moreover, RAID scores are higher for patients whose symptoms meet *DSM-IV* criteria for GAD, and a cutoff score of 11 provides a sensitivity of 0.90 and a specificity of 0.79 (Shankar et al., 1999). Because these findings are based on a single study (Shankar et al.) with a relatively small sample size (N=83), they should be interpreted cautiously. The RAID correlates with some but not all measures of anxiety, with correlations ranging from 0.16 to 0.62 (Gibbons et al., 2006; Shankar et al., 1999). Its correlation with the CSDD (Alexopoulos et al., 1988) is of a similar magnitude or even higher, ranging from 0.66 to 0.69 (Gibbons et al., 2006; Shankar et al., 1999). The substantial correlation between the RAID and the CSDD may be due to poor validity of one or both measures, symptom overlap and/or co-morbidity (Gibbons et al., 2006). Thus, none of the existing instruments is entirely adequate, particularly as it pertains to convergent and divergent validity; but three instruments (the NPI, BEHAVE-AD and RAID) have some preliminary support. The NPI or, alternatively, the BEHAVE-AD, can be used to assess neuropsychiatric symptoms in general, including anxiety. For studies for which anxiety is a primary focus, Seignourel et al. concluded that the RAID, although imperfect, has the best support at this point (Seignourel et al., 2008).

9.7.3.2 Evidence-Based Treatment (Brief and Intensive Approaches)

Nonpharmacological Treatments

Very little is known about the treatment of anxiety in patients with dementia, and no randomized controlled studies have been conducted so far. Existing data are very sparse and suggest that behavioral and environmental approaches might be beneficial (Seignourel et al., 2008). Two case reports have shown CBT to be effective in reducing anxiety and depression in patients with dementia (Koder, 1998; Teri & Gallagher-Thompson, 1991). The nature of dementia and cognitive impairment makes it particularly challenging to apply CBT to older individuals who might have difficulties comprehending and applying the instructions/homework, and clinicians might have to rely greatly on caregivers (Kraus et al., 2008). A recent case study looked at results of two patients treated with a version of CBT especially modified for anxiety in dementia (CBT-AD). In this study, efforts were made to facilitate learning by simplifying the skills usually used, such as education and awareness treatment, diaphragmatic breathing, coping self-statements and behavioral activation. In an attempt to improve understanding, patients were actively involved, repeating the information given and helping in creating their own reminder cues (e.g., reminder cards, calendars). Caregivers were present in the sessions to learn the procedure so they could act as "coaches" to patients between sessions as needed.

Spaced retrieval was used to enhance encoding and retrieval. This evidence-based method was chosen because it is a function of procedural memory, which is relatively preserved in later stages of dementia. It has also been successful in teaching patients with dementia to engage in occupational therapy and to remember the way to their room (Bourgeois et al., 2003; Camp, 2006). It entails progressively increasing the intervals of time between questions every time the patient gives the right answer to the question and going back to the previous interval of time whenever the patient gives a wrong answer. Another advantage of spaced retrieval is that caregivers were able to use it with good results (Arkin, 1991; McKitrick, Camp, & Black, 1992). Each CBT-AD session was limited to 30–40 min and to one to two skills. The clinician would also give concrete and simplified instruction for the homework. Baseline anxiety levels were assessed, using the RAID and the NPI. After completion of treatment, both patients had significantly reduced anxiety, as measured with the RAID (19 pretreatment and 10 post-treatment for patient A and 12 pretreatment and 8 post-treatment for patient B) and the NPI (no change for patient A but a decrease in 7 points for patient B [8 pre vs. 1 post]); and both deep breathing and increasing activity might have been particularly useful. This study suggests that modified CBT is a potentially promising treatment for anxiety in dementia. The authors are still working on further modifications, but more studies and a broader application as well as RCTs are needed before reaching definite conclusions (Kraus et al., 2008). Other nondrug interventions that show promising results in case series or small pilot studies include milieu therapy, addressing patients' specific environmental needs, and caregiver psychoeducation (Haupt, Karger, & Janner, 2000; Qazi, Shankar, & Orrell, 2003). Milieu therapy is a form of psychotherapy that encourages the patient, while in the "milieu" or residential environment, including peers and staff members, to actively participate in group psychotherapy and structured practical activities and to take responsibility for him/herself and others (Dulcan, 1994).

Pharmacological Treatment

Although pharmacological interventions are most frequently used (Wetherell, Gatz, & Craske, 2003), no randomized clinical trials have evaluated the use of medication for treating anxiety disorders in persons with dementia. Thus, drug therapy must be used cautiously. Among the different options, SSRIs may be useful. A small prospective controlled study showed citalopram to be superior to placebo for elderly but cognitively intact patients with GAD (Lenze et al., 2005). The high co-morbidity of depression with anxiety in dementia patients may further justify a trial of an SSRI (Shub & Kunik, 2009). However in older individuals with potential polypharmacy, we should be very cautious not to combine serotoninergic drugs to prevent development of the serotonin syndrome, which is highly dangerous and includes delirium, autonomic instability and increased neuromuscular activity (Kalapatapu & Neugroschl, 2009). Benzodiazepines may have an unacceptably high risk of cognitive adverse effects and falls in patients with dementia.

9.8 Sleep Disorders

Insomnia is an important problem in older adults. In addition to sleep changes that normally occur with aging, the neurodegenerative changes of dementia further compound the problem by increasing the frequency and severity of sleep disturbances and associated behavioral disruptions (Shub, Darvishi, & Kunik, 2009). Sleep disturbances can be a significant contributor to caregiver burden, and they are often a reason caregivers cite for their decision to institutionalize (Pollak & Perlick, 1991). Chronic insomnia in older patients is also an independent predictor of cognitive decline, falls, and increased 2-year mortality (Brassington, King, & Bliwise, 2000; Cricco, Simonsick, & Foley, 2001; Manabe et al., 2000).

9.8.1 Epidemiology

A community-residing, population-based study of individuals with AD suggests that 35% of subjects are affected by sleep disturbances (McCurry et al., 1999). Patients with more severe dementia have increased sleep disturbances (Lyketsos, Lindell Veiel, et al., 1999). Patients in nursing home have poorer sleep quality, more disturbed sleep onset, more advanced sleep-wake cycles, and higher use of sedative-hypnotics than those in the community (Colenda, Cohen, McCall, & Rosenquist, 1997). In a population-based sample of AD patients, the most common sleep-related behavior problems reported by caregivers were sleeping more than usual (40%) and awakening early (31%), whereas being awakened at night (24%) was the most distressing problem for caregivers (McCurry et al., 1999; Shub et al., 2009).

9.8.2 Pathophysiology

In patients with dementia, sleep disturbances are multifactorial (Deschenes & McCurry, 2009). Sleep architecture changes normally with aging, and the changes are accentuated in dementia (Shub et al., 2009). Patients spend less time in stages 3 and 4 (slow-wave sleep), in rapid-eye-movement (REM) sleep and in total sleep time but spend more time in stages 1 and 2 (light sleep) (Ancoli-Israel, 2000; Vitiello & Borson, 2001). These changes in sleep structure manifest in increased sleep fragmentation and arousals, with resultant excessive daytime sleepiness and napping. Damage of neuronal pathways in the suprachiasmatic nucleus of the hypothalamus, the area believed to initiate and maintain sleep as well as changes in the circadian rhythm, may further disrupt sleep in persons with dementia and lead to shifts or complete day/night sleep-pattern reversals (Vitiello & Borson). Primary sleep disorders such as sleep apnea and restless leg syndrome can also exacerbate sleep disturbances in patients with dementia. The side-effects of some medications used to treat the cognitive and behavioral co-morbidities of dementia should be monitored (Deschenes & McCurry, 2009). For example, olanzapine and risperdal can cause daytime sleepiness, whereas acetylcholinesterase inhibitors such as donepezil have been found to be associated with dream disturbances (Dauvilliers, 2007) and night-time stimulation. Patients with dementia often have age-related medical co-morbidities that can affect sleep, such as diabetes, ischemic heart disease, pulmonary disorders, and renal failure (National Institutes of Health, 2005).

Chronic pain syndromes, including arthritis, also interfere with sleep. Lack of sleep decreases the pain threshold, which will exacerbate pain, as well as insomnia (Blay, Andreoli, & Gastal, 2007). Medications used to treat pain are often sedating and increase daytime napping. Depression and anxiety are frequent psychiatric comorbid conditions in patients with dementia, are well known to cause sleep disturbances and, in return, worsen with lack of sleep (Cole & Dendukuri, 2003). Although psychotropic medications used to treat them can improve insomnia, they can also decrease the quality of sleep in patients with untreated obstructive sleep apnea (Smith, Dingwall, Jorgenson, & Douglas, 2006), and they have several serious side-effects, such as daytime sleepiness and increased risk for falls in adults with cognitive impairment.

Sleep can also be affected by environmental factors, such as noise, excessive light exposure at night, poor sleep hygiene and uncomfortable bedding (Deschenes & McCurry, 2009). In clinical practice, a combination of these factors can be found in patients with dementia suffering from sleep disturbances (McCurry, Reynolds, Ancoli-Israel, Teri, & Vitiello, 2000).

Patients with Lewy's body dementia also experience prolonged sleep latency, increased sleep fragmentation, nightmares, and increases in early-morning awakenings. Sleep disturbances are very frequent in this subpopulation (Bhatt, Podder, & Chokroverty, 2005; Dauvilliers, 2007); and some, such as REM-sleep behavior disorder, can be dangerous for patients. In REM-sleep behavior disorder, as a consequence of the disruption of normal-sleep paralytic mechanisms, patients physically act out their dreams, usually in the second half of the night (Boeve, Silber, & Ferman, 2004). Most of the time patients do not remember the behaviors upon awakening; but the behaviors can be very violent, causing harm to patients or their bed partners. One should also keep in mind that the extrapyramidal symptoms associated with Lewy's body dementia and the medications prescribed to these patients are additional factors causing sleep disturbance. For example, persistent movements and muscle stiffness make it more difficult to initiate and maintain sleep. Dopamine agonists have nighttime stimulating effects and can cause sudden daytime sleep attacks that can be very dangerous for the patient's physical safety (Dauvilliers, 2007), whereas levodopa reduces REM sleep while increasing REM sleep latency.

9.8.3 Clinical Care

9.8.3.1 Assessment

Clinical assessment of individuals with insomnia must always include screening for secondary causes, including medical (e.g., heart failure, nycturia) and psychiatric conditions (e.g., depression, anxiety) and medication side-effects, as well as specific sleep disorders. Objective baseline measure of the patient's sleep disturbance may be helpful in identifying specific target areas and gauging the efficacy of a proposed intervention. Because performing a sleep study with polysomnography is impractical and self-report is unreliable in this patient population, a sleep diary filled out by the caregiver is often the best alternative (Shub et al., 2009). The diary can include bedtime and rising time, frequency and duration of daytime naps, use of sleep medications, frequency and duration of sleep disturbances and subjective sleep-quality ratings (McCurry et al., 2005).

For research purposes, wrist-movement recorders are used; but their use might not be practical for clinical practice. They are matchbox-sized devices worn on the wrist that use software to score sleep/wake time after incorporating maximum activity measures and daily levels of light exposure (McCurry et al., 2005). Standardized ratings of sleep include the Pittsburgh Sleep Quality Index (Buysse, Reynolds, Monk, Berman, & Kupfer, 1989), a 19-item instrument that indicates poor sleep with scores of 5 or greater, as well as the Epworth Sleepiness Scale (Johns, 1991), an eight-item scale that rates daytime sleepiness when scores are higher than 16. As mentioned previously, it might be more accurate for caregivers to complete these scales (McCurry et al., 2005).

9.8.3.2 Evidence-Based Treatment (Brief and Intensive Approaches)

Nonpharmacological Treatment

Although there are little data, clinical experience suggests that it is prudent to consider nonpharmacologic treatments as a first-line intervention when initial evaluation fails to identify another medical or psychiatric condition as the cause of insomnia (Rabins et al., 2007; Shub et al., 2009).

Light Therapy

Exposure to light of sufficient intensity and duration can have marked effects on an individual's mood and sleep. Bright-light therapy has a proven indication for treatment of winter depression, or seasonal affective disorders (McCurry et al., 2005), and is also one of the most widely studied nonpharmacologic interventions for sleep and behavioral symptoms in dementia patients (Shub et al., 2009). Light exposure is usually best in the mornings and evenings to be in concordance with the human photoperiod. Patients who suffer from sleep-maintenance problems or those who awake very early in the morning because they fall asleep early in the evening benefit from exposure to light in the evening, whereas exposure in the morning is more helpful to patients whose sleep onset and morning rising are delayed (Deschenes & McCurry, 2009). NITE-AD, the first clinical trial to date funded by the National Institute of Mental Health to have examined the efficacy of nonpharmacologic therapies for treating sleep disturbances in community-dwelling patients with AD (McCurry et al., 2005), demonstrated significant, 32% reductions from baseline in nighttime awakenings and total time awake at night compared with control subjects who worsened on both measures (McCurry et al., 2005; Shub et al., 2009). Patients and caregivers found this treatment feasible, with high compliance with the daily light-box recommendation during two 3-week active-treatment periods and at 6-month follow-up (Shub et al.).

Providers must, however, overcome several challenges in recommending and implementing home-based light treatment. First, light therapy requires a light source of sufficient luminosity to affect circadian phase-shift. Although there is currently not a gold standard for intensity of light exposure, its frequency, duration or best modality of delivery (Deschenes & McCurry, 2009), most studies expose patients to 1,000–10,000 lux for 30–90 min, far greater than can be achieved with ordinary home lighting. Thus, it is necessary to purchase specialized light equipment, i.e., a "light box." Readily available from online retailers, the cost of a light box ranges from around $130 for a small lamp to $300 for the unit used in the NITE-AD study. Although this may seem prohibitive to some patients and caregivers, it is comparable to costs of pharmacologic treatment, given that a month's supply of zolpidem (Ambien) costs $130 (Shub et al., 2009).

Another potential limitation is that a demented patient may not be able to understand and follow instructions for light-therapy treatment. A caregiver is usually necessary to ensure that the patient remains seated and faces the light source, which should be placed 2–3 ft away within a 45° visual field. It is important that the patient not sleep or nap during treatment because light must fall onto the retina to influence the circadian system. Patients can do other things during the treatment session (such as read, eat, converse or watch television – the light box can be placed on top of the television) during light-treatment sessions. Light-exposure treatment should be within 3 h before the patient's habitual bedtime, except for patients who already have extremely late bedtimes. In the NITE-AD study, patients used a light box delivering approximately 2,500 lux of full-spectrum light for 1 h each day (Shub et al., 2009). Caregivers who have difficulty ensuring at least a 30 min seated treatment time may need help in identifying and planning sedentary activities to help keep patients in position during light-therapy sessions. Resources are available from the Alzheimer's Association and the Alzheimer's Disease Education and Referral Center of the National Institute on Aging (Shub et al.). In a recent controlled trial Sloane et al. (2007) demonstrated that exposure to ceiling-mounted bright light in a nursing home, whether for 4-h intervals in the mornings and evenings or for 11 h during the day, significantly improved total nighttime sleep. A recent RCT (Riemersma-van der Lek et al., 2008) found that irritability, dizziness and headaches can be side-effects of whole day, bright light exposure but still concluded that it is safe for use in long-term care settings. If the results are replicated, this technique will likely improve adherence to light therapy.

Exercise

Physical exercise is an important component of nonpharmacologic therapy for sleep disturbances. PCP clearance on the patient's physical condition and tolerance for exercise is prudent, especially for elderly patients with dementia, as well as those with several medical co-morbidities.

A home-based exercise program combined with behavioral management can, in addition to the benefit of phase shifting of circadian rhythms (Baehr et al., 2003; King, Oman, Brassington, Bliwise, & Haskell, 1979) and improving quality of sleep, reduce functional dependence, improve physical health and depression, and delay institutionalization among patients with AD, according to evidence from an RCT (McCurry et al., 2005; Teri et al., 2003).

A supervised exercise program is feasible for community-dwelling individuals. Most persons with dementia could walk for 30 or more min per day in one study (McCurry et al., 2005). Several other exercise protocols have been used in clinical trials for patients with dementia. These range from walking to more comprehensive programs, including aerobic/endurance activities, strength training, balance, and flexibility training. The main challenge to implementing these, as with all behavioral interventions, is the time required of the caregiver. Nevertheless, a primary care clinic can be an ideal setting for encouraging patients to increase their physical activity level. Tailored exercise prescriptions delivered in the primary care practice setting have been shown to improve physical fitness and exercise adherence in older (age>65 years), community-dwelling adults (Petrella, Koval, Cunningham, & Paterson, 2003). Patients with dementia and their caregivers should be instructed to walk for exercise daily for 30 min, preferably outside in natural light, weather permitting (McCurry et al., 2005). Frail patients can start with shorter walking intervals and gradually build up over time (Shub et al., 2009). Information regarding exercise safety, as well as sample endurance, strength, balance, and stretching exercises, is available in the Exercise Guide distributed by the National Institute on Aging. PCPs can encourage patients to try a new exercise from the guide every day (Shub et al.).

Sleep Hygiene

Sleep hygiene refers to an individual's sleep habits and routines. Establishing good sleep practices is the first-line treatment for all patients with insomnia. There is now ample clinical and empirical evidence to suggest that behavioral interventions aimed at improving sleep hygiene can be helpful in treating sleep and nighttime disturbances in dementia patients (McCurry et al., 2004, 2005; McCurry, Gibbons, Logsdon, Vitiello, & Teri, 2003). The feasibility of changing sleep routines in community-dwelling dementia patients hinges on the provider's help in developing an individualized behavioral plan tailored to the caregiver's particular situation. In the NITE-AD study, compared with patients whose caregivers received only educational materials, patients whose caregivers received active assistance in setting up and implementing a sleep hygiene program were more likely to maintain a consistent bedtime (83 vs. 38%) and rising time (96 vs. 59%) schedule and were less likely to nap during the daytime (70 vs. 28%, McCurry et al., 2004). Before formulating an individualized sleep hygiene program, it is useful to screen for patients who would benefit the most from intensive behavioral intervention. Providers can begin by obtaining details on the patient's baseline sleeping habits, using either caregiver reports or, ideally, a sleep-data diary kept for at least a week (Shub et al., 2009). Patients who need to make changes in their bedtime, rising time, or daytime napping schedules are candidates for sleep-hygiene changes and should receive further instruction (McCurry et al., 2004).

Caregivers may require assistance in identifying desirable bed and rising times and in adhering to these within a 30-min leeway. They should be encouraged to limit patients' naps to 30 min or less and to eliminate naps after 1 PM altogether. Effort should also be devoted to identifying triggers for nighttime awakenings and to devising strategies for eliminating them. Common problems include nighttime noise and light and incontinence. Helpful behavioral strategies to address these are keeping sleeping areas dark, turning off the television at night, avoiding excessive fluid intake, and restricting caffeinated beverages in the evening. A more comprehensive list of educational information on sleep hygiene, including environmental, dietary, and health guidelines such as that given to all subjects participating in the NITE-AD project, can be found in McCurry et al. (2003, 2004).

The main obstacle to implementing sleep-hygiene changes in persons with dementia is the requirement for significant time and effort from caregivers, which may contribute to caregiver burden. As already alluded to, it is crucial for providers to make specific suggestions and to troubleshoot problems that arise in caregivers' attempts to change sleep and activity routines, as opposed to having them rely on written educational materials alone. For example, it could be very challenging to keep individuals from napping without a concrete plan for keeping them occupied, active, and awake during daytime. Scheduling a long walk or another type of physical activity in the afternoon might be helpful, but any plan must take into account the caregiver's ability to follow through with the recommendation; and there must be collaboration on possible alternatives (Shub et al., 2009).

Pharmacological Treatment

Pharmacological treatment should be considered only after nonpharmacological interventions have failed and after having carefully pondered potential benefits and side-effects (Rabins et al., 2007). They should be used only for a short time because little data exist on their long-term safety and use in cognitively impaired individuals (Deschenes & McCurry, 2009).

Sedative hypnotics, including benzodiazepines, are the most commonly used class of medications (Deschenes & McCurry, 2009). Benzodiazepines have several potential undesirable effects, such as tolerance, daytime somnolence, rebound insomnia, worsening cognition, falls, disinhibition, confusion and delirium. Triazolam is associated with amnesia and should therefore be avoided. Benzodiazepines affect the respiratory drive and should be used only once sleep apnea has been ruled out, given its prevalence in the dementia population. They improve sleep quality by decreasing sleep latency. They also decrease the amount of time spent in stage 2 sleep and, depending on their duration of action, they can reduce intermittent wakefulness, increasing time of total sleep (Roehrs & Roth, 2009). Nonbenzodiazepine hypnotics such as zolpidem (5–10 mg at bedtime) or zaleplon (5–10 mg at bedtime) and eszopiclone can also be used, as they have fewer side-effects, but more studies are needed (Deschenes & McCurry, 2009; Rabins et al., 2007).

If a patient has a comorbid psychiatric condition such as depression, antidepressants such as SSRIs or those with sedative side-effects (mirtazapine, trazodone) can be prescribed at bedtime to treat insomnia, especially because it is often difficult to distinguish primary sleep disturbances from those secondary to depression (Rabins et al., 2007). Trazodone is frequently prescribed, but one should keep in mind that no evidence-based data exist to support its use in the elderly (Mendelson, 2005). Antidepressants act by decreasing sleep latency and have a relatively safe side-effect profile; but they can also cause sedation, weight gain and dizziness in the elderly population (Deschenes & McCurry, 2009). The sedating effect of atypical antipsychotics can be useful if a patient also exhibits psychotic symptoms (Rabins et al., 2007).

Diphenhydramine, an antihistamine found in most over-the-counter sleep aids, should be avoided in elderly patients because of its side-effect profile, especially anticholinergic effects (Rabins et al., 2007). Products containing diphenhydramine are highly sedative and increase the rate of cognitive decline (Deschenes & McCurry, 2009). Although melatonin supplementation might be expected to promote sleep, studies have failed to prove its efficacy as a primary treatment for treating insomnia (Serfaty, Kennell-Webb, Warner, Blizard, & Raven, 2002; Singer et al., 2003). It has been found, however, to enhance the effects of light therapy (Deschenes & McCurry, 2009; Dowling et al., 2008). In 2005, the FDA approved the use of melatonin agonists for the treatment of sleep disturbances. Ramelteon acts on the MT1 and MT2 receptors and acts to shorten latency, increase total sleep time and improve sleep efficiency (Borja & Daniel, 2006). It has been approved for the long-term treatment of insomnia, as it has a favorable side-effect profile (Deschenes & McCurry, 2009).

Very few evidence-based guidelines exist to address insomnia in AD. The few existing data are encouraging for behavioral treatments such as light therapy, exercise and sleep hygiene; but more RCTs are still needed, especially to compare behavioral and pharmacological treatments. A combination of behavioral and pharmacological treatments might yield the most efficacious results (Shub et al., 2009).

9.9 Conclusion

Behavioral and/or psychological co-morbidities of dementia affect 90% of patients during the course of their illness. Not only do these co-morbidities increase the financial burden patients and caregivers face, they are also a major cause of distress and decreased QoL for both patients and caregivers and a major factor leading to patient institutionalization. More research is needed, however, to better understand differences across the different stages and subtypes of dementia. Diagnosis and treatment of psychological co-morbidities of AD are challenging. The use of standardized assessment instruments in clinical practice is helpful. Although strong evidence for many treatments is limited, a great deal of reasonable pharmacological and behavioral options exists. The general principle is to initially identify and treat reversible medical or environmental causes such as pain, physiological needs, or strained caregiver relationships. Then, whenever possible, nonpharmacological interventions should be attempted first. In many countries, healthcare professionals, patients and family members are advocating to make dementia a national priority; and hope abounds for more research in this field that would result in stronger evidence-based guidelines for the treatment of dementia in general and its behavioral and psychological co-morbidities in particular.

References

Aalten, P., van Valen, E., Clare, L., Kenny, G., & Verhey, F. (2005). Awareness in dementia: A review of clinical correlates. *Aging & Mental Health, 9*, 414–422.

Aalten, P., Verhen, F. R., Boziki, M., Brugnolo, A., Bullock, R., Byrne, E. J., et al. (2008). Consistency of neuropsychiatric syndromes across dementias: Results from the European Alzheimer Disease Consortium. *Dementia and Geriatric Cognitive Disorders, 25*, 1–8.

Agronin, M. E. (2004). *Practical guides in psychiatry: Dementia*. Philadelphia: Lippincott Williams & Wilkins.

AGS Panel on Persistent Pain in Older Persons. (2002). The management of persistent pain in older persons. *Journal of the American Geriatrics Society, 50*(6 Suppl), S205–S224.

Aguero-Torres, H., von Strauss, E., Viitanen, M., Winblad, B., & Fratiglioni, L. (2001). Institutionalization in the elderly: The role of chronic diseases and dementia. Cross-sectional and longitudinal data from a population-based study. *Journal of Clinical Epidemiology, 54*, 795–801.

Alexopoulos, G. S., Abrams, R. C., Young, R. C., & Shamoian, C. A. (1988). Cornell scale for depression in dementia. *Biological Psychiatry, 23*, 271–284.

Alexopoulos, G. S., Jeste, D. V., Chung, H., Carpenter, D., Ross, R., & Docherty, J. P. (2005). The expert consensus guideline series: Treatment of dementia and its behavioral disturbances. *Postgraduate Medicine Special Report, 2005*, 1–108.

Alzheimer's Society. (2007). *Dementia UK: The full report*. London: Alzheimer's Society.

American Association for Geriatric Psychiatry. (2005). Comment on the US Food and Drug Administration's (FDA) advisory on off-label use of atypical antipsychotics in the elderly [online]. Available from URL: http://www.aagponline.org/prof/antipsychstat_0705.asp. Accessed October 31, 2005.

American Psychiatric Association. (2000). Diagnostic and statistical manual of mental disorders (4th ed., text revision). Washington: American Psychiatric Association.

American Psychiatric Association Work Group on Alzheimer's Disease and Other Dementias. (2007). Practice guideline for the treatment of patients with Alzheimer's disease and other dementias of late life. *The American Journal of Psychiatry, 51*(3), S121–S131.

Ancoli-Israel, S. (2000). Insomnia in the elderly: A review for the primary care practitioner. *Sleep, 23*(Suppl 1), S23–S30.

Arkin, S. M. (1991). Memory training in early Alzheimer's disease: An optimistic look at the field. *American Journal of Alzheimer's Disease and Other Dementias, 6*, 17–25.

Baehr, E. K., Eastman, C. I., Revelle, W., Olson, S. H., Wolfe, L. F., & Zee, P. C. (2003). Circadian phaseshifting effects of nocturnal exercise in older compared with young adults. *American*

Journal of Physiology. Regulatory, Integrative and Comparative Physiology, 284, R1542–R1550.

Baker, R., Holloway, J., Holtkamp, C. C. M., Larson, A., Hartman, L. C., Pearce, R., et al. (2003). Effects of multi-sensory stimulation for people with dementia. *Journal of Advanced Nursing, 43*, 465–477.

Bakker, T. J. E. M., Duivenvoorden, H. J., van der Lee, J., & Trijsburg, R. W. (2005). Prevalence of psychiatric function disorders in psychogeriatric patients at referral to nursing home care – The relation to cognition, activities of daily living and general details. *Dementia and Geriatric Cognitive Disorders, 20*, 215–224.

Ballard, C. (2006). The effectiveness of atypical antipsychotics for the treatment of aggression and psychosis in Alzheimer's disease. *Cochrane Database of Systematic Reviews, 1*, 1–108.

Bass, D. M., McClendon, G., Deimling, G. T., & Mukherjee, S. (1994). The influence of diagnosed mental impairment on family caregiver strain. *Journal of Gerontology, 49*, S146–S155.

Bass, D. M., Noelker, L. S., & Rechlin, L. R. (1996). The moderating influence of service use on negative caregiving consequences. *The Journals of Gerontology, Series B, Psychological Sciences and Social Sciences, 51*, S121–S131.

Bassuk, S. S., Berkman, L. F., & Wypij, D. (1998). Depressive symptomatology and incident cognitive decline in an elderly community sample. *Archives of General Psychiatry, 55*, 1073–1081.

Beaudreau, S. A., & O'Hara, R. (2008). Late-life anxiety and cognitive impairment: A review. *The American Journal of Geriatric Psychiatry, 16*, 790–803.

Beck, C. K., Vogelpohl, T. S., Rasin, H. J., Uriri, J. T., O'Sullivan, P., Walls, R., et al. (2002). Effects of behavioral interventions on disruptive behavior and affect in demented nursing home residents. *Nursing Research, 51*, 219–228.

Benson, H., & Klipper, M. (1975). *The relaxation response*. New York: Avon Books.

Bharani, N., & Snowden, M. (2005). Evidence-based interventions for nursing home residents with dementia-related behavioral symptoms. *The Psychiatric Clinics of North America, 28*, 985–1005.

Bhatt, M. H., Podder, N., & Chokroverty, S. (2005). Sleep and neurodegenerative disorders. *Seminars in Neurology, 25*, 39–51.

Blay, S. L., Andreoli, S. B., & Gastal, F. L. (2007). Chronic painful physical conditions, disturbed sleep and psychiatric morbidity: Results from an elderly survey. *Annals of Clinical Psychiatry, 19*, 169–174.

Boeve, B. F., Silber, M. H., & Ferman, T. J. (2004). REM sleep behavior disorder in Parkinson's disease and dementia with Lewy bodies. *Journal of Geriatric Psychiatry and Neurology, 17*, 146–157.

Bondareff, W. (1996). Neuropathology of psychotic symptoms in Alzheimer's disease. *International Psychogeriatrics, 8*(Suppl 3), 233–237.

Borja, N. L., & Daniel, K. L. (2006). Ramelteon for the treatment of insomnia. *Clinical Therapeutics, 28*, 1540–1555.

Bourgeois, M. S., Camp, C., Rose, M., White, B., Malone, M., Carr, J., et al. (2003). A comparison of training strategies to enhance use of external aids by persons with dementia. *Journal of Communication Disorders, 36*, 361–378.

Boyle, P. A., & Malloy, P. F. (2004). Treating apathy in Alzheimer's disease. *Dementia and Geriatric Cognitive Disorders, 17*, 91–99.

Brassington, G. S., King, A. C., & Bliwise, D. L. (2000). Sleep problems as a risk factor for falls in a sample of community-dwelling adults aged 64–99 years. *Journal of the American Geriatrics Society, 48*, 1234–1240.

Braun, U. K., & Kunik, M. E. (2004). Behavioral disturbances in dementia: Finding the cause(s). *Geriatrics, 59*, 32–33.

Brodaty, H., & Luscombe, G. (1996). Depression in persons with dementia. *International Psychogeriatrics, 8*, 609–622.

Buettner, L. L., & Fitzsimmons, S. (2002). AD-venture program: Therapeutic biking for the treatment of depression in long-term care residents with dementia. *American Journal of Alzheimer's Disease and Other Dementias, 17*, 121–127.

Bungener, C., Jouvent, R., & Derouesne, C. (1996). Affective disturbances in Alzheimer's disease. *Journal of the American Geriatrics Society, 44*, 1066–1071.
Burns, A., & Iliffe, S. (2009). Dementia. *British Medical Journal, 338*, b75.
Burton, L. C., German, P. S., Rovner, B. W., & Brant, L. J. (1992). Physical restraint use and cognitive decline among nursing home residents. *Journal of the American Geriatrics Society, 40*, 811–816.
Buysse, D. J., Reynolds, C. F., Monk, T. H., Berman, S. R., & Kupfer, D. J. (1989). The Pittsburgh sleep quality index: A new instrument for psychiatric practice and research. *Psychiatry Research, 28*, 193–213.
Callahan, C. M., Boustani, M. A., Unverzagt, F. W., Austrom, M. G., Damush, T. M., Perkins, A. J., et al. (2006). Effectiveness of collaborative care for older adults with Alzheimer disease in primary care. *Journal of the American Medical Association, 295*, 2148–2157.
Camberg, L., Woods, P., Ooi, W. L., Hurley, A., Volicer, L., Ashley, J., et al. (1999). Evaluation of simulated presence: A personalized approach to enhance well-being in persons with Alzheimer's disease. *Journal of the American Geriatrics Society, 47*, 446–452.
Camp, C. J. (2006). Spaced retrieval: A case study in dissemination of a cognitive intervention for persons with dementia. In D. K. Attix & K. A. Welsh-Bohmer (Eds.), *Geriatric neuropsychology: Assessment and intervention* (pp. 275–292). New York: Guilford.
Chapman, S. B., Weiner, M. F., Rackley, A., Hynan, L. S., & Zientz, J. (2004). Effects of cognitive-communication stimulation for Alzheimer's disease patients treated with donepezil. *Journal of Speech, Language, and Hearing Research, 47*, 1149–1163.
Chatterjee, A., Anderson, K. E., Moskowitz, C. B., Hauser, W. A., & Marder, K. S. (2005). A comparison of self-report and caregiver assessment of depression, apathy, and irritability in Huntington's disease. *The Journal of Neuropsychiatry and Clinical Neurosciences, 17*, 378–383.
Chemerinski, E., Petracca, G., Manes, R., Leiguarda, R., & Starkstein, S. E. (1998). Prevalence and correlates of anxiety in Alzheimer's disease. *Depression and Anxiety, 7*, 166–170.
Chow, T. W., Binns, M. A., Cummings, J. L., Lam, I., Black, S. E., Miller, B. L., et al. (2009). Apathy symptom profile and behavioral associations in frontotemporal dementia vs dementia of Alzheimer type. *Archives of Neurology, 66*, 888–893.
Cohen-Mansfield, J. (2000). Theoretical frameworks for behavioral problems in dementia. *Alzheimers Care Quarterly, 1*, 8–21.
Cohen-Mansfield, J., Marx, M. S., & Rosenthal, A. S. (1989). A description of agitation in a nursing home. *Journal of Gerontology, 44*, M77–M84.
Cole, M. G., & Dendukuri, N. (2003). Risk factors for depression among elderly community subjects: A systematic review and metaanalysis. *The American Journal of Psychiatry, 160*, 1147–1156.
Colenda, C. C., Cohen, W., McCall, W. V., & Rosenquist, P. B. (1997). Phototherapy for patients with Alzheimer disease with disturbed sleep patterns: Results of a community-based pilot study. *Alzheimer Disease and Associated Disorders, 11*, 175–178.
Coon, D. W., & Evans, B. (2009). Empirically based treatments for family caregiver distress: What works and where do we go from here? *Geriatric Nursing, 30*, 426–436.
Craig, A. H., Cummings, J. L., Fairbanks, L., Itti, L., Miller, B. L., Li, J., et al. (1996). Cerebral blood flow correlates of apathy in Alzheimer disease. *Archives of Neurology, 53*, 1116–1120.
Cricco, M., Simonsick, E. M., & Foley, D. J. (2001). The impact of insomnia on cognitive functioning in older adults. *Journal of the American Geriatrics Society, 49*, 1185–1189.
Cummings, J. L. (1997). The Neuropsychiatric Inventory: Assessing psychopathology in dementia patients. *Neurology, 48*(Suppl 6), S10–S16.
Cummings, J. L. (2000). Cholinesterase inhibitors: A new class of psychotropic compounds. *The American Journal of Psychiatry, 157*, 4–15.
Cummings, J. L. (2003). Use of cholinesterase inhibitors in clinical practice: Evidence-based recommendations. *The American Journal of Geriatric Psychiatry, 11*, 131–145.
Cummings, J. L., Mega, M., Gray, K., Rosenberg-Thompson, S., Carusi, D. A., & Gornbein, J. (1994). The Neuropsychiatric Inventory: Comprehensive assessment of psychopathology in dementia. *Neurology, 44*, 2308–2314.
Dauvilliers, Y. (2007). Insomnia in patients with neurodegenerative conditions. *Sleep Medicine, 4*(Suppl 4), S27–S34.

Derouesné, C., Thibault, S., Lagha-Pierucci, S., Baudouin-Madec, V., Ancri, D., & Lacomblez, L. (1999). Decreased awareness of cognitive deficits in patients with mild dementia of the Alzheimer type. *International Journal of Geriatric Psychiatry, 14*, 1019–1103.
Deschenes, C. L., & McCurry, S. M. (2009). Current treatments for sleep disturbances in individuals with dementia. *Current Psychiatry Reports, 11*, 20–26.
Devanand, D. P., Jacobs, D. M., Tang, M. X., Del Castillo-Castaneda, C., Sano, M., Marder, K., et al. (1997). The course of psychopathologic features in mild to moderate Alzheimer disease. *Archives of General Psychiatry, 54*, 257–263.
Dowling, G. A., Burr, R. L., Van Someren, E. J., Hubbard, E. M., Luxenberg, J. S., Mastick, J., et al. (2008). Melatonin and bright-light treatment for rest-activity disruption in institutionalized patients with Alzheimer's disease. *Journal of the American Geriatrics Society, 56*, 239–246.
Dulcan, M. K. (1994). Treatment of children and adolescents. In R. E. Hales, S. C. Yudofsky, & J. A. Talbott (Eds.), *Textbook of psychiatry* (2nd ed., p. 1241). Washington: American Psychiatric Press.
Fahim, S., van Duijn, C. M., Baker, F. M., Launer, L., Breteler, M. M., Schudel, W. J., et al. (1998). A study of familial aggregation of depression, dementia and Parkinson's disease. *European Journal of Epidemiology, 14*, 233–238.
Ferretti, L., McCurry, S. M., Logsdon, R., Gibbons, L., & Teri, L. (2001). Anxiety and Alzheimer's disease. *Journal of Geriatric Psychiatry and Neurology, 14*, 52–58.
Ferri, C. P., Prince, M., Brayne, C., Brodaty, H., Fratiglioni, L., Ganguli, M., et al. (2005). Global prevalence of dementia: A Delphi consensus study. *The Lancet, 366*, 2112–2117.
Finkel, S. I., Burns, A., & Cohen, G. D. (2000). Overview, behavioral and psychological symptoms of dementia (BPSD): A clinical and research update. *International Psychogeriatrics, 12*(S1), 13–18.
Forsell, Y., Jorm, A. F., Fratiglioni, L., Grut, M., & Winblad, B. (1993). Application of DSM-III-R criteria for major depressive episode to elderly subjects with and without dementia. *The American Journal of Psychiatry, 150*, 1199–1202.
Förstl, H., Burns, A., Luthert, P., Cairns, N., Lantos, P., & Levy, R. (1992). Clinical and neuropathological correlates of depression in Alzheimer's disease. *Psychological Medicine, 22*, 877–884.
Fuh, J. L., Liu, C. K., Meg, M. S., Wang, S. J., & Cummings, J. L. (2001). Behavioral disorders and caregivers' reaction in Taiwanese patients with Alzheimer's disease. *International Psychogeriatrics, 13*, 121–128.
Gibbons, L. E., Teri, L., & Logsdon, R. (2002). Anxiety symptoms as predictors of nursing home placement in patients with Alzheimer's disease. *Journal of Clinical Geropsychology, 8*, 335–342.
Gibbons, L. E., Teri, L., Logsdon, R. G., & McCurry, S. M. (2006). Assessment of anxiety in dementia: An investigation into the association of different methods of measurement. *Journal of Geriatric Psychiatry and Neurology, 19*, 202–208.
Gilley, D. W., Wilson, R. S., Bennett, D. A., & Fox, J. H. (1991). Predictors of behavioral disturbance in Alzheimer's disease. *Journal of Gerontology, 46*, P362–P371.
González-Salvador, T., Lyketsos, C. G., Baker, A., Hovanec, L., Roques, C., Brandt, J., et al. (2000). Quality of life in dementia patients in long-term care. *International Journal of Geriatric Psychiatry, 15*, 181–189.
Graeff, F. G., Guimaraes, F. S., De Andrade, T. G., & Deakin, J. F. (1996). Role of 5-HT instress, anxiety, and depression. *Pharmacology Biochemistry and Behavior, 54*, 129–141.
Greenspan, A., Eerdekens, M., & Mahmoud, R. (2004). Is there an increased rate of cerebrovascular events among dementia patients? *Presented at the 24th congress of the collegium internationale neuropsychopharmacologicum (CINP)*, June 20–24, Paris.
Hadjistavropoulos, T., & Hadjistavropoulos, H. D. (2008). *Pain management for older adults: A self-help guide*. Seattle: IASP Press.
Harwood, D. G., Ownby, R. L., & Barker, W. W. (1998). The behavioral pathology in Alzheimer's disease scale (BEHAVE-AD): Factor structure among community-dwelling Alzheimer's disease patients. *International Journal of Geriatric Psychiatry, 13*, 793–800.

Haupt, M., Karger, A., & Janner, M. (2000). Improvement of agitation and anxiety in demented patients after psychoeducative group intervention with their caregivers. *International Journal of Geriatric Psychiatry, 15*, 1125–1129.

Haw, C., Harwood, D., & Hawton, K. (2009). Dementia and suicidal behavior: A review of the literature. *International Psychogeriatrics, 21*, 440–453.

Herrmann, N. (1998). Valproic acid treatment of agitation in dementia. *Canadian Journal of Psychiatry, 43*, 69–72.

Heun, R., Papassotiropoulos, A., Jessen, F., Maier, W., & Breitner, J. C. (2001). A family study of Alzheimer disease and early and late-onset depression in elderly patients. *Archives of General Psychiatry, 58*, 190–196.

Hoe, J., Hancock, G., Livingston, G., & Orrell, M. (2006). Quality of life of people with dementia in residential care homes. *The British Journal of Psychiatry, 188*, 460–464.

Holmes, C., Arranz, M., Collier, D., Powell, J., & Lovestone, S. (2003). Depression in Alzheimer's disease: The effect of serotonin receptor gene variation. *American Journal of Medical Genetics Part B, Neuropsychiatric Genetics, 119B*(1), 40–43.

Hwang, T. J., Masterman, D. L., Ortiz, F., Fairbanks, L. A., & Cummings, J. L. (2004). Mild cognitive impairment is associated with characteristic neuropsychiatric symptoms. *Alzheimer Disease and Associated Disorders, 18*, 17–21.

Jeste, D. V., Sanford, I., & Finkel, S. I. (2000). Psychosis of Alzheimer's disease and related dementias: Diagnostic criteria for a distinct syndrome. *The American Journal of Geriatric Psychiatry, 8*, 1.

Johns, M. W. (1991). A new method for measuring daytime sleepiness. The Epworth Sleepiness Scale. *Sleep, 14*, 540–545.

Kalapatapu, R. K., & Neugroschl, J. A. (2009). Update on neuropsychiatric symptoms of dementia: Evaluation and management. *Geriatrics, 64*, 20–26.

Kang, S. J., Choi, S. H., Lee, B. H., Jeong, Y., Hahm, D. S., Han, I. W., et al. (2004). Caregiver-administered Neuropsychiatric Inventory (CGA-NPI). *Journal of Geriatric Psychiatry and Neurology, 17*, 32–35.

Kaplan, H. I., & Sadock, B. J. (2007). *Kaplan and Sadock's synopsis of psychiatry* (10th ed., pp. 1117–1124). Philadelphia: Lippincott, Williams & Wilkins.

Kapp, M. B. (2000). Increasing liability risks among nursing homes: Therapeutic consequences, costs, and alternatives. *Journal of the American Geriatrics Society, 48*(1), 97–99.

Kaufer, D. I., Cummings, J. L., Ketchel, P., Smith, V., MacMillan, A., Shelley, T., et al. (2000). Validation of the NPI-Q, a brief clinical form of the Neuropsychiatric Inventory. *The Journal of Neuropsychiatry and Clinical Neurosciences, 12*, 233–239.

Keefe, F. J. (1996). Cognitive behavioral therapy for managing pain. *Clinical Psychology, 49*(3), 4–5.

Kim, D. H., Payne, M. E., Levy, R. M., MacFall, J. R., & Steffens, D. C. (2002). APOE genotype and hippocampal volume change in geriatric depression. *Biological Psychiatry, 51*, 426–429.

King, A. C., Oman, R. F., Brassington, G. S., Bliwise, D. L., & Haskell, W. L. (1979). Moderate-intensity exercise and self-rated quality of sleep in older adults. A randomized controlled trial. *Journal of the American Medical Association, 277*, 32–37.

Koder, D. A. (1998). Treatment of anxiety in the cognitively impaired elderly: Can cognitive-behavior therapy help? *International Psychogeriatrics, 10*, 173–182.

Kraus, C. A., Seignourel, P., Balasubramanyam, V., Snow, A. L., Wilson, N. L., Kunik, M. E., et al. (2008). Cognitive-behavioral treatment for anxiety in patients with dementia: Two case studies. *Journal of Psychiatric Practice, 14*, 186–192.

Krishnan, K. R., Tupler, L. A., Ritchie, J. C. J., McDonald, W. M., Knight, D. L., Nemeroff, C. B., et al. (1996). Apolipoprotein E-epsilon 4 frequency in geriatric depression. *Biological Psychiatry, 40*, 69–71.

Kunik, M. E., Huffman, J. C., Bharani, N., Hillman, S. L., Molinari, V. A., & Orengo, C. A. (2000). Behavioral disturbances in geropsychiatric inpatients across dementia types. *Journal of Geriatric Psychiatry and Neurology, 13*, 49–52.

Kunik, M. E., Martinez, M., Snow, A. L., Beck, C. K., Cody, M., Rapp, C. G., et al. (2003). Determinants of behavioral symptoms in dementia patients. *Clinical Gerontologist, 26*, 83–89.

Kunik, M. E., Snow, A. L., Davila, J. A., Steele, A. B., Balasubramanyam, V., Doody, R. S., et al. (2010). Causes of aggressive behavior in patients with dementia. *The Journal of Clinical Psychiatry, 71*(9), 1145–1152.

Kunik, M. E., Snow, L., Davila, J. A., Steele, A. B., Balasubramanyam, V., Doody, R. S., et al. (2008). High incidence of aggression in persons with dementia. In *Presented at the American association for geriatric psychiatry 2008 annual meeting*, March 14–17, Orlando, FL.

LaBarge, E. (1993). A preliminary scale to measure the degree of worry among mildly demented Alzheimer disease patients. *Physical and Occupational Therapy in Geriatrics, 11*, 43–57.

Lanctot, K. I., Best, T. S., Mittman, N., Liu, B. A., Oh, P. I., Einarson, T. R., et al. (1998). Efficacy and safety of 33 neuroleptics in behavioral disorders associated with dementia. *The Journal of Clinical Psychiatry, 59*, 550–561.

Landes, A. M., Sperry, S. D., Milton, E., Strauss, M. E., & Geldmacher, D. S. (2001). Apathy in Alzheimer's disease. *Journal of the American Geriatrics Society, 49*, 1700–1707.

Lawton, M. P., Van Haitsma, K., Klapper, J., Kleban, M. H., Katz, I. R., & Corn, J. (1998). A stimulation-retreat special care unit for elders with dementing illness. *International Psychogeriatric 10*, 379–95.

Lenze, E. J., Mulsant, B. H., Shear, M. K., Dew, M. A., Miller, M. D., Pollock, B. G., et al. (2005). Efficacy and tolerability of citalopram in the treatment of late-life anxiety disorders: Results from an 8-week randomized, placebo-controlled trial. *The American Journal of Psychiatry, 162*(1), 146–150.

Lerner, A. J., Strauss, M., & Sami, S. A. (2007). Recognizing apathy in Alzheimer's disease. *Geriatrics, 62*(11), 14–17.

Lesser, J. M., & Hughes, S. V. (2006). Psychosis-related disturbances. Psychosis, agitation, and disinhibition in Alzheimer's disease: Definitions and treatment options. *Geriatrics, 61*, 14–20.

Luppa, M., Luck, T., Brähler, E., König, H. H., & Riedel-Heller, S. G. (2008). Prediction of institutionalisation in dementia. *Dementia and Geriatric Cognitive Disorders, 26*, 65–78.

Lyketsos, C. G., DelCampo, L., Steinberg, M., Miles, Q., Steele, C. D., Munro, C., et al. (2003). Treating depression in Alzheimer disease: Efficacy and safety of sertraline therapy, and the benefits of depression reduction: The DIADS. *Archives of General Psychiatry, 60*, 737–746.

Lyketsos, C. G., & Lee, H. B. (2004). Diagnosis and treatment of depression in Alzheimer's disease. *Dementia and Geriatric Cognitive Disorders, 17*, 1–4.

Lyketsos, C. G., Lindell Veiel, L., Baker, A., & Steele, C. (1999). A randomized, controlled trial of bright light therapy for agitated behaviors in dementia patients residing in long-term care. *International Journal of Geriatric Psychiatry, 14*, 520–525.

Lyketsos, C. G., Sheppard, J. M., Steinberg, M., Tschanz, J. A., Norton, M. C., Steffens, D. C., et al. (2001). Neuropsychiatric disturbance in Alzheimer's disease clusters into three groups: The Cache County study. *International Journal of Geriatric Psychiatry, 16*, 1043–1053.

Lyketsos, C. G., Steele, C., Baker, L., Galik, E., Kopunek, S., Steinberg, M., et al. (1997). Major and minor depression in Alzheimer's disease: Prevalence and impact. *The Journal of Neuropsychiatry and Clinical Neurosciences, 1997*(9), 556–561.

Lyketsos, C. G., Steele, C., Galik, E., Rosenblatt, A., Steinberg, M., Warren, A., et al. (1999). Physical aggression in dementia patients and its relationship to depression. *The American Journal of Psychiatry, 156*, 66–71.

Lyketsos, C. G., Steinberg, M., Tschanz, J. T., Norton, M. C., Steffens, D. C., & Breitner, J. C. (2000). Mental and behavioral disturbances in dementia: Findings from the Cache County Study on Memory in Aging. *The American Journal of Psychiatry, 157*, 708–714.

Lyketsos, C. G., & Olin, J. T. (2002). Depression in Alzheimer's disease: Overview and treatment. *Biological Psychiatry, 52*, 243–252.

Macdonald, A. J. (1999). Can delirium be separated from dementia? *Dementia and Geriatric Cognitive Disorders, 10*, 386–388.

Mack, J. L., & Patterson, M. B. (1994). The evaluation of behavioral disturbances in Alzheimer's disease: The utility of three rating scales. *Journal of Geriatric Psychiatry Neurology, 7*, 101–117.

Madhusoodanan, S., Shah, P., Brenner, R., & Gupta, S. (2007). Pharmacological treatment of the psychosis of Alzheimer's disease: What is the best approach? *CNS Drugs, 21*, 101–115.

Manabe, K., Matsui, T., Yamaya, M., Sato-Nakagawa, T., Okamura, N., Arai, H., et al. (2000). Sleep patterns and mortality among elderly patients in a geriatric hospital. *Gerontology, 46*, 318–322.

Mathew, S. J., Mao, X., Coplan, J. D., Smith, E. L., Sackeim, H. A., Gorman, J. M., et al. (2004). Dorsolateral prefrontalcortical pathology in generalized anxiety disorder: A proton magnetic resonance spectroscopic imaging study. *The American Journal of Psychiatry, 161*, 1119–1121.

Mayer, L. S., Bay, R. C., Politis, A., Steinberg, M., Steele, C., Baker, A. S., et al. (2006). Comparison of three rating scales as outcome measures for treatment trials of depression in Alzheimer disease: Findings from DIADS. *International Journal of Geriatric Psychiatry, 21*, 930–936.

McCurry, S. M., Gibbons, L. E., Logsden, R. E., Logsdon, R. G., Vitiello, M. V., & Teri, L. (2005). Nighttime insomnia treatment and education for Alzheimer's disease: A randomized, controlled trial. *Journal of the American Geriatrics Society, 53*, 793–802.

McCurry, S. M., Gibbons, L. E., Logsdon, R. G., Vitiello, M., & Teri, L. (2003). Training caregivers to change the sleep hygiene practices of patients with dementia: The NITE-AD project. *Journal of the American Geriatrics Society, 51*, 1455–1460.

McCurry, S. M., Logsdon, R. G., Teri, L., Gibbons, L. E., Kukull, W. A., Bowen, J. D., et al. (1999). Characteristics of sleep disturbance in community-dwelling Alzheimer's disease patients. *Journal of Geriatric Psychiatry and Neurology, 12*, 53–59.

McCurry, S. M., Logsdon, R. G., Vitiello, M. V., & Teri, L. (2004). Treatment of sleep and nighttime disturbances in Alzheimer's disease: A behavioral management approach. *Sleep Medicine, 5*, 373–377.

McCurry, S. M., Reynolds, C. F., Ancoli-Israel, S., Teri, L., & Vitiello, M. C. (2000). Treatment of sleep disturbance in Alzheimer's disease. *Sleep Medicine Reviews, 4*, 603–608.

McKitrick, L. A., Camp, C. J., & Black, F. W. (1992). Prospective memory intervention in Alzheimer's disease. *Journal of Gerontology, 47*, 337–343.

Mega, M. S., Cummings, J. L., Fiorello, T., & Gornbein, J. (1996). The spectrum of behavioral changes in Alzheimer's disease. *Neurology, 46*, 130–135.

Mendelson, W. B. (2005). A review of the evidence for the efficacy and safety of trazodone in insomnia. *The Journal of Clinical Psychiatry, 66*, 469–476.

Millan, M. J. (2003). The neurobiology and control of anxious states. *Progress in Neurobiology, 70*, 83–244.

Mintzer, J. E., & Brawman-Mintzer, O. (1996). Agitation as a possible expression of generalized anxiety disorder in demented elderly patients: Toward a treatment approach. *The Journal of Clinical Psychiatry, 57*(Suppl 7), 55–63.

Mukaetova-Ladinska, E. B., Harrington, C. R., Xuereb, J., Roth, M., & Wischik, C. M. (1995). Treating Alzheimer's and other dementias. In M. Bergene & S. I. Finkel (Eds.), *Treating Alzheimer's and other dementias* (pp. 57–80). New York: Springer.

Mulsant, B., Sweet, R., & Rifal, H. (1994). The use of Hamilton Depression Scale for depression in elderly patients with cognitive impairment and physical illness. *The American Journal of Geriatric Psychiatry, 2*, 220–229.

National Institutes of Health. (2005). National Institutes of Health State of the science conference statement on manifestations and management of chronic insomnia in adults, June 13–15, 2005. *Sleep, 28*, 1049–1057.

Nguyen, V. T., Love, A. R., & Kunik, M. E. (2008). Preventing aggression in persons with dementia. *Geriatrics, 63*, 21–26.

Olin, J. T., Katz, I. R., Meyers, B. S., Schneider, L. S., & Lebowitz, B. D. (2002). Provisional diagnostic criteria for depression of Alzheimer disease: Rationale and background. *The American Journal of Psychiatry, 10*, 129–141.

Olin, J. T., Shneider, L. S., Katz, I. R., Meyers, B. S., Alexopoulos, G. S., Breitner, J. C., et al. (2002). Provisional diagnostic criteria for depression of Alzheimer disease. *American Journal of Geriatric Psychiatry, 10*, 125–128.

Onyike, C. U., Sheppard, J. M., Tschanz, J. T., Norton, M. C., Green, R. C., Steinberg, M., et al. (2007). Epidemiology of apathy in older adults: The Cache County study. *The American Journal of Geriatric Psychiatry, 15*, 365–375.

Patterson, M. B., Schnell, A. H., Martin, R. J., Mendez, M. F., Smyth, K. A., & Whitehouse, P. J. (1990). Assessment of behavioral and affective symptoms in Alzheimer's disease. *Journal of Geriatric Psychiatry and Neurology, 3*, 21–30.

Paulsen, J. S., Salmon, D. P., Thal, L. J., Romero, R., Weisstein-Jenkins, C., Galasko, D., et al. (2000). Incidence of and risk factors for hallucinations and delusions in patients with probable AD. *Neurology, 54*, 1965–1971.

Payne, J. L., Lyketsos, C. G., Steele, C., Baker, L., Galik, E., Kopunek, S., et al. (1998). Relationship of cognitive and functional impairment to depressive features in Alzheimer's disease and other dementias. *The Journal of Neuropsychiatry and Clinical Neurosciences, 10*(4), 440–447.

Petrella, R. J., Koval, J. J., Cunningham, D. A., & Paterson, D. H. (2003). Can primary care doctors prescribe exercise to improve fitness? The Step Test Exercise Prescription (STEP) project. *American Journal of Preventive Medicine, 24*, 316–322.

Plassman, B. L., Langa, K. M., Fisher, G. G., Heerringa, S. G., Weir, D. R., Ofstedal, M. B., et al. (2007). Prevalence of dementia in the United States: The aging, demographics, and memory study. *Neuroepidemiology, 29*, 125–132.

Politis, A. M., Vozzella, S., Mayer, L. S., Onyike, C. U., Baker, A. S., & Lyketsos, C. G. (2004). A randomized, controlled, clinical trial of activity therapy for apathy in patients with dementia residing in long-term care. *International Journal of Geriatric Psychiatry, 19*, 1087–1094.

Pollak, C. P., & Perlick, D. (1991). Sleep problems and institutionalization of the elderly. *Journal of Geriatric Psychiatry and Neurology, 4*, 204–210.

Pollock, B. G., Muisant, B. H., Rosen, J., Mazumdar, S., Blakesley, R. E., Houck, P. R., et al. (2007). A double-blind comparison of citaiopram and risperidonefor treatment of behavioral and psychotic symptoms associated with dementia. *The American Journal of Geriatric Psychiatry, 15*, 942–952.

Pollock, B. G., Mulsant, B. H., Rosen, J., Sweet, R. A., Mazumdar, S., Bharucha, A., et al. (2002). Comparison of citalopram, perphenazine, and placebo for the acute treatment of psychosis and behavioral disturbances in hospitalized, demented patients. *The American Journal of Psychiatry, 159*, 460–465.

Porter, V. R., Buxton, W. G., Fairbanks, L. A., Strickland, T., O'Connor, S. M., Rosenberg-Thompson, S., et al. (2003). Frequency and characteristics of anxiety among patients with Alzheimer's disease and related dementias. *The Journal of Neuropsychiatry and Clinical Neurosciences, 15*, 180–186.

Qazi, A., Shankar, K., & Orrell, M. (2003). Managing anxiety in people with dementia. A case series. *Journal of Affective Disorders, 76*, 261–265.

Rabins, P. V., Blacker, D., Rovner, B. W., Rummans, T., Schneider, L. S., Tariot, P. N., et al. (2007). American Psychiatric Association practice guideline for the treatment of patients with Alzheimer's disease and other dementias. *The American Journal of Psychiatry, 164*(Suppl 12), 5–56.

Rao, V., & Lyketsos, C. G. (2000). The benefits and risks of ECT for patients with primary dementia who also suffer from depression. *International Journal of Geriatric Psychiatry, 15*, 729–735.

Rayner, A., O'Brien, J., & Schoenbachier, B. (2006). Behavior disorders of dementia: Recognition and treatment. *American Family Physician, 73*, 647–652.

Reisberg, B., Auer, S. R., & Monteiro, I. M. (1996). Behavioral pathology in Alzheimer's disease (BEHAVE-AD) rating scale. *International Psychogeriatrics, 8*(Suppl 3), 301–308.

Reisberg, B., Borenstein, J., Salob, S. P., Ferris, S. H., Franssen, E., & Georgotas, A. (1987). Behavioral symptoms in Alzheimer's disease: Phenomenology and treatment. *The Journal of Clinical Psychiatry, 48*(Suppl), 9–15.

Rimersma-van der Lek, R. F., Swaab, D. F., Tiwsk, J., Hol, E. M., Hoogendijk, W. J., & Van Someren, E. J. (2008). Effect of bright light and melatonin on cognitive and noncognitive function in elderly residents of group care facilities: A randomized controlled trial. *Journal of the American Medical Association, 299*, 2642–2655.

Roehrs, T. R., & Roth, T. (2009). *The effect of drugs on sleep quality and architecture*. UpTo Date. Available from www.uptodate.com/patients/content/topic.do?topicKey=~91BE3rs_xppRr958. Accessed September 28, 2009.

Ropacki, S. A., & Jeste, D. V. (2005). Epidemiology of and risk factors for psychosis of Alzheimer's disease: A review of 55 studies published from 1990 to 2003. *The American Journal of Psychiatry, 162*, 2022–2030.

Schneider, L. S., & Dagerman, K. S. (2004). Psychosis of Alzheimer's disease: Clinical characteristics and history. *Journal of Psychiatric Research, 38*, 105–111.

Schneider, L. S., Dagerman, K. S., & Insel, P. (2005). Risk of deaths with atypical antipsychotic treatment for dementia: Meta analysis of randomized placebo controlled trials. *Journal of the American Medical Association, 294*, 1934–1943.

Schneider, L. S., Pollack, V. E., & Lyness, S. A. (1990). A meta analysis of controlled trials of neuroleptic treatment in dementia. *Journal of the American Geriatrics Society, 38*, 553–563.

Sclan, S. G., Saillon, A., Franssen, L., Hugonot-Diener, L., Saillon, A., Reisberg, B., et al. (1996). The behavioral pathology in Alzheimer's Disease Rating Scale (BEHAVE-AD): Reliability and analysis of symptom category scores. *International Journal of Geriatric Psychiatry, 11*, 819–830.

Seignourel, P., Kunik, M. E., Snow, L., Wilson, N., & Stanley, M. (2008). Anxiety in dementia: A critical review. *Clinical Psychology Review, 28*, 1071–1082.

Serfaty, M., Kennell-Webb, S., Warner, J., Blizard, R., & Raven, P. (2002). Double blind randomised placebo controlled trial of low dose melatonin for sleep disorders in dementia. *International Journal of Geriatric Psychiatry, 17*, 1120–1127.

Shankar, K. K., Walker, M., & Frost, D. (1999). The development of a valid and reliable scale for rating anxiety in dementia (RAID). *Aging & Mental Health, 3*, 39–49.

Shub, D., Darvishi, R., & Kunik, M. E. (2009). Non-pharmacologic treatment of insomnia in persons with dementia. *Geriatrics, 64*, 22–26.

Shub, D., & Kunik, M. E. (2009). Psychiatric comorbidity in persons with dementia. *Psychiatric Times, 26*, 32–35.

Siddique, H., Hynan, L. S., & Weiner, M. F. (2009). Effect of a serotonin reuptake inhibitor on irritability, apathy, and psychotic symptoms in patients with Alzheimer's disease. *The Journal of Clinical Psychiatry, 70*, 915–918.

Singer, C., Tractenberg, R. E., Kaye, J., Schafer, K., Gamst, A., Grundman, M., et al. (2003). A multicenter, placebo-controlled trial of melatonin for sleep disturbance in Alzheimer's disease. *Sleep, 26*, 893–901.

Sink, K. M., Holden, K. L., & Yaffe, K. (2005). Pharmacological treatment of neuropsychiatric symptoms in dementia: A review of the evidence. *Journal of the American Medical Association, 293*, 596–608.

Skinner, B. (1953). *Science and human behavior*. New York: The Free Press.

Sloane, P. D., Williams, C. S., Mitchell, C. M., Preisser, J. S., Wood, W., Barrick, A. L., et al. (2007). High-intensity environmental light in dementia: Effect on sleep and activity. *Journal of the American Geriatrics Society, 55*, 1524–1533.

Smith, S. S., Dingwall, K., Jorgenson, G., & Douglas, J. (2006). Associations between the use of common medications and sleep architecture in patients with untreated obstructive sleep apnea. *Journal of Clinical Sleep Medicine, 2*, 156–162.

Snow, A. L., Weber, J. B., O'Malley, K. J., Cody, M., Beck, C., Bruera, E., et al. (2004). NOPPAIN: A nursing assistant administered pain assessment instrument for use in dementia. *Dementia and Geriatric Cognitive Disorders, 17*, 240–246.

Staal, J., Pinkney, L., & Roane, D. (2003). Assessment of stimulus preferences in multisensory environment therapy for older people with dementia. *British Journal of Occupational Therapy, 66*, 542–549.

Staal, J. A., Sacks, A., Matheis, R., Collier, L., Calia, T., Hanif, H., et al. (2007). The effects of snoezelen (multi-sensory behavior therapy) and psychiatric care on agitation, apathy, and activities of daily living in dementia patients on a short term geriatric psychiatric inpatient unit. *International Journal of Psychiatry in Medicine, 37*, 357–370.

Starkstein, S., Ingram, L., Garau, M., & Mizrahi, R. (1983). On the overlap between apathy and depression in dementia. *Journal of Neurology Neurosurgery Psychiatry Research, 17*, 37–49.

Starkstein, S. E., Jorge, R., Petracca, G., & Robinson, R. G. (2007). The construct of generalized anxiety disorder in Alzheimer disease. *The American Journal of Geriatric Psychiatry, 15*, 42–49.
Stern, Y., Albert, M., Brandt, J., Jacobs, D. M., Tang, M. X., Marder, K., et al. (1994). Utility of extrapyramidal signs and psychosis as predictors of cognitive and functional decline, nursing home admission, and death in Alzheimer's disease: Prospective analyses from the predictors study. *Neurology, 44*, 2300–2307.
Stone, M. (2005). Deaths in controlled trials of atypical antipsychotics in patients with behavioral disturbances from dementia. In *Presented at the 45th annual New Clinical Drug Evaluation Unit (NCDEU) meeting*, June 6–9, Boca Raton, FL.
Strauss, M. E., & Sperry, S. D. (2002). An informant-based assessment of apathy in Alzheimer disease. *Neuropsychiatry, Neuropsychology, and Behavioral Neurology, 15*(3), 176–183.
Stuss, D. T., van Reekum, R., & Murphy, K. J. (2000). Differentiation of states and causes of apathy. In J. Borod (Ed.), *The neuropsychology of emotion* (pp. 340–363). New York: Oxford University Press.
Sultzer, D. L., Brown, C. V., Mandelkern, M. D., Mahler, M. E., Mendez, M. F., Chen, S. T., et al. (2003). Delusional thoughts and regional frontal/temporal cortex metabolism in Alzheimer's disease. *The American Journal of Psychiatry, 160*, 341–349.
Sultzer, D. L., Davis, S. M., Tariot, P. N., Dagerman, K. S., Lebowitz, B. D., Lyketsos, C. G., et al. (2008). Clinical symptom responses to atypical antipsychotic medications in Alzheimer's disease: Phase 1 outcomes from the CATIE-AD effectiveness trial. *The American Journal of Psychiatry, 165*, 844.
Sultzer, D. L., Gray, K. F., Gunay, I., Berisford, M. A., & Mahler, M. E. (1997). A double-blind comparison of trazodone and haloperidol for treatment of agitation in patients with dementia. *The American Journal of Geriatric Psychiatry, 5*, 60–69.
Sultzer, D. L., Mahler, M. E., Mandelkern, M. A., Cummings, J. L., Van Gorp, W. G., Hinkin, C. H., et al. (1995). The relationship between psychiatric symptoms and regional cortical metabolism in Alzheimer's disease. *The Journal of Neuropsychiatry and Clinical Neurosciences, 7*, 476–484.
Tariot, P. N. (1999). Treatment of agitation in dementia. *The Journal of Clinical Psychiatry, 60*(Suppl 8), 11–20.
Teri, L. (1994). Behavioral treatment of depression in patients with dementia. Alzheimer's Disease and *Associated Disorders, 8,* suppl 3, 66–74.
Teri, L., Ferretti, L. E., Gibbons, L. E., Logsdon, R. G., McCurry, S. M., Kukull, W. A., et al. (1999). Anxiety in Alzheimer's disease: Prevalence and comorbidity. *The Journals of Gerontology Series A, Biological Sciences and Medical Sciences, 54*, M348–M352.
Teri, L., & Gallagher-Thompson, D. (1991). Cognitive-behavioral interventions for treatment of depression in Alzheimer's patients. *The Gerontologist, 31*, 413–416.
Teri, L., Gibbons, L. E., McCurry, S. M., Logsdon, R. G., Buchner, D. M., Barlow, W. E., et al. (2003). Exercise plus behavioral management in patients with Alzheimer disease. *Journal of the American Medical Association, 290*, 2015–2022.
Teri, L., McKenzie, G., & La Fazia, D. (2005). Psycho-social treatment of depression in older adults, with dementia. *Clinical Psychology: Science and Practice, 12*, 303–16.
van Reekum, R., Stuss, D. T., & Ostrander, L. (2005). Apathy: Why care? *The Journal of Neuropsychiatry and Clinical Neurosciences, 17*, 7–19.
Vaughan, M., & Michael, J. (1982). Automatic reinforcement: An important but ignored concept. *Behaviorism, 10*(212), 217–227.
Vitiello, M. V., & Borson, S. (2001). Sleep disturbances in patients with Alzheimer's disease. *CNS Drugs, 15*, 777–796.
Wands, K., Merskey, H., Hachinski, V. C., Fisman, M., Fox, H., & Boniferro, M. (1990). A questionnaire investigation of anxiety and depression in early dementia. *Journal of the American Geriatrics Society, 38*, 535–538.
Wang, J. J. (2007). Group reminiscence therapy for cognitive and affective function of dementia elderly in Taiwan. *International Journal of Geriatric Psychiatry, 22*, 1235–1240.

Weintraub, D., & Hurtig, H. (2007). Presentation and management of psychosis in Parkinson's disease and dementia with Lewy bodies. *The American Journal of Psychiatry, 164*, 1491.

Wetherell, J. L., Gatz, M., & Craske, M. G. (2003). Treatment of generalized anxiety disorder in older adults. *Journal of Consulting and Clinical Psychology, 71*, 31–40.

Wick, J. Y., & Zanni, O. R. (2005). Sundowning: Disruptive behavior with many causes. *The Consultant Pharmacist, 20*(947–50), 957–961.

Wilson, R. S., Arnold, S. E., Schneider, J. A., & Bennett, D. A. (2007). Chronic distress, age related neuropathology, and late-life dementia. *Psychosomatic Medicine, 69*, 47–53.

Wimo, A., Winblad, B., & Jonsson, L. (2007). An estimate of the total worldwide societal costs of dementia in 2005. *Alzheimers Dementia, 3*, 81–91.

Yesavage, J. A., Brink, T. L., Rose, T. L., Lum, O., Huang, V., Aday, M., et al. (1983). Development and validation of a geriatric depression screening scale: A preliminary report. *Journal of Psychiatric Research, 17*, 37–49.

Yesavage, J. A., & Taylor, B. (1991). Anxiety and dementia. In C. Salzman & B. D. Lebowitz (Eds.), *Anxiety in the elderly: Treatment and research* (pp. 79–85). New York: Springer.

Zanetti, O., Vallotti, B., Frisoni, G. B., Geroldi, C., Bianchetti, A., Pasqualetti, P., et al. (1999). Insight in dementia: When does it occur? Evidence for a nonlinear relationship between insight and cognitive status. *The Journals of Gerontology Series B, Psychological Sciences and Social Sciences, 54*, P100–P106.

Zill, P., Padberg, F., de Jonge, S., Hampel, H., Burger, K., Stubner, S., et al. (2000). Serotonin transporter (5-HTT) gene polymorphism in psychogeriatric patients. *Neuroscience Letters, 284*(1–2), 113–115.

Zubenko, G. S., Moossy, J., Martinez, A. J., Rao, G., Claassen, D., Rosen, J., et al. (1991). Neuropathologic and neurochemical correlates of psychosis in primary dementia. *Archives of Neurology, 48*, 619–624.

Zubenko, G. S., Zubenko, W. N., McPherson, S., Spoor, E., Marin, D. B., Farlow, M. R., et al. (2003). A collaborative study of the emergence and clinical features of the major depressive syndrome of Alzheimer's disease. *The American Journal of Psychiatry, 160*, 857–866.

Zuidema, S., Koopmans, R., & Verhey, F. (2007). Prevalence and predictors of neuropsychiatric symptoms in cognitively impaired nursing home patients. *Geriatric Psychiatry Neurology, 20*, 41–49.

Chapter 10
Psychological Co-morbidities of Irritable Bowel Syndrome

Laurie Keefer, Jennifer L. Kiebles, and Tiffany H. Taft

10.1 Introduction: Definition and Prevalence

Irritable bowel syndrome (IBS) is a chronic abdominal pain condition associated with diarrhea, constipation, or an alternation of both (Longstreth et al., 2006; Remes-Troche et al., 2009). It is diagnosed according to the Rome Criteria for Functional Bowel Disorders (Longstreth et al., 2006) and requires:

Recurrent abdominal pain or discomfort ("Discomfort" means an uncomfortable sensation not described as pain) at least 3 days/month in the last 3 months associated with two or more of the following:

1. Improvement with defecation
2. Onset associated with a change in frequency of stool
3. Onset associated with a change in form (appearance) of stool

Criterion fulfilled for the last 3 months with symptom onset at least 6 months prior to diagnosis.

A common medical condition that accounts for a significant portion of missed work days, triple that of healthy adults (Spiegel, 2009), IBS rivals cardiovascular disease and diabetes as one of the most financially burdensome conditions for employers, the health care system, and individuals (Spiegel). IBS affects between 15 and 22% of North American adults (Drossman, Corrazziari, Talley, Thompson, & Whitehead, 2006) with nearly twice as many women as men reporting symptoms (Heitkemper & Jarrett, 2008; Heitkemper, Jarrett, & Bond, 2004). IBS is most prevalent in the 4th and 5th decades of life, but can occur at any time during the lifespan (Hungin, Chang, Locke, Dennis, & Barghout, 2005; Hungin, Whorwell,

L. Keefer (✉)
Northwestern University, Feinberg School of Medicine, Division of Gastroenterology, Center for Psychosocial Research, 676 N. St. Clair, Suite 1400, Chicago, IL 60611, USA
e-mail: laurie.keefer@northwestern.edu

S. Pagoto (ed.), *Psychological Co-morbidities of Physical Illness: A Behavioral Medicine Perspective*, DOI 10.1007/978-1-4419-0029-6_10,

Tack, & Mearin, 2003). Prevalence rates of IBS are remarkably similar across various ethnic groups around the world; however, methodological concerns and differences in access to health care limit these findings (Sperber, 2009).

IBS can be further categorized by predominant stool consistency subtype, diarrhea-predominant (IBS-D), constipation predominant (IBS-C), mixed (IBS-M) or unspecified (IBS-U) (Longstreth et al., 2006). The Bristol Stool Scale (Riegler & Esposito, 2001) is often used by physicians to clarify what is meant by stool consistency – scores of 1 and 2 are indicative of constipation, scores of 6 and 7 are indicative of diarrhea/urgency, and scores of 3 and 4 are considered "ideal" in terms of ease in passing. This tool is widely used by physicians to facilitate communication with the patient, who may or may not have an understanding of "normal" stool consistency. Further, the tool can help the physician subtype the patient's IBS. To date, there is limited data discriminating between subtypes on most variables of interest. That said, it is still common practice to limit clinical trials to one IBS subtype only, thereby limiting the generalizability of results.

10.2 Etiology

The cause of IBS is largely unknown, but research supports its classification as a *functional gastrointestinal disorder* (Longstreth et al., 2006; Remes-Troche et al., 2009). In other words, the altered pain perception and disturbed colonic motility characteristic of IBS cannot be explained by a visible organic or structural abnormality. IBS is distinct from more serious diseases such as inflammatory bowel diseases (IBD; e.g., ulcerative colitis and Crohn's disease) or colorectal cancer (Longstreth et al., 2006). The diagnosis of IBS can be made with a fair amount of certainty from the Rome Criteria (Longstreth et al.). Only when "alarm signs" including blood in the stool, anemia, fever, significant weight loss, or a family history of colorectal cancer are present should patients with suspected IBS undergo additional workup with a gastroenterologist (Remes-Troche et al., 2009).

IBS is characterized by its subjective symptom profile, marked heterogeneity among patients, significant overlap with other medically unexplained symptoms including fibromyalgia, chronic fatigue syndrome, and chronic pelvic pain (Riedl et al., 2008), and the lack of a reliable biomarker. As such, the experience of IBS, dominated by chronic abdominal pain and embarrassing GI symptoms, can be a consequence as well as a cause of psychological distress, and which comes first remains unknown (Sykes, Blanchard, Lackner, Keefer, & Krasner, 2003). Only about half of the individuals with symptoms of IBS seek medical treatment; this group reports the most psychological distress and poorest quality of life (QOL) (Cremonini & Talley, 2005; Talley, Boyce, & Jones, 1997).

10.3 The Biopsychosocial Model of IBS

The predominant conceptual model for the assessment and treatment of IBS rests on the assumption that experiences throughout life affect the biology of the gut and overall sensitivity to normal gut functions. More specifically, the onset or maintenance of IBS occurs through one or more interactions between biology and genetics, early life experiences, cognitive processes, learned behaviors, and societal reinforcements (Drossman, Camilleri, Mayer, & Whitehead, 2002; Halpert & Drossman, 2005) (see Fig. 10.1).

10.3.1 Stress and IBS

Consistent with many psychiatric conditions, a physiological susceptibility to the *negative effects of stress* can lead to the development or worsening of IBS (Sapolsky, 1996a, 1996b, 2004). The occurrence of major life events and the experience of minor daily hassles have been shown to affect gastrointestinal (GI) functioning; however, the data are mixed as to whether persons with IBS experience more stressors than a variety of

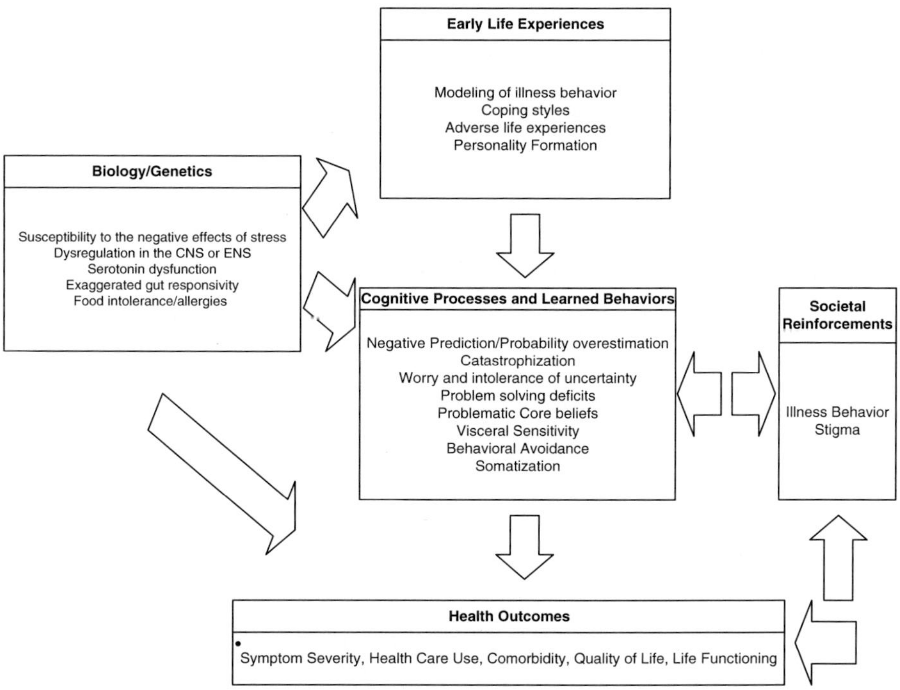

Fig. 10.1 The biopsychosocial model of IBS

healthy and disease control groups (Blanchard et al., 2008). One reason for the lack of clarity on this issue is that the impact of stressful events on the body is mediated by a variety of other factors such as core beliefs, cognitive appraisals, coping behaviors, and access to social support and therefore varies widely across individuals.

10.3.2 Brain-Gut Connection

Biological predisposition towards dysregulation in the central and/or enteric nervous systems might explain the overlap between IBS, depression, and anxiety. Indeed, the gut has been called "the second brain" given the significance of the brain-gut connection, regulated through the hypothalamic-pituitary-adrenal (HPA) axis, on the perception of pain and GI function. Serotonin dysfunction has also been implicated in the brain-gut dysregulation commonly noted in IBS (Camilleri, 2005), with individuals who have weaker serotonin transporter systems responding to signals from their gut more readily in the emotion-regulating brain regions (Fukudo et al., 2009). IBS patients may also have an exaggerated gut response to psychological stress, food and other stressors (Fukudo, Nomura, Muranaka, & Taguchi, 1993), identify pain in their rectum earlier and at lower levels of pressure than healthy controls due to sensitive nerve endings (Spetalen, Sandvik, Blomhoff, & Jacobsen, 2009; Whitehead & Palsson, 1998), and exhibit visceral sensitivity to normal gut sensations such as hunger, satiety, bowel sounds, and digestion (Delvaux, 2002; Spetalen et al., 2009; Whitehead, Palsson, & Jones, 2002).

10.3.3 The Nature vs. Nurture Debate

Although a genetic link for IBS has been implied (Kalantar, Locke, Zinsmeister, Beighley, & Talley, 2003; Levy et al., 2001; Morris-Yates, Talley, Boyce, Nandurkar, & Andrews, 1998; Saito & Talley, 2008), it is also likely that modeling of illness behavior contributes to the onset of IBS. Individuals who grew up in a household where a parent had IBS or "stomach problems" are more likely to develop IBS – this seems to be most profound when a parent received excessive attention for somatic symptoms or generally demonstrated poor physical functioning (Levy et al., 2001; Levy & Langer, 2007; Levy, Langer, & Whitehead, 2007).

Early learning around pain, bowel habits, coping, and healthcare seeking also seems to influence the onset or maintenance of IBS (Chitkara et al., 2009; Chitkara, van Tilburg, Blois-Martin, & Whitehead, 2008). Finally, psychological processes including dysfunctional core beliefs, negative cognitive appraisals, maladaptive coping, suppression of emotion, and alexithymia can also be transmitted within the family environment and contribute to IBS (Chitkara et al.). Some evidence suggests that individuals with IBS may use confrontative, escape-avoidance, and self-controlling coping strategies to manage stress, including their IBS symptoms (Jones, Wessinger, & Crowell, 2006).

The multifactorial nature of IBS and the poorly understood etiology limit the ability of any one medical or psychological therapy to effectively treat the entire range of symptoms. Thus, careful assessment of initiating and maintaining factors is critical to treatment planning.

10.4 Practical Assessment Tools

In addition to a comprehensive psychological intake, the therapist must do a thorough history of the patient's IBS symptoms and the context in which IBS occurs. Therapist comfort with discussing bowel habits is critical at the first interview. IBS patients often experience stigma and discomfort around these sensitive issues, even from their gastroenterologist, which has also been linked to outcomes (Jones et al., 2009). To augment the clinical interview, several reliable and valid measures of IBS symptom severity, symptom tracking, health-related quality of life, and pain experiences are available to help guide treatment planning. Proper diagnosis of IBS via established Rome III criteria is an obvious important first step in determining treatment. However, patients may present to psychotherapy reporting that they have been diagnosed with IBS, but do not actually meet Rome criteria. The Rome III Questionnaire for IBS is available via the Rome Foundation website[1] and may be useful in confirming/classifying IBS and educating patients about the syndrome.

10.4.1 Symptom Monitoring

Daily symptom diaries serve as useful assessment tools throughout treatment. Ideally, an IBS patient should complete 2–3 weeks of symptom diaries at the beginning of treatment to establish baseline symptoms and identify any potential symptom patterns. Symptom diaries should include patient ratings of abdominal pain, bloating, number of bowel movements per day, and urgency. Patients should complete symptom diaries at the same time each day to avoid recall bias or inaccurate reporting of their experience. In addition to symptom diaries, it may be helpful to use food logs and stressful situation records that are modified to include IBS symptoms as they relate to eating or stressful situations. A standardized IBS Daily Diary is available through the International Foundation of Functional Gastrointestinal Disorders.

10.4.2 Pain Assessment

Abdominal pain, improved with a bowel movement at least some of the time, is critical to the IBS diagnosis (Longstreth et al., 2006). A useful tool for evaluating

[1] http://www.romecriteria.org/questionnaires.

psychological factors affecting the experience of pain is the *Pain Catastrophizing Scale* (PCS) (Sullivan, Bishop, & Pivik, 1995). The PCS can identify ruminative thoughts and the inability to control worries. Magnification of any pain experiences, expectations for negative outcomes, and a sense of helplessness to cope with IBS-related pain can also be assessed (Sullivan et al.). Previous research has suggested that catastrophizing partly mediates the association between depression and pain in patients with severe IBS (Lackner, Jaccard, & Blanchard, 2005) and directly contributes to interpersonal difficulties (Lackner & Gurtman, 2004). Other pain scales, such as the *McGill Pain Questionnaire* (Melzack, 1975), which considers affective and sensory experiences and pain suffering, are useful in assessing IBS patient-reported pain.

10.4.3 Quality of Life

Understanding the impact IBS has on the patient's health-related quality of life (HRQOL) is another important component in a thorough assessment. Patients with more severe symptoms will likely report poorer HRQOL (Palsson, Turner, Johnson, Burnett, & Whitehead, 2002). The most widely accepted HRQOL measure is the Irritable Bowel Syndrome-Quality of Life (IBS-QOL) questionnaire (Drossman et al., 2000). This measure evaluates how much IBS symptoms have impacted the patient's life over the past month and is a useful cognitive measure of symptom perception. Other questionnaires that address HRQOL in IBS patients include the Functional Digestive Disorders Quality of Life Questionnaire (FDDQL) (Chassany et al., 1999), the IBS Questionnaire (IBSQ) (Wong, Guyatt, Cook, Griffith, & Irvine, 1998), and the IBS-36 (Groll et al., 2002).

10.5 Treatment of IBS

Three types of interventions have been considered for IBS: pharmacological, dietary, and psychological.

10.5.1 Pharmacological Treatment

The American College of Gastroenterologists issued 2010 guidelines (Schmulson et al., 2009) based on a series of meta-analyses, suggesting that medical therapy for IBS is largely ineffective for its full range of symptoms (Camilleri & Mayer, 2009). A few classes of medications have demonstrated small effects on specific symptoms of IBS in randomized controlled trials (RCTs), including *antispasmodics* (Ford et al., 2008), *antidiarrheals* (Schmulson et al., 2009), *nonabsorbable antibiotics* such as rifaximin, (Fumi & Trexler, 2008; Pimentel, Park, Mirocha, Kane, & Kong, 2006), *probiotics* (Brenner & Chey, 2009; Brenner, Moeller, Chey, & Schoenfeld, 2009; Moayyedi et al., 2010), *5HT receptor antagonists and agonists* (Camilleri, 2005), *C-2 chloride channel activators*, (Chey, Drossman, Scott, Panas, Ueno, 2008), and *antidepressants*, including tricyclics (Clouse, 2003; Ford, Talley, Schoenfeld, Quigley, & Moayyedi, 2009; Spiller et al., 2007) and SSRIs (Creed et al., 2003, 2008).

10.5.2 Dietary Therapy

There are no established dietary guidelines for IBS despite the rapid growth of diet-based websites for IBS (Heizer, Southern, & McGovern, 2009). Further, meta-analyses considered in the 2010 IBS treatment guidelines confirm the lack of support for the use of *fiber* (Ford et al., 2008; Schmulson et al., 2009) or *laxatives* (Schmulson et al.) for IBS. Of note, long-term laxative use and laxative abuse can have significant physiological consequences (Kudo et al., 1998; Motola et al., 2002).

10.5.3 Psychotherapy

The relevance of psychosocial factors to IBS is further supported by several lines of research that demonstrate the efficacy of psychotropic medications (Clouse, 1994, 2003) and the benefit of a variety of psychological therapies (Lackner, Mesmer, Morley, Dowzer, & Hamilton, 2004; Mayer, 2008) on IBS symptoms. A recent meta-analysis suggested that psychotherapy as a class of treatment for IBS is modestly effective when compared to wait list control conditions, but not necessarily superior to active control conditions (Lackner et al., 2004). Results from two systematic reviews (Ford et al., 2009; Zijdenbos, de Wit, van der Heijden, Rubin, & Quartero, 2009) suggest that psychological interventions may be slightly superior to usual care or wait list controls condition (Zijdenbos et al.) and that psychological therapies are likely comparable to use of antidepressants in the treatment of IBS (106) – however, psychological and medical therapy have never been compared directly. Three broad classes of psychotherapy have demonstrated efficacy via RCTs – these include brief psychodynamic therapy, gut-directed hypnotherapy, and cognitive-behavior therapy.

10.5.3.1 Brief Psychodynamic Therapy for IBS

Brief psychodynamic therapy for IBS involves helping the patient develop insight into their experiences with IBS, including relationships with others, and to identify feelings about their illness. RCTs from independent groups have supported this treatment approach (Guthrie, Creed, Dawson, & Tomenson, 1993; Hislop, 1980; Svedlund, 1983; Svedlund, Sjodin, Ottosson, & Dotevall, 1983), especially in the case of interpersonal difficulties (Hyphantis, Guthrie, Tomenson, & Creed, 2009) and somatization (Creed et al., 2008), both of which are common to this patient group (Choung, Locke, Zinsmeister, Schleck, & Talley, 2009; Jones et al., 2006; Lackner & Gurtman, 2005; Riedl et al., 2008). Further, results from a cost-effectiveness study suggested that interpersonal psychotherapy was equivalent to paroxetine in reducing IBS symptoms (Creed et al., 2003).

10.5.3.2 Gut-Directed Hypnotherapy

Gut-directed hypnotherapy is an effective self-management technique for IBS, particularly in refractory cases (Blanchard, 2001; Galovski & Blanchard, 2002; Miller & Whorwell, 2009). Two models of gut-directed hypnotherapy have been put forth, the Manchester Model (Whorwell, 2006) and the North Carolina Protocol (Palsson, 2006).[2] Both have demonstrated efficacy; patient preference and clinician judgment should inform protocol choice. In a study examining at the efficacy of hypnosis on refractory IBS, Whorwell and colleagues (Whorwell, Prior, & Faragher, 1984) observed significant reductions in abdominal pain, bloating, and dysfunctional bowel habits for the treatment group beyond that of the two control arms (medication placebo and supportive therapy). In a somewhat larger sample of refractory IBS patients, 95% of cases had minimal to no symptoms following a hypnosis intervention compared to wait list control (Whorwell, Prior, & Colgan, 1987). Several other case studies and RCTs (Gonsalkorale, Miller, Afzal, & Whorwell, 2003; Lea et al., 2003; Palsson et al., 2002; Palsson, Turner, & Whitehead, 2006; Palsson & Whitehead, 2002) support the efficacy of gut-directed hypnotherapy. Underlying mechanisms of hypnosis remain unknown, but reductions in rectal sensitivity (Lea et al., 2003), somatization and depression (Palsson et al., 2002), and cognitive change have been reported (Gonsalkorale, Toner, & Whorwell, 2004). Further, gut-directed hypnotherapy seems to have an effect on both colonic and noncolonic symptoms (Whorwell, 2008) and has maintained its effects up to 5 years posttreatment (Gonsalkorale et al., 2003). The typical course of gut-directed hypnotherapy is between 7 and 12 weekly to biweekly hour-long sessions. Therapists administering gut-directed hypnotherapy must be trained in hypnosis and competent in the psychological treatment of IBS more generally.

10.5.3.3 Cognitive-Behavioral Therapy

Cognitive behavior therapy (CBT) is the most extensively tested and efficacious form of psychotherapy for IBS (Lackner et al., 2004; Mayer, 2008). There is also some preliminary data suggesting that cognitive therapy for IBS is associated with

[2] The North Carolina Protocol can be obtained by licensed therapists through www.ibshypnosis.com.

limbic system changes as evidenced with brain imaging (Lackner et al., 2006). As a collaborative, goal-oriented, and problem-focused psychotherapeutic intervention, CBT for IBS targets maladaptive cognitions and associated behaviors, particularly as they relate to the experience of physical symptoms and their impact on QOL (Blanchard et al., 2007; Lackner et al., 2007, 2008). Treatment is applied within 8–10 weeks in a multicomponent fashion. Treatment may include a variety of established techniques such as relaxation training, exposure, reducing behavioral avoidance, problem-solving, coping, stress management, assertiveness training, and cognitive monitoring, restructuring, and reframing.

CBT for IBS has yielded fairly consistent results favoring CBT over control conditions with regard to anxiety (Bennett & Wilkinson, 1985), bowel symptoms (Neff & Blanchard, 1987; Lynch et al., 2008), reducing depression and perceived stress (Lynch et al., 2008), and reducing pain and bowel distress, depression, negative self-talk, and increasing the use of positive self-talk (Greene & Blanchard, 1994). Durability of CBT was also noted in a RCT for both CBT and medical control group on stomach pain, constipation, irritability, and headache; the only significant group difference was that the CBT group showed improvement with respect to avoidance behaviors (Corney, Stanton, Newell, Clare, & Fairclough, 1991).

Cognitive behavior therapy (CBT) is the most well-supported behavioral treatment for IBS to date, although both hypnotherapy and interpersonal psychotherapy have also demonstrated efficacy in certain patient groups. No study to our knowledge has examined patient preference for type of behavioral intervention in IBS. For example, it would be interesting to know whether gut-directed hypnotherapy might be as appealing as CBT with nearly as much evidence. Further, data are insufficient to answer questions around treatment matching and/or the role of clinical judgment in choice of approach to IBS. When considering co-morbidity, the clinician may choose CBT over other interventions given its flexibility across psychiatric disorders. However, in cases where IBS and a co-morbid psychiatric disorder should be treated independently, gut-directed hypnotherapy may be an excellent adjunct. Finally, in the case of trauma history without posttraumatic stress disorder (PTSD), interpersonal therapy for IBS may be particularly useful. Some patients in a psychologist's treatment center will not be interested in traditional psychotherapy. In these cases, gut-directed hypnotherapy can be a compromise between an IBS-directed intervention and a broader psychological approach.

10.6 Psychiatric Co-morbidities of IBS

IBS is often associated with co-morbid psychiatric disorders, the most common being depression and generalized anxiety disorder (GAD) (Blanchard et al., 2004). Anxiety disorders as a group are the most common Axis I disorder, present in about 50% of patients with IBS, followed by mood disorders (Blanchard, 2000; Blanchard, Keefer, Payne, Turner, & Galovski, 2002; Ford, 2009) and Somatization Disorders

Table 10.1 Lifetime prevalence of psychiatric co-morbidity in IBS

DSM-IV axis I disorder	Lifetime prevalence in IBS
Mood disorders	34%
Major depressive disorder	12–28%
Dysthymic disorder	7%
Bipolar disorder	Unknown
Anxiety disorders	58%
Panic disorder	15–41%
Specific phobia	13%
Social phobia	7–26%
Obsessive-compulsive disorder	35%
Posttraumatic stress disorder	10–12%
Generalized anxiety disorder	4–58%
Somatoform disorders	15%
Somatization disorder	3–25%
Conversion disorder	Unknown
Pain disorder	13%
Hypochondriasis	Unknown
Body dysmorphic disorder	Unknown

Ballenger et al. (2001); Blanchard et al. (1990); Canavan, Bennett, Feely, O'Morain, & O'Connor (2009); Choung et al. (2009); Dewsnap, Gomborone, Libby, & Farthing (1996); Ford (2009); Gros, Antony, McCabe, & Swinson (2009); Guthrie, Creed, & Whorwell (1990); Irwin et al. (1996); Kirmayer, Robbins, Dworkind, & Yaffe (1993); Lee et al. (2009); Lydiard, Fosset, Marsh, & Ballenger (1993); Masand et al. (1995, 2006); Miller et al. (2001); North & Alpers (2000); North, Alpers, Thompson, & Spitznagel (1996); North et al. (2004); Porcelli, Leandro, & De Carne (1998); Riedl et al. (2008); Sykes et al. (2003); Whitehead et al. (2002)

(Riedl et al., 2008). Most of the evidence points to the stability of co-morbid Axis I disorders over time, with an onset before the occurrence of IBS and a persistence of symptoms even after IBS has improved (Sykes et al., 2003). Psychotherapy for IBS tends to work most effectively when psychiatric co-morbidity is absent (Reme, Kennedy, Jones, Darnley, & Chalder, 2010). Current recommendations for treatment of IBS and co-morbid psychiatric diagnoses are to treat them independently while acknowledging that they impact each other (North, Hong, & Alpers, 2007). See Table 10.1 for the most recent estimates of the lifetime prevalence of co-morbid IBS and psychiatric diagnosis.

10.6.1 IBS and Depression

Numerous studies have documented the association between IBS and depression (Addolorato et al., 2008; Kovacs & Kovacs, 2007b; Sugaya, Kaiya, Kumano, & Nomura, 2008; Sugaya & Nomura, 2008), which occurs in about 10% of patients with IBS (Blanchard et al., 2002). In an age- and gender-matched sample of patients with IBS and IBD and healthy controls, IBS and IBD patients had higher depressive and anxiety symptoms compared to controls, with IBS patients reporting the most symptoms (Kovacs & Kovacs, 2007a). A recent study of primary care patients suggested an overlap of 27% between GI disorders and clinical depression (Addolorato et al., 2008). In an epidemiological study of more than 3,000 community subjects, the estimated prevalence of major depressive disorder using symptom cut-off scores was 17%, with 54% of those with self-reported depressive symptoms of low mood and anhedonia reporting frequent abdominal pain, diarrhea, constipation, dyspepsia, or IBS symptoms (Hillila, Hamalainen, Heikkinen, & Farkkila, 2008).

10.6.1.1 Assessment

Evaluation for depression should begin with a clinical interview to determine if diagnostic criteria are met and in what context. Additional screening via standardized measures is also recommended. The Beck Depression Inventory (BDI-II) (Beck, Steer, & Brown, 1996) is a widely used tool to supplement diagnosis of depression within clinical practice. However, when diagnosing depression in patients with IBS, the therapist may also want to use a measure that clearly differentiates depression from somatic symptoms. For example, alternative measures to the BDI-II that are more useful in medical populations include the Hospital Anxiety and Depression Index (HADS) (Zigmond & Snaith, 1983) and the Brief Symptom Inventory-18 (BSI-18) (Derogatis, 2000; Derogatis & Melisaratos, 1983). Both the HADS and the BSI-18 provide subscale scores of depression and anxiety. The BSI-18 also provides a separate subscale to gauge the patient's level of somatization. IBS patients should be screened for current or past suicidal ideation given the high association between suicide and chronic pain conditions (Ratcliffe, Enns, Belik, & Sareen, 2008).

Suicidal ideation has been estimated to be present in between 15 and 38% of patients with IBS and has been linked to hopelessness associated with symptom severity, interference with life, and inadequacy of treatment (Miller, Hopkins, & Whorwell, 2004).

The extent to which IBS symptoms contribute to the patient's depression, including cognitions about their illness and the associated emotions and behaviors, is an important component of assessment when depression and IBS are co-morbid. For example, IBS patients appear to have more dysfunctional attitudes and depressogenic coping styles when compared to IBD and other control groups (Kovacs & Kovacs, 2007b). Further, in a large sample of college students with IBS, depression was negatively correlated with perceptions of the controllability of GI symptoms (Sugaya & Nomura, 2008).

10.6.1.2 Treatment

Treatment of depression in the IBS patient is dependent on the severity and duration of the depressive symptoms and should follow standard evidence-based depression treatment guidelines which include a combined approach of pharmacotherapy and psychotherapy (Davidson, 2010; Isometsa et al., 2009). No studies have tested interventions specifically targeting co-morbid depression and IBS. However, interpersonal psychodynamic therapy, cognitive-behavioral therapy, and hypnotherapy have all demonstrated reductions in depressive and anxiety symptoms when they were present in IBS outcome studies (Kearney & Brown-Chang, 2008; Lackner et al., 2004); however, improvements in bowel symptoms appear to be independent from improvement in psychological distress (Lackner et al., 2007).

Cognitive behavior strategies to treat depression in IBS patients include cognitive restructuring of negative automatic thoughts about their illness, activity scheduling and reduction of rumination and other avoidance behaviors, and identification of core beliefs as they relate to the patient's understanding of having a chronic, incurable condition.

Antidepressant medication, often prescribed in low dose for IBS management (Clouse, 1994), may be indicated for co-morbid depression with dosing commensurate with the treatment for depression. This is particularly a desirable option for patients who are not interested in psychotherapy.

Examples of Maladaptive Core Beliefs in IBS:

Patients with a *need for approval* will experience stress over their symptoms largely because they feel they are inconveniencing others.

> I don't want to offend Rachel by not eating her homemade lasagna, even though I know it will make me sick.

Patients with a *sense of overresponsibility* experience stress around the unpredictable and uncontrollable nature of symptoms, expressing anxiety about their performance suffering when they are sick, at work, with parenting or family.

> I don't want to say yes to the vacation because if I can't go, I'll ruin it for everyone

Perfectionism is particularly problematic in this population as it has the most chance of alienating care providers and limits a patient's ability to accept the nature of IBS. Perfectionists also tend to blame themselves or others for continued symptoms.

> I can't believe the doctor missed a polyp during my colonoscopy (outward focus) or I ate something I shouldn't have and now I am paying for it (inward focus)

Group therapy may also be a useful approach to treating co-morbid depression and IBS. To reduce cost and resources associated with individual psychotherapy, nurse-led patient education groups and community support groups are often a useful way to engage patients in self-management of their illness and have demonstrated some efficacy in reducing IBS symptoms and improving QOL in RCTs (Colwell, Prather, Phillips, & Zinsmeister, 1998; Hungin, 2006; Saito et al., 2004). Social support may be operating in these programs; IBS patients often have difficulty finding support for their symptoms, which can also influence their symptom experience (Lackner & Gurtman, 2005; Lackner et al., 2010). IBS also has many characteristics that make it susceptible to stigmatization, including its unalterable course, limited treatment options, lack of clear etiology, unpredictability and uncontrollability, social disruption of bowel disorders, and an association with psychopathology. Patients also report feelings that IBS is not taken seriously and is poorly understood and perceive that others imply that their symptoms are their fault or are "all in their head" (Jones et al., 2009). Approximately half of patients with IBS perceive themselves as being stigmatized due to their condition, with the most perceived stigma coming from coworkers and employers, followed by healthcare providers and friends (Jones et al., 2009). Although not previously investigated, social support groups may help with reducing shame and stigma associated with a chronic bowel disorder.

10.6.1.3 Clinical Considerations

In cases where IBS is determined to be the main source of a patient's depression, treatment might be most effective if IBS symptoms are targeted first. Symptoms of depression associated with IBS might include social withdrawal and isolation, perceived stigma, feelings of hopelessness about successfully managing their condition, and loss of roles or change in personal identity (e.g., adopting the sick role). The three most common core beliefs reported among IBS patients are (1) need for approval, (2) feelings of overresponsibility, and (3) perfectionism (Lackner et al., 2008). However, depression may not always be entirely related to or at all related to IBS, so it is important to evaluate all potential sources of depressive symptoms and the role of IBS in those symptoms.

10.6.2 IBS and Anxiety Disorders

10.6.2.1 Generalized Anxiety Disorder

The most common anxiety disorder among patients with IBS is GAD, estimated to occur in as many as 58% of patients (Blanchard, Scharff, Schwarz, Suls, & Barlow, 1990; Ford, 2009; Lee et al., 2009). Worry and intolerance of uncertainty are significant predictors of IBS symptom onset and maintenance (Keefer et al., 2005). Although co-morbid GAD is often present prior to the diagnosis of IBS (Sykes et al., 2003), the predisposition to chronic worry may be directed toward IBS symptoms, with patients focusing on the possibility that they have a more serious illness and that their symptoms are out of their control (Crane & Martin, 2002). Because IBS is often unpredictable and can be difficult to treat, intolerance to uncertainty can exacerbate worry, thereby increasing anxiety and IBS symptoms. The result may be a self-perpetuating cycle of anticipatory anxiety about having IBS symptoms, symptom hypersensitivity, increased anxiety and autonomic nervous system arousal, and increased IBS symptoms. Worries may differ for patients depending on their predominant symptom type (Keefer et al., 2005). Patients with constipation are more likely to exhibit socially focused worries such as spending too much time in the bathroom, passing gas, or appearing bloated. They may also fixate on the timing of their next bowel movement or worry about whether or not they should use a laxative. Diarrhea-predominant patients may be more worried about having a bowel accident, becoming dehydrated, or eating out. They may also express concern that their diarrhea is indicative of a parasite or other pathologic process (Keefer et al.).

Assessment

Evaluating anxiety disorders in IBS patients may be done via diagnostic interview and supplemented with standardized measures such as the Beck Anxiety Inventory (BAI) (Beck, Epstein, Brown, & Steer, 1988), the Hospital Anxiety and Depression Scale (HADS) (Zigmond & Snaith, 1983), or the Brief Symptom Inventory-18 (Derogatis, 2000). As with depression, understanding the relationship between IBS symptoms and anxiety is vital. Because IBS patients have a tendency for chronic worry and intolerance of uncertainty prior to their diagnosis, the clinician should obtain a thorough history of sources of anxiety and its symptoms. Many IBS patients will describe themselves as chronic worriers, but may not associate this worry with their condition.

The Penn State Worry Questionnaire (PSWQ) (Meyer, Miller, Metzger, & Borkovec, 1990) is an instrument that can be helpful in measuring the degree of generalized worry vs. IBS-specific worry. Worry has been linked with affective experience (as opposed to sensory) of pain and suffering in patients with IBS, with patients who experience uncontrollable worry, commonly seen in GAD, experiencing the most suffering (Lackner & Quigley, 2005). Interestingly, catastrophizing appears to fully mediate the association between worry and painful suffering in IBS patients (Lackner & Quigley), underscoring the need to assess and address this cognitive distortion early in treatment.

Treatment

No studies have tested interventions specifically targeting co-morbid GAD and IBS, thus psychological treatment of GAD in IBS patients should follow standard evidence-based anxiety treatment guidelines for GAD (Cape, Whittington, Buszewicz, Wallace, & Underwood, 2010). Many patients with co-morbid GAD and IBS find value in initially targeting the source and nature of worry about IBS symptoms. Because of the role of the heightened stress response in IBS physiology, using relaxation techniques to reduce arousal is critical in treating anxiety in these patients. In IBS, almost all relaxation techniques are beneficial and have adequate evidence to support themselves as stand-alone treatments, including meditation (Keefer & Blanchard, 2001), progressive muscle relaxation (Blanchard, Greene, Scharff, & Schwarz-McMorris, 1993), and EMG biofeedback (Radnitz & Blanchard, 1988).

Studies suggests that IBS patients tend to approach all problems in the same way regardless of whether they are controllable or uncontrollable (Cheng, Chan, Hui, & Lam, 2003). This inflexibility and inability to adapt behavior facilitates unhelpful worry and experiential avoidance. One study demonstrated that IBS patients were unique in comparison to other chronic illnesses (e.g., arthritis) and healthy controls in this regard (Cheng et al.); hence, new CBT protocols for IBS rely heavily on flexible problem solving (Lackner et al., 2008). Rather than having a problem-solving deficit, patients with IBS often have a mismatch between solvability of a problem and their chosen problem-solving strategy. A subset of patients may apply faulty problem solving to their IBS in general, becoming fixated on a "cure" or solution such as diet, medication, or procedures at the expense of self-management. Given the high rate of co-morbidity and intertwining symptomatology, further research is needed on the optimal approach to treating co-morbid GAD and IBS.

10.6.2.2 Panic Disorder

The prevalence of panic disorder in IBS patients is estimated to be between 15 and 41%, with a positive correlation between the severity of panic disorder and IBS symptoms (Lydiard et al., 1994). Recent evidence suggests that health anxiety in particular may be a vulnerability factor for the development of Panic Disorder (Rudaz, Craske, Becker, Ledermann, & Margraf, 2010). Individuals with IBS and panic symptoms share the tendency to catastrophize normal bodily sensations. This tendency leads to a heightened stress response (including GI distress), increased anxiety and/or depression, and a higher likelihood of selecting other maladaptive-coping strategies (Folkman, Lazarus, Dunkel-Schetter, DeLongis, & Gruen, 1986; Folkman, Lazarus, Gruen, & DeLongis, 1986; Lazarus, DeLongis, Folkman, & Gruen, 1985). As with generalized anxiety, the subtype of IBS plays a role in the risk of co-morbid panic disorder with individuals with diarrhea-predominant IBS at greater risk of panic symptoms and subsequent avoidance behavior. IBS combined with panic symptoms or disorder often leads to the most significant impairments in QOL including increased social withdrawal, feelings of isolation, and a sense of helplessness and hopelessness in some cases (Lydiard et al., 1994).

Assessment

Evaluating IBS patients for panic disorder should be done via diagnostic interview, including obtaining a thorough history of panic attack onset, symptoms, duration, and severity and confirming that panic symptoms are not solely GI in nature (e.g., nausea, vomiting, diarrhea, abdominal cramps). IBS patients often report increased levels of visceral sensitivity, or a heightened awareness of common GI symptoms (bowel sounds, hunger pangs, bloating) typically ignored by people who do not have IBS. Enhanced perceptual responses to normal visceral events can lead to symptom-specific anxiety and selective attention to these sensations (Whitehead & Palsson, 1998). Subsequently, this process will promote fear of visceral stimuli and mislabeling of internal sensations as dangerous, a construct known as visceral sensitivity. The Visceral Sensitivity Index (VSI) is designed to measure increased pain sensitivity and GI symptom-specific anxiety (Labus et al., 2004). Anxiety specific to GI symptoms consists of: (1) obsessive or catastrophic thoughts; (2) learned fear responses; (3) increased vigilance and sensitivity; and (4) avoidance behaviors. The VSI provides an overall score of visceral sensitivity that reflects these areas of anxiety often found in IBS patients. High visceral sensitivity associated with IBS is further supported in brain imaging studies (Mayer et al., 2009; Naliboff et al., 2006, 2008).

Individuals with IBS may have such a heightened awareness of sensations from their digestive tract that they become unable to divert their attention to other things and consequently become fixated on gut sensations and attempts to understand what dietary or other environmental factors may contribute to their presence. This can lead to severe dietary restrictions or other behaviors that may appear out of proportion to reported symptom severity (Whitehead et al., 2002; Whitehead & Palsson, 1998). Often these patients will express frustration in others' inability to fully understand the alarming nature of these sensations, which can further contribute to alienation and isolation (Whitehead et al., 2002).

Sensitivity to bodily sensations can make treatment of IBS patients challenging. For example, the sensations of increased fullness, bloating, or looser stools associated with increased fiber intake may be perceived as a worsening of IBS or an intolerance of the intervention. There is also evidence that the subtype of IBS may influence the relationship between cognitive appraisals and degree of reported negative emotions, symptom exacerbation, and psychological distress. Specifically, a patient with IBS-D is more likely than an IBS-C patient to demonstrate increased anxiety related to negative cognitive appraisals of their illness (Sugaya & Nomura, 2008).

Treatment

Psychological treatment of panic disorder in IBS patients should follow standard evidence-based treatment guidelines which include CBT featuring interoceptive exposure (Barlow, Gorman, Shear, & Woods, 2000; Cape et al., 2010). Evidence suggests that when therapists are overly flexible in the administration of panic disorder techniques, simultaneously addressing more than one problem or implementing more than one technique in a session, efficacy of exposure therapy may be reduced (Craske et al., 2007).Therefore, panic should be addressed before IBS. However, evidence shows that treatment for panic disorder may well have a positive effect on IBS (Tsao, Mystkowski, Zucker, & Craske, 2005) and IBS is unlikely to interfere with the efficacy of panic disorder treatment (Allen et al., 2010).

Other targets in treatment of co-morbid IBS and panic with agoraphobia might include negative prediction, also called probability overestimation. Probability overestimation is the tendency to overestimate the likelihood that a negative event will occur, treating it as probable regardless of its actual likelihood. IBS patients overestimate the likelihood of symptoms occurring or causing them negative consequences (Lackner et al., 2007, 2008).

Another noteworthy characteristic of co-morbid panic and IBS is catastrophizing, that is, when patients maximize the awfulness or potential awfulness of a situation while simultaneously minimizing their ability to cope. IBS patients in particular have a tendency to perceive the consequences of having symptoms as much worse than they actually are (Lackner & Quigley, 2005). Catastrophization of the social and functional ramifications of GI symptoms is higher in IBS patients than in those with other chronic GI conditions such as IBD (Lackner & Quigley), underscoring the central role of catastrophizing in the manifestation of IBS behavior.

10.6.2.3 Posttraumatic Stress Disorder

Between 10 and 30% of patients with IBS have met diagnostic criteria for lifetime PTSD (Irwin et al., 1996). A recent study demonstrated a substantially increased risk for IBS among female veterans with PTSD (Savas et al., 2009). Trauma is not typically the cause of IBS symptoms; however, unresolved PTSD can contribute to worsening of IBS symptoms due to the chronic hyperarousal of the autonomic nervous system associated with PTSD.

Assessment

Diagnostic interview will be necessary to make the formal diagnosis of PTSD. Screening for PTSD in IBS patients is important because relaxation strategies such as gut-directed hypnotherapy may be contraindicated in individuals with a significant trauma history given the degree of dissociation required to achieve the hypnotic state (Mott & Hammond, 1998). Several screening measures are available including the Primary Care PTSD Screen (PC-PTSD), which is recommended for medical and other settings that are not conducive to performing complete diagnostic interviews (Prins et al., 2004). This is a 4-item measure that identifies core symptoms associated with PTSD (nightmares, avoidance behaviors, hypervigilance, and emotional numbing), and although it does not provide a diagnosis of PTSD, it can be used to inform referrals.

As is the case in many physical disorders, early adverse life experiences can predispose an individual to IBS (Chitkara et al., 2008) through multiple pathways including central response systems, such as the HPA axis (Videlock et al., 2009), psychological distress, and somatization (Choung et al., 2009; Savas et al., 2009). Childhood physical and sexual abuse has been reported in 20–60% of patients with IBS, with this particular subset of patients reporting more severe symptoms, increased healthcare use (Leserman, Drossman, & Hu, 1998; Leserman et al., 1996), and a higher rate of psychiatric co-morbidity (Blanchard et al., 2004). Sexual abuse may lower the threshold at which people experience symptoms or, alternatively, increase intestinal motility (Drossman, 1997; Drossman et al., 1990; Drossman, Talley, Olden, & Barreiro, 1995). There is also evidence that IBS and early abuse may be connected through the general sensitization of the central nervous system (Ringel et al., 2003; Scarinci et al., 1994).

Treatment

Treatment of co-morbid PTSD and IBS should follow evidence-based treatment guidelines, which include cognitive processing therapy (Foa et al., 2005; Resick et al., 2008; Resick, Nishith, Weaver, Astin, & Feuer, 2002; Resick & Schnicke, 1992) and/or prolonged exposure (Foa et al., 2005; Foa & Rauch, 2004). Interestingly, the subset of IBS patients with a trauma history generally have had a positive response to interpersonal psychodynamic psychotherapy for their IBS (Creed et al., 2005), although a direct comparison between therapies has not been made.

10.6.2.4 Somatization Disorders

Despite the overlap of IBS with several other medical complaints, IBS should not be considered a somatization disorder (Riedl et al., 2008). Somatization disorders are characterized by a pathological process in which a person reports multiple symptoms of unknown or limited physiological etiology across several organ systems over an extended period of time (DSM-IV-TR; Bankier et al., 2000). It is not uncommon for individuals with features of somatization to make inaccurate attributions about symptoms or to seek medical attention for benign medical problems (Lipowski, 1988). Co-morbidity between IBS and somatization disorders is estimated to be as high as 25% (Lydiard et al., 1993; Miller et al., 2001), considerably higher than the general population (Whitehead, Palsson, Levy, Feld, Turner, & Von Korff, 2007). In an effort to classify and understand IBS, researchers have evaluated it within the broader context of physical symptoms that are "medically unexplained" or "disproportionate" to the severity of an underlying medical disorder – a concept central to the diagnosis of somatoform disorder. Due to the nature of functional conditions such as IBS, which often lack satisfactory treatment by medical providers, patients may solicit medical advice from multiple specialist physicians. This often leads to unnecessary (and repeated) testing, hospitalizations, or cumulative diagnoses that may only serve to further enhance the individual's level of health-related anxiety (Creed et al., 2008; Riedl et al., 2008). IBS patients are often likely to report other somatic conditions such as chronic headaches, fibromyalgia, chronic fatigue syndrome, and chronic pelvic pain (Riedl et al.). Despite this, somatization disorder does not entirely explain the overlap of IBS with these other somatic conditions.

Assessment

Screening for somatization, if suspected, should include questions about the history and duration of the multiple, unexplained medical complaints as these are an important diagnostic criterion. The therapist should also seek to understand the patterns of illness behaviors and possible secondary gains for identifying with and remaining in the sick role. Illness behavior can be adaptive (asking for help when you need it;

calling an ambulance if something is life-threatening) or maladaptive (staying home sick from school when you have a pimple). Maladaptive illness behavior has been identified in a subset of patients with IBS and has origins in childhood (Levy et al., 2001, 2004). Alexithymia or the inability to identify, experience, and express emotions has also been linked to somatization and illness behavior (Taylor, Parker, Bagby, & Acklin, 1992) with some data to support its role in IBS (Jones et al., 2006). The Toronto Alexithymia Scale (TAS-20) (Taylor, Bagby, & Parker, 1992) is a useful measure of alexithymia in IBS patients. The BSI-18 (Derogatis, 2000) is another useful measure to use to gauge degree of somatization, though it is not diagnostic of somatization disorder.

Treatment

Evidence-based treatments for somatization disorder are similar to those for IBS and include cognitive therapy to address catastrophic thinking about physical sensations; behavioral interventions to gradually increase activities and reduce social withdrawal; communication skills training to help the patient work better with their medical providers and improve interpersonal relationships that may be strained as a result of chronic medical complaints; and emotion-focused therapy to help the patient better identify and understand emotional responses should alexithymia be present (Kroenke & Swindle, 2000). The goal of treatment when somatization occurs with IBS is to control illness behaviors that are excessive and detrimental to the patient's QOL. Treatment should broadly focus on somatic behaviors rather than IBS symptoms exclusively. Care should be taken to ensure that the patient does not feel stigmatized by being given the message that "it's all in your head" (Jones et al., 2009). Treatment should focus on reducing the interference in personal activities and responsibilities, such as school, work, family, or social life. It is also important to address the role of GI symptom anxiety and hypersensitivity in the development and maintenance of somatization disorder (Labus, Mayer, Chang, Bolus, & Naliboff, 2007).

10.6.2.5 Personality Disorders

Although a fair amount of research has explored personality characteristics and IBS, most notably neuroticism (Farnam, Somi, Sarami, & Farhang, 2008; Tkalcic, Hauser, & Stimac, 2010), only one study to our knowledge has examined the prevalence of Axis II personality disorders in IBS (E. B. Blanchard et al., 2004). Findings suggested that as many as 30% of patients meet criteria for an DSM-IV criteria for an Axis II disorder following a structured clinical interview, with the most common being Cluster C disorders: obsessive-compulsive (12%) and avoidant personality disorder (5%). Fewer patients met criteria for Cluster A personality disorder (8%), and only very few presented with Cluster B personality disorder (1.5%). The primary limitation of this study was that patients were self-referred to psychological treatment for their IBS and therefore the prevalence of Axis II disorders may be overestimated – however, these findings may have important treatment implications. To date, no trials have examined the efficacy of treatments for co-morbid IBS and a personality disorder. As with other co-morbidities, personality disorders should be treated independently of IBS while acknowledging that they may influence each other with respect to severity or outcome.

10.7 Summary and Conclusions

IBS is a common, painful GI condition associated with several common psychiatric co-morbidities and often significant psychological distress (Whitehead et al., 2007). The most common psychiatric co-morbidities are anxiety disorders, somatization, and mood disorders. Very little research has tested the efficacy of psychological interventions specifically in co-morbid samples. Psychological interventions, described above, have demonstrated modest efficacy in treating IBS (Kearney & Brown-Chang, 2008). This is not surprising given the overlap in cognitive and affective processes between patients with IBS and patients with mood and anxiety disorders. In fact, psychotherapy for both conditions targets hyperarousal, cognitive distortions, problem solving, remediation of skills deficits, and/or interpersonal relationship difficulties.

In most cases, it is recommended that co-morbid conditions be treated independently unless there is an apparent relationship between the two (e.g., one causes the other). Further, a reasonable amount of evidence suggests that high psychological distress often weakens the efficacy of psychological interventions for IBS symptoms. This recommendation plays out most intuitively in panic disorder when: (1) the presence of panic attacks is likely to make IBS worse while the presence of IBS will not likely make treatment for panic more difficult (Roy-Byrne et al., 1999); (2) when therapists administer interoceptive exposure while simultaneously addressing other co-morbidities in the session, efficacy of exposure therapy may be reduced (Craske et al., 2007); and (3) treatment of panic disorder will likely improve IBS concomitantly (Craske et al.). PTSD is another co-morbidity in which treating the psychiatric disorder first will demonstrate an improvement in IBS, but not vice versa.

When IBS seems to be a central feature in the co-morbidity, psychotherapy for IBS may be helpful for both disorders. For example, if depression is caused by the isolation and behavioral avoidance associated with IBS, then addressing IBS may help to improve depressive symptoms. Alternatively, if IBS is one aspect of a disorder that has multiple determinants, then treatment blending may be helpful. For example, when a patient with GAD presents with IBS, the clinician might choose to focus on GI symptom worries initially, blending CBT strategies of IBS with those of GAD. More research is needed on the optimal approach to treating IBS in the context of the various psychiatric co-morbidities.

10.8 Books for Therapists and Patients

Gershon, M. D. (1998). *The second brain: A groundbreaking new understanding of nervous disorders of the stomach and intestine* (p. 312). New York: HarperCollins.

Lackner, J. M. (2007). *Controlling IBS the drug-free way: A 10-step plan for symptom relief* (p. 240). New York: STC Healthy Living.

Acknowledgments The authors would like to thank Darren M. Brenner, MD, and Bethany Doerfler, RD, for their assistance ensuring accuracy with respect to the medical and dietary information reviewed in this chapter.

References

Addolorato, G., Mirijello, A., D'Angelo, C., Leggio, L., Ferrulli, A., Abenavoli, L., et al. (2008). State and trait anxiety and depression in patients affected by gastrointestinal diseases: Psychometric evaluation of 1641 patients referred to an internal medicine outpatient setting. *International Journal of Clinical Practice, 62*(7), 1063–1069.

Allen, L. B., White, K. S., Barlow, D. H., Shear, M. K., Gorman, J. M., & Woods, S. W. (2010). Cognitive-behavior therapy (CBT) for panic disorder: Relationship of anxiety and depression comorbidity with treatment outcome. *Journal of Psychopathology and Behavioral Assessment, 32*(2), 185–192.

Ballenger, J., Davidson, J. R., Lecrubier, Y., Nutt, D. J., Lydiard, R. B., & Mayer, E. A. (2001). Consensus statement on depression, anxiety, and functional gastrointestinal disorders. *Journal of Clinical Psychiatry, 62*(Suppl 8), 48–51.

Bankier, B., Aigner, M., Krones, S., & Bach, M. (2000). Screening for DSM-IV somatoform disorders in chronic pain patients, *Psychopathology, 33*(3), 115–118.

Barlow, D. H., Gorman, J. M., Shear, M. K., & Woods, S. W. (2000). Cognitive-behavioral therapy, imipramine, or their combination for panic disorder: A randomized controlled trial. *JAMA, 283*(19), 2529–2536.

Beck, A., Steer, R. A., & Brown, G. K. (1996). *Beck Depression Inventory* (2nd ed.). San Antonio: The Psychological Corporation.

Beck, A. T., Epstein, N., Brown, G., & Steer, R. A. (1988). An inventory for measuring clinical anxiety: Psychometric properties. *Journal of Consulting and Clinical Psychology, 56*(6), 893–897.

Bennett, P., & Wilkinson, S. (1985). A comparison of psychological and medical treatment of the irritable bowel syndrome. *British Journal of Clinical Psychology, 24*(Pt 3), 215–216.

Blanchard, E. (2000). *Irritable bowel syndrome: Psychosocial assessment and treatment*. Washington DC: American Psychological Association.

Blanchard, E. (2001). *Irritable bowel syndrome: Psychosocial assessment and treatment*. Washington: American Psychological Association.

Blanchard, E., Lackner, J. M., Jaccard, J., Rowell, D., Carosella, A. M., Powell, C., et al. (2008). The role of stress in symptom exacerbation among IBS patients. *Journal of Psychosomatic Research, 64*(2), 119–128.

Blanchard, E. B., Greene, B., Scharff, L., & Schwarz-McMorris, S. P. (1993). Relaxation training as a treatment for irritable bowel syndrome. *Biofeedback and Self-Regulation, 18*(3), 125–132.

Blanchard, E. B., Keefer, L., Lackner, J. M., Galovski, T. E., Krasner, S., & Sykes, M. A. (2004). The role of childhood abuse in Axis I and Axis II psychiatric disorders and medical disorders of unknown origin among irritable bowel syndrome patients. *Journal of Psychosomatic Research, 56*(4), 431–436.

Blanchard, E. B., Keefer, L., Payne, A., Turner, S. M., & Galovski, T. E. (2002). Early abuse, psychiatric diagnoses and irritable bowel syndrome. *Behaviour Research and Therapy, 40*(3), 289–298.

Blanchard, E. B., Lackner, J. M., Sanders, K., Krasner, S., Keefer, L., Payne, A., et al. (2007). A controlled evaluation of group cognitive therapy in the treatment of irritable bowel syndrome. *Behaviour Research and Therapy, 45*(4), 633–648.

Blanchard, E. B., Scharff, L., Schwarz, S., Suls, J. M., & Barlow, D. H. (1990). The role of anxiety and depression in the irritable bowel syndrome. *Behavior Research and Therapy, 28*(5), 401–405.

Brenner, D. M., & Chey, W. D. (2009). Bifidobacterium infantis 35624: A novel probiotic for the treatment of irritable bowel syndrome. *Reviews in Gastroenterological Disorders, 9*(1), 7–15.

Brenner, D. M., Moeller, M. J., Chey, W. D., & Schoenfeld, P. S. (2009). The utility of probiotics in the treatment of irritable bowel syndrome: A systematic review. *American Journal of Gastroenterology, 104*(4), 1033–1049; quiz 1050.

Camilleri, M. (2005). Pharmacogenomics and functional gastrointestinal disorders. *Pharmacogenomics, 6*(5), 491–501.

Camilleri, M., & Mayer, E. A. (2009). Developing irritable bowel syndrome guidelines through meta-analyses: Does the emperor really have new clothes? *Gastroenterology, 137*(3), 766–769.

Canavan, J. B., Bennett, K., Feely, J., O'Morain, C. A., & O'Connor, H. J. (2009). Significant psychological morbidity occurs in irritable bowel syndrome: A case-control study using a pharmacy reimbursement database. *Alimentary Pharmacology and Therapeutics, 29*(4), 440–449.

Cape, J., Whittington, C., Buszewicz, M., Wallace, P., & Underwood, L. (2010). Brief psychological therapies for anxiety and depression in primary care: Meta-analysis and meta-regression. *BMC Medicine, 8*(1), 38.

Chassany, O., Marquis, P., Scherrer, B., Read, N. W., Finger, T., Bergmann, J. F., et al. (1999). Validation of a specific quality of life questionnaire for functional digestive disorders. *Gut, 44*(4), 527–533.

Cheng, C., Chan, A. O., Hui, W. M., & Lam, S. K. (2003). Coping strategies, illness perception, anxiety and depression of patients with idiopathic constipation: A population-based study. *Alimentary Pharmacology and Therapeutics, 18*(3), 319–326.

Chey, W., Drossman, D. A., Scott, C., Panas, R. M., & Ueno, R. (2008). What symptoms drive global symptom improvement with lubiprostone in patients with irritable bowel syndrome and constipation: Data from two multicenter, randomized, placebo-controlled trials. *Gastroenterology, 134*, A28.

Chitkara, D. K., Talley, N. J., Schleck, C., Zinsmeister, A. R., Shah, N. D., & Locke, G. R., III. (2009). Recollection of childhood abdominal pain in adults with functional gastrointestinal disorders. *Scandinavian Journal of Gastroenterology, 44*(3), 301–307.

Chitkara, D. K., van Tilburg, M. A., Blois-Martin, N., & Whitehead, W. E. (2008). Early life risk factors that contribute to irritable bowel syndrome in adults: A systematic review. *American Journal of Gastroenterology, 103*(3), 765–774; quiz 775.

Choung, R. S., Locke, G. R., III, Zinsmeister, A. R., Schleck, C. D., & Talley, N. J. (2009). Psychosocial distress and somatic symptoms in community subjects with irritable bowel syndrome: A psychological component is the rule. *American Journal of Gastroenterology, 104*(7), 1772–1779.

Clouse, R. E. (1994). Antidepressants for functional gastrointestinal syndromes. *Digestive Diseases and Sciences, 39*(11), 2352–2363.

Clouse, R. E. (2003). Managing functional bowel disorders from the top down: Lessons from a well-designed treatment trial. *Gastroenterology, 125*(1), 249–253.

Colwell, L. J., Prather, C. M., Phillips, S. F., & Zinsmeister, A. R. (1998). Effects of an irritable bowel syndrome educational class on health-promoting behaviors and symptoms. *American Journal of Gastroenterology, 93*(6), 901–905.

Corney, R. H., Stanton, R., Newell, R., Clare, A., & Fairclough, P. (1991). Behavioural psychotherapy in the treatment of irritable bowel syndrome. *Journal of Psychosomatic Research, 35*(4–5), 461–469.

Crane, C., & Martin, M. (2002). Perceived vulnerability to illness in individuals with irritable bowel syndrome. *Journal of Psychosomatic Research, 53*(6), 1115–1122.

Craske, M. G., Farchione, T. J., Allen, L. B., Barrios, V., Stoyanova, M., & Rose, R. (2007). Cognitive behavioral therapy for panic disorder and comorbidity: More of the same or less of more? *Behaviour Research and Therapy, 45*(6), 1095–1109.

Creed, F., Fernandes, L., Guthrie, E., Palmer, S., Ratcliffe, J., Read, N., et al. (2003). The cost-effectiveness of psychotherapy and paroxetine for severe irritable bowel syndrome. *Gastroenterology, 124*(2), 303–317.

Creed, F., Guthrie, E., Ratcliffe, J., Fernandes, L., Rigby, C., Tomenson, B., et al. (2005). Reported sexual abuse predicts impaired functioning but a good response to psychological treatments in patients with severe irritable bowel syndrome. *Psychosomatic Medicine, 67*(3), 490–499.

Creed, F., Tomenson, B., Guthrie, E., Ratcliffe, J., Fernandes, L., Read, N., et al. (2008). The relationship between somatisation and outcome in patients with severe irritable bowel syndrome. *Journal of Psychosomatic Research, 64*(6), 613–620.

Cremonini, F., & Talley, N. J. (2005). Irritable bowel syndrome: Epidemiology, natural history, health care seeking and emerging risk factors. *Gastroenterology Clinics of North America, 34*(2), 189–204.

Davidson, J. R. (2010). Major depressive disorder treatment guidelines in America and Europe. *Journal of Clinical Psychiatry, 71*(Suppl E1), e04.

Delvaux, M. (2002). Role of visceral sensitivity in the pathophysiology of irritable bowel syndrome. *Gut, 51*(Suppl 1), i67–i71.

Derogatis, L. (2000). *Brief Symptom Inventory 18*. Minneapolis: National Computer Systems Pearson, Inc.

Derogatis, L. R., & Melisaratos, N. (1983). The brief symptom inventory: An introductory report. *Psychological Medicine, 13*, 595–605.

Dewsnap, P., Gomborone, J., Libby, G., & Farthing, M. (1996). The prevalence of symptoms of irritable bowel syndrome among acute psychiatric inpatients with an affective diagnosis. *Psychosomatics, 37*(4), 385–389.

Drossman, D., Camilleri, M., Mayer, E., & Whitehead, W. (2002). AGA technical review on irritable bowel syndrome. *Gastroenterology, 123*, 2108–2131.

Drossman, D. A. (1997). Irritable bowel syndrome and sexual/physical abuse history. *European Journal of Gastroenterology and Hepatology, 9*, 327–330.

Drossman, D. A., Corrazziari, E., Talley, N. J., Thompson, W. G., & Whitehead, W. E. (2006). *The functional gastrointestinal disorders* (3rd ed.). McLean: Degnon Associates.

Drossman, D. A., Leserman, J., Nachman, G., Li, Z., Gluck, H., Toomey, T. C., et al. (1990). Sexual and physical abuse in women with functional or organic gastrointestinal disorders. *Annals of Internal Medicine, 113*, 828–833.

Drossman, D. A., Patrick, D. L., Whitehead, W. E., Toner, B. B., Diamant, N. E., Hu, Y., et al. (2000). Further validation of the IBS-QOL: A disease-specific quality-of-life questionnaire. *American Journal of Gastroenterology, 95*(4), 999–1007.

Drossman, D. A., Talley, N. J., Olden, K. W., & Barreiro, M. A. (1995). Sexual and physical abuse and gastrointesintal illness: Review and recommendations. *Annals of Internal Medicine, 123*(10), 782–794.

Farnam, A., Somi, M. H., Sarami, F., & Farhang, S. (2008). Five personality dimensions in patients with irritable bowel syndrome. *Neuropsychiatric Disease and Treatment, 4*(5), 959–962.

Foa, E. B., Hembree, E. A., Cahill, S. P., Rauch, S. A., Riggs, D. S., Feeny, N. C., et al. (2005). Randomized trial of prolonged exposure for posttraumatic stress disorder with and without cognitive restructuring: Outcome at academic and community clinics. *Journal of Consulting and Clinical Psychology, 73*(5), 953–964.

Foa, E. B., & Rauch, S. A. (2004). Cognitive changes during prolonged exposure versus prolonged exposure plus cognitive restructuring in female assault survivors with posttraumatic stress disorder. *Journal of Consulting and Clinical Psychology, 72*(5), 879–884.

Folkman, S., Lazarus, R. S., Dunkel-Schetter, C., DeLongis, A., & Gruen, R. J. (1986). Dynamics of a stressful encounter: Cognitive appraisal, coping, and encounter outcomes. *Journal of Personality and Social Psychology, 50*(5), 992–1003.

Folkman, S., Lazarus, R. S., Gruen, R. J., & DeLongis, A. (1986). Appraisal, coping, health status, and psychological symptoms. *Journal of Personality and Social Psychology, 50*(3), 571–579.

Ford, A. C. (2009). Generalized anxiety disorder and irritable bowel syndrome. *Alimentary Pharmacology and Therapeutics, 30*(10), 1087–1088; author reply 1088–1089.

Ford, A. C., Talley, N. J., Schoenfeld, P. S., Quigley, E. M., & Moayyedi, P. (2009). Efficacy of antidepressants and psychological therapies in irritable bowel syndrome: Systematic review and meta-analysis. *Gut, 58*(3), 367–378.

Ford, A. C., Talley, N. J., Spiegel, B. M., Foxx-Orenstein, A. E., Schiller, L., Quigley, E. M., et al. (2008). Effect of fibre, antispasmodics, and peppermint oil in the treatment of irritable bowel syndrome: Systematic review and meta-analysis. *British Medical Journal, 337*, a2313.

Fukudo, S., Kanazawa, M., Mizuno, T., Hamaguchi, T., Kano, M., Watanabe, S., et al. (2009). Impact of serotonin transporter gene polymorphism on brain activation by colorectal distention. *NeuroImage, 47*(3), 946–951.

Fukudo, S., Nomura, T., Muranaka, M., & Taguchi, F. (1993). Brain-gut response to stress and cholinergic stimulation in irritable bowel syndrome. A preliminary study. *Journal of Clinical Gastroenterology, 17*(2), 133–141.

Fumi, A. L., & Trexler, K. (2008). Rifaximin treatment for symptoms of irritable bowel syndrome. *The Annals of Pharmacotherapy, 42*(3), 408–412.

Galovski, T. E., & Blanchard, E. B. (2002). Hypnotherapy and refractory irritable bowel syndrome: A single case study. *American Journal of Clinical Hypnosis, 45*(1), 31–37.

Gonsalkorale, W. M., Miller, V., Afzal, A., & Whorwell, P. J. (2003). Long term benefits of hypnotherapy for irritable bowel syndrome. *Gut, 52*(11), 1623–1629.

Gonsalkorale, W. M., Toner, B. B., & Whorwell, P. J. (2004). Cognitive change in patients undergoing hypnotherapy for irritable bowel syndrome. *Journal of Psychosomatic Research, 56*(3), 271–278.

Greene, B., & Blanchard, E. B. (1994). Cognitive therapy for irritable bowel syndrome. *Journal of Consulting and Clinical Psychology, 62*(3), 576–782.

Groll, D., Vanner, S. J., Depew, W. T., DaCosta, L. R., Simon, J. B., Groll, A., et al. (2002). The IBS-36: A new quality of life measure for irritable bowel syndrome. *American Journal of Gastroenterology, 97*(4), 962–971.

Gros, D. F., Antony, M. M., McCabe, R. E., & Swinson, R. P. (2009). Frequency and severity of the symptoms of irritable bowel syndrome across the anxiety disorders and depression. *Journal of Anxiety Disorders, 23*(2), 290–296.

Guthrie, E., Creed, F., Dawson, D., & Tomenson, B. (1993). A randomised controlled trial of psychotherapy in patients with refractory irritable bowel syndrome. *The British Journal of Psychiatry, 163*, 315–321.

Guthrie, E. A., Creed, F. H., & Whorwell, P. J. (1990). Eating disorders in patients with irritable bowel syndrome: A comparison with inflammatory bowel disease and peptic ulceration. *European Journal of Gastroenterology and Hepatology, 2*, 471–473.

Halpert, A., & Drossman, D. (2005). Biopsychosocial issues in irritable bowel syndrome. *Journal of Clinical Gastroenterology, 39*(8), 665–669.

Heitkemper, M., & Jarrett, M. (2008). Irritable bowel syndrome: Does gender matter? *Journal of Psychosomatic Research, 64*(6), 583–587.

Heitkemper, M., Jarrett, M., & Bond, E. F. (2004). Irritable bowel syndrome in women: A common health problem. *The Nursing Clinics of North America, 39*(1), 69–81.

Heizer, W. D., Southern, S., & McGovern, S. (2009). The role of diet in symptoms of irritable bowel syndrome in adults: A narrative review. *Journal of the American Dietetic Association, 109*(7), 1204–1214.

Hillila, M. T., Hamalainen, J., Heikkinen, M. E., & Farkkila, M. A. (2008). Gastrointestinal complaints among subjects with depressive symptoms in the general population. *Alimentary Pharmacology and Therapeutics, 28*(5), 648–654.

Hislop, I. G. (1980). Effect of very brief psychotherapy on the irritable bowel syndrome. *The Medical Journal of Australia, 2*(11), 620–623.

Hungin, A. P. (2006). Self-help interventions in irritable bowel syndrome. *Gut, 55*(5), 603–604.

Hungin, A. P., Chang, L., Locke, G. R., Dennis, E. H., & Barghout, V. (2005). Irritable bowel syndrome in the United States: Prevalence, symptom patterns and impact. *Alimentary Pharmacology and Therapeutics, 21*(11), 1365–1375.

Hungin, A. P., Whorwell, P. J., Tack, J., & Mearin, F. (2003). The prevalence, patterns and impact of irritable bowel syndrome: An international survey of 40,000 subjects. *Alimentary Pharmacology and Therapeutics, 17*(5), 643–650.

Hyphantis, T., Guthrie, E., Tomenson, B., & Creed, F. (2009). Psychodynamic interpersonal therapy and improvement in interpersonal difficulties in people with severe irritable bowel syndrome. *Pain, 145*(1–2), 196–203.

Irwin, C., Falsetti, S. A., Lydiard, R. B., Ballenger, J. C., Brock, C. D., & Brener, W. (1996). Comorbidity of postraumatic stress disorder and irritable bowel syndrome. *The Journal of Clinical Psychiatry, 57*(12), 576–581.

Isometsa, E., Jousilahti, P., Lindfors, O., Luutonen, S., Marttunen, M., Pirkola, S., et al. (2009). [Update on current care guidelines. Depression, current care guideline]. *Duodecim, 125*(16), 1755–1756.

Jones, M. P., Keefer, L., Bratten, J., Taft, T. H., Crowell, M. D., Levy, R., et al. (2009). Development and initial validation of a measure of perceived stigma in irritable bowel syndrome. *Psychology, Health & Medicine, 14*(3), 367–374.

Jones, M. P., Wessinger, S., & Crowell, M. D. (2006). Coping strategies and interpersonal support in patients with irritable bowel syndrome and inflammatory bowel disease. *Clinical Gastroenterology and Hepatology, 4*(4), 474–481.

Kalantar, J. S., Locke, G. R., III, Zinsmeister, A. R., Beighley, C. M., & Talley, N. J. (2003). Familial aggregation of irritable bowel syndrome: A prospective study. *Gut, 52*(12), 1703–1707.

Kearney, D. J., & Brown-Chang, J. (2008). Complementary and alternative medicine for IBS in adults: Mind-body interventions. *Nature Clinical Practice. Gastroenterology & Hepatology, 5*(11), 624–636.

Keefer, L., & Blanchard, E. B. (2001). The effects of relaxation response meditation on the symptoms of irritable bowel syndrome: Results of a controlled treatment study. *Behaviour Research and Therapy, 39*(7), 801–811.

Keefer, L., Sanders, K., Sykes, M. A., Blanchard, E. B., Lackner, J. M., & Krasner, S. (2005). Towards a better understanding of anxiety in irritable bowel syndrome: A preliminary look at worry and intolerance of uncertainty. *Journal of Cognitive Psychotherapy, 19*(2), 163–173.

Kirmayer, L., Robbins, J., Dworkind, M., & Yaffe, M. (1993). Somatization and the reocgnition of depression and anxiety in primary care. *The American Journal of Psychiatry, 150*, 734–741.

Kovacs, Z., & Kovacs, F. (2007a). Depressive and anxiety symptoms, coping strategies in patients with irritable bowel syndrome and inflammatory bowel disease. *Psychiatria Hungarica, 22*(3), 212–221.

Kovacs, Z., & Kovacs, F. (2007b). Depressive and anxiety symptoms, dysfunctional attitudes and social aspects in irritable bowel syndrome and inflammatory bowel disease. *International Journal of Psychiatry in Medicine, 37*(3), 245–255.

Kroenke, K., & Swindle, R. (2000). Cognitive-behavioral therapy for somatization and symptom syndromes: A critical review of controlled clinical trials. *Psychotherapy and Psychosomatics, 69*(4), 205–215.

Kudo, K., Miyazaki, C., Kadoya, R., Imamura, T., Jitsufuchi, N., & Ikeda, N. (1998). Laxative poisoning: Toxicological analysis of bisacodyl and its metabolite in urine, serum, and stool. *Journal of Analytical Toxicology, 22*(4), 274–278.

Labus, J. S., Bolus, R., Chang, L., Wiklund, I., Naesdal, J., Mayer, E. A., et al. (2004). The Visceral Sensitivity Index: Development and validation of a gastrointestinal symptom-specific anxiety scale. *Alimentary Pharmacology and Therapeutics, 20*(1), 89–97.

Labus, J. S., Mayer, E. A., Chang, L., Bolus, R., & Naliboff, B. D. (2007). The central role of gastrointestinal-specific anxiety in irritable bowel syndrome: Further validation of the visceral sensitivity index. *Psychosomatic Medicine, 69*(1), 89–98.

Lackner, J., & Gurtman, M. B. (2005). Patterns of interpersonal problems in irritable bowel syndrome patients: A circumplex analysis. *Journal of Psychosomatic Research, 58*(6), 523–532.

Lackner, J. M., Brasel, A. M., Quigley, B. M., Keefer, L., Krasner, S. S., Powell, C., et al. (2010). The ties that bind: Perceived social support, stress, and IBS in severely affected patients. *Neurogastroenterology and Motility, 22*, 893–900.
Lackner, J. M., & Gurtman, M. B. (2004). Pain catastrophizing and interpersonal problems: A circumplex analysis of the communal coping model. *Pain, 110*(3), 597–604.
Lackner, J. M., Jaccard, J., & Blanchard, E. B. (2005). Testing the sequential model of pain processing in irritable bowel syndrome: A structural equation modeling analysis. *European Journal of Pain, 9*(2), 207–218.
Lackner, J. M., Jaccard, J., Krasner, S. S., Katz, L. A., Gudleski, G. D., & Blanchard, E. B. (2007). How does cognitive behavior therapy for irritable bowel syndrome work? A mediational analysis of a randomized clinical trial. *Gastroenterology, 133*(2), 433–444.
Lackner, J. M., Jaccard, J., Krasner, S. S., Katz, L. A., Gudleski, G. D., & Holroyd, K. (2008). Self-administered cognitive behavior therapy for moderate to severe irritable bowel syndrome: Clinical efficacy, tolerability, feasibility. *Clinical Gastroenterology and Hepatology, 6*(8), 899–906.
Lackner, J. M., Lou Coad, M., Mertz, H. R., Wack, D. S., Katz, L. A., Krasner, S. S., et al. (2006). Cognitive therapy for irritable bowel syndrome is associated with reduced limbic activity, GI symptoms, and anxiety. *Behaviour Research and Therapy, 44*(5), 621–638.
Lackner, J. M., Mesmer, C., Morley, S., Dowzer, C., & Hamilton, S. (2004). Psychological treatments for irritable bowel syndrome: A systematic review and meta-analysis. *Journal of Consulting and Clinical Psychology, 72*(6), 1100–1113.
Lackner, J. M., & Quigley, B. M. (2005). Pain catastrophizing mediates the relationship between worry and pain suffering in patients with irritable bowel syndrome. *Behaviour Research and Therapy, 43*(7), 943–957.
Lazarus, R. S., DeLongis, A., Folkman, S., & Gruen, R. (1985). Stress and adaptational outcomes. The problem of confounded measures. *The American Psychologist, 40*(7), 770–785.
Lea, R., Houghton, L. A., Calvert, E. L., Larder, S., Gonsalkorale, W. M., Whelan, V., et al. (2003). Gut-focused hypnotherapy normalizes disordered rectal sensitivity in patients with irritable bowel syndrome. *Alimentary Pharmacology and Therapeutics, 17*(5), 635–642.
Lee, S., Wu, J., Ma, Y. L., Tsang, A., Guo, W. J., & Sung, J. (2009). Irritable bowel syndrome is strongly associated with generalized anxiety disorder: A community study. *Alimentary Pharmacology and Therapeutics, 30*(6), 643–651.
Leserman, J., Drossman, D. A., & Hu, Y. J. B. (1998). Selected symptoms associated with sexual and physical abuse history among female patients with gastrointestinal disorders: The impact on subsequent health care visits. *Psychological Medicine, 28*, 417–425.
Leserman, J., Drossman, D. A., Zhiming, L., Toomey, T. C., Nachman, G., & Glogau, L. (1996). Sexual and physical abuse history in gastroenterology practice: How types of abuse impact health status. *Psychosomatic Medicine, 58*, 4–15.
Levy, R. L., Jones, K. R., Whitehead, W. E., Feld, S. I., Talley, N. J., & Corey, L. A. (2001). Irritable bowel syndrome in twins: Heredity and social learning both contribute to etiology. *Gastroenterology, 121*(4), 799–804.
Levy, R. L., & Langer, S. L. (2007). Pain, disability, and symptoms among siblings of children with functional abdominal pain. *Journal of Developmental and Behavioral Pediatrics, 28*(1), 45–46.
Levy, R. L., Langer, S. L., & Whitehead, W. E. (2007). Social learning contributions to the etiology and treatment of functional abdominal pain and inflammatory bowel disease in children and adults. *World Journal of Gastroenterology, 13*(17), 2397–2403.
Levy, R. L., Whitehead, W. E., Walker, L. S., Von Korff, M., Feld, A. D., Garner, M., et al. (2004). Increased somatic complaints and health-care utilization in children: Effects of parent IBS status and parent response to gastrointestinal symptoms. *American Journal of Gastroenterology, 99*(12), 2442–2451.
Lipowski, Z. J. (1988). Somatization: The concept and its clinical application. *The American Journal of Psychiatry, 145*(11), 1358–1368.
Longstreth, G. F., Thompson, W. G., Chey, W. D., Houghton, L. A., Mearin, F., & Spiller, R. C. (2006). Functional bowel disorders. *Gastroenterology, 130*, 1480–1491.

Lydiard, R. B., Fosset, M. D., Marsh, W., & Ballenger, J. C. (1993). Prevalence of psychiatric disorders in patients with irritable bowel syndrome. *Psychosomatics, 34*(3), 229–233.
Lydiard, R. B., Greenwald, S., Weissman, M. M., Johnson, J., Drossman, D. A., & Ballenger, J. C. (1994). Panic disorder and gastrointestinal symptoms: Findings from the NIMH Epidemiologic Catchment Area Project. *The American Journal of Psychiatry, 151*, 64–70.
Lynch, A., Webb, C. et al. (2008). "Clinical inquiries. What are the most effective nonpharmacologic therapies for irritable bowel syndrome?" *J Fam Pract 57* (1), 57–58.
Masand, P. S., Kaplan, D. S., Gupta, S., Bhandary, A. N., Nasra, G. S., Kline, M. D., et al. (1995). Major depression and irritable bowel syndrome: Is there a relationship. *The Journal of Clinical Psychiatry, 56*(8), 363–367.
Masand, P. S., Keuthen, N. J., Gupta, S., Virk, S., Yu-Siao, B., & Kaplan, D. (2006). Prevalence of irritable bowel syndrome in obsessive-compulsive disorder. *CNS Spectrums, 11*(1), 21–25.
Mayer, E. A. (2008). Clinical practice. Irritable bowel syndrome. *The New England Journal of Medicine, 358*(16), 1692–1699.
Mayer, E. A., Aziz, Q., Coen, S., Kern, M., Labus, J. S., Lane, R., et al. (2009). Brain imaging approaches to the study of functional GI disorders: A Rome working team report. *Neurogastroenterology and Motility, 21*(6), 579–596.
Melzack, R. (1975). McGill pain questionnaire: Major properties and scoring methods. *Pain, 1*, 277–299.
Meyer, T. J., Miller, M. L., Metzger, R. L., & Borkovec, T. D. (1990). Development and validation of the Penn State Worry Questionnaire. *Behavior Research and Therapy, 28*(6), 487–495.
Miller, A. R., North, C. S., Clouse, R. E., Wetzel, R. D., Spitznagel, E. L., & Alpers, D. H. (2001). The association of irritable bowel syndrome and somatization disorder. *Annals of Clinical Psychiatry, 13*(1), 25–30.
Miller, V., Hopkins, L., & Whorwell, P. J. (2004). Suicidal ideation in patients with irritable bowel syndrome. *Clinical Gastroenterology and Hepatology, 2*(12), 1064–1068.
Miller, V., & Whorwell, P. J. (2009). Hypnotherapy for functional gastrointestinal disorders: A review. *International Journal of Clinical and Experimental Hypnosis, 57*(3), 279–292.
Moayyedi, P., Ford, A. C., Talley, N. J., Cremonini, F., Foxx-Orenstein, A. E., Brandt, L. J., et al. (2010). The efficacy of probiotics in the treatment of irritable bowel syndrome: A systematic review. *Gut, 59*(3), 325–332.
Morris-Yates, A., Talley, N. J., Boyce, P. M., Nandurkar, S., & Andrews, G. (1998). Evidence of a genetic contribution to functional bowel disorder. *American Journal of Gastroenterology, 93*(8), 1311–1317.
Motola, G., Mazzeo, F., Rinaldi, B., Capuano, A., Rossi, S., Russo, F., et al. (2002). Self-prescribed laxative use: A drug utilization review. *Advances in Therapy, 19*(5), 203–208.
Mott, T., Hammond DC. (1998). Adverse reaction in the use of hypnosis. In D. C. Hammond (Ed.), *Hypnotic induction and suggestion*. Chicago: American Society of Clinical Hypnosis.
Naliboff, B. D., Berman, S., Suyenobu, B., Labus, J. S., Chang, L., Stains, J., et al. (2006). Longitudinal change in perceptual and brain activation response to visceral stimuli in irritable bowel syndrome patients. *Gastroenterology, 131*(2), 352–365.
Naliboff, B. D., Waters, A. M., Labus, J. S., Kilpatrick, L., Craske, M. G., Chang, L., et al. (2008). Increased acoustic startle responses in IBS patients during abdominal and nonabdominal threat. *Psychosomatic Medicine, 70*(8), 920–927.
Neff, D. F., & Blanchard, E. B. (1987). A multi-component treatment for irritable bowel syndrome. *Behavior Therapy, 18*, 70–76.
North, C., Alpers, D., Thompson, S., & Spitznagel, E. (1996). Gastrointestinal symptoms and psychiatric disorders in the general population. Findings from the NIMH Epidemiological Catchment Area Project. *Digestive Diseases and Sciences, 41*(4), 633–640.
North, C. S., & Alpers, D. H. (2000). Irritable bowel syndrome in a psychiatric patient population. *Comprehensive Psychiatry, 41*(2), 116–122.
North, C. S., Downs, D., Clouse, R. E., Alrakawi, A., Dokucu, M. E., Cox, J., et al. (2004). The presentation of irritable bowel syndrome in the context of somatization disorder. *Clinical Gastroenterology and Hepatology, 2*(9), 787–795.

North, C. S., Hong, B. A., & Alpers, D. H. (2007). Relationship of functional gastrointestinal disorders and psychiatric disorders: Implications for treatment. *World Journal of Gastroenterology, 13*(14), 2020–2027.

Palsson, O. S. (2006). Standardized hypnosis treatment for irritable bowel syndrome: The North Carolina protocol. *International Journal of Clinical and Experimental Hypnosis, 54*(1), 51–64.

Palsson, O. S., Turner, M. J., Johnson, D. A., Burnett, C. K., & Whitehead, W. E. (2002). Hypnosis treatment for severe irritable bowel syndrome: Investigation of mechanism and effects on symptoms. *Digestive Diseases and Sciences, 47*(11), 2605–2614.

Palsson, O. S., Turner, M. J., & Whitehead, W. E. (2006). Hypnosis home treatment for irritable bowel syndrome: A pilot study. *International Journal of Clinical and Experimental Hypnosis, 54*(1), 85–99.

Palsson, O. S., & Whitehead, W. E. (2002). The growing case for hypnosis as adjunctive therapy for functional gastrointestinal disorders. *Gastroenterology, 123*(6), 2132–2135.

Pimentel, M., Park, S., Mirocha, J., Kane, S. V., & Kong, Y. (2006). The effect of a nonabsorbed oral antibiotic (rifaximin) on the symptoms of the irritable bowel syndrome: A randomized trial. *Annals of Internal Medicine, 145*(8), 557–563.

Porcelli, P., Leandro, G., & De Carne, M. (1998). Functional gastrointestinal disorders and eating disorders. Relevance of the association in clinical management. *Scandinavian Journal of Gastroenterology, 33*(6), 577–582.

Prins, C. & Schellekens, M. (2004). The chilling-effect of liability law on initiatives to enhance the reliability of on-line health-related information. *Eur J Health Law 11*(2), 201–208.

Radnitz, C. L., & Blanchard, E. B. (1988). Bowel sound biofeedback as a treatment for irritable bowel syndrome. *Biofeedback and Self-Regulation, 13*(2), 169–179.

Ratcliffe, G. E., Enns, M. W., Belik, S. L., & Sareen, J. (2008). Chronic pain conditions and suicidal ideation and suicide attempts: An epidemiologic perspective. *The Clinical Journal of Pain, 24*(3), 204–210.

Reme, S. E., Kennedy, T., Jones, R., Darnley, S., & Chalder, T. (2010). Predictors of treatment outcome after cognitive behavior therapy and antispasmodic treatment for patients with irritable bowel syndrome in primary care. *Journal of Psychosomatic Research, 68*(4), 385–388.

Remes-Troche, J., Bernal-Reyes, R., Valladares-Lepine, M., Alonso-Larraga, O., Gomez-Escudero, O., & Melendez-Mena, D. (2009). Gastroenterology diagnosis and treatment guidelines of irritable bowel syndrome; clinical features and diagnostic criteria. *Revista de Gastroenterologia de Mexico, 74*(1), 58–62.

Resick, P. A., Galovski, T. E., O'Brien Uhlmansiek, M., Scher, C. D., Clum, G. A., & Young-Xu, Y. (2008). A randomized clinical trial to dismantle components of cognitive processing therapy for posttraumatic stress disorder in female victims of interpersonal violence. *Journal of Consulting and Clinical Psychology, 76*(2), 243–258.

Resick, P. A., Nishith, P., Weaver, T. L., Astin, M. C., & Feuer, C. A. (2002). A comparison of cognitive-processing therapy with prolonged exposure and a waiting condition for the treatment of chronic posttraumatic stress disorder in female rape victims. *Journal of Consulting and Clinical Psychology, 70*(4), 867–879.

Resick, P. A., & Schnicke, M. K. (1992). Cognitive processing therapy for sexual assault victims. *Journal of Consulting and Clinical Psychology, 60*(5), 748–756.

Riedl, A., Schmidtmann, M., Stengel, A., Goebel, M., Wisser, A. S., Klapp, B. F., et al. (2008). Somatic comorbidities of irritable bowel syndrome: A systematic analysis. *Journal of Psychosomatic Research, 64*(6), 573–582.

Riegler, G., & Esposito, I. (2001). Bristol scale stool form. A still valid help in medical practice and clinical research. *Techniques in Coloproctology, 5*(3), 163–164.

Ringel, Y., Drossman, D. A., Turkington, T. G., Bradshaw, B., Hawk, T. C., Bangdiwala, S., et al. (2003). Regional brain activation in response to rectal distension in patients with irritable bowel syndrome and the effect of a history of abuse, *Dig Dis Sci, 48*(9), 1774–1781.

Roy-Byrne, P. P., Stein, M. B., Russo, J., Mercier, E., Thomas, R., McQuaid, J., et al. (1999). Panic disorder in the primary care setting: Comorbidity, disability, service utilization, and treatment. *Journal of Clinical Psychiatry, 60*(7), 492–499; quiz 500.

Rudaz, M., Craske, M. G., Becker, E. S., Ledermann, T., & Margraf, J. (2010). Health anxiety and fear of fear in panic disorder and agoraphobia vs. social phobia: A prospective longitudinal study. *Depression and Anxiety, 27*(4), 404–411.

Saito, Y. A., Prather, C. M., Van Dyke, C. T., Fett, S., Zinsmeister, A. R., & Locke, G. R., III. (2004). Effects of multidisciplinary education on outcomes in patients with irritable bowel syndrome. *Clinical Gastroenterology and Hepatology, 2*(7), 576–584.

Saito, Y. A., & Talley, N. J. (2008). Genetics of irritable bowel syndrome. *American Journal of Gastroenterology, 103*(8), 2100–2104; quiz 2105.

Sapolsky, R. M. (1996a). Stress, glucocorticoids, and damage to the nervous system: The current state of confusion. *Stress, 1*(1), 1–19.

Sapolsky, R. M. (1996b). Why stress is bad for your brain. *Science, 273*(5276), 749–750.

Sapolsky, R. M. (2004). Organismal stress and telomeric aging: An unexpected connection. *Proceedings of the National Academy of Sciences of the United States of America, 101*(50), 17323–17324.

Savas, L. S., White, D. L., Wieman, M., Daci, K., Fitzgerald, S., Laday Smith, S., et al. (2009). Irritable bowel syndrome and dyspepsia among women veterans: Prevalence and association with psychological distress. *Alimentary Pharmacology and Therapeutics, 29*, 115–125.

Scarinci, I. C., McDonald-Haile, J. M., Bradley, L. A. et al. (1994). Altered pain perception and psychosocial features among women with gastrointestinal disorders and history of abuse: A preliminary model. *Amercian Journal of Medicine, 97*, 108–118.

Schmulson, M., Noble-Lugo, A., Valenzuela-de la Cueva, V., De Arino-Suarez, M., Guillermo-Denis, L., & Ramos-Narvaez, F. (2009). [Gastroenterology diagnosis and treatment guidelines of Irritable Bowel Syndrome; Treatment.]. *Revista Gastroenterologia de Mexico, 74*(1), 63–70.

Sperber, A. D. (2009). The challenge of cross-cultural, multi-national research: Potential benefits in the functional gastrointestinal disorders. *Neurogastroenterology and Motility, 21*, 351–360.

Spetalen, S., Sandvik, L., Blomhoff, S., & Jacobsen, M. B. (2009). Rectal visceral sensitivity in women with irritable bowel syndrome without psychiatric comorbidity compared with healthy volunteers. *Gastroenterology Research and Practice, 2009*, 130684.

Spiegel, B. M. (2009). The burden of IBS: Looking at metrics. *Current Gastroenterology Reports, 11*(4), 265–269.

Spiller, R., Aziz, Q., Creed, F., Emmanuel, A., Houghton, L., Hungin, P., et al. (2007). Guidelines on the irritable bowel syndrome: Mechanisms and practical management. *Gut, 56*(12), 1770–1798.

Sugaya, N., Kaiya, H., Kumano, H., & Nomura, S. (2008). Relationship between subtypes of irritable bowel syndrome and severity of symptoms associated with panic disorder. *Scandinavian Journal of Gastroenterology, 43*(6), 675–681.

Sugaya, N., & Nomura, S. (2008). Relationship between cognitive appraisals of symptoms and negative mood for subtypes of irritable bowel syndrome. *Biopsychosocial Medicine, 2*, 9.

Sullivan, M. J. L., Bishop, S. R., & Pivik, J. (1995). The pain catastrophizing scale: Development and validation. *Psychological Assessment, 7*(4), 524–532.

Svedlund, J. (1983). Psychotherapy in irritable bowel syndrome. A controlled outcome study. *Acta Psychiatrica Scandinavica. Supplementum, 306*, 1–86.

Svedlund, J., Sjodin, I., Ottosson, J. O., & Dotevall, G. (1983). Controlled study of psychotherapy in irritable bowel syndrome. *Lancet, 2*(8350), 589–592.

Sykes, M. A., Blanchard, E. B., Lackner, J., Keefer, L., & Krasner, S. (2003). Psychopathology in irritable bowel syndrome: Support for a psychophysiological model. *Journal of Behavioral Medicine, 26*(4), 361–372.

Talley, N. J., Boyce, P. M., & Jones, M. (1997). Predictors of health care seeking for irritable bowel syndrome: A population based study. *Gut, 41*, 394–398.

Taylor, G. J., Bagby, R. M., & Parker, J. D. (1992). The Revised Toronto Alexithymia Scale: Some reliability, validity, and normative data. *Psychotherapy and Psychosomatics, 57*(1–2), 34–41.

Taylor, G. J., Parker, J. D., Bagby, R. M., & Acklin, M. W. (1992). Alexithymia and somatic complaints in psychiatric out-patients. *Journal of Psychosomatic Research, 36*(5), 417–424.

Tkalcic, M., Hauser, G., & Stimac, D. (2010). Differences in the health-related quality of life, affective status, and personality between irritable bowel syndrome and inflammatory bowel disease patients. *European Journal of Gastroenterology and Hepatology, 22*, 862–867.

Tsao, J. C., Mystkowski, J. L., Zucker, B. G., & Craske, M. G. (2005). Impact of cognitive-behavioral therapy for panic disorder on comorbidity: A controlled investigation. *Behaviour Research and Therapy, 43*(7), 959–970.

Videlock, E. J., Adeyemo, M., Licudine, A., Hirano, M., Ohning, G., Mayer, M., et al. (2009). Childhood trauma is associated with hypothalamic-pituitary-adrenal axis responsiveness in irritable bowel syndrome. *Gastroenterology, 137*(6), 1954–1962.

Whitehead, W. E., Palsson, O. S., Levy, R. R., Feld, A. D., Turner, M., & Von Korff, M. (2007). Comorbidity in irritable bowel syndrome. *American Journal of Gastroenterology, 102*, 2767–2776.

Whitehead, W. E., Palsson, O., & Jones, K. R. (2002). Systematic review of the comorbidity of irritable bowel syndrome with other disorders: What are the causes and implications? *Gastroenterology, 122*(4), 1140–1156.

Whitehead, W. E., & Palsson, O. S. (1998). Is rectal pain sensitivity a biological marker for irritable bowel syndrome: Psychological influences on pain perception. *Gastroenterology, 115*(5), 1263–1271.

Whorwell, P. J. (2006). Effective management of irritable bowel syndrome–the Manchester Model. *International Journal of Clinical and Experimental Hypnosis, 54*(1), 21–26.

Whorwell, P. J. (2008). Hypnotherapy for irritable bowel syndrome: The response of colonic and noncolonic symptoms. *Journal of Psychosomatic Research, 64*(6), 621–623.

Whorwell, P. J., Prior, A., & Colgan, S. M. (1987). Hypnotherapy in severe irritable bowel syndrome: Further experience. *Gut, 28*(4), 423–425.

Whorwell, P. J., Prior, A., & Faragher, E. B. (1984). Controlled trial of hypnotherapy in the treatment of severe refractory irritable-bowel syndrome. *Lancet, 2*(8414), 1232–1234.

Wong, E., Guyatt, G. H., Cook, D. J., Griffith, L. E., & Irvine, E. J. (1998). Development of a questionnaire to measure quality of life in patients with irritable bowel syndrome. *The European Journal of Surgery. Supplement, 583*, 50–56.

Zigmond, A., & Snaith, R. P. (1983). The hospital anxiety and depression scale. *Acta Psychiatry Scandanavia, 67*(6), 361–370.

Zijdenbos, I. L., de Wit, N. J., van der Heijden, G. J., Rubin, G., & Quartero, A. O. (2009). Psychological treatments for the management of irritable bowel syndrome. *Cochrane Database Systemic Reviews* (1), CD006442.

Chapter 11
Psychological Co-morbidities of COPD

Susan McCrone and Heidi Putnam-Casdorph

11.1 Introduction

Chronic obstructive pulmonary disease (COPD) is a debilitating disease characterized by progressive and irreversible airflow limitations that result in significant morbidity and mortality (Nazir & Erbland, 2009). The Global Initiative for Obstructive Lung Disease (GOLD) report released by the National Institutes of Health, National Heart, Lung and Blood Institute (NHLBI), and World Health Organization (WHO) estimates that the economic burden of COPD in the United States was $32.1 billion dollars in direct and indirect costs in 2004. In a matched cohort study of Medicare beneficiaries, patients with COPD were more likely to utilize healthcare services and had significantly higher healthcare costs than a comparison cohort. Physical co-morbidities were high in the COPD group, which accounted for 46% of the observed excess cost (Menzin et al., 2008). This chapter will review the pathophysiology of COPD, the prevalence of both the disease and its psychological co-morbidities, and explore evidence-based treatment options.

11.2 Definition of COPD

The term COPD encompasses a heterogeneous group of conditions that involve both the airways and lung parenchyma, which includes chronic bronchitis and emphysema (Nazir & Erbland, 2009). According to the GOLD guidelines, COPD is defined as:

> a preventable and treatable disease with some significant extrapulmonary effects that may contribute to the severity of individual patients. Its pulmonary component is characterized

S. McCrone (✉)
School of Nursing, West Virginia University, PO Box 6201, Morgantown, WV 26506, USA
e-mail: smccrone@hsc.wvu.edu

S. Pagoto (ed.), *Psychological Co-morbidities of Physical Illness: A Behavioral Medicine Perspective*, DOI 10.1007/978-1-4419-0029-6_11,

by airflow limitation that is not fully reversible. The airflow limitation is usually progressive and associated with an abnormal inflammatory response of the lung to noxious particles or gases (GOLD, 2009, p. 1).

Chronic airflow limitation in COPD is caused by a combination of small airway disease (obstructive bronchiolitis) and parenchymal destruction (emphysema), which varies from person to person (GOLD, 2009). Symptoms of COPD include: cough, sputum production, wheezing, and dyspnea.

11.2.1 Diagnostic Criteria for COPD

The COPD severity classification is based on lung function as measured by spirometry (pulmonary function testing). Obstruction is most commonly defined as a ratio of forced expiratory volume in one second (FEV_1) to forced vital capacity (FVC) less than 70% after administration of an inhaled bronchodilator. Staging of COPD is based on the percent of predicted values for FEV_1, which accounts for age, sex, height, weight, race, and ethnicity. Staging of COPD includes the following: Stage I (mild) ≥80% predicted, with or without symptoms of dyspnea, cough, or sputum production; Stage II (moderate) $50\% \leq FEV_1 < 80\%$ predicted; Stage III (severe) $30\% \leq FEV_1 < 50\%$ predicted; Stage IV (very severe) $FEV_1 < 30\%$ predicted or $FEV_1 < 50\%$ plus chronic respiratory failure. In Stage I, the individual is usually unaware that his or her lung function is abnormal. In Stage II, the individual typically seeks medical attention because of chronic respiratory symptoms or an exacerbation of his or her disease. Stage III is characterized by worsening of airflow limitations, greater shortness of breath, reduced exercise capacity, fatigue, and repeated exacerbations often leading to a decrease in the patient's quality of life. Stage IV is characterized by severe airflow limitation and chronic respiratory failure (GOLD, 2009). Overall treatment recommendations based on the GOLD guidelines include: assessing and monitoring the disease, reducing risk factors for the development of COPD, managing stable COPD, and managing exacerbations (GOLD, 2009; Rabe et al., 2007).

Several authors have suggested that a more comprehensive evaluation would better predict outcomes (Celli et al., 2004; Cote & Celli, 2009; Funk, Kirchheiner, Burghuber, & Hartl, 2009). Investigators noted that a composite index incorporated the most important predictors of mortality, a more comprehensive way to evaluate COPD. In a prospective study of 207 patients with COPD, investigators identified four variables that predicted an elevated risk for mortality: "BMI (B), degree of airflow obstruction as measured by FEV_1 (O), dyspnea as measured by the Medical Research Council (MRC) Index dyspnea scale (D), and exercise capacity as measured by the 6 minute walk distance (6MWD) test (E)" (Cote & Celli, 2009, p. 310). The researchers incorporated these variables into a multidimensional scale, the BODE index.

11.3 Epidemiology of COPD

COPD is the fourth leading cause of death in the world and is projected to be the third by the year 2020 (Rabe et al., 2007). Globally, COPD is the only leading cause of death that is increasing in prevalence (Hurd, 2000). Although rates of death from heart disease and stroke have decreased by 52 and 63%, respectively, from 1970 to 2002, death rates from COPD have increased by 103% (Jemal, Ward, Hao, & Thun, 2005), and the death rate in women has more than doubled in the past 30 years (O'Neill, 2002). Treatment for other chronic illnesses such as cancer and cardiovascular disease is advancing to improve the health status of patients, but little progress has been made in decreasing the morbidity and mortality associated with COPD (O'Neill).

COPD is a highly prevalent, underdiagnosed, and undertreated disease (Celli, 2008). About 16 million people in the United States are currently diagnosed with COPD, and according to the WHO, in 2006 an estimated 80 million people globally had moderate-to-severe COPD. An additional 14 million or more cases in the United States likely remain undiagnosed, due to early stage, minimal symptoms, and access to care (COPD International, 2010, www.copd-international.com; World Health Organization, 2010). The global prevalence of COPD in males ranges from 9.8 to 23% and in females ranges from 5.6 to 11.6% (Han et al., 2007).

In a systematic review and meta-analysis, investigators identified the prevalence of physiologically defined COPD globally in adults 40 and older as 9–10% (Halbert et al., 2006). In the BOLD (Burden of Obstructive Lung Disease) study, the overall prevalence of COPD GOLD stage II or higher across 12 countries was 11.8% for men and 8.5% for women. The study confirmed that the prevalence of COPD has been shown to increase with age with the highest prevalence in men and women ≥70 years, 19–47 and 6–33%, respectively (Buist et al., 2007). Although the overall prevalence is somewhat lower in women than men, rates are increasing in both higher- and lower-income women as tobacco use among women in higher-income countries has increased, as has exposure to indoor air pollution for women living in low-income countries. COPD is a disease that affects men and women in almost equal numbers, and yet remains largely underdiagnosed (Damarla, Celli, Mullerova, & Pinto-Plata, 2006; Talamo et al., 2007; World Health Organization, 2010).

11.4 Pathophysiology of COPD

The most prevalent cause of COPD is smoking (80–90% of cases), (Mikkelsen, Middelboe, Pisinger, & Stage, 2004) as it produces accelerated decreases in FEV_1 (Global Obstructive Lung Initiative (GOLD), 2009). The diagnosis of COPD is based upon data from medical history, physical examination, and results from pulmonary function testing (Kumar & Gross, 2002). One barrier to accurate diagnosis in older patients is that age seems to reduce the perception of bronchoconstriction leading to less reporting of milder symptoms and thus underdiagnosis (Ottanelli et al., 2001).

A second diagnostic issue is the cut point used by the Global Initiative for Chronic Obstructive Lung Disease (GOLD) guidelines of an FEV_1/FVC ratio of 0.7, below which a diagnosis of COPD is made (GOLD, 2009). With normal aging, some loss of lung elasticity and increased airway collapsibility occurs leading to a normal decrease in the FEV_1/FVC ratio (Gelb & Zamel, 1975). When a fixed ratio of 0.7 is used as a cut-off for older adults, there is a risk of overdiagnosis (Nazir & Erbland, 2009). While COPD affects the lungs, it also produces significant systemic effects. Systemic inflammatory markers are elevated in patients with COPD, and may play a role in the pathogenesis of smoking-related conditions such as muscle wasting, cardiovascular disease, and osteoporosis (Gan, Man, Senthilselvan, & Sin, 2004; Gerhardsson de Verdier, 2008). Although it may be overdiagnosed in older adults, it is often underdiagnosed in younger adults.

Dyspnea or breathlessness tends to be the most prominent and disabling symptom, the major symptom associated with acute exacerbations, and the most common reason that patients seek medical care. Despite extensive research on the pathophysiology and affective components of dyspnea, the precise physical mechanism of breathlessness is not known (Bailey, 2004). In a qualitative study by Bailey (2004) involving ten patient-family units interviewed during an acute episode, dyspnea as an experience was described as "inextricably related to anxiety and emotional functioning" (p. 760). The investigator identified a "dyspnea-anxiety-dyspnea cycle" where dyspnea results in anxiety which further exacerbates dyspnea. Functional dyspnea suffered by those with COPD can severely affect daily activities and quality of life.

11.4.1 Acute Exacerbations

COPD is characterized by acute exacerbations often leading to hospitalization. Acute exacerbations represent a major burden for patients and healthcare systems (Puhan, Scharplatz, Trooster, & Steurer, 2005). Acute exacerbations are associated with: further impairment of health status (Seemungal et al., 1998), decreased health-related quality of life (Quint, Baghai-Ravary, Donaldson, & Wedzicha, 2008), increased healthcare expenditures worldwide (Almagro et al., 2006; Anderson et al., 2002), and increased mortality (Connors et al., 1996). Studies on mortality after hospitalization for an acute exacerbation of COPD (AECOPD) have identified 1-year mortality from 22 to 43%, and 2-year mortality of 36–49% (Almagro et al., 2002; Connors et al., 1996; Groenewegen, Schols, & Wouters, 2003; Yohannes, Baldwin, & Connolly, 2005). In some studies, anxiety and/or depression were related to readmissions and mortality, while in others they were not. In addition, some studies found a relationship of anxiety and depression in bivariate analyses that did not remain in multivariate analyses. These differences appear to be the result of the use of different tools to measure anxiety and depression and varying sample sizes.

In a study of 100 patients admitted for AECOPD, presence of a depressive illness, level of disability, and impairment of quality of life were all significant predictors of

1-year mortality in bivariate analyses, but age, sex, smoking status, social class, FEV_1, body mass index, co-morbidity, arterial blood gas levels, and pack years smoked were not predictors. In multivariate analyses, perception of breathing problems was the only significant predictor of 1-year mortality (Yohannes et al., 2005). In a study by Almagro et al. (2002), greater mortality was observed among older patients, women, and unmarried patients. Hospital admission during the previous year, functional dependence, greater co-morbidity, depression, quality of life, and hypercapnia at discharge were also significant predictors of mortality. Unlike the study by Yohannes et al. (2005), depression along with quality of life (activity scale), co-morbidity, hospital readmissions, and marital status remained independent predictors of mortality when using multivariate analyses. As identified by Almagro et al. (2002), sex appears to play a role in predicting mortality among patients with COPD.

11.5 Sex-Related Differences in COPD

Until recently, there has been a lack of information regarding sex and COPD. Most previous studies were completed with largely male samples. In a cross-sectional, multicenter study examining co-morbidity and gender-related differences in patients hospitalized for COPD exacerbation, the investigators found significant differences in number of co-morbidities between males and females. Female patients had a lower prevalence of ischemic heart disease and alcoholism, but a higher prevalence of chronic heart failure, osteoporosis, and diabetes without complications. Mortality (5%) was related to FEV_1, but not age, gender, co-morbidities, or number of previous hospitalizations (Almagro et al., 2009).

In an FEV_1-matched study of men and women attending a pulmonary clinic (de Torres et al., 2005), investigators found that women were younger (mean aged 57 vs. 65 years), smoked less, had better partial pressure of oxygen, lower partial pressure of carbon dioxide in arterial blood, lower BMI, more exacerbations in the last year, and fewer co-morbidities. Despite the fact that women had the same FEV_1 levels, had better partial pressure of oxygen, lower partial pressure of carbon dioxide in arterial blood, and fewer co-morbidities, they performed poorly in walking distance, reported a worse quality of life, and reported a higher degree of dyspnea. Although women had more exacerbations than men, there were no differences in the rate of hospitalizations. The investigators noted that more attention needs to be given to the way in which exposure to inhaled particles (from cigarette smoke or from biomass fuels) affects women.

In a second study by the same group of investigators (de Torres et al., 2006), 146 men and women with moderate-to-severe COPD from a pulmonary clinic were examined for differences in factors associated with quality of life. Exercise capacity, dyspnea, and co-morbidity had the highest independent association with quality of life for men, while dyspnea and oxygenation had the highest independent association with quality of life for women. Although factors like dyspnea, exercise capacity, degree of hyperinflation, and co-morbidities explained almost 90% of the variation in quality of life for males, dyspnea and level of oxygenation only explained 50% of the variation for females. Clearly other factors are impacting the quality of life for female patients with COPD.

The high prevalence of death in women with COPD has been attributed to the increased number of smoking women, exposure to toxins, and overall longer female lifespan compared to men. Research has shown significant differences in the numbers and types of co-morbidities in men and women with COPD. Differences were also found in physical performance and FEV_1 between men and women. Women reported more acute exacerbations than men. These differences have been attributed to how exposure to and inhalation of particulate matter affects the female physiology differently than men. Research has also found that women have a decreased quality of life at an earlier age than men with possible noninvestigated psychological factors explaining the difference.

11.6 Medications for COPD

Medications recommended by the GOLD guidelines to treat COPD include bronchodilators and glucocorticoids. Long-term pharmacological treatment of COPD may also include vaccines (both pneumococcal and influenza), antibiotics as needed, mucolytics, and antitussives. Several pharmacologic agents that are often used in the treatment of COPD can cause central nervous system side effects that can put the patient at higher risk for developing psychiatric co-morbidities. Inhaled bronchodilators, such as short- or long-acting beta-agonists or anticholinergics, can cause patients to experience feelings of restlessness, apprehension, anxiety, fear, and irritability. Inhaled or systemic corticosteroids, used for long-term treatment or acute exacerbations, can possibly cause irritability, restlessness, and mood changes. However, systemic corticosteroids are more likely to cause psychiatric symptoms when compare to inhaled corticosteroids (Physician's Desk Reference, 2009). Research related to mood and cognitive changes during systemic steroid therapy in chronic illness identified the side effects of mania, depression, memory loss, and psychoses, as well as physical manifestations such as weight gain (Brown & Chandler, 2001). A cross-sectional analysis of patients with chronic respiratory disease ($N=395$) found that patients perceived and identified at least 57 different side effects while taking a daily dose of inhaled steroids. These side effects ranged from psychological manifestations to physical symptoms (Foster et al., 2006).

11.7 Psychological Co-morbidities

Depression in patients with COPD is often characterized by feelings of hopelessness and pessimism, reduced sleep, decreased appetite, increased lethargy, difficulty with concentration, and social isolation (Emery, Green, & Suh, 2008). Symptoms of anxiety may include physiological arousal with tachycardia, sweating, and dyspnea (Emery et al.). The presence of psychiatric co-morbidities, most frequently depression, anxiety, and panic disorder, has been linked to: decreased functional status, decreased quality of life, increased social isolation, increased episodes of exacerbations, longer hospital lengths of stay, lower compliance with treatment, and increased mortality (Bosley, Corden, Rees, & Cochrane, 1996; Brenes, 2003; Celli & MacNee, 2004; Cully et al., 2006; Kim et al., 2000; Ng et al., 2007; Quint et al., 2008; Yellowlees, Alpers, Bowden, Bryant, & Ruffin, 1987).

One study found that anxiety and depression contributed significantly to the overall variance in functional status of patients with COPD, but neither medical burden nor COPD severity contributed to the variance (Kim et al., 2000). The relationship of anxiety and depression to quality of life was examined in a sample of 179 veterans with COPD. Anxiety and depression symptoms, as measured by the Beck Depression and Anxiety Inventories, were both significantly related to negative health-related quality of life outcomes (anxiety with both mental and physical health-related outcomes, and depression primarily with mental health outcomes) (Cully et al., 2006). The impact, scope, and prevalence of COPD warrant an exploration of current research focusing on patients suffering from psychological co-morbidities. These include anxiety, panic disorder, major depressive disorder, and depressive symptoms. It is important to explore prevalence, symptomatology, and evidence-based treatments.

11.7.1 Prevalence of Psychological Co-morbidities

Prevalence rates of psychological co-morbidities in patients with COPD vary across reports with the most commonly reported co-morbidities including panic disorder, major depressive disorder, as well as elevated symptoms of anxiety and depression. The prevalence of these psychological disorders and elevated symptoms are significantly higher in patients with COPD than in the general population (Wagena, Arrindell, Wouters, & van Schayck, 2005; Wagena, Knipschild, Huibers, Wouters, & van Schayck, 2005).

Very few population-based studies have examined the prevalence of mental disorders in patients with chronic respiratory conditions. In a large national health survey conducted in Canada (Patten & Williams, 2007), chronic respiratory conditions were significantly associated with major depressive disorder, bipolar disorder, panic disorder, social phobia, and substance abuse. Despite the significant associations, prevalence rates were lower than reports from clinical samples (Patten & Williams, 2007). In a large, population-based study, investigators found that the prevalence of major depressive disorder was higher in those diagnosed with COPD (23.1%) than in people with no diagnosis of COPD (16.8%) (Schneider, Jicks, Bothner, & Meier, 2010). Patients with severe COPD had the highest risk of developing depression.

A cross-sectional study reported the overall prevalence of psychiatric disorders in a sample of patients with COPD attending a respiratory clinic was 49%, with 24%

having two or more mood and anxiety disorders and 14% having both an anxiety and mood disorder (Laurin et al., 2007). Women were more likely to meet the diagnostic criteria for anxiety disorders than men (56 vs. 35%), panic disorder specifically (29 vs. 9%), but the sex difference in rates of major depression (18 vs. 7%) was not significant. These findings are consistent with Wagena et al. (2005) who reported significantly higher anxiety sensitivity and depressive symptoms in women than men in a sample of inpatients and outpatients with COPD. Despite having comparable COPD severity, dyspnea scores, and exacerbation rates, women reported being less confident in their ability to control respiratory symptoms and having more daily physical limitations.

Among patients with severe COPD on and off long-term oxygen (LTOH), investigators found 25% scored in the "definite" case range for anxiety on the Hospital Anxiety and Depression Scale (HADS $\geq$ 11; Sigmond & Snaith, 1983). Thirty-seven percent of patients off oxygen and 33% of patients on oxygen scored in the "definite" case range for depression (HADS > 11). In both groups, only 11% of patients with "definite" anxiety or depression were prescribed anxiolytics and/or antidepressants. The relationship between anxiety and depression is likely bidirectional with anxiety and depression increasing susceptibility to developing COPD perhaps through increased risk of smoking and difficulty quitting and also being a result of it (developing anxiety and depression from physical limitations) (Lewis et al., 2007). Although some studies evaluated risk for developing anxiety and/or depression, other studies measured general psychological distress.

In a study designed to evaluate the level of psychological distress in a heterogeneous group of patients with COPD (N = 118) as compared to the general population and psychiatric outpatients, investigators found that patients with COPD experienced significantly more psychological distress than the general population and significantly less than psychiatric outpatients. Although no significant association was found between the level of psychological distress and severity of pulmonary disease, patients with severe or very severe COPD seemed to be at increased risk for developing depression. No significant differences on any of the subscales of the Symptom Checklist 90 Revised (SCL-90-R) were found by sex. Although the prevalence of moderate-to-severe depression was higher in females than males (36 vs. 25%) and may be clinically relevant, it was not statistically significant (Wagena et al., 2005).

11.7.1.1 Prevalence of Anxiety Disorders and Anxiety Symptoms

Lifetime prevalence for anxiety disorders in patients with COPD ranged from 2 to 96% with the highest rates in inpatient samples and lowest rates in population samples (Aghanwa & Erhabor, 2001; Dowson et al., 2001; Guell et al., 2006; Mikkelsen et al., 2004; Yellowlees et al., 1987). Elevated prevalence of anxiety disorders has been observed in studies from Western countries as well as developing countries (Aghanwa & Erhabor, 2001). In a sample of 1,334 U.S. veterans with COPD, 80% screened positive for depression, anxiety, or both (Kunik et al., 2005). Although some studies examined prevalence of elevated anxiety symptoms, other studies looked more specifically at the prevalence of specific anxiety disorders. Lifetime prevalence rates for GAD ranged from 10 to 20% in patients with COPD (Karajgi, Rifkin, Doddi, & Kolli, 1990; Porzelius, Vest, & Nochomovitz, 1992; Yellowlees et al., 1987). These rates are higher than the general population for GAD (i.e., 3.1%) (Kessler, Chiu, Demler, & Walters, 2005). In an early intervention study on dyspnea and anxiety, patients with COPD have significantly higher levels of anxiety during episodes of high dyspnea as compared to episodes of low dyspnea (Gift, Moore, & Soeken, 1992).

Prevalence of Panic Attacks and Panic Disorder

Panic is a common experience in pulmonary disease (Smoller, Pollack, Otto, Rosenbaum, & Kradin, 1996). A large number of patients with COPD experience panic attacks, which are episodes of intense anxiety accompanied by dyspnea and other symptoms of physical arousal (American Psychiatric Association, 2000). The central feature of panic disorder is the recurrence of unexpected panic attacks accompanied by persistent fears or worries about having additional attacks and significant change in behavior related to the attack (American Psychiatric Association). In multiple studies exploring inpatients and outpatients, lifetime rates for Panic Disorder ranged from 8 to 37% (Karajgi et al., 1990; Porzelius et al., 1992; Yellowlees et al., 1987). These rates are greater than the general population rate of 2–4% for Panic Disorder (Kessler et al., 1994). In large US community samples of patients with COPD, estimated lifetime prevalence has ranged from 10 to 15% for panic attacks (Eaton, Kessler, Wittchen, & Magee, 1994; Kessler et al., 1994).

A study of 50 patients with chronic obstructive airway disease referred to a respiratory unit reported that 34% of the patients met DSM-III criteria for anxiety disorder and 24% met criteria for panic disorder. Panic disorder was the single most common psychiatric disorder in the sample (Yellowlees et al., 1987). Two studies reported a 32 and 37% prevalence of panic disorder in patients with COPD (Moore & Zebb, 1999; Yohannes, Baldwin, & Connolly, 2000), which is ten times higher than the general public (3.4% panic disorder and 4.1% panic attacks without a diagnosis of panic disorder) (Kessler et al., 1994).

While high rates of panic are observed in COPD patients, studies have also reported high rates of respiratory diseases in people with panic disorder. For example, in a study of psychiatric outpatients, the lifetime prevalence of respiratory disorders was 47% in patients with panic disorder as compared with 13% in patients with obsessive compulsive or eating disorders (Zandbergen et al. 1991). In a retrospective case-control study of 150 patients with anxiety disorders, 42.7% of patients with a history of panic disorder also had a history of respiratory disease that predated their panic disorder (Verburg et al., 1995). Respiratory diseases may increase risk for the development of panic disorders.

Pathophysiology of Co-morbid Panic and COPD

The interrelationship of dyspnea, hyperventilation, and panic has been interpreted within the context of three conceptual models: the hyperventilation model, the carbon dioxide hypersensitivity/suffocation false alarm model, and the cognitive-behavioral model (Smoller et al., 1996). The hyperventilation model postulates that hyperventilation leads to dyspnea and anxiety. The carbon dioxide model is based upon the idea that some patients with COPD may have a neurobiological sensitivity to CO_2, lactate, or other signals of suffocation. The cognitive-behavioral model suggests that some patients may have a catastrophic misinterpretation of respiratory symptoms. In a study examining panic attacks and the perception of inspiratory resistive loads, investigators found that patients with COPD and panic attacks showed heightened sensitivity to inspiratory loads, thus supporting the influence of psychological factors (cognitive-behavioral model) on symptom perception with COPD (Livermore et al., 2010). The investigators note that although there appears to be a relationship among anxiety, depression, and perceived dyspnea, the direction of causality has not been established and thus may indicate a reciprocal interaction. In a second study describing illness perception and panic in chronic obstructive disease, investigators identified that panic was unrelated to level of disease severity, but illness perception (beliefs related to illness identity, timeline, consequences, and emotional representations) was important in differentiating patients with and without panic attacks (Howard, Hallas, Wray, & Carby, 2009). Some empirical support exists for the cognitive-behavioral model to explain the interrelationship between hyperventilation, dyspnea, and panic in the context of COPD.

11.7.1.2 Prevalence of Depressive Symptoms and Major Depressive Disorder

The prevalence of depressive symptoms and/or major depressive disorder in patients with COPD has been reported to range from 6 to 88.4%, which is higher than the rates of depression found in older adults in primary care (i.e., 2.8–35%) (Beekman, Copeland, & Prince, 1999; Schane, Woodruff, Dinno, Covinsky, & Walter, 2008). In a study of 290 subjects with irreversible airway obstruction, the prevalence of depression as identified by a self-report questionnaire was significantly higher in patients with COPD who were under the age of 55 and had a mild airway obstruction (van Manen et al., 2001). Another study comparing age-matched patients with a registered diagnosis of COPD in general practice to a random sample of subjects without a diagnosis of asthma or COPD reported prevalence rates of depression of 25% in patients with severe disease, 19.6% in patients with mild-to-moderate disease, and 17.5% in healthy controls. When the results were adjusted for demographic variables and co-morbidities, the risk for depression was 2.5 times greater for patients with severe COPD, but no greater for those patients with mild-to-moderate disease than for healthy controls. Factors predictive of depression were: living alone, reversibility of FEV_1, and physical impairment. Age, sex, education,

FEV_1, and co-morbidities were not predictive of depression (van Manen et al., 2002). In contrast, younger age, sex, education, and co-morbidities were risk factors for depression among COPD patients in the 2004 Health and Retirement Survey (N=1,736 subjects with self-reported COPD), along with marital status, smoking, dyspnea, and difficulty walking (Schane et al., 2008). In a review of the literature on COPD and depression, higher incidence of depression was reported among the elderly (Borson, Claypoole, & McDonald, 1998). Despite the fact that the depressive symptoms and major depressive disorder are common in patients with COPD, few patients are treated who have this co-morbidity (Fan et al., 2007).

11.7.1.3 Prevalence of Co-morbid Anxiety and Depression

Although studies have cited the independent prevalence rates of depression and anxiety, a large percentage of COPD patients report both anxiety and depression (22–48%) and anxiety and depression are highly correlated in patients with COPD (Kunik et al., 2005, 2007; Lenfant, 2005; Roundy et al., 2005; Yohannes et al., 2000). In a large, age-matched study of patients of COPD and healthy controls, DiMarco et al. (2006) found that prevalence of anxiety symptoms (as measured by the State Trait Anxiety Inventory [STAI]) and depressive symptoms (as measured by the Zung Self-Rated Depression Scale) was high (28.2 and 18.8%, respectively) compared to a healthy control group (6.1 and 3.5%, respectively) even when patients had only mild COPD. Prevalence rates of anxiety and depression are likely to be underestimated given underdiagnosis and sampling bias. Anxiety and depression may co-occur in COPD given that both are related to smoking, a major risk factor for COPD (Norwood & Balkissoon, 2005). Causal paths linking smoking, depression, and anxiety are complex and likely reciprocal. Anxiety and depression are associated with higher risk of smoking and greater difficulty quitting (Wamboldt, 2005). In support of the reciprocal path, smoking appears to promote anxiety and depression through direct CNS toxicity arising from constituents of cigarette smoke as well as the consequences of nicotine withdrawal (Wamboldt). COPD, as a systemic disease, can possibly cause CNS dysfunction that could, in turn, lead to symptoms of anxiety and depression (Nazir & Erbland, 2009; Norwood & Balkissoon, 2005).

11.7.1.4 Sex Differences in Prevalence Rates of Anxiety and Depression

Female patients with COPD reported higher levels of anxiety, depression, and dyspnea, and worse symptom-related quality of life than males (DiMarco et al., 2006). In addition, dyspnea was more strongly associated with depression in women than in men.

In a study of primary care patients (Chavannes et al., 2005), depressive symptoms in patients with COPD were related to female gender and the presence of dyspneic complaints. Based upon these findings and those of other studies, the investigators hypothesized that females with COPD may utilize a different disease coping pattern and experience more depressive symptoms. There is strong support for a relationship between dypsnea and psychological co-morbidities in women. In a subsample of 58 patients recruited for a randomized controlled trial of cognitive-behavioral therapy in patients with COPD and co-morbid anxiety and/or depression, women had better FEV_1 values, were younger, scored higher on the anxiety scale, and had more co-morbid medical conditions than their male counterparts (Hynninen, Pallesen, & Nordhaus, 2007). Given that female patients with COPD have higher rates of depression and anxiety, clinical approaches to address the assessment of depression and anxiety in men and women with COPD need to be differentiated and carefully considered.

11.7.1.5 Impact of Depression and Anxiety on COPD

Anxiety and depression impede pulmonary rehabilitation, exacerbate problems with dyspnea, and impact smoking cessation (Borson, 1998). The presence of anxiety and panic in patients with COPD is important as it is associated with greater restrictions on mobility, decreased energy, difficulties with activities of daily living, greater dependence on others for care, and impaired functional status (Moore & Zebb, 1998; Weaver, Richmond, & Narsavage, 1997). Depression has also been found to negatively impact exercise capacity, health perception/well-being, the utilization of inpatient and outpatient health services, and hospital admissions both first admission and total number of admissions in patients with COPD (Koenig & Kuchibhatla, 1998; Ng et al., 2007; Ormel et al., 1998; Weaver & Narsavage, 1992; Weaver et al., 1997) and a variety of other acute and chronic conditions (Ormel et al.; Koenig & Kuchibhatla). Despite the greater number of days spent in the hospital by patients with co-morbid depression, the frequency of mental health visits was no higher in medically ill patients with depression than in patients without depression (Koenig & Kuchibhatla). Patients with COPD and depression have been shown to have worse compliance with medical treatment (Sirey, Raue, & Alexopoulos, 2007), experience more impaired functional status (Sirey et al.), have greater symptom burden, and report lower quality of life (COPD International, 2007; DiMatteo, Lepper, & Croghan, 2000; Seung-Kim et al., 2000). Major depression can significantly interfere with an individual's ability to adhere to treatment recommendations and is associated with increasing impairment (Sirey et al., 2007).

Although some studies reported an increased mortality rate in patients with COPD and depression (Almagro et al., 2002), others reported a decreased rate of mortality (Ng et al., 2007; Stage, Middleboe, & Pisinger, 2005). In a prospective cohort study, increased risk was not observed for respiratory hospitalizations or 1-year mortality, but was observed for 3-year mortality between patients in the lowest quintile for depression and those in the highest. Anxiety was not associated with either increased hospitalizations or mortality (Fan et al., 2007).

In a study of COPD patients in five Nordic countries, among patients with low perceived health status, the risk of readmission was also increased in subjects with anxiety. No significant relationship between depression and risk of readmission was found regardless of health status (Gudmundsson et al., 2005). In a study with a similar 1-year readmission rate (58.5%) conducted in Spain, investigators found readmission was associated with previous year hospitalization, dyspnea scale score, hypercapnia at discharge, depression, cor pulmonale, chronic domiciliary oxygen, and quality of life. In multivariate analysis, the best predictor of readmission was the combination of hospitalization for COPD in the previous year, the total score on the quality of life scale, and hypercapnia at discharge.

In contrast, in a study examining whether psychological factors predicted outcome after emergency treatment for acute COPD exacerbation, investigators found that anxiety and depression were related to the outcome of the emergency treatment. After adjusting for age, gender, allergy status, treatment, and pack years, a significant association remained between treatment failure and anxiety and/or depression (Dahlen & Jansen, 2002). Similarly, Yohannes et al. (2000) found that anxiety was a major predictor for frequency of hospital admissions for acute exacerbations of COPD in older patients. Narsavage and chen (2008) examined factors that predicted depressed mood at discharge and 3 months post discharge for patients with COPD. They found that after controlling for FEV_1, anxiety, preserved health competence daily functioning and family emotional coping predicted depressed mood.

A study conducted in China identified that probable depression (HADS depression score ≥ 11) was associated with an increased risk of symptom-based exacerbations, event-based exacerbations, and hospitalizations. Patients with an elevated anxiety score experienced a longer duration of event-based exacerbations. Depressed patients had a significantly higher mortality than nondepressed patients, but there was no significant difference in mortality between anxious and nonanxious patients (Xu et al., 2008).

Findings of the impact of anxiety and depression on COPD are mixed. Reasons for the mixed literature include that different anxiety and depression tools were utilized and studies used varying sample characteristics and sizes. The literature does appear to support the association between depression and/or anxiety and hospital readmissions after an AECOPD (Almagro et al., 2006). Research also suggests that depressed patients with COPD have a significantly higher mortality rate compared to nondepressed patients with COPD (Almagro et al., 2002; Yohannes et al., 2005). Given the impact of depression and anxiety on complications and mortality, the diagnosis and treatment of depression and anxiety in patients with COPD is paramount.

11.8 Assessment

11.8.1 Diagnostic Tools

Controversy exists regarding the appropriate diagnostic procedures for depression and anxiety disorders in patients with serious medical illnesses. The gold standard has always been the diagnostic interview based upon a specific set of diagnostic criteria generally from the ICD-10 or DSM-IV-TR. Several concerns have been raised about this method of diagnosis. Some studies suggest that patients with subsyndromal depression appear similar to patients diagnosed with full blown syndromes in terms of subjective distress, course of depressive symptoms, functional impairment, and history of and response to psychiatric treatment (Barbee, Billings, Bologna, & Townsend, 2003; Judd et al., 1998; Rapaport and Judd, 1998; Roy-Byrne et al., 1994; Yohannes, Baldwin, & Connolly, 2003). Wamboldt (2005) suggests that future research needs to investigate whether excluding patients with subsyndromal depression underestimates the number of depressed patients who could benefit from treatment. As psychiatric interviews were not included in many studies, a review of the instruments used to evaluate anxiety and depression is warranted.

11.8.1.1 Anxiety Measures

The instruments most frequently used to measure anxiety or anxious symptoms in patients with COPD were the Beck Anxiety Inventory (BAI), the Spielberger STAI, The Hamilton Anxiety Rating Scale (HAM-A), and The Profile of Mood States (POMS). The BAI consists of 21-items scaled from 0 (absence of symptoms) to 3 (most severe symptoms) (Beck, Emery, & Greenberg, 2005). These items are summed to a total score. Items are descriptive of subjective, somatic, or panic-related symptoms of anxiety. The score range is 0–60 with a score >20 indicating moderate anxiety (Beck et al., 2005). In psychometric testing, the scale demonstrated excellent internal consistency and good test-retest reliability (Beck, Epstein, Brown, & Steer, 1988; Beck, Steer, & Garbin, 1988).

The Spielberger STAI measures anxiety in adults and helps to distinguish between an individual's feelings of anxiety and depression (Spielberger, 1966). There are two scales: one measuring state anxiety (the way that the respondent feels at the moment) and trait anxiety (the way that the respondent generally feels). Each scale of the STAI consists of 20-items, each rated on a 4-point Likert-type scale ranging from 1 (not at all) to 4 (very much so). The items within the instrument focus on examining feelings of apprehension, tension, nervousness, and worry (Spielberger). Both the BAI and the STAI are useful in evaluating changes in symptoms of anxiety over time.

The HAM-A is an instrument that quantifies the severity of anxiety symptoms and assesses the response to therapeutic interventions. It can be administered in 10–15 min (Hamilton, 1959). There are 14-items covering mood and physical complaints scored on a scale of 0 (not present) to 4 (present most of the time) (Hamilton).

The POMS measures acute mood states (McNair & Lorr, 1964). The instrument consists of 65 adjectives rated on a 5-point Likert Scale from 1 (not at all) to 5 (extremely). The POMS has been found to be a reliable measure of mood (McNair & Lorr). It consists of six subscales including: tension-anxiety, anger-hostility, fatigue-inertia, depression-dejection, vigor-activity, and confusion-bewilderment (McNair & Lorr).

Of the four studies that specifically differentiated panic disorder or attacks from anxiety disorders, three based the diagnosis on the DSM-III or DSM-IV diagnostic criteria (Karajgi et al., 1990; Livermore et al., 2010; Moore & Zebb, 1999) and one used a self-report frequency of panic attacks in the last 3 weeks (Porzelius et al., 1992).

11.8.1.2 Assessment of Depressive Symptoms/Depression in COPD

The instruments most frequently used to measure depressive symptoms or depression in patients with COPD were the Center for Epidemiological Studies Depression Scale (CES-D) (Radloff, 1977), the Hospital Anxiety and Depression Scale (HAD-S) (Zigmond & Snaith, 1983), the Beck Depression Inventory (BDI) (Beck, 1978), and the Patient Health Questionnaire Depression Scale (PHQ) (Spitzer et al., 1999).

The CES-D was developed to assess depressive symptoms in the general population. It has been found to be a reliable measure of depressive symptoms across many populations and settings (Hann, Winter, & Jacobson, 1999; Radloff, 1991). The CES-D has 20 items scored on a scale of 0 (rarely or none, less than 1 day) to 3 (most or all of the time, 5–7 days). The score range is 0–60 with a score >16 indicating depression that may be clinically significant. CES-D items are based on a recall interval of 1 week (Radloff, 1977).

The BDI is a 21-item survey used to measure the severity of depression focusing on depressive symptoms such as hopelessness, irritability, guilt, and feelings of being punished. The BDI also measures some physical symptoms such as fatigue, weight loss, and lack of libido (Beck, 1961). The score range is 0–63 with a score >20 indicating moderate depression. It has excellent psychometric properties (Beck, Epstein, et al., 1988; Beck, Steer, et al., 1988). The BDI has been used in clinical settings to document changes in depressive symptoms (Johnson & Heather, 1974).

The PHQ Depression Scale is a 9-item self-report measure to screen and diagnose depressive disorders in primary care. In psychometric testing, it has demonstrated good reliability and validity (Kroenke, Spitzer, & Williams, 2001) and has been used to evaluate changes in depressive symptoms. Recently, an ultrabrief screening scale for anxiety and depression, the PHQ-4 was validated for detecting both anxiety and depressive disorders. Scores on the tool were strongly associated with functional impairment, disability days, and healthcare utilization (Kroenke, Spitzer, Williams, & Lowe, 2009). This measure may be particularly useful in settings where very little time is available to assess depression symptoms.

The HAD-S was developed to identify possible and probable anxiety disorders and depression among patients in nonpsychiatric acute care hospitals (Bejelland, Dahl, Haug, & Neckelmann, 2002). The HAD-S is a self-report questionnaire that has 14 items and 2 subscales, anxiety and depression. Each item is scored on a 4-point scale of 0 (not at all) to 3 (definitely) (Zigmond & Snaith, 1983). None of the 14 items focus on somatic symptoms, hence it is particularly well suited for identifying depression and anxiety in patient with chronic illnesses.

The Brief Assessment Schedule Depression Cards (BASDEC) (Adshead, Cody, & Pitt, 1992) is based upon the Brief Assessment Schedule. It was developed for use with older medical inpatients and thus has few somatic items. It is composed of 19 cards with statements related to depression. The scale is administered by an interviewer, takes 2–8 min to complete, and requires a true or false response. The tool was found to have high sensitivity and specificity when the recommended cut-off of 7 was used (Yohannes et al., 2000). Since no individual self-report instrument to assess depression or anxiety has been found to provide superior objective measurement, the choice of screening instrument is often a function of accessibility, time, and familiarity on the part of the assessor (Schane et al., 2008).

11.9 Treatment

Thirty-five studies from 1992 to 2009 were identified that examined the effect of interventions such as pharmacology, psychotherapy, or pulmonary rehabilitation on anxiety and/or depression in patients with COPD.

11.9.1 Pharmacologic Interventions

Selective serotonin-reuptake inhibitors, tricyclic antidepressants, and anxiolytics have been found to reduce symptoms of anxiety and/or depression in patients with COPD (Argyropoulou, Patakas, Koukou, Vasiliadis, & Georgopoulos, 1993; Borson et al., 1992; Eiser, Harte, Karvounis, Phillips, & Isaac, 2005; Evans, Hammond, Wilson, Lye, & Copeland, 1997; Lacasse, Beaudoin, Rousseau, & Maltais, 2004; Silvertooth et al., 2004; Smoller, Pollack, Systrom, & Kradin, 1998; Yohannes, Connolly, & Baldwin, 2001). See Table 11.1 for specific study descriptions.

11.9.1.1 Pharmacotherapy for Anxiety in COPD

Two small randomized trials tested buspirone for anxiety in patients with COPD with mixed findings. In a double-blind, crossover, randomized clinical trial of 16 patients with COPD, researchers found that 14-day treatment with 20 mg of buspirone produced clinically and statistically significant decreases in anxiety and dyspnea and improvement in exercise tolerance. Although the sample size was small ($N=16$) and the length of treatment short (14 days), there was a significant treatment effect (Argyropoulou et al., 1993). Another small double-blind, placebo-controlled randomized study of buspirone, with a crossover design ($N=11$), revealed no significant effects either in anxiety or physical parameters when buspirone 10–20 mg was administered three times a day for 6 weeks to patients with mild-to-moderate anxiety (Singh et al., 1993). The small sample with no power calculation

Table 11.1 Pharmacologic interventions

References	Patients	Study design/intervention	Outcomes
Borson et al. (1992)	$N=30$; pulmonary clinics; moderate-to-severe COPD and co-morbid depressive disorder	Randomized controlled trial; nortriptyline over 12 weeks	Marked improvement in depression, anxiety, certain respiratory symptoms, overall physical comfort, day-to-day function
Argyropoulou et al. (1993)	$N=16$; chronic airway obstruction	Double-blind, crossover "randomized way"; 14 days of buspirone (20 mg daily)	Significant improvement in anxiety, depression, and obsessive compulsive symptoms and complaints. Improvement in exercise tolerance and sensation of dyspnea
Singh, Despars, Stansbury, Avalos, and Light (1993)	$N=11$; outpatient pulmonary clinic; mild-to-moderate anxiety and chronic airway obstruction	Double-blind, placebo-controlled, randomized study, crossover design, buspirone 10–20 mg, 3 times per day; 6 week trial	No significant differences in anxiety scores or physical parameters including dyspnea
Papp et al. (1995)	$N=6$ consecutive patients; outpatient pulmonary clinic	Descriptive study; sertraline 12.5 mg/day increased to 100 mg/day over 2 weeks; remained on dosage 6 weeks	Medication tolerated well with minimal side effects; at week 6, 5/6 showed improvement on scale of daily living; ½ with psychiatric diagnoses reported marked subjective improvement; no significant changes in spirometric indices or arterial blood gases
Evans (1997)	$N=82$; depressed, physically ill older adults; 42 completed 8 week trial	Double-blind, randomized, parallel-group study; fluoxetine 20 mg/day for 8 weeks	No significant response rate found between the groups; patients with serious physical illness who completed 5 or more weeks showed significant improvement in mood
Smoller et al. (1998)	$N=7$ obstructive airway disease	Case series (6 retrospective, 1 prospective); sertraline 25–100 mg/day cases ranged from 2 months to a year in duration	Decrease in breathlessness and in some cases subjective improvement in exercise tolerance
Yohannes et al. (2001)	$N=57$; outpatients; moderate-to- severe COPD and depression	Single-blinded (open) study; fluoxetine 20 mg/day over 6 months	Patient acceptance of fluoxetine was poor; only seven patients completing the trial; of the 7, 4 responded to the drug; depression remained in 86% of untreated patients

(continued)

Table 11.1 (continued)

References	Patients	Study design/intervention	Outcomes
Lacasse et al. (2004)	$N=23$; end-stage COPD started the trial and 15 completed	Double-blind, randomized, placebo-controlled trial; paroxetine (dosage not specified) conducted over 12 weeks	Statistically and clinically significant improvement in emotional function and mastery (quality of life measures); dyspnea and fatigue improved but not significantly; no worsening of respiratory symptoms
Eiser et al. (2005)	$N=28$ COPD patients	Double-blind, randomized, placebo-controlled trial with paroxetine 20 mg over 6 weeks, and all unblinded on Paroxetine for 3 months	No significant differences in depression, quality of life, or 6 minute walk distance (6MWD) at 6 weeks, but the 3 month unblinded treatment significantly improved depression scores
Silvertooth et al. (2004)	$N=19$ COPD patients	Double-blind, random assignment, placebo-controlled trial with citalopram 20 mg/day, increased to 40 mg/day at 6 weeks, if tolerated for 12 weeks	No significant differences in depression, anxiety, or physical function, but effect depended upon initial severity; citalopram more effective in patients with mild-to-moderate initial levels of depression, anxiety, and physical function; no different than placebo in patients with severe depression, anxiety, or impaired physical function
Wagena et al. (2005)	$N=225$ adults at risk for COPD or with COPD	Placebo-controlled double-dummy randomized trial; buproprion SR 150 mg twice daily or nortriptyline 75 mg once a day for 12 weeks	In patients with COPD, Buproprion SR and nortriptyline resulted in higher prolonged (no cigarettes from week 4 to 52) abstinence rates compared to placebo, only buproprion SR was statistically different from placebo

makes the findings difficult to interpret. Additional studies with larger samples are needed to determine whether buspirone is effective in reducing anxiety symptoms, including panic in patients with COPD.

The effect of sertraline on anxiety was evaluated in two uncontrolled studies of patients with COPD, a case series and a descriptive study (Papp et al., 1995; Smoller et al., 1998). Sertraline appeared to be well tolerated in patients with COPD for the treatment of anxiety symptoms, although randomized controlled trials testing its efficacy on anxiety are lacking.

11.9.1.2 Pharmacotherapy for Depression in COPD

Two randomized trials examined the effect of fluoxetine in COPD patients with major depressive disorder (Evans et al., 1997; Yohannes et al., 2001). Reductions in depressive symptoms were observed in both trials, but both had high attrition rates (50%). One of the studies reported a 72% refusal rate. Reasons for refusal included: denial of depression, fear about antidepressant medications, embarrassment, and reluctance to take an additional medication. This suggests that many people who are in need of treatment for their depression may not be interested in receiving it. Patient education about depression and the importance of treatment may be necessary to increase treatment engagement.

In a 12-week, randomized, placebo-controlled trial of paroxetine in COPD patients with co-morbid depression, emotional functioning and feelings of mastery improved and respiratory symptoms were not adversely affected (Lacasse et al., 2004). In another randomized placebo-controlled trial ($N=28$) of paroxetine, no significant differences were found in depression at 6 weeks, but when the study was unblinded and continued for 3 months, significant improvement in depression scores was observed. The authors noted that perhaps a longer trial is needed to see improvements in COPD patients (Eiser et al., 2005). In general, some limited support exists for depression pharmacotherapy in COPD patients, but additional trials are needed and on a broader range of outcomes, including COPD symptoms, functioning, and quality of life.

11.9.1.3 Pharmacotherapy for Co-morbid Anxiety and Depression

Two studies examined pharmacotherapy in COPD patients with mixed anxiety and depression given that depression and anxiety more often co-occur than occur independently in COPD patients. One small, placebo-controlled randomized controlled trial of nortriptyline, a tricyclic antidepressant, in 30 patients with COPD, co-morbid depression, and anxiety revealed significant reductions in depression, anxiety, certain respiratory symptoms, and overall physical discomfort (Borson et al., 1992). The second study was a small double-blind placebo-controlled randomized trial ($N=19$) of citalopram in COPD patients with mild-to-moderate levels of anxiety and/or depression (Silvertooth et al., 2004). Patients with mild-to-moderate depression and/or anxiety symptoms but not those with more severe symptoms benefited from citalopram in terms of anxiety and physical functioning. Attrition was much higher (40 vs. 17% placebo group) for patients assigned to citalopram.

11.9.1.4 Additional Benefits of Antidepressant Therapy

Studies provide some evidence that selected antidepressants (e.g., sertraline, paroxetine, fluoxetine, and citalopram) and buspirone are tolerated in some patients with COPD and may relieve anxiety and depressive symptoms, at least over relatively brief treatment periods. Antidepressants have also been shown to reduce tobacco cravings (particularly with bupropion) (Tashkin et al., 2001), improve subjective dyspnea (Smoller et al., 1998), and improve appetite and weight. In a randomized trial testing the efficacy of bupropion SR and nortriptyline for smoking cessation among people at risk for or with chronic obstructive disease, investigators found that in patients with COPD, bupropion SR and nortriptyline were effective relative to placebo in achieving prolonged abstinence from week 4 to 26 (Wagena et al., 2005). Twenty-eight percent of the participants on bupropion SR and 25% on nortriptyline remained abstinent as compared to 15% of the participants on placebo. As smoking is the most frequent etiology of COPD and continued smoking after the diagnosis tends to exacerbate symptoms, pharmacologic interventions to improve abstinence have the potential to make a large contribution to the prevention and treatment of COPD. Trials examining the impact of antidepressants on quality of life and survival in COPD are greatly needed (Raji, 2006).

11.9.2 Cognitive and Behavioral Interventions

Ten studies were identified that evaluated the efficacy of cognitive-behavioral interventions on anxiety, panic attacks, and/or depression in patients with COPD with discrepant results. See Table 11.2 for study descriptions.

11.9.2.1 CBT for Anxiety and Panic Disorder

In an early randomized trial of a taped progressive muscle relaxation program on physiologic and psychological variables, Gift et al. (1992) found that the intervention group significantly decreased in anxiety severity and dyspnea and increased in peak flow. In a randomized trial of exercise, stress management, and education, the exercise, stress management group, and education group improved in endurance, and cognitive performance (verbal fluency) and had a reduction in anexity. These improvements were not found in the education and stress management group without exercise or waiting list groups (Emery et al., 1998).

A 2002 systematic review of the efficacy of behavioral treatments to reduce anxiety and panic in patients with COPD noted a lack of evidence for behavioral interventions for anxiety in COPD (Rose et al., 2002). In addition, several deficiencies were identified in the studies: failure to measure lung function, large variations in attrition, lack of blinding in assessing treatment outcomes, and inconsistent use of standardized instruments to measure anxiety. Since that review, one randomized trial has examined CBT on the development of or worsening of panic spectrum psychopathology and anxiety symptoms compared to routine care in patients with COPD. At 18 months, 60% of the patients in the routine care group had experienced at least one panic attack in the past 6 months with 17% of the patients being diagnosed with a panic disorder. In contrast, none of the patients in the CBT intervention group experienced a panic attack. In addition, the CBT group experienced reductions in anxiety symptoms, catastrophic cognitions, and a lower number of hospital admissions. Limitations of the study included small sample size ($N=41$) and lack of blinding to the treatment condition (Livermore et al., 2010). As in previous trials, lung function was not assessed, thus it is unknown whether CBT for anxiety and panic has the ability to affect lung function in COPD patients.

11.9.2.2 CBT for Anxiety and Depression

In a randomized, controlled trial of CBT for $N=56$ individuals were randomly assigned to either the CBT group involving 2 h of group cognitive therapy with workbooks, audiotapes and weekly calls, or the education group, which met with an internist and discussed the process, etiology, and treatment of COPD (Kunik et al., 2001). Participants in the CBT group had significantly lower scores than the education group on self-report measures of anxiety and depressive symptoms after 6 weeks of intervention.

A randomized controlled trial ($N=30$) compared psychotherapy in conjunction with pulmonary rehabilitation to usual care on anxiety and depression in patients with COPD (de Godoy & de Godoy, 2003). The psychotherapy group participated in an enhanced pulmonary rehabilitation program which included the addition of 12 psychotherapy sessions. Only the psychotherapy group had significant reductions in anxiety and depression with statistically significant differences between groups on the anxiety and depression measures. In addition, the psychotherapy group improved twice as much as the control group on the 6MWD. Limitations of the study include the small sample size, and the possibility that the improvement in physical health may have affected psychological health as well.

In a recent, small nonrandomized study ($N=10$) of individualized CBT conducted by a respiratory nurse with CBT training, significant improvements were observed in anxiety, depression, and hospitalizations after an average of four sessions. Limitations of the study included a small sample size and no randomization or blinding (Heslop et al., 2009).

A systematic review of CBT in COPD found limited evidence that CBT when used in conjunction with exercise and education contributed to significant reductions in anxiety and depression in patients with mild-to-moderate COPD (Coventry & Gellatly, 2008). Further randomized, controlled trials are needed to evaluate the

Table 11.2 Cognitive and behavioral interventions

References	Patients	Study design/intervention	Outcomes
Gift et al. (1992)	$N=6$; COPD with dyspnea	Convenience sample; randomly assigned to intervention or control group; relaxation group used a prerecorded tape, four sessions over 4 weeks	Dyspnea, anxiety, and airway obstruction were reduced in intervention group; control group remained the same or became worse
Lisansky and Hendel-Clough (1996)	$N=8$; COPD	Descriptive study; convenience sample; 8-week cognitive-behavioral self-help educational program	Significant decrease in disability as measured by the psychosocial and total Sickness Impact Profile scores; decrease in cognitive distortion; no change in depression or anxiety
Eiser, West, Evans, Jeffers, and Quirk (1997)	$N=10$; moderately severe COPD	Descriptive study; 6-week, 90 min sessions of cognitive-behavioral psychotherapy	Sustained improvement in exercise tolerance; improvement sustained 3 months later; no change in anxiety
Emery, Schein, Hauck, and MacIntyre (1998)	$N=79$; COPD	Preposttest, random assignment; 3 group (exercise, stress management and education, education and stress management, waiting list); 10-week duration of program	Patients in exercise and stress management group experienced improvement in endurance, reduced anxiety, and improved cognitive performance (verbal fluency); significant changes in depression found in the exercise, stress management, and education group and in the wait list group
Kunik et al. (2001)	$N=56$; COPD	Two group single blind, randomized controlled clinical trial; one 2 h session of cognitive-behavioral therapy (CBT) followed by homework and weekly calls for 6 weeks vs. one 2 h session of COPD education and weekly calls	CBT group decreased depressive and anxious symptoms, but no change in physical functioning
de Godoy and de Godoy (2003)	$N=33$; COPD	Two groups, blind, randomized, controlled trial, all attending pulmonary rehab; Group 1, 24 sessions of physical exercise and physiotherapy, 12 psychologic sessions, 3 educational sessions Group 2, no psychotherapy sessions	Psychotherapy in a pulmonary rehab program reduced anxiety and depression levels, but did not improve the 6-min walk test

McGeoch et al. (2006)	N=159 COPD	Prospective, unblinded, randomized controlled trial of unusual care vs. usual care with structured education on COPD action plan	Self-management knowledge higher in intervention group, but no differences in groups for quality of life or mental health
Kunik et al. (2008)	N=181 Older adults with COPD and moderate anxiety and/or depression symptoms treated by a primary care provider or pulmonologist	Eight group sessions of group CBT or COPD education; assessments: baseline, 4, 8 weeks, 4, 8, and 12 months	Both treatment groups significantly improved quality of life, 6MWD, symptoms of anxiety, and depression over 8 weeks with no significant differences between the groups; the improvement was maintained with no significant change during the entire follow-up period
Heslop, De Soyza, Baker, Stenton, and Burns (2009)	N=10 COPD outpatient clinic	Convenience sample of patients with anxiety or depression as identified by their treating doctor; individualized sessions of CBT with a respiratory nurse implementing the intervention; an average of four sessions (range 2–13)	Significant decrease in anxiety, depression, and number of hospital admission from baseline to completion of CBT sessions
Livermore, Sharpe, and McKenzie (2010)	N=41 (21 CBT 20 routine care) COPD postpulmonary rehabilitation	Random assignment to 4-session CBT or routine care; assessments: baseline, postintervention, and at 6, 12, and 18 month follow-up	By 18-month follow-up, 60% of routine care had experienced at least one panic attack with 17% being diagnosed with a panic disorder, no CBT participants experienced a panic attack; CBT group experienced significant reductions in anxiety symptoms and catastrophic cognitions, a lower number of hospital admissions between 6 and 12 month follow-up

effectiveness of CBT in patients with COPD who are experiencing anxiety and depression (Brenes, 2003). In addition, research is needed to establish the most effective and appropriate model of CBT for use with patients with COPD and co-morbid anxiety and depression (Coventry & Gellatly, 2008). To date, no studies have compared the efficacy of antidepressants, CBT, and COPD education (Kunik et al., 2008).

11.9.3 Pulmonary Rehabilitation

Pulmonary rehabilitation is an evidence-based, comprehensive, multidisciplinary intervention designed to reduce COPD symptoms, increase functional performance, increase participation and health-related quality of life, and reduce healthcare costs through stabilizing or reversing systemic manifestations of disease. Programs generally involve patient assessment, exercise training, education, nutritional interventions, and psychosocial support (Nici et al., 2006). Pulmonary rehabilitation has been found to impact depression and anxiety possibly by reducing symptoms of COPD, providing psychosocial support, and increasing quality of life but the exact mechanism of effect is not known.

In a systematic review of respiratory rehabilitation after acute exacerbations of COPD, investigators identified that rehabilitation reduced the risk for hospital admissions, improved quality of life, emotional functioning, and exercise capacity, and decreased mortality (Puhan et al., 2005). The Joint American Thoracic Society/European Respiratory Society guidelines recommended that initial assessment before pulmonary rehabilitation should include screening for anxiety and depression. They note that mild-to-moderate levels of anxiety or depression may improve with pulmonary rehabilitation, but patients with more severe symptoms require referral (Nici, p. 1400). Unfortunately, patients with depressive and anxiety symptoms have lower adherence to pulmonary rehabilitation than those patients without these co-morbidities (Fan, Giardino, Blough, Kaplan, & Ramsey, 2008) which underscores the importance of assessment and special care for patients with these co-morbidities.

Although pulmonary rehabilitation for COPD focuses on physical conditioning, some programs include behavioral interventions that may address depressive symptoms (Alexopoulos et al., 2006). Fourteen trials tested the efficacy of pulmonary rehabilitation on anxiety, depression, and/or emotional functioning in patients with COPD with mixed results (Alexopoulos et al., 2006; de Godoy, Teixeira, Junior, Michellli, & de Godoy, 2009; Elci, Borekci, Ovayolu, & Elbek, 2008; Griffiths et al., 2000; Guell et al., 2000, 2006; Kayahan, Karapolat, Atyntoprak, Atasever, & Ozturk, 2006; Kozora, Tran, & Make, 2002; Lolak, Connors, Sheridan, & Wise, 2009; Nguyen & Carrieri-Kohlman, 2005; Paz-Diaz, de Oca, Lopez, & Celli, 2007; Ries, Kaplan, Limberg, & Prewitt, 1995; Sassi-Dambron, Eakin, Ries, & Kaplan, 1995; Withers, Rudkin, & White, 1999) (see Table 11.3).

Table 11.3 Pulmonary rehabilitation

References	Patients	Study design/intervention	Outcomes
Sassi-Dambron et al. (1995)	$N=89$; COPD	Randomized clinical trial; 6-week treatment of progressive muscle relaxation (PMR), breathing retraining, pacing, self-talk, and panic control or general health education	No significant difference between the treatment and control group on any physical parameters, quality of life, anxiety, or depression
Ries et al. (1995)	$N=119$; outpatients; stable COPD	Randomized clinical trial; 8-week comprehensive pulmonary rehabilitation: 12, 4 h sessions of education, physical and respiratory care instruction, psychosocial support, and supervised exercise training with monthly reinforcement sessions for 1 year or education: 4, 2 h sessions including videotapes, lectures, and discussions but not individual instruction or exercise training	Comprehensive rehabilitation group showed significantly greater increases in maximal exercise tolerance, exercise endurance, shortness of breath, and self-efficacy for walking. Lung function, depression, and quality of life did not differ between groups.
Withers et al. (1999)	$N=95$ outpatients severe COPD	Longitudinal study; one group pre- and postdesign; convenience sample 6-week outpatient rehabilitation program: supervised exercise training, education, and psychosocial support; posttesting at 3 months	Pulmonary rehabilitation led to significant decreases in depressive and anxious symptoms; both anxiety and depression remained lower at 6-month follow-up; anxious patients showed significantly greater improvement in exercise capacity
Guell et al. (2000)	$N=60$ moderate-to-severe COPD (30 patients intervention, 30 control)	Randomized, controlled trial with blinding of outcome assessment and follow-up; 3 months outpatient breathing retraining and chest physiotherapy, 3 months supervised, daily exercise, 6 months of weekly supervised breathing exercises, control group received standard care	Significant differences between groups in perception of dyspnea, in 6MWD, reduction of exacerbations, and in day-to-day dyspnea, fatigue, and emotional function; improvements were evident by the third month and continued though diminished until the 2-year follow-up
Griffiths et al. (2000)	$N=180$ (92 intervention, 88 standard medical management) outpatients with disabling, chronic lung disease	Randomized, controlled trial, 6-week, outpatient pulmonary rehabilitation; evaluation baseline, post-PR, and at 1 year	Improvements in exercise tolerance, health-related quality of life, anxiety and depression post-PR that remained significant but declined at 1-year follow-up

(continued)

Table 11.3 (continued)

References	Patients	Study design/intervention	Outcomes
Kozora (2002)	$N=80$; 59 with COPD; 21 healthy subjects	Three group, prepost test design; convenience sample; 3-week rehabilitation program: exercise, psychosocial and educational sessions, medical comparison group and healthy adults	Rehabilitation group had significantly decreased depressive symptoms and increased 6-min walk; clinically significant improvement in visual attention, verbal retention, and visuospatial ability also noted in the most impaired patients in the rehabilitation group
Nguyen and Carrieri-Kohlman (2005)	$N=100$ moderate-to-severe COPD	Randomized clinical trial of 3 dyspnea management programs; programs differed in the amount of supervised exercise (none, 4 or 24 sessions)	All three versions of the intervention equally and significantly improved depressed mood and social functioning with no difference between the groups
Kayahan et al. (2006)	$N=45$ COPD 26 rehabilitation patients and 19 control patients	Randomized clinical trial; 2-month pulmonary rehabilitation program (PRP): education, relaxation exercise, bronchial hygiene program, breathing retraining, and exercise; control group received standard care	Pulmonary rehabilitation led to significant improvement in anxiety both across time and between groups. Dyspnea, health status, and exercise tolerance improved significantly in the rehabilitation group. No change in the depression scores either across time or between groups
Guell et al. (2006)	$N=40$ COPD	Prospective, randomized, controlled trial with blinding of outcome assessment and data analysis, 16 weeks of pulmonary rehab, evaluated psychosocial morbidity using the MBHI and the SCL-90-R questionnaires and 6MWD and the CRQ	Pulmonary rehab may decrease psychosocial morbidity in COPD patients even when no specific psychological intervention is performed
Alexopoulos et al. (2006)	$N=63$ COPD	Convenience sample of consecutive admissions to an inpatient pulmonary rehabilitation unit. Treatment regime tailored by a multidisciplinary team for each patient. Offered 10 mg of escitalopram or continued on admission antidepressant regimen. Median length of stay was 16 days	51% met criteria for response (50% or greater reduction) in depressive scores from baseline and 39% met criteria for remission (final Hamilton D score ≤ 10). Social support and satisfaction with treatment predicted improvement. All disability domains were lower at discharge

Paz-Diaz et al. (2007)	$N=24$ severe COPD	Prospective, randomized study examining benefits of pulmonary rehab on scores of objective psychological tests, dyspnea, and quality of life	After pulmonary rehab, a significant improvement noted in the severity of depression, decrease in symptoms, increase in daily living activities, and an improvement on the dyspnea scale
Elci et al. (2008)	$N=78$ (39 intervention 39 control) COPD secondary-care community hospital	Randomized, controlled, prospective study; pulmonary rehabilitation including exercise and education over 3 months (24 sessions of up to 90 min twice a week)	Significant differences in 6MWD, SF-36 quality of life scale, SGRQ and HADS total score at second and third month; no significant differences in FEV_1 or dyspnea scale
Lolak et al. (2009)	$N=66$ (31 intervention, 35 standard care) chronic breathing disorders	Prospective, randomized controlled trial; 8 week PR; standard care included 2 days/week exercise, education, and psychosocial support from multidisciplinary team; intervention group received additional sessions of PMR therapy using prerecorded tape for 25 min/week during weeks 2–8	Anxiety and depression significantly improved in both groups over time; no statistical difference between groups in anxiety and depression, results favored the PMR group for depression for weeks 5–8
de Godoy et al. (2009)	$N=30$ severe and extreme COPD who had completed pulmonary rehabilitation 2 years before and were not currently monitored	12-week PRP, 24 exercise sessions, 24 respiratory rehabilitation sessions, 12 psychotherapy sessions, and 3 educational sessions; evaluations at baseline, post-PRP, and 2 years later	Significant decreases in anxiety and depression and improvement in quality of life and 6 MWD were sustained for 2 years with no significant differences between post-PRP and 2 years later

Some studies found significant improvements in anxiety and depression but not physical symptoms. Other studies found improvement in physical symptoms but not anxiety and depression, yet others found improvements in both psychological and physical symptoms. One early study (Sassi-Dambron et al., 1995) found no improvement in any of these dimensions.

Multidisciplinary and multimodal pulmonary rehabilitation appears to be among the leading nonpharmacological approaches to effectively managing anxiety and depression in patients with COPD. A systematic review and meta-analysis of the effect of pulmonary rehabilitation (with or without education) on self-reported symptoms of anxiety and depression showed that comprehensive pulmonary rehabilitation is associated with small-to-moderate and significant reductions in symptoms of anxiety and depression. Although the components of the programs differed, all included supervised and incremental exercise and education or psychosocial support or both at least 3 times a week for a minimum of 6 weeks (Coventry, 2009; Coventry & Hind, 2007). Coventry raises several issues about the heterogeneity of the trials of pulmonary rehabilitation. The professional composition, treatment components, and program duration vary widely, making it difficult to identify which elements are associated with improvement in anxiety and depression. Most studies have not specifically recruited patients with a diagnosed anxiety disorder and/or major depression, as such the efficacy of PR in patients with clinically diagnosed depression and anxiety is yet to be determined. Also, findings on the long-term efficacy of PR have been equivocal. While some studies showed diminishing effects over time, others demonstrated maintenance for up to 2 years. Very little data are available on how pulmonary rehabilitation improves symptoms of anxiety and depression. Coventry & Hind (2007) call for future trials that test strategies to improve maintenance and stepped care approaches for COPD in the context of a psychological co-morbidity.

11.9.4 Clinical Considerations

A number of issues should be considered in the clinical management of COPD in the context of psychological co-morbidities. Six major challenges were identified in the treatment of depression in patients with COPD (Sirey et al., 2007). These include patients' misconceptions about COPD, depression, what depression treatment is, and when it is needed. Denial of depression symptoms is also common. Psychoeducation could be helpful to overcome these barriers. Also, cost of medications and access to treatment are significant logistical barriers, especially for low-income patients and those who are disengaged from the healthcare system. Finally, guilt and stigma associated with having COPD and depression, hopelessness and helplessness, and poor mobility and functioning are all significant treatment barriers. The negative spiral of guilt, hopelessness, and helplessness associated with depression and COPD may contribute to a fatalistic attitude that causes inactivity and nonadherence with treatment (Sirey et al.).

The clinician should also note that anxiety, panic, and depression are largely overlooked, underdiagnosed, and undertreated. In light of the overall evidence regarding the prevalence and negative impact of anxiety, panic, and depression on patients, a routine assessment and screening for anxiety, panic, and depression in all patients diagnosed with COPD should be considered. Clinicians should consider several options to assist persons with COPD suffering from anxiety, panic, and/or depression. Physical aids such as pursed lip breathing, oxygen therapy, and pharmacological intervention may bring patients a degree of relief. However, based on the studies reviewed, this may not be enough. Even after identification of co-morbid anxiety, panic, or depression through self-report questionnaires, patients with COPD may be reluctant to enter into treatment (Sirey et al., 2007). Studies of antidepressant medications have found mixed results for the treatment of both anxiety and depression with many patients choosing to discontinue the medication due to side effects (Evans et al., 1997; Yohannes et al., 2001). As most patients with COPD are older adults, starting with low dosages and increasing the dosage slowly may alleviate some of the problems with side effects.

Patients scoring in the high range for anxiety and depression should be referred to a mental health professional for assessment and treatment. Ultimately, one standard modality of treatment will not be sufficient or appropriate for all patients, but rather each patient should be approached on an individual basis considering all techniques shown to help alleviate both the symptoms of COPD as well as anxiety, panic, and/or depression and balancing this consideration with patient preferences for treatment.

11.10 Summary

A review of the literature on COPD with co-morbid anxiety, panic, and/or depression has yielded several key areas for consideration. The prevalence of anxiety, panic, and depression in patients with COPD is well above the general population. The literature shows a significant impact of anxiety, panic, and depression on patients with COPD. For example, depression has been found to negatively impact exercise capacity, health perception/well-being, the utilization of inpatient and outpatient health services, and hospital stays (Koenig & Kuchibhatla, 1998; Ng et al., 2007; Ormel et al., 1998; Weaver & Narsavage, 1992; Weaver et al., 1997). Patients with COPD and depression are more often noncompliant with medical treatment and have more impaired functional status, increased symptom burden, decreased quality of life and, in some studies, higher mortality rates (COPD International, 2007; DiMatteo et al., 2000; Ng et al., 2007; Seung-Kim et al., 2000). The presence of anxiety and panic in patients with COPD is associated with greater restrictions on mobility, decreased energy, difficulties with activities of daily living, greater dependence on others for care, and impaired functional status (Moore & Zebb, 1998; Weaver et al., 1997).

COPD is characterized by acute exacerbations often leading to hospitalization and associated with further impairment of health status, decreased health-related quality of life, increased healthcare expenditures worldwide, and increased mortality (Almagro et al., 2006; Anderson et al., 2002; Connors et al., 1996; Quint et al., 2008; Seemungal et al., 1998).

Women appear to report higher levels of anxiety and depression and lower quality of life (de Torres et al., 2005; DiMarco et al., 2006; Hynninen et al., 2007). Researchers have identified sex-related differences in the symptoms of COPD, co-morbidities, and death rates. As described earlier, COPD mortality rates for women have significantly increased probably due to more women smoking cigarettes, exposure to toxins, and women's longer life span. It has been postulated that females cope differently with their disease (Chavannes et al., 2005), and thus, interventions may need to address gender differences. Both depression and anxiety have been found to negatively impact COPD treatment modalities such as pulmonary rehabilitation and smoking cessation efforts (Kayahan et al., 2006; Nguyen et al. 2005).

Results are mixed regarding the efficacy of pharmacological interventions for anxiety, depression, respiratory symptoms, and physical comfort. Antidepressant medication in particular has been found to decrease tobacco cravings, facilitate smoking cessation, dyspnea, increase appetite, and decrease anxiety (Roundy et al., 2005; Smoller et al., 1998; Tashkin et al., 2001; Versiani, Moreno, Ramakers-van Moorsel, & Schutte, 2005). As smoking is the most frequent etiology of COPD and continued smoking tends to exacerbate symptoms, pharmacologic agents to improve abstinence while improving mood have tremendous potential in the treatment of COPD.

Studies examining cognitive-behavioral interventions for anxiety and depression in COPD patients yielded mixed results. In some studies, relaxation techniques were found to be helpful (Emery et al., 1998; Gift et al., 1992; Sassi-Dambron et al., 1995). Pulmonary rehabilitation studies in patients with COPD and co-morbid depression also produced mixed results. Some studies found overall physical improvements, but no psychological benefits (Ries et al., 1995; Sassi-Dambron et al., 1995), but others found significant improvements in overall health status, exercise tolerance, dyspnea, and anxiety symptoms (Guell et al., 2006; Kayahan et al., 2006; Kozora et al., 2002; Nguyen et al. 2005; Paz-Diaz et al., 2007; Withers et al., 1999).

11.11 Conclusions and Future Research Recommendations

The prevalence of anxiety, panic, and depression among patients with COPD is significantly higher than in the general population; however, there are serious barriers to the recognition and treatment of these co-morbid conditions at the patient, provider, and system levels. Patients may fear the stigma of mental illness and may focus on somatic complaints rather than emotional problems. Providers, who are limited by time constraints with patients, focus on treating the physiologic symptoms of COPD rather than emotional symptoms. Some providers believe that depression and anxiety are simply part of the symptom profile of patients with airway obstructions and do not assess or treat these co-morbidities. At a system level, mental health care is not well integrated into primary care. If patients need to be referred to mental health centers, often patients will not accept either the diagnosis of depression and/or anxiety or a referral for psychiatric services (Maurer et al., 2008). Based on a long-term, mounting body of evidence, future research needs to include large-scale randomized controlled trials of both pharmacological and psychological interventions to determine which interventions are most efficacious for COPD in the context of psychological co-morbidities.

References

Adshead, F., Cody, D., & Pitt, B. (1992). BASDEC: A novel screening instrument for depression in elderly medical patients. *British Medical Journal, 305*(6854), 648.

Aghanwa, H. S., & Erhabor, G. E. (2001). Specific psychiatric morbidity among patients with chronic obstructive pulmonary disease in a Nigerian general hospital. *Journal of Psychosomatic Research, 50*, 179–183.

Alexopoulos, G. S., Sirey, J. A., Raue, P. J., Kanellopoulos, D., Clark, T. E., & Novitch, R. (2006). Outcomes of depressed patients undergoing inpatient pulmonary rehabilitation. *American Journal of Geriatric Psychiatry, 14*, 466–475.

Almagro, P., Barreiro, B., Ochoa de Echaguen, A., Quintana, S., Carballeira, M., Heredia, J., et al. (2006). Risk factors for hospital readmission in patients with chronic obstructive pulmonary disease. *Respiration, 73*, 311–317.

Almagro, P., Calbo, E., Ochoa de Echaguen, A., Barreiro, B., Quintana, S., Heredia, J., et al. (2002). Mortality after hospitalization in COPD. *Chest, 121*(5), 1441–1448.

Almagro, P., Garcia, F., Cabrera, F., Montero, L., Morchon, D., Diez, J., et al. (2009). Comorbidity and gender-related differences in patients hospitalized for COPD, The ECCO study. *Respiratory Medicine, 20*, 1–7.

American Psychiatric Association. (2000). *Quick reference to the diagnostic criteria from the DSM-IV-TR*. Washington: American Psychiatric Association.

Anderson, F., Borg, S., Jansson, S. A., Jonsson, A. C., Ericsson, A., Prutz, C., et al. (2002). The costs of exacerbations in chronic obstructive pulmonary disease. *Respiratory Medicine, 96*, 700–708.

Argyropoulou, P., Patakas, D., Koukou, A., Vasiliadis, P., & Georgopoulos, D. (1993). Buspirone effect on breathlessness and exercise performance in patients with chronic obstructive pulmonary disease. *Respiration, 60*, 216–220.

Bailey, P. H. (2004). The dyspnea-anxiety-dyspnea cycle-COPD patients' stories of breathlessness: "It's scary/when you can't breathe". *Qualitative Health Research, 14*(6), 760–778.

Barbee, J. G., Billings, C. K., Bologna, N. B., & Townsend, M. H. (2003). A follow-up study of DSM-III-R generalized anxiety disorder with syndromal and subsyndromal major depression. *Journal of Affective Disorders, 73*(3), 229–236.

Beck, A. T. (1961). A systematic investigation of depression. *Comprehensive Psychiatry, 2*, 163–170.

Beck, A. T. (1978). *Depression inventory*. Philadelphia: Center for Cognitive Therapy.

Beck, A. T., Emery, G., & Greenberg, R. (2005). *Anxiety disorders and phobias: Cognitive perspective*. New York: Basic Books.

Beck, A. T., Epstein, N., Brown, G., & Steer, R. A. (1988). An inventory for measuring clinical anxiety: Psychometric properties. *Journal of Consulting and Clinical Psychology, 56*(6), 893–897.

Beck, A. T., Steer, R. A., & Garbin, M. G. (1988). Psychometric properties of the Beck depression inventory twenty-five years of evaluation. *Clinical Psychology Review, 8*, 77–100.

Beekman, A. T., Copeland, J. R., & Prince, M. J. (1999). Review of community prevalence of depression in later life. *British Journal of Psychiatry, 174*, 307–311.

Bejelland, I., Dahl, A., Haug, T., & Neckelmann, D. (2002). The validity of the hospital anxiety and depression scale: An updated literature review. *Journal of Psychiatric Research, 52*, 69–77.

Borson, S., Claypoole, K., & McDonald, G. (1998). Depression and chronic obstructive pulmonary disease: Treatment trials. *Seminars in Clinical Neuropsychiatry, 3*, 115–130.

Borson, S., McDonald, G. J., Gayle, T., Deffebach, M., Lakshminarayan, S., & VanTuinen, C. (1992). Improvement in mood, physical symptoms, and function with nortriptyline for depression in patients with chronic obstructive pulmonary disease. *Psychomatics, 33*(2), 190–201.

Bosley, C. M., Corden, Z. M., Rees, P. J., & Cochrane, G. M. (1996). Psychological factors associated with use of home nebulized therapy for COPD. *The European Respiratory Journal, 9*(11), 2346–2350.

Brenes, G. A. (2003). Anxiety and chronic obstructive pulmonary disease: Prevalence, impact, and treatment. *Psychosomatic Medicine, 65*, 963–970.

Brown, E. S., & Chandler, P. A. (2001). Mood and cognitive changes during systemic corticosteroid therapy. *Primary Care Companion to The Journal of Clinical Psychiatry, 3*, 17–21.

Buist, A. S., McBurnie, M. A., Vollmer, W. M., Gillespie, S., Burney, P., Mannino, D. M., et al. (2007). International variations in the prevalence of COPD (the BOLD study): A population-based prevalence study. *The Lancet, 370*(9589), 741–750.

Celli, B. R., Cote, C. G., Marin, J. M., Casanova, C., de Oca, M. M., Mendez, R. A., et al. (2004). The body-mass index, airflow obstruction, dyspnea, and exercise capacity index in chronic obstructive pulmonary disease. *The New England Journal of Medicine, 350*(10), 1005–1012.

Celli, B. R., & MacNee, W. (2004). Standards for the diagnosis and treatment of patients with COPD: A summary of the ATS/ERS Task Force. *The European Respiratory Journal, 23*, 932–946.

Chavannes, N. H., Huibers, M. J., Schermer, T. R., Hendriks, A., van Weel, C., Wouters, E., et al. (2005). Associations of depressive symptoms with gender, body mass index, and dyspnea in primary care COPD patients. *Family Practice, 22*, 604–607.

Chronic Obstructive Pulmonary Disease Fact Sheet. August 2006. American Lung Association. Accessed March 8, 2007, www.lungusa.org

Connors, A. F., Dawson, N. V., Thomas, C., Harrell, F. F., Desbiens, N., Fulkerson, W. J., et al. (1996). Outcomes following acute exacerbation of severe chronic obstructive disease. *American Journal of Respiratory and Critical Care Medicine, 154*, 959–967.

COPD International. Accessed February 7, 2010, www.copd-international.com

Cote, C. G., & Celli, B. R. (2009). BODE index: A new tool to stage and monitor progression of chronic obstructive pulmonary disease. *Pneumonologia i Alergologia Polska, 77*, 305–313.

Coventry, P. A. (2009). Does pulmonary rehabilitation reduce anxiety and depression in chronic obstructive pulmonary disease? *Current Opinion in Pulmonary Medicine, 15*, 143–149.

Coventry, P. A., & Gellatly, J. L. (2008). Improving outcomes for COPD patients with mild-to-moderate anxiety and depression: A systematic review of cognitive behavioral therapy. *British Journal of Health Psychology, 13*, 381–400.

Coventry, P. A., & Hind, D. (2007). Comprehensive pulmonary rehabilitation for anxiety and depression in adults with chronic obstructive pulmonary disease: A systematic review and meta-analysis. *Journal of Psychosomatic Research, 63*, 551–565.

Cully, J. A., Graham, D. P., Stanley, M. A., Ferguson, C. J., Sharafkhaneh, A., Souchek, J., et al. (2006). Quality of life in patients with chronic obstructive pulmonary disease and comorbid anxiety or depression. *Psychosomatics, 47*(4), 312–319.

Dahlen, I., & Jansen, C. (2002). Anxiety and depression are related to the outcome of emergency treatment in patients with obstructive pulmonary disease. *Chest, 122*, 1633–1637.

Damarla, M., Celli, R., Mullerova, H., & Pinto-Plata, V. (2006). Discrepancy in the use of confirmatory tests in patients hospitalized with the diagnosis of chronic obstructive pulmonary disease or congestive heart failure. *Respiratory Care, 51*, 1120–1124.

de Godoy, D., & de Godoy, R. (2003). A randomized controlled trial of the effect of psychotherapy on anxiety and depression in chronic obstructive pulmonary disease. *Archives of Physical Medicine and Rehabilitation, 84*, 1154–1157.
de Godoy, R. F., Teixeira, P. J., Junior, B. B., Michellli, M., & de Godoy, D. V. (2009). Long-term repercussions of a pulmonary rehabilitation program on the indices of anxiety, depression, quality of life and physical performance in patients with COPD. *Jornal Brasileiro de Pneumologia, 35*(2), 129–136.
de Torres, J., Casanova, C., Hernandez, C., Abreu, J., Aquirre-Jaime, A., & Celli, B. (2005). Gender and COPD in patients attending a pulmonary clinic. *Chest, 128*, 2012–2016.
de Torres, J., Casanova, C., Hernandez, C., Abreu, J., Montejo de Garcini, A., & Aquirre-Jaime, A. (2006). Gender associated differences in determinants of quality of life in patients with COPD: A case series study. *Health and Quality of Life Outcomes, 4*, 72.
DiMarco, F., Verga, M., Reggente, M., Casanova, F., Santus, P., Blasi, F., et al. (2006). Anxiety and depression in COPD patients: The roles of gender and disease severity. *Respiratory Medicine, 100*, 1767–1774.
DiMatteo, M. R., Lepper, H. S., & Croghan, T. W. (2000). Depression is a risk factor for noncompliance with medical treatment: Meta-analysis of the effects of anxiety and depression on patient adherence. *Archives of Internal Medicine, 160*, 2101–2107.
Dowson, C., Laing, R., Barraclough, R., Town, I., Mulder, R., Norris, K., et al. (2001). The use of the Hospital Anxiety and Depression scale (HADS) in patients with chronic obstructive pulmonary disease: A pilot study. *The New Zealand Medical Journal, 114*, 447–449.
Eaton, W. W., Kessler, R. C., Wittchen, H. U., & Magee, W. J. (1994). Panic and panic disorder in the United States. *The American Journal of Psychiatry, 151*, 413–420.
Eiser, N., Harte, R., Karvounis, S., Phillips, C., & Isaac, M. (2005). Effect of treating depression on quality of life and exercise tolerance in severe COPD. *Chronic Obstructive Pulmonary Disease, 2*, 233–241.
Eiser, N., West, C., Evans, S., Jeffers, A., & Quirk, F. (1997). Effects of psychotherapy in moderately severe COPD: A pilot study. *The European Respiratory Journal, 10*, 1581–1584.
Elci, A., Borekci, S., Ovayolu, N., & Elbek, O. (2008). The efficacy and applicability of a pulmonary rehabilitation programme for patients with COPD in a secondary-care community hospital. *Respirology, 13*, 703–707.
Emery, C. F., Green, M. R., & Suh, S. (2008). Neuropsychiatric function in chronic lung disease: The role of pulmonary rehabilitation. *Respiratory Care, 53*(9), 1208–1216.
Emery, C. F., Schein, R. L., Hauck, E. R., & MacIntyre, N. R. (1998). Psychological and cognitive outcomes of a randomized trial of exercise among patients with chronic obstructive pulmonary disease. *Journal of Health Psychology, 17*, 232–240.
Evans, M., Hammond, M., Wilson, K., Lye, M., & Copeland, J. (1997). Placebo controlled treatment trial of depression in elderly physically ill patients. *International Journal of Geriatric Psychiatry, 12*, 817–824.
Fan, V. S., Giardino, N. D., Blough, D. K., Kaplan, R. M., & Ramsey, S. D. (2008). Costs of pulmonary rehabilitation and predictors of adherence in the National Emphysema Treatment Trial. *Chronic Obstructive Pulmonary Disease, 5*, 105–116.
Fan, V. S., Ramsey, S. D., Giardino, N. D., Make, B. J., Emery, C. F., Diaz, P. T., et al. (2007). Sex, depression, and risk of hospitalization and mortality in chronic obstructive pulmonary disease. *Archives of Internal Medicine, 167*(21), 2345–2353.
Foster, J. M., Aucott, L., van der Werf, R. H., van der Meijden, M. S., Schraa, G., Postma, D. S., et al. (2006). High patient perceived side effects related to higher daily doses of inhaled corticosteroids in the community: A cross-sectional analysis. *Respiratory Medicine, 100*, 1318–1336.
Funk, G., Kirchheiner, K., Burghuber, O. C., & Hartl, S. (2009). BODE index versus GOLD classification for explaining anxious and depressive symptoms in patients with COPD – A cross sectional study. *Respiratory Research, 10*, 1.
Gan, W. Q., Man, S. F., Senthilselvan, A., & Sin, D. D. (2004). Association between chronic obstructive pulmonary disease and systemic inflammation: A systematic review and meta-analysis. *Thorax, 59*(7), 574–580.

Gelb, A. F., & Zamel, N. (1975). Effect of aging on lung mechanics in healthy nonsmokers. *Chest, 68*(4), 538–541.
Gerhardsson de Verdier, M. (2008). The big three concept: A way to tackle the health care crisis? *Proceedings of the American Thoracic Society, 5*(8), 800–805.
Gift, A. G., Moore, T., & Soeken, K. (1992). Relaxation to reduce dyspnea and anxiety in COPD patients. *Nursing Research, 41*, 242–246.
Global Obstructive Lung Initiative (GOLD), updated 2009. Accessed February 7, 2010, www.goldcopd.com
Griffiths, T. L., Burr, M. L., Campbell, I. A., Lewis-Jenkins, V., Mullins, J., Shiels, K., et al. (2000). Results at 1 year of outpatient multidisciplinary pulmonary rehabilitation: A randomized controlled trial. *The Lancet, 355*, 362–368.
Groenewegen, K. H., Schols, A. M., & Wouters, E. F. (2003). Mortality and mortality-related factors after hospitalization for acute exacerbation of COPD. *Chest, 124*, 459–467.
Gudmundsson, G., Gislason, T., Janson, C., Lindberg, E., Hallin, R., Ulrik, C., et al. (2005). Risk factors rehospitalization in COPD: Role of health status, anxiety and depression. *The European Respiratory Journal, 26*, 414–419.
Guell, R., Casan, P., Belda, J., Sangenis, M., Morante, F., Guyatt, G., et al. (2000). Long-term effect of outpatient rehabilitation of COPD. *Chest, 117*, 976–983.
Guell, R., Resqueti, V., Sangenis, M., Morante, F., Martorell, B., Casan, P., et al. (2006). Impact of pulmonary rehabilitation on psychosocial morbidity in patients with severe COPD. *Chest, 129*, 899–904.
Halbert, R. J., Natoli, J. L., Gano, A., Badamgarav, E., Buist, A. S., & Mannino, D. M. (2006). Global burden of COPD: Systematic review and meta-analysis. *The European Respiratory Journal, 28*, 523–532.
Hamilton, M. (1959). The assessment of anxiety states by rating. *The British Journal of Medical Psychology, 32*, 50–55.
Han, M. K., Postma, D., Mannino, D. M., Giardino, N. D., Buist, S., Curtis, J. L., et al. (2007). Gender and chronic obstructive pulmonary disease: Why it matters. *American Journal of Respiratory and Critical Care Medicine, 176*, 1179–1184.
Hann, D., Winter, K., & Jacobson, P. (1999). Measurement of depressive symptoms in cancer patients: Evaluation of the Center for Epidemiological Studies Depression scale (CES-D). *Journal of Psychiatric Research, 46*, 437–443.
Heslop, K., De Soyza, A., Baker, C., Stenton, C., & Burns, G. (2009). Using individualized cognitive behavioral therapy as a treatment for people with COPD. *Nursing Times, 105*(14), 14–17.
Howard, C., Hallas, C., Wray, J., & Carby, M. (2009). The relationship between illness perceptions and panic in chronic obstructive pulmonary disease. *Behaviour Research and Therapy, 47*, 71–76.
Hurd, S. (2000). The impact of COPD on lung health worldwide: Epidemiology and incidence. *Chest, 117*(2 Suppl.), 1S–4S.
Hynninen, M. J., Pallesen, S., & Nordhaus, I. (2007). Factors affecting health status in COPD patients with co-morbid anxiety or depression. *International Journal of Chronic Obstructive Pulmonary Disease, 2*(3), 323–328.
Jemal, A., Ward, E., Hao, Y., & Thun, M. (2005). Trends in leading causes of death in the United States, 1970–2002. *Journal of the American Medical Association, 294*(10), 1255–1259.
Johnson, D. A., & Heather, B. B. (1974). The sensitivity of the Beck Depression Inventory to changes in symptomatology. *The British Journal of Psychiatry, 125*, 184–185.
Judd, L. L., Akiskal, H. S., Maser, J. D., Zeller, P. J., Endicott, J., Coryell, W., et al. (1998). A prospective 12-year study of subsyndromal and syndromal depressive symptoms in unipolar major depressive disorders. *Archives of General Psychiatry, 55*(8), 694–700.
Karajgi, B., Rifkin, A., Doddi, S., & Kolli, R. (1990). The prevalence of anxiety disorders in patients with chronic obstructive pulmonary disease. *The American Journal of Psychiatry, 147*, 200–201.
Kayahan, B., Karapolat, H., Atyntoprak, E., Atasever, A., & Ozturk, O. (2006). Psychological outcomes of an outpatient pulmonary rehabilitation program in patients with chronic obstructive pulmonary disease. *Respiratory Medicine, 100*, 1050–1057.

Kessler, R. C., Chiu, W. T., Demler, O., & Walters, E. E. (2005). Prevalence, severity, and comorbidity of twelve-month DSM-IV disorders in the National Comorbidity Survey Report (NCS-R). *Archives of General Psychiatry, 62*(6), 612–627.

Kessler, R. C., McGonagle, K. A., Zhao, S., Nelson, C. B., Hughes, M., Eshleman, S., et al. (1994). Lifetime and 12-month prevalence of DSM-III-R psychiatric disorders in the United States. *Archives of General Psychiatry, 51*, 8–19.

Kim, H. F., Kunik, M. E., Molinari, V. A., Hillman, S. L., Lalani, S., Orengo, C., et al. (2000). Functional impairment in COPD patients: The impact of anxiety and depression. *Psychosomatics, 41*, 465–471.

Koenig, H. G., & Kuchibhatla, M. (1998). Use of health services by hospitalized medically ill depressed elderly patients. *The American Journal of Psychiatry, 155*, 871–877.

Kozora, E., Tran, Z. V., & Make, B. (2002). Neurobehavioral improvement after brief rehabilitation in patients with chronic obstructive pulmonary disease. *Journal of Cardiopulmonary Rehabilitation, 22*, 426–430.

Kroenke, K., Spitzer, R. L., & Williams, J. B. (2001). The PHQ-9: Validity of a brief depression screening measure. *Journal of General Internal Medicine, 16*(9), 606–613.

Kroenke, K., Spitzer, R. L., Williams, J. B., & Lowe, B. (2009). An ultra- brief screening tool for anxiety and depression: The PHQ-4. *Psychosomatics, 50*(6), 613–621.

Kumar, S., & Gross, N. J. (2002). The global initiative for COPD: What you need to know; smoking cessation is still the most effective way to reduce risk (chronic obstructive pulmonary disease). *Journal of Respiratory Disease, 23*(11), 549–556.

Kunik, M., Azzam, P., Souchek, J., Cully, J., Wray, N., Krishnan, L., et al. (2007). A practical screening tool for anxiety and depression in patients with chronic breathing disorders. *Psychosomatics, 48*, 16–21.

Kunik, M. E., Braun, U., Stanley, M. A., Wristers, K., Molinari, V., Stoebner, D., et al. (2001). One session cognitive behavioral therapy for elderly patients with chronic pulmonary disease. *Psychological Medicine, 31*, 717–723.

Kunik, M. E., Roundy, K., Veazey, C., Souchek, J., Richardson, P., Wray, N. P., et al. (2005). Surprisingly high prevalence of anxiety and depression in chronic breathing disorders. *Chest, 127*, 1205–1211.

Kunik, M. E., Veazey, C., Cully, J. A., Soucek, J., Graham, D. P., Hopko, D., et al. (2008). COPD education and cognitive behavioral therapy group treatment for clinically significant symptoms of depression and anxiety in COPD patients: A randomized controlled trial. *Psychological Medicine, 38*, 385–396.

Lacasse, Y., Beaudoin, L., Rousseau, L., & Maltais, F. (2004). Randomized trial of paroxetine in end-stage COPD. *Monaldi Archives for Chest Disease, 61*, 140–147.

Laurin, C., Lavoie, K., Bacon, S., Dupuis, G., Lacoste, G., Cartier, A., et al. (2007). Sex differences in the prevalence of psychiatric disorders with psychological distress in patients with COPD. *Chest, 132*, 148–155.

Lenfant, C. (2005). Medical and psychiatric illness: Different but concurrent! *Metabolism, Clinical and Experimental, 54*, 53–54.

Lewis, K. E., Annandale, J. A., Sykes, R. N., Hurlin, C., Owen, C., & Harrison, N. K. (2007). Prevalence of anxiety and depression in patients with severe COPD: Similar high levels with and without LTOT. *Chronic Obstructive Pulmonary Disease, 4*, 305–312.

Lisansky, D., & Hendel-Clough, D. (1996). A cognitive-behavioral self-help educational program for patients with COPD: A pilot study. *Psychotherapy and Psychosomatics, 65*, 97–101.

Livermore, N., Butler, J. E., Sharpe, L., McBain, R. A., Gandevia, S. C., & McKenzie, D. K. (2008). Panic attacks and perception of inspiratory resistive loads in chronic obstructive pulmonary disease. *American Journal of Respiratory and Critical Care Medicine, 178*, 7–12.

Livermore, N., Sharpe, L., & McKenzie, D. (2010). Prevention of panic attacks and panic disorder in chronic obstructive pulmonary disease. *The European Respiratory Journal, 35*(3), 557–563.

Lolak, S., Connors, G., Sheridan, M., & Wise, T. (2009). Effects of progressive muscle relaxation training on anxiety and depression in patients enrolled in an outpatient pulmonary rehabilitation program. *Psychotherapy and Psychosomatics, 77*, 119–125.

Maurer, J., Rebbapragada, V., Borson, S., Goldstein, R., Kunik, M., Yohannes, A. M., et al. (2008). Anxiety and depression in COPD: Current understanding, unanswered questions, and research needs. *Chest, 134*, 43S–56S.

McGeoch, G., Willsman, K., Dowson, C., Town, G., Frampton, C., & McCartin, F. (2006). Self management plans in the primary care of patients with chronic obstructive pulmonary disease. *Respirology, 11*, 611–618.

McNair, D. M., & Lorr, M. (1964). An analysis of mood in neurotics. *Journal of Abnormal and Social Psychology, 69*, 620–627.

Menzin, J., Boulanger, L., Marton, J., Guadagno, L., Dastani, H., Dirani, R., et al. (2008). The economic burden of chronic obstructive pulmonary disease (COPD) in a U.S. Medicare population. *Respiratory Medicine, 102*, 1248–1256.

Mikkelsen, R. L., Middelboe, T., Pisinger, C., & Stage, K. B. (2004). Anxiety and depression in patients with chronic obstructive disease (COPD). *Nordic Journal of Psychiatry, 58*, 65–70.

Moore, M. C., & Zebb, B. J. (1998). Functional status in chronic obstructive pulmonary disease: The moderating effect of panic. *International Journal of Rehabilitation and Health, 42*(2), 83–93.

Moore, M. C., & Zebb, B. J. (1999). The catastrophic misinterpretation of physiological distress. *Behaviour Research and Therapy, 37*, 1105–1118.

Narsavage, G. L., & Chen, K. Y. (2008). Factors related to depressed mood in adults with chronic obstructive pulmonary diseases after hospitalization. *Home Health care nurse, 26*(8), 447–482.

Nazir, S. A., & Erbland, M. L. (2009). Chronic obstructive pulmonary disease: An update on diagnosis and management issues in older adults. *Drugs & Aging, 26*(10), 813–831.

Ng, T. P., Niti, M., Tan, W. C., Cao, Z., Ong, K. C., & Eng, P. (2007). Depressive symptoms and chronic obstructive pulmonary disease: Effect on mortality, hospital readmission symptom burden, functional status, and quality of life. *Archives of Internal Medicine, 167*, 60–67.

Nguyen, H. Q., & Carrieri-Kohlman, V. (2005). Dyspnea self-management in patients with chronic obstructive pulmonary disease: Moderating effects of depressed mood. *Psychosomatics, 46*, 402–410.

Nici, L., Donner, D., Wouters, E., Zuwallack, R., Ambrosino, N., Bourbeau, J., et al. (2006). American Thoracic Society/European Respiratory Society statement on pulmonary rehabilitation. *American Journal of Respiratory and Critical Care Medicine, 173*, 1390–1413.

Norwood, R., & Balkissoon, R. (2005). Current perspectives on management and co-morbid depression in COPD. *Chronic Obstructive Pulmonary Disease, 2*, 185–193.

O'Neill, E. S. (2002). Illness representation and coping of women with chronic obstructive pulmonary disease: A pilot study. *Heart & Lung, 31*, 295–302.

Ormel, J., Kempen, G., Deeg, D., Brilman, E., Sondersen, E., & Relyveld, J. (1998). Functioning, well-being, and health perception in late middle-age and older people: Comparing the effects of depressive symptoms and chronic medical conditions. *Journal of the American Geriatrics Society, 46*, 39–48.

Ottanelli, R., Rosi, E., Ronchi, M. C., Grazzini, M., Lanini, B., Stendardi, L., et al. (2001). Perception of bronchoconstriction in smokers with airflow limitation. *Clinical Science, 101*(5), 515–522.

Papp, L. A., Weiss, J. R., Greenberg, H. E., Rifkin, A., Scharf, S. M., Gorman, J. M., et al. (1995). Sertraline for chronic obstructive pulmonary disease and co-morbid anxiety and mood disorders (letter to the editor). *The American Journal of Psychiatry, 152*, 1531.

Patten, S. B., & Williams, J. V. (2007). Chronic obstructive lung diseases and prevalence of mood, anxiety, and substance-use disorders in a large population sample. *Psychosomatics, 48*(6), 496–501.

Paz-Diaz, H., de Oca, M., Lopez, J., & Celli, B. (2007). Pulmonary rehabilitation improves depression, anxiety, dyspnea, and health status in patients with COPD. *American Journal of Physical Medical & Rehabilitation, 86*, 30–36.

Physician's desk reference. (2009). 63rd, Florence, KY: Thomson Healthcare.

Porzelius, J., Vest, M., & Nochomovitz, M. (1992). Respiratory function, cognitions, and panic in chronic obstructive pulmonary patients. *Behaviour Research and Therapy, 30*, 75–77.

Puhan, M. A., Scharplatz, M., Trooster, T., & Steurer, J. (2005). Respiratory rehabilitation after acute exacerbation of COPD may reduce risk for readmission and mortality – A systematic review. *Respiratory Research, 6*, 54.

Quint, J. K., Baghai-Ravary, R., Donaldson, G. C., & Wedzicha, J. A. (2008). Relationship between depression and exacerbations in COPD. *The European Respiratory Journal, 32*(1), 53–60.

Rabe, K. F., Hurd, S., Anzueto, A., Barnes, P. J., Buist, S. A., Calverley, P., et al. (2007). Global strategy for the diagnosis, management, and prevention of chronic obstructive pulmonary disease: Gold executive summary. *American Journal of Respiratory and Critical Care Medicine, 174*, 532–555.

Radloff, L. S. (1977). The CES-D scale: A self-report depression scale for research in the general population. *Applied Psychological Measurement, 1*, 385–401.

Radloff, L. S. (1991). The use of the Center for Epidemiologic Studies Depression Scale on adolescents and your adults. *Journal of Youth & Adolescence, 20*, 149–166.

Raji, M. A. (2006). On depression, antidepressant medications, and resuscitation preferences in COPD patients. *Chest, 129*, 211.

Rapaport, M. H., & Judd, L. L. (1998). Minor depressive disorder and subsyndromal depressive symptoms: Functional impairment and response to treatment. *Journal of Affective Disorder, 48*(2–3), 227–232.

Ries, A. L., Kaplan, R. M., Limberg, T. M., & Prewitt, L. M. (1995). Effects of pulmonary rehabilitation on physiologic and psychosocial outcomes in patients with chronic obstructive pulmonary disease. *Annals of Internal Medicine, 122*, 823–832.

Rose, C., Wallace, L., Dickson, R., Ayres, J., Lehman, R., Searle, Y., et al. (2002). The most effective psychologically-based treatments to reduce anxiety and panic in patients with chronic obstructive pulmonary disease (COPD): A systematic review. *Patient Education and Counseling, 47*, 311–318.

Roundy, K., Cully, J., Stanley, M., Veazey, C., Souchek, J., Wray, N., et al. (2005). Are anxiety and depression addressed in primary care patients with chronic obstructive pulmonary disease? A chart review. *The Journal of Clinical Psychiatry, 7*, 213–220.

Roy-Byrne, P., Katon, W., Broadhead, W. E., Lepine, J. P., Richards, J., Brantley, P. J., et al. (1994). Subsyndromal ("mixed") anxiety-depression in primary care. *Journal of General Internal Medicine, 9*(9), 507–512.

Sassi-Dambron, D. E., Eakin, E. G., Ries, A. L., & Kaplan, R. M. (1995). Treatment of dyspnea in COPD: A controlled clinical trial of dyspnea management strategies. *Chest, 107*, 724–729.

Schane, R. E., Woodruff, P. G., Dinno, A., Covinsky, M. D., & Walter, L. C. (2008). Prevalence and risk factors for depressive symptoms in persons with chronic obstructive pulmonary disease. *Journal of General Internal Medicine, 23*(11), 1757–1762.

Schneider, C., Jicks, S., Bothner, U., & Meier, C. R. (2010). Chronic obstructive pulmonary disease and the risk of depression. *Chest, 137*, 341–347.

Seemungal, T. A., Donaldson, N. V., Paul, E. A., Bestall, J. C., Jeffries, D. J., & Wedzicha, J. A. (1998). Effects of exacerbations on quality of life in patients with chronic obstructive pulmonary disease. *American Journal of Respiratory and Critical Care Medicine, 157*, 1418–1422.

Seung-Kim, H. F., Kunik, M. E., Molinari, V. A., Hillman, S. L., Lalani, S., Orengo, C. A., et al. (2000). Functional impairment in COPD patients: The impact of anxiety and depression. *Psychosomatics, 41*, 465–471.

Sigmond, A. S., & Snaith, R. P. (1983). The hospital anxiety and depression scale. *Acta Psychiatrica Scandinavica, 67*(6), 361–370.

Silvertooth, E. J., Doraiswamy, P. M., Clary, G. L., Babyak, M. A., Wilkerson, N., Hellegars, C., et al. (2004). Citalopram and quality of life in lung transplant recipients. *Psychosomatics, 45*, 271–272.

Singh, N. P., Despars, J. A., Stansbury, D. W., Avalos, K., & Light, R. W. (1993). Effects of buspirone on anxiety levels and exercise tolerance in patients with chronic airflow obstruction and mild anxiety. *Chest, 103*, 800–804.

Sirey, J. A., Raue, P. J., & Alexopoulos, G. S. (2007). An intervention to improve depression care in older adults with COPD. *International Journal of Geriatric Psychiatry, 22*, 154–159.

Smoller, J. W., Pollack, M. H., Otto, M. W., Rosenbaum, J. F., & Kradin, R. L. (1996). Panic anxiety, dyspnea, and respiratory disease: Theoretical and clinical considerations. *American Journal of Respiratory and Critical Care Medicine, 154*, 6–17.

Smoller, J. W., Pollack, M. H., Systrom, D., & Kradin, R. L. (1998). Sertraline effects on dyspnea in patients with obstructive airways disease. *Psychosomatics, 39*, 24–29.

Spielberger, C. D. (1966). *Theory and research on anxiety*. New York: Academic.

Spitzer, R. L., Kroenke, K., & Williams, J. B. (1999). Validation and utility of a self-report version of Prime-MD: The PHQ primary care study. Primary Care Evaluative of Mental Disorder. Patient Health Questionnaire. *Journal of the American Medical Association. 282*(18), 1737–1744.

Stage, K. B., Middleboe, T., & Pisinger, C. (2005). Depression and chronic obstructive pulmonary disease (COPD). Impact on survival. *Acta Psychiatrica Scandinavica, 111*, 320–323.

Talamo, C., de Oca, M. M., Halbert, R., Perez-Padilla, R., Jardim, J., Muino, A., et al. (2007). Diagnostic labeling of COPD in five Latin American cities. *Chest, 131*, 60–67.

Tashkin, D., Kanner, R., Bailey, W., Buist, S., Anderson, P., Nides, M., et al. (2001). Smoking cessation in patients with chronic obstructive pulmonary disease: A double-blind, placebo-controlled, randomized trial. *The Lancet, 357*, 1571–1575.

van Manen, J. G., Bindels, P. J., Dekker, F. W., Ijzermans, C. J., van der Zee, J. S., & Schade, E. (2002). Risk of depression in patients with chronic obstructive pulmonary disease and its determinants. *Thorax, 57*, 412–416.

van Manen, J. G., Bindels, P. J. E., IJzermans, C. J., van der Zee, J. S., Bottems, B. J. A. M., & Schade, E. (2001). Prevalence of comorbidity in patients with chronic airway obstruction and controls over the age of 40. *Journal of Clinical Epidemiology, 54*, 287–293.

Verburg, K., Griez, E., Meijer, J., Pois, H. (1995). Respiratory disorders as a possible predisposed factor for panic disorder. *Journal of Affective Disorders, 33*(2), 129–13.

Versiani, M., Moreno, R., Ramakers-van Moorsel, C. J., & Schutte, A. J. (2005). Comparison of the effects of mirtazapine and fluoxetine in severely depressed patients. *CNS Drugs, 19*, 137–146.

Wagena, E. J., Arrindell, W. A., Wouters, E. F., & van Schayck, C. P. (2005). Are patients with COPD psychologically distressed? *The European Respiratory Journal, 26*, 242–248.

Wagena, E. J., Knipschild, P. G., Huibers, M. J., Wouters, E. F., & van Schayck, C. P. (2005). Efficacy of bupropion and nortriptyline for smoking cessation among people at risk for or with chronic obstructive pulmonary disease. *Archives of Internal Medicine, 165*, 2286–2292.

Wamboldt, F. S. (2005). Anxiety and depression in COPD: A call (and need) for further research. *Chronic Obstructive Pulmonary Disease, 2*, 199–201.

Weaver, T. E., & Narsavage, G. L. (1992). Physiological variables related to functional status in chronic obstructive pulmonary disease. *Nursing Research, 41*, 286–291.

Weaver, T. E., Richmond, T. S., & Narsavage, G. L. (1997). An explanatory model of functional status in chronic obstructive pulmonary disease. *Nursing Research, 46*, 26–31.

Withers, N. J., Rudkin, S. T., & White, R. J. (1999). Anxiety and depression in severe chronic obstructive pulmonary disease: The effects of pulmonary rehabilitation. *Journal of Cardiopulmonary Rehabilitation, 19*, 362–365.

World Health Organization. (2010). *Chronic respiratory diseases: Burden*. Accessed February 7, 2010, http://www/who.int/respiratory/copd/burden/en

Xu, W., Collet, J., Shapiro, S., Lin, Y., Yang, T., Platt, R. W., et al. (2008). Independent effect of depression and anxiety on chronic obstructive pulmonary disease exacerbations and hospitalizations. *American Journal of Respiratory and Critical Care Medicine, 178*, 913–920.

Yellowlees, P. M., Alpers, J. H., Bowden, J. J., Bryant, G. D., & Ruffin, R. E. (1987). Psychiatric morbidity in patients with chronic airflow obstruction. *The Medical Journal of Australia, 146*, 305–307.

Yohannes, A. M., Baldwin, R. C., & Connolly, M. J. (2000). Depression and anxiety in elderly outpatients with chronic obstructive pulmonary disease: Prevalence and validation of the BASDEC screening questionnaire. *International Journal of Psychiatry, 15*, 1090–1096.

Yohannes, A. M., Baldwin, R. C., & Connolly, M. J. (2003). Prevalence of subthreshold depression in elderly patients with chronic obstructive pulmonary disease. *Journal of Geriatric Psychiatry, 18*(5), 412–416.

Yohannes, A. M., Baldwin, R. C., & Connolly, M. J. (2005). Predictors of 1-year mortality in patients discharged from hospital following acute exacerbation of chronic obstructive disease. *Age and Ageing, 34*, 491–496.

Yohannes, A. M., Connolly, M. J., & Baldwin, R. C. (2001). A feasibility study of antidepressant drug therapy in depressed elderly patients with chronic obstructive pulmonary disease. *International Journal of Psychiatry, 16*, 451–454.

Zandbergen, G., Bright, M., Pots, H., Fernandez, I., Dehoof, C., Gricz, E.G. (1991). Higher lifetime prevalence of respiratory diseases in panic disorder? *American Journal of Psychiatry, 148*(11), 1583–1585.

Zigmond, A. S., & Snaith, R. P. (1983). The hospital anxiety and depression scale. *Acta Psychiatrica Scandinavica, 67*, 361–370.

Index

A
Acquired immunodeficiency syndrome (AIDS). *See* Human immunodeficiency virus (HIV)
Addressing tobacco through organizational change (ATTOC), 224
Adrenocorticotropic hormone (ACTH), 3, 25
Aggressive disorder. *See* Behavioral disorder, dementia
Alprazolam, 87, 222
American Diabetes Association (ADA), 74, 103
American Psychiatric Association (APA), 215
Antidepressants
  cancer, 187
  cardiovascular disease, 130–133, 142
  chronic obstructive pulmonary disease, 434, 435
  dementia, 346–347
  generalized anxiety disorder, 15
  IBS, 396
  multiple sclerosis, 324
  obesity, 5, 8
  tobacco addiction, 218
  type 2 diabetes, 80, 107
Anxiety
  cancer
    clinical assessment, 171–172
    cognitive-behavioral therapy, 186–188
    collaborative depression, 187–188
    diagnostic criteria, 169–170
    etiology, 170–171
    evidence-based recommendations, 183–185
    meta-analysis, 180–181
    prevalence and course, 168–170
  cardiovascular disease
    autonomic imbalance, 140–141
    behavioral risk factors, 141
    clinical assessment, 142–143
    generalized anxiety disorder, 137
    panic disorder, 138
    pharmacology, 142
    pharmacotherapy, 144
    prevalence, 137
    psychotherapy, 144
    PTSD, 138–139
    symptoms, 139–140
  chronic obstructive pulmonary disease
    clinical impacts, 426–427
    cognitive and behavioral interventions, 434–435
    diagnostic tools, 428–429
    panic attacks and disorder, 423–424
    pharmacotherapy, 430–434
    prevalence, 422–423
    sex differences, 425–426
  dementia
    definition, 360
    epidemiology, 360
    nonpharmacological treatments, 364–365
    NPI/the BEHAVE-AD correlation, 362–363
    pathophysiology, 360–361
    patients assessment, 362
    pharmacological treatments, 365
    RAID/Worry Scale, 363–364
    symptoms, 362
  HIV, 246, 249
    adherence medication, 250
    clinical assessment, 251–252

S. Pagoto (ed.), *Psychological Co-morbidities of Physical Illness: A Behavioral Medicine Perspective*, DOI 10.1007/978-1-4419-0029-6,

Anxiety (*cont.*)
clinical recommendations and treatment, 253–254
evidence-based treatment, 252–253
GAD, 248
linkage and retention, 250–251
mood disorder, 249
panic disorder, 248
post traumatic stress disorder, 246–248
stress and immune functioning, 249–250
IBS
clinical assessment, 398
GAD, 397–398
treatment, 398–399
nicotine dependence, 213
obesity
GAD, 15
panic disorder, 16–17
social phobia, 17–18
specific phobia, 18–19
pain
medical treatment outcome, 284
prevalence, 283–284
type 2 diabetes mellitus
clinical assessment, 84–85
diagnostic issues, 84–85
epidemiology, 81–83
evidence-based treatment, 85–87
pathophysiology, 83–84
prevalence, 81
symptoms, 81
treatment decision-making issues, 88
Apathy
clinical assessment, 338–339
definition, 336
depression, 339
epidemiology, 337
neurochemical disturbances, 337–338
neuropathological disturbances, 337
pharmacological therapy, 339–341
Atripla, 238
Attention deficit hyperactivity disorder (ADHD)
atomoxetine, 49
clinical assessment, 48
decision making, 50–51
depression, 48
hyperactivity, 44
impulsivity, 47
inattention, 46
prevalence, 44–45
psychological interventions, 50
psychotropic medications, 49–50
reward sensitivity, 46–47
weight regulation, 46–47
ATTOC. *See* Addressing tobacco through organizational change

B

Beck Anxiety Inventory (BAI), 428
Beck Depression Inventory (BDI), 429
BED. *See* Binge-eating disorder (BED)
Behavioral disorder, dementia
caregiver burden/relationship, 351
caregiver care approach, 353
caregiver factors, 349
clinical assessment, 350–351
environmental factors, 349
epidemiology, 347
nonpharmacological treatment, 352–354
patient behavioral approach, 352
patient factors, 348–349
pharmacotherapy, 354–355
sundowning, 349
Behavioral inhibition system/behavioral activation system (BIS/BAS), 46
Behavioral Pathology in Alzheimer's Disease Rating Scale (BEHAVE-AD), 350
Benzodiazepines
anxiety and CVD, 140, 143–144
dementia
behavioral disorder, 355
sleep disorder, 371
Binge-eating disorder (BED), 21
ADHD, 45, 47
obesity
behavioral treatments, 28–29
clinical assessment, 27–28
decision making, 30
neurobiological mechanisms, 26
pharmacotherapy, 29
prevalence, 24–25
psychological factors, 26–27
stress, 25–26
T2DM, 89, 106
Bipolar disorder
cardiovascular disease
clinical assessment, 136
lifestyle factors, 135
prevalence, 134
psychotropic medication, 135
treatment issues, 136–137
multiple sclerosis, 313
obesity
behavioral interventions, 13–14
clinical assessment, 12
HPA axis dysregulation, 11–12

medication augmentation and switching, 12–13
prevalence, 10–11
psychopharmacology, 11
type 2 diabetes mellitus
adherence medications, 98
clinical care assessment, 98–99
epidemiology, 94–95
evidence-based treatment, 99–101
prevalence, 95
treatment decision-making issues, 101
Brief Assessment Schedule Depression Cards (BASDEC), 430
Bupropion
apathy, 340
COPD, 434
tobacco addiction, 215–217, 220–221

C

Cancer
anxiety
clinical assessment, 171–172
cognitive-behavioral therapy, 186–188
collaborative depression, 187–188
diagnostic criteria, 169–170
etiology, 170–171
evidence-based recommendations, 183–185
meta-analysis, 180–181
prevalence and course, 168–170
depression
clinical assessment, 167–168
etiology, 166–167
prevalence and course, 164–165
systematic reviews and meta-analyses, 172–179
diagnosis and treatment, 163
future aspects, 197
psychological interventions, 197
sexual problems
clinical assessment, 193–194
etiology, 193
evidence-supported intervention, 196
prevalence, 192–193
research literature, 194–195
sleep problems
clinical assessment, 190
etiology, 189–190
evidence-supported intervention, 191–192
prevalence, 189
research, 190–191
Cardiovascular disease (CVD)
anxiety disorders
autonomic imbalance, 140–141
behavioral risk factors, 141
clinical assessment, 142–143
generalized anxiety disorder, 137
panic disorder, 138
pharmacology, 142
pharmacotherapy, 144
prevalence, 137
psychotherapy, 144
PTSD, 138–139
symptoms, 139–140
mood disorders
bipolar disorder (*see* Bipolar disorder)
major depressive disorder (*see* Major depressive disorder)
psychotic disorders
antipsychotic medication, 146–147
autonomic dysfunction, 147–148
lifestyle factors, 148–149
prevalence, 145–146
schizophrenia, 149–151
Catastrophization
IBS and anxiety disorders, 401
pain, 390
assessment, 292
treatment, 293
CBT for adherence and depression (CBT-AD), 79
Center for Epidemiological Studies Depression Scale (CES-D), 429
Centers for disease control and prevention (CDC), 233
Cholinesterase inhibitors, 340, 355
Chronic obstructive pulmonary disease (COPD)
anxiety
clinical impacts, 426–427
cognitive and behavioral interventions, 434–435
diagnostic tools, 428–429
panic attacks and disorder, 423–424
pharmacotherapy, 430–434
prevalence, 422–423
sex differences, 425–426
symptoms, 420–421
clinical considerations, 442–443
definition, 415–416
depression, 420
antidepressant therapy, 435
clinical impacts, 426–427
cognitive and behavioral interventions, 435, 438
diagnostic tools, 429–430

Chronic obstructive pulmonary disease (COPD) (*cont.*)
- major depressive disorder, 424–425
- pharmacotherapy, 433–434
- prevalence, 425
- sex differences, 425–426
- symptoms, 424–425

diagnostic criteria, 416
epidemiology, 417
medications, 420
pathophysiology
- acute exacerbations, 418–419
- diagnosis issues, 417–418
- dyspnea/breathlessness, 418

pharmacotherapy, 431–432
pulmonary rehabilitation
- efficacy, test trials, 438–441
- nonpharmacological approach, 442
- patient assessment, 438

quality of life, 421

Cognitive-behavioral therapy (CBT), 79, 353
- cardiovascular disease, 132–133, 144
- COPD, 434–438
- dementia, 353, 364
- diabetes mellitus, 78, 79, 93, 107
- HIV, 244, 253, 258, 261
- irritable bowel syndrome, 392, 393, 399, 400, 404
- obesity, 7, 28–30, 34, 50
- obesity, MDD, 7
- pain, 287, 291, 293, 295, 297
- psychiatric disorder, 325, 326
- somatoform disorders, 286–287
- T2DM, 86

Cohen-Mansifield Agitation Inventory, 350
COPD. *See* Chronic obstructive pulmonary disease (COPD)
Corticotrophin-releasing hormone (CRH), 3, 4
CVD. *See* Cardiovascular disease (CVD)
Cytochrome P450 1A2 (CYP1A2), nicotine, 211

D

Dementia
- Alzheimer's disease, 335
- anxiety disorder
  - definition, 360
  - epidemiology, 360
  - nonpharmacological treatments, 364–365
  - NPI/the BEHAVE-AD correlation, 362–363
  - pathophysiology, 360–361
  - patients assessment, 362
  - pharmacological treatments, 365
  - RAID/Worry Scale, 363–364
  - symptoms, 362
- apathy
  - clinical assessment, 338–339
  - definition, 336
  - depression, 339
  - epidemiology, 337
  - neurochemical disturbances, 337–338
  - neuropathological disturbances, 337
  - pharmacological therapy, 339–341
- behavioral/aggressive disorder
  - caregiver burden/relationship, 351
  - caregiver care approach, 353
  - caregiver factors, 349
  - clinical assessment, 350–351
  - environmental factors, 349
  - epidemiology, 347
  - nonpharmacological treatment, 352–354
  - patient behavioral approach, 352
  - patient factors, 348–349
  - pharmacotherapy, 354–355
  - sundowning, 349
- cognitive impairment, 335
- depressive disorders
  - antidepressants, 346–347
  - caregivers approach, 345
  - clinical assessment, 343–344
  - ECT, 347
  - epidemiology, 341–342
  - pathophysiology, 342–343
  - psychosocial modalities, 344–346
- memory impairment, 335
- prevalence, 336
- psychiatric axis I diagnosis, 335
- psychotic disorders, 355
  - clinical care assessment, 357
  - epidemiology, 356
  - nonpharmacological treatment, 357–358
  - pathophysiology, 356–357
  - pharmacological treatment, 358–360
- sleep disorders
  - clinical care assessment, 367–368
  - definition, 366
  - epidemiology, 366
  - light therapy, 368–369
  - mirtazapine, 372
  - pathophysiology, 366–367
  - pharmacological treatment, 371–372
  - physical exercise, 369–370
  - sleep hygiene, 370–371
- substance abuse, 335
- types, 336

Depression
cancer
clinical assessment, 167–168
etiology, 166–167
prevalence and course, 164–165
systematic reviews and meta-analyses, 172–179
chronic obstructive pulmonary disease, 420
antidepressant therapy, 435
clinical impacts, 426–427
cognitive and behavioral interventions, 435, 438
diagnostic tools, 429–430
major depressive disorder, 424–425
pharmacotherapy, 433–434
prevalence, 425
sex differences, 425–426
symptoms, 424–425
dementia
antidepressants, 346–347
caregivers approach, 345
clinical assessment, 343–344
ECT, 347
epidemiology, 341–342
pathophysiology, 342–343
psychosocial modalities, 344–346
HIV
antiretroviral adherence, 240–241
clinical assessment, 242–243
diagnosis, 238–239
effects, 239
epidemiology, 236
evidenced-based interventions, 244
immune function, 239–240
infection or transmission, 237–238
intravenous drug users, 236–237
linkage and retention, 241–242
survival, 240
treatment, 244–246
IBS
antidepressant medication, 396
clinical assessment, 395
clinical considerations, 397
cognitive behavior, 396
group therapy, 396–397
perfectionism, 396
treatment guidelines, 396
irritable bowel syndrome
antidepressant medication, 396
clinical assessment, 395
clinical considerations, 397
cognitive behavior, 396
group therapy, 396–397
treatment guidelines, 396
multiple sclerosis
antidepressant medications, 324
anxiety, 327–328
CBT, 325–326
physician care, 324–325
response and relapse prediction, 326–327
secondary outcomes, 327
stress and exacerbation, 319–320
obesity, MDD
antidepressant medication, 5
appetite suppressants, 8
buproprion, 8
characterization, 2
class I/II and III, 2
clinical assessment, 6
decision making, 9
HPA axis dysregulation, 3–4
inflammatory markers, 5
obese adults *vs* non-obese adults, 2
prevalence, 2
psychological mechanisms, 5–6
psychotherapy, 7
racial and ethnic minorities, 9–10
pain
diagnosis, 279–280
medical treatment outcome, 280–281
reciprocal improvements, 281–282
type 2 diabetes mellitus
CBT, CBT-AD, 79
clinical assessment, 77–78
diagnostic issues, 77–78
epidemiology, 75–76
evidence-based treatment, 78–80
pathophysiology, 76–77
prevalence, 75
symptoms, 76
treatment decision-making issues, 80
Diabetes mellitus. *See* Type 2diabetes mellitus (T2DM)
Diphenhydramine, 372
Disease-modifying treatments (DMTs), 317
Distal symmetrical polyneuropathy (DSP), 258
Dopaminergic agents, 340
Dysthymia
CVD, 134
depression
HIV, 236
MDD, 75–76
pain, 282
multiple sclerosis, 313

E

Eating disorders
obesity (*see* BED; Night eating syndrome)
type 2 diabetes mellitus
anorexia, 89
BED, 89
CBT and NPT, 93
clinical care assessment, 92–93
EAT, 92
evidence-based treatment, 93–94
insulin omission, 89–90
maladaptive eating behaviors, 91
night eating syndrome, 90
overweight patients, 89
pathophysiology, 91–92
poorer metabolic control, 90
prevalence, 88
treatment decision-making issues, 94
European Respiratory Society, 438

F

Fear Avoidance Belief Questionnaire (FABQ), 291
Fear of Pain Questionnaire (FPQ), 291
Fludiazepam, 87

G

Galantamine, 340
Generalized anxiety disorder (GAD), 393
HIV, 248
obesity, 15
type 2 diabetes, 81

H

Hamilton Anxiety Rating Scale (HAM-A), 428
Harm Avoidance scale, 290
Highly active antiretroviral therapy (HAART), 234
HIV Cost and Services Utilization Study (HCSUS), 236
Hospital Anxiety and Depression Scale (HADS), 422, 429
Human immunodeficiency virus (HIV)
acute stress disorder, 247
antiretroviral therapy, 234, 235
anxiety, 246, 249
clinical assessment, 251–252
clinical recommendations and treatment, 253–254
evidence-based treatment, 252–253
generalized anxiety disorder, 248
linkage and retention, 250–251
medication adherence, 250
mood disorder, 249
panic disorder, 248
post traumatic stress disorder, 246–248
stress and immune functioning, 249–250
cultural considerations
evidence-based interventions, 261
HIV-positive patients, 260–261
mental illness, 259–260
treatment recommendations, 261
treatment utilization and retention, 260
depression
antiretroviral adherence, 240–241
clinical assessment, 242–243
diagnosis, 238–239
epidemiology, 236–237
evidenced-based interventions, 244
HIV progression, 239
immune function, 239–240
infection and transmission, 236–237
linkage and retention, 241–242
survival, 240
treatment, 244–246
pain disorder, 258–259
schizophrenia
pathophysiology, 254–255
prevalence, 254
treatment, 255–256
self-care behavior, 234
sexual disorder, 257–258
sleep disorders, 256–257
Hypercortisolism, 4
Hypothalamic pituitary adrenal (HPA) axis dysregulation
anxiety disorders, 84
multiple sclerosis, 320
obesity
bipolar disorder, 11–12
depression, 3–4
night eating syndrome, 32
Hypothyroidism, 96, 344

I

Insulin omission, 89–90
Irritable bowel syndrome (IBS)
anxiety disorders
clinical assessment, 398
GAD, 393, 397–398
treatment, 398–399
assessment tools
pain, 389–390
quality of life, 390
symptom monitoring, 389

biopsychosocial model
brain-gut connection, 388
nature *vs.* nurture debate, 388–389
stress, 386–387
categorization, 386
chronic abdominal pain, 385
clinical considerations, 397
depression
antidepressant medication, 396
clinical assessment, 395
clinical considerations, 397
cognitive behavior, 396
group therapy, 396–397
treatment guidelines, 396
etiology, 386
lifetime prevalence, 394
panic disorder
clinical assessment, 399–400
heightened stress, 399
treatment, 400–401
personality disorders, 403–404
posttraumatic stress disorder
clinical assessment, 401
treatment, 402
somatization disorders
clinical assessment, 402–403
medical disorder, 402
pathological process, 402
treatment, 403
treatment
dietary therapy, 391
pharmacology, 390–391
psychotherapy (*See* Psychotherapy)

J

Joint American Thoracic Society, 438

K

Ketoacidosis, 102
Kinesiophobia
Fear Avoidance Belief Questionnaire, 291
Fear of Pain Questionnaire, 291
functional disability, 291
physical activity, 290
Tampa Scale for Kinesiophobia, 291
treatment, 291

M

Major depressive disorder (MDD)
cardiovascular disease
autonomic nervous system imbalance, 126
clinical assessment, 129–130
genetic factors, 127–128
inflammation, 127
lifestyle factors, 125
pharmacological treatments, 130–131
platelet activation, 126–127
prevalence, 124
psychotherapy, 132–133
stroke, 128
symptoms, 129
COPD, 421, 424–425
multiple sclerosis, 313, 324
obesity
antidepressant medication, 5
appetite suppressants, 8
buproprion, 8
characterization, 2
class I/II and III, 2
clinical assessment, 6
decision making, 9
HPA axis dysregulation, 3–4
inflammatory markers, 5
obese adults *vs* non-obese adults, 2
prevalence, 2
psychological mechanisms, 5–6
psychotherapy, 7
racial and ethnic minorities, 9–10
type 2 diabetes, 75–76
Medically unexplained symptoms (MUS), 286, 298
Minnesota Multidimensional Personality Inventory (MMPI), 288–289
Mirtazapine, 372
Mood disorder
CVD (*see* Bipolar disorder; Major depressive disorder)
nicotine dependence, 213–214
obesity (*see* Obesity)
Multiple sclerosis (MS)
co-morbidity, biobehavioral mechanisms
genetic factors, 314–315
MS pathogenesis, 315–316
MS pathology, 316
MS treatment, 317
physical and cognitive symptom severity, 316–317
psychosocial factors, 318–319
diagnosis, 323
epidemiology, 312–313
exacerbation, 311–312
progression, 312
psychological disorders
anxiety, life-time history, 313
bipolar disorder, 313
dysregulation of affect, 313–314

Multiple sclerosis (MS) (*cont.*)
neuropsychological functioning, 314
prevalence, 313
relapsing-remitting course, 312
stress and depression (*see* Depression; Stress)
Multisensory behavioral therapy (MSBT), 341

N
National Comorbidity Survey Replication (NCSR), 88
NEO Personality Inventory (NEO-PI), 288–289
Neuropsychiatric Inventory (NPI), 338
Nicotine dependence. *See* Tobacco addiction
Nicotine gum, 217
Nicotine nasal spray, 217
Nicotine replacement therapies (NRT), 216–218
Nicotinic acetylcholine receptors (nAChRs), 213
Night eating syndrome (NES)
obesity
behavioral approaches, 33–34
circadian rhythm disruption, 32
clinical assessment, 33
decision making, 34
HPA axis functioning, 32
pharmacotherapy, 33
prevalence, 30–31
type 2 diabetes, 90
Nonnucleoside reverse transcriptase inhibitors (NNRTIs), 238
Non-prescriptive therapy (NPT), 93

O
Obesity
anxiety disorders
GAD, 15
panic disorder, 16–17
social phobia, 17–18
specific phobia, 18–19
attention deficit hyperactivity disorder
atomoxetine, 49
clinical assessment, 48
decision making, 50–51
depression, 48
hyperactivity, 44
impulsivity, 47
inattention, 46
prevalence, 44–45
psychological interventions, 50
psychotropic medications, 49–50
reward sensitivity, 46–47
weight regulation, 46–47
binge-eating disorder
behavioral treatments, 28–29
clinical assessment, 27–28
decision making, 30
neurobiological mechanisms, 26
pharmacotherapy, 29
prevalence, 24–25
psychological factors, 26–27
stress, 25–26
bipolar disorder
behavioral interventions, 13–14
clinical assessment, 12
HPA axis dysregulation, 11–12
medication augmentation and switching, 12–13
prevalence, 10–11
psychopharmacology, 11
eating disorders (*see* BED; Night eating syndrome)
major depressive disorders
antidepressant medication, 5
appetite suppressants, 8
buproprion, 8
characterization, 2
class I/II and III, 2
clinical assessment, 6
decision making, 9
HPA axis dysregulation, 3–4
inflammatory markers, 5
obese adults *vs.* non-obese adults, 2
prevalence, 2
psychological mechanisms, 5–6
psychotherapy, 7
racial and ethnic minorities, 9–10
night eating syndrome
behavioral approaches, 33–34
circadian rhythm disruption, 32
clinical assessment, 33
decision making, 34
HPA axis functioning, 32
pharmacotherapy, 33
prevalence, 30–31
psychotic disorders
adjunctive pharmacological intervention, 42–43
bariatric surgery, 43
lifestyle factors, 37–38
lifestyle interventions, 38–40
medication switching, 40–42
schizophrenia, 35
second-generation antipsychotic medication, 36–37
PTSD
clinical considerations, 22–23

depression and eating disorder, 21
inhibitory control, 21–22
neurobiological mechanisms, 20
prevalence, 19–20
psychological mechanisms, 21
Oral inhaler, 216, 218

P
Pain
anxiety
medical treatment outcome, 284
prevalence, 283–284
axis II personality disorders
diathesis-stress framework, 289–290
DSM-IV, 288
emotional pain, 288
Harm Avoidance scale, 290
MMPI, 288–289
NEO-PI, 288–289
organic and nonorganic pain, 288
prevalence, 289
temperament and character dimensions, 290
biopsychosocial nature, 275–276
catastrophizing
assessment, 292
treatment, 293
dementia, 350–351
depression
diagnosis, 279–280
medical treatment outcome, 280–281
reciprocal improvements, 281–282
epidemiology, 277
fear-avoidance
Fear Avoidance Belief Questionnaire, 291
Fear of Pain Questionnaire, 291
functional disability, 291
physical activity, 290
Tampa Scale for Kinesiophobia, 291
treatment, 291
HIV, 258–259
psychological treatment
cognitive-behavioral therapy, 295
patient-centered outcomes, 294–295
psychodynamic therapy, 296
psychosocial variables, 297
somatoform disorders, 298
pain disorder, 285–286
somatization disorder, 284–285
treatment, 286–287
treatment outcome goals, 297
Panic disorder
HIV, 248
IBS
clinical assessment, 399–400
heightened stress, 399
treatment, 400–401
obesity, 16–17
Patient Health Questionnaire Depression Scale (PHQ), 429
Perfectionism, 396
Personality disorder not otherwise specified (PDNOS), 288
Personality disorders
IBS, 403–404
pain
diathesis-stress framework, 289–290
DSM-IV, 288
emotional pain, 288
Harm Avoidance scale, 290
MMPI, 288–289
NEO-PI, 288–289
organic and nonorganic pain, 288
prevalence, 289
temperament and character dimensions, 290
Pharmacotherapy
anxiety
cardiovascular disease, 144
chronic obstructive pulmonary disease, 430–434
behavioral disorder, dementia, 354–355
COPD
antidepressant therapy, 434
anxiety, 430–434
depression, 434
dementia, 354–355
obesity, 29, 33
PHQ Depression Scale, 429
Polycyclic aromatic hydrocarbons, 211
Posttraumatic stress disorder (PTSD), 81, 138–139
cardiovascular disease, 138–139
HIV, 246–248
IBS
clinical assessment, 401
treatment, 402
nicotine dependence, 213, 219
obesity
clinical considerations, 22–23
depression and eating disorder, 21
inhibitory control, 21–22
neurobiological mechanisms, 20
prevalence, 19–20
psychological mechanisms, 21
type 2 diabetes mellitus, 81

Profile of Mood States (POMS), 428
Psychotherapy
anxiety, 144
IBS
CBT, 392–393
gut-directed hypnotherapy, 392
IBS, 391–392
major depressive disorder
cardiovascular disease, 132–133
obesity, 7
Psychotic disorders
CVD
antipsychotic medication, 146–147
autonomic dysfunction, 147–148
CVD preventive care, 150–151
CVD risk factors screening, 149
lifestyle factors, 148–149
prevalence, 145–146
dementia, 355
clinical care assessment, 357
epidemiology, 356
nonpharmacological treatment, 357–358
pathophysiology, 356–357
pharmacological treatment, 358–360
obesity
adjunctive pharmacological intervention, 42–43
bariatric surgery, 43
lifestyle factors, 37–38
lifestyle interventions, 38–40
medication switching, 40–42
schizophrenia, 35
second-generation antipsychotic medication, 36–37
type 2 diabetes mellitus
adherence medications, 98
clinical care assessment, 98–99
epidemiology, 94–95
evidence-based treatment, 99–101
prevalence, 95
treatment decision-making issues, 101
Pulmonary rehabilitation, COPD
efficacy, test trials, 438–441
nonpharmacological approach, 442
patient assessment, 438

R
Randomized controlled trial (RCT), 339
Rating for Anxiety in Dementia (RAID), 363

S
Schizophrenia. *See also* Psychotic disorders
CVD
management, 149–151
risk factors screening, 149
HIV, 254–255
nicotine dependence, 212
Selective serotonin reuptake inhibitors (SSRIs)
CVD, 127, 131
obesity, 5, 33, 339
pain, 281
Self-Injection Anxiety (SIA), 327–328
Sexual disorder
cancer
clinical assessment, 193–194
etiology, 193
evidence-supported intervention, 196
prevalence, 192–193
research literature, 194–195
HIV, 257–258
SIA counseling (SIAC), 328
Sleep disorder
cancer
assessment, 190
etiology, 189–190
intervention effective, 191–192
prevalence, 189
research, 190–191
dementia
clinical care assessment, 367–368
definition, 366
epidemiology, 366
light therapy, 368–369
mirtazapine, 372
pathophysiology, 366–367
pharmacological treatment, 371–372
physical exercise, 369–370
sleep hygiene, 370–371
HIV, 256–257
Social phobia, 17–18
Somatization disorder
IBS
clinical assessment, 402–403
medical disorder, 402
pathological process, 402
treatment, 403
pain
medically unexplained symptoms, 286
pain disorder, 285–286
somatization disorder, 284–285
treatment, 286–287
Specific phobia, 18–19
Spielberger STAI, 428

Stress, multiple sclerosis
attributional style, 321
biological models, 322
coping, 321–322
depression, 321
social support, 322
Substance use disorders. *See also* Tobacco addiction
nicotine dependence, 214–215
type 2 diabetes mellitus
clinical care assessment, 103
epidemiology, 101–102
evidence-based treatment, 103–104
pathophysiology, 102–103
treatment decision-making issues, 104–105

T
Tampa Scale for Kinesiophobia (TSK), 291
Tardive dyskenesia, 222
Telephone-administered CBT (T-CBT) intervention, 325
Telephone-administered supportive emotion-focused therapy (T-SEFT), 325
Tobacco addiction
bio-behavioral mechanisms, 209
cultural considerations, 211–212
genetic and neurobiological factors, 209–211
characterization, 207
cigarettes, 207
clinical symptoms
addiction treatment settings, 223–224
alcohol and other drug, 220
clinical considerations, 221–222
ethnic population, 222–223
self-sustaining treatment culture, 224
smoking cessation, 223–224
epidemiology, 208
smoking and symptoms
anxiety, 213
mood disorders, 213–214
placebo effects, 214
schizophrenia, 212
substance use disorders, 214–215
treatment
behavioral therapy approach, 218–220
evidence-based medications, 215–216
nonnicotine medication, 217–218
NRT medications, 216–217
Trazodone, 355
Triazolam, 371
Tricyclic antidepressants (TCAs)
cardiovascular disease, 126
COPD, 430, 433
obesity, 4
pain, 281–282
type 2 diabetes, 80
Type 2 diabetes mellitus (T2DM)
anxiety disorders
clinical assessment, 84–85
diagnostic issues, 84–85
epidemiology, 81–83
evidence-based treatment, 85–87
pathophysiology, 83–84
prevalence, 81
symptoms, 81
treatment decision-making issues, 88
depression
CBT, CBT-AD, 79
clinical assessment, 77–78
diagnostic issues, 77–78
epidemiology, 75–76
evidence-based treatment, 78–80
pathophysiology, 76–77
prevalence, 75
symptoms, 76
treatment decision-making issues, 80
eating disorders
anorexia, 89
BED, 89
CBT and NPT, 93
clinical care assessment, 92–93
EAT, 92
evidence-based treatment, 93–94
insulin omission, 89–90
maladaptive eating behaviors, 91
night eating syndrome, 90
overweight patients, 89
pathophysiology, 91–92
poorer metabolic control, 90
prevalence, 88
treatment decision-making issues, 94
glucose management, 74
obesity, insulin resistance, 73
prevalence, 73
psychotic disorders and bipolar disorders
adherence medications, 98
clinical care assessment, 98–99
epidemiology, 94–95
evidence-based treatment, 99–101
prevalence, 95
treatment decision-making issues, 101
race and ethnicity
cookie cutter, 107
hispanics, 106

Type 2 diabetes mellitus (T2DM) (*cont.*)
hypoglycemics, 108
prevalence, 106
racial disparities, 105
socioeconomic disparities, 106
self-care deficience, 74
substance use disorders
clinical care assessment, 103
epidemiology, 101–102
evidence-based treatment, 103–104
pathophysiology, 102–103
treatment decision-making issues, 104–105
treatment, 74–75

V

Varenicline, 215–217

MIX
Papier aus verantwortungsvollen Quellen
Paper from responsible sources
FSC® C105338

Printed by Books on Demand, Germany